Exercise and Sport Sciences Reviews

Volume 17, 1989

EXERCISE AND SPORT SCIENCES REVIEWS

Volume 17, 1989

Edited by KENT B. PANDOLF, Ph.D.

Director, Military Ergonomics Division
U.S. Army Research Institute of Environmental Medicine
Natick, Massachusetts

Adjunct Professor of Health Sciences
Sargent College of Allied Health Professions
Boston University
Boston, Massachusetts

Adjunct Professor of Environmental Medicine
Springfield College
Springfield, Massachusetts

American College of Sports Medicine Series

WILLIAMS & WILKINS
Baltimore • Hong Kong • London • Sydney

Editor: John P. Butler
Associate Editor: Marjorie Kidd Keating
Copy Editor: Debbie Klenotic
Design: Dan Pfisterer
Illustration Planning: Lorraine Wrzosek
Production: Theda Harris

RC
1200
. E94
V 17
July 1999

Printed in the United States of America

Library of Congress Cataloging in Publication Data

ISSN No. 72-12187
ISBN No. 0-683-00046-2

89 90 91 92 93
1 2 3 4 5 6 7 8 9 10

Preface

Exercise and Sport Sciences Reviews is an annual publication sponsored by the American College of Sports Medicine that reviews current research concerning behavioral, biochemical, biomechanical, clinical, physiological, and rehabilitational topics involving exercise science. The Editorial Board for this series currently consists of 12 recognized authorities each of whom has assumed the responsibility for one of the following general topics: biochemistry, exercise physiology, psychology, motor control, athletic medicine, rehabilitation, sociology of sport, environmental physiology, biomechanics, growth and development, epidemiology, and physical fitness. The areas of epidemiology and physical fitness are new additions to this series commencing with this volume. The organization of the Editorial Board should help foster the commitment of the American College of Sports Medicine to publish timely reviews in broad areas of interest to clinicians, educators, exercise scientists, and students. The goal for this Editorial Board is to provide at least one review in each of these 12 areas for each issue of *Exercise and Sport Sciences Reviews*. Further, the Editor shall select three or four additional topics to be developed into chapters based on current interest, timeliness, and importance to the above audience.

The contributors for each volume are selected by the Editorial Board members and the Editor. Although the majority of these reviews are invited, unsolicited manuscripts or potential chapter topics will be received by the Editor and reviewed by him and/or various members of the Editorial Board for possible inclusion in future volumes. Correspondence should be directed to Kent B. Pandolf, Ph.D., U.S. Army Research Institute of Environmental Medicine, Natick, MA 01760-5007, who assumed the role of Editor of *Exercise and Sport Sciences Reviews* beginning with Volume 14.

Kent B. Pandolf, Ph.D.
Editor

Guest Referee Editors

The Editor of *Exercise and Sport Sciences Reviews* gratefully acknowledges the services of the following Guest Referee Editors who assisted the Editorial Board in the review of these chapters.

Raul Artal

Lee E. Baker

Deborah L. Feltz

James D. Garrick

Norman Gledhill

Michael C. Hogan

Howard G. Knuttgen

John T. Reeves

Brenda R. Bigland-Ritchie

Michael N. Sawka

Hugh G. Welch

Andrew J. Young

Contributors

Jack W. Berryman, Ph.D.
Department of Medical History and Ethics
School of Medicine
University of Washington
Seattle, Washington

Mark Parry-Billings, B.Sc.
Department of Biochemistry
University of Oxford
Oxford, United Kingdom

Frank W. Booth, Ph.D., F.A.C.S.M.
Department of Physiology and Cell Biology
University of Texas
Health Science Center at Houston
Houston, Texas

Carl J. Caspersen, Ph.D., M.P.H.
Behavioral Epidemiology and Evaluation Branch
Division of Health Education
Center for Health Promotion and Education
Centers for Disease Control
Atlanta, Georgia

Richard H.T. Edwards, M.D.
Department of Medicine
University of Liverpool
Liverpool, United Kingdom

Henry Gibson, Ph.D.
Department of Medicine
University of Liverpool
Liverpool, United Kingdom

L. Bruce Gladden, Ph.D., F.A.C.S.M.
Exercise Physiology Laboratory
University of Louisville
Louisville, Kentucky

Michael E. Gordon, M.S.
Rehabilitation Research and Development Center
Veterans Administration Medical Center
Palo Alto, California

Robert W. Gotshall, Ph.D.
Departments of Physiology/Biophysics and Pediatrics
School of Medicine
Wright State University
Dayton, Ohio

Ronald G. Haller, M.D.
Neurology Service
Veterans Administration Medical Center
Dallas, Texas

John McA. Harris, M.D.
Department of Orthopedics
Boston Veterans Administration Medical Center
Boston, Massachusetts

Bruce H. Jones, M.D.
Exercise Physiology Division
U.S. Army Research Institute of Environmental Medicine
Natick, Massachusetts

Steven F. Lewis, Ph.D., F.A.C.S.M.
Department of Physiology
University of Texas
Southwestern Medical Center
Dallas, Texas

Don P. MacLaren, M.Sc.
School of Health Sciences
Liverpool Polytechnic
Liverpool, United Kingdom

Penny McCullagh, Ph.D.
Department of Kinesiology
University of Colorado at Boulder
Boulder, Colorado

Michael J. McGrath, M.D.
Department of Obstetrics and Gynecology
Queens University
Kingston, Ontario, Canada

Daniel S. Miles, Ph.D., F.A.C.S.M.
Graduate Hospital
Human Performance and Sports Medicine Center
Wayne, Pennsylvania

Michelle F. Mottola, Ph.D.
Department of Anatomy
University of Western Ontario
London, Ontario, Canada

Patricia J. Ohtake, M.Sc.
Department of Physiology
Queens University
Kingston, Ontario, Canada

Alan D. Rogol, M.D., Ph.D.
Division of Endocrinology and Metabolism
Department of Pediatrics
School of Medicine
University of Virginia
Charlottesville, Virginia

Diane Ross, Ph.D.
Department of Physical Education
California State University–Fullerton
Fullerton, California

Clint Rubin, Ph.D.
Department of Orthopedics
State University of New York at Stony Brook
Health Sciences Center
Stony Brook, New York

Michael N. Sawka, Ph.D., F.A.C.S.M.
Physiology Branch, Military Ergonomics Division
U.S. Army Research Institute of Environmental Medicine
Natick, Massachusetts

William T. Stauber, Ph.D., F.A.C.S.M.
Departments of Physiology and Neurology
West Virginia University
Health Sciences Center North
Morgantown, West Virginia

Tuyethoa M. Vinh, M.D.
Department of Orthopedic Pathology
Armed Forces Institute of Pathology
Washington, D.C.

Maureen R. Weiss, Ph.D.
Department of Physical Education and Human Movement Studies
University of Oregon
Eugene, Oregon

Larry A. Wolfe, Ph.D., F.A.C.S.M.
School of Physical and Health Education
Queens University
Kingston, Ontario, Canada

Andrew J. Young, Ph.D., F.A.C.S.M.
Physiology Branch, Military Ergonomics Division
U.S. Army Research Institute of Environmental Medicine
Natick, Massachusetts

Felix E. Zajac, Ph.D.
Design Division
Mechanical Engineering Department
Stanford University
Stanford, California

Contents

1
Application of Molecular Biology in Exercise Physiology

FRANK W. BOOTH, Ph.D.

It is generally accepted that application of scientifically based information to training techniques can improve athletic performance. Examples are numerous: The use of physical laws to enhance biomechanical techniques in various sports and the employment of blood glucose assays to document an association between hypoglycemia and physical exhaustion are but a few of the applications. The recent technical revolution in the field of molecular biology offers another opportunity to make use of scientific information for the improvement of human physical performance.

This review is divided into three major parts. The first section describes some background and defines some technical terms used in molecular biology. The second section reports results of research employing molecular biological techniques to questions in exercise physiology. The third part discusses potential future applications of molecular biological procedures to the investigation of additional questions in exercise biochemistry.

TERMS IN MOLECULAR BIOLOGY

The purpose of this section is to define some basic terminology employed by molecular biologists which will be helpful for understanding the principles of certain techniques and experiments described later in this review.

Deoxyribonucleic acid (DNA) is the component in our cells that forms the structural backbone of chromosomes and holds the hereditary blueprint that determines the protein composition in our cells and body. *Genes* are distinct segments of the DNA, each of which possesses the functional information to make a specific protein. The DNA of a gene stores the information to produce protein in the form of an "alphabetic" code. The "letters" of this alphabet consist of the four deoxynucleotides—deoxyadenosine (dA), deoxycytidine (dC), deoxyguanosine (dG), and deoxythymidine (dT)—that are part of the basic structural units of DNA. Just as in a real alphabet, these letters can be used to form words; however, in the case of DNA the "words" are restricted to three-letter combinations (codons) that represent amino acids, the building blocks

1

of protein. This code can be likened to the dots and dashes used in Morse code. For example, the letter sequence dT-dC-dG "spells" the code word for the amino acid serine. The words (amino acids) can also be strung together to form "sentences" (proteins). A string of three-letter DNA words (codons) necessary to form one "sentence" (protein) is a gene, and the amino acid sequence that is derived from this DNA "sentence" is the gene product or protein. However, the DNA "sentence" cannot be decoded directly into a protein. The DNA must first be "copied" into a form of a messenger that delivers the information in the DNA to the cell to be translated (decoded) by the ribosomes (protein assemblers) into a protein. The "copy" from the DNA that is made is called messenger ribonucleic acid (mRNA) and the "copying" process is termed *transcription*. The "letters" that compromise mRNA molecules are similar to those of DNA with the exceptions that mRNA has one more OH^- group in its nucleotide letters than does DNA and the nucleotide uridine (U) is substituted for deoxythmidine in mRNA molecules. Thus the letters in the mRNA alphabet are designated adenosine (A), cytidine (C), guanosine (G), and uridine (U). The mRNA is copied from DNA by using the existing DNA nucleotide sequence as a template or guide. Mammalian DNA consists of two strings of letters (deoxynucleotides). These two strands of DNA are connected in parallel to one another by hydrogen bonding in a manner analogous to the legs of a ladder (nucleotide sequence) held together by its rungs (hydrogen bonds). The biochemical properties of nucleotides are such that deoxyadenosine (dA) binds specifically to deoxythymidine (dT) by two hydrogen bonds and deoxyguanosine (dG) binds exclusively to deoxycytidine (dC) with three hydrogen bonds. That is, whenever the letter "dA" appears in one strand of DNA, the opposite strand must have a "dT" and vice versa. A pair of nucleotides that bind with each other are termed *complementary nucleotides*. The same rule applies to "dG" and "dC" as well as to the RNA "letters" (U binds A and G binds C). DNA letters (deoxynucleotides) are also complementary to RNA letters (nucleotides). Thus, when a mRNA copy of DNA is made, the cell follows the complementary nucleotide rule using one of the two DNA strands as a template. However, instead of "printing" the image of the template (dA prints dT), the DNA "prints" the complementary RNA nucleotide to its template DNA nucleotide. That is, dA prints U, dG prints C, etc. The cell is specific as to which DNA strand is used as the template. One of the two DNA strands possesses a deoxynucleotide sequence that is complementary to the mRNA nucleotide sequence. This strand is used as the template to copy the mRNA and is designated the noncoding strand because its nucleotide sequence "code" is not the same as the mRNA nucleotide sequence "code." For example if the mRNA nucleotide sequence is A-G-C-C-U then the template strand will be dT-dC-dG-dG-dA. The second or nontemplate

FIGURE 1.1

Schematic of gene structure. See text for description.

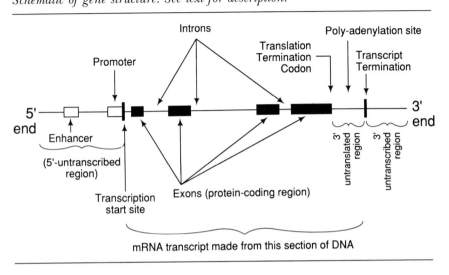

DNA strand possesses a noncomplentary nucleotide sequence to the mRNA. This strand is termed the *coding strand* because its nucleotide "code" (sequence) is identical to the mRNA nucleotide "code." That is, in reference to the mRNA sequence above, the nontemplate DNA strand sequence is dA-dG-dC-dC-dT. Therefore, the resulting mRNA copy is simply a copy of the "coding" strand but is made with RNA (ribonucleic acid) "letters" (A, U, G, C) instead of DNA (deoxyribonucleic acid) "letters" (dA, dT, dG, dC). This distinction is very important since only the mRNA can be decoded (translated) by the cell machinery and formed into a protein.

Before the mRNA can be translated into a string of amino acid words (protein), the mRNA molecule must be "edited" similar to how written sentences are edited by publishers. The "unedited" mRNA at this stage is termed precurser or *heterogeneous mRNA*. To fully understand editing, a knowledge of basic gene structure may be helpful (Fig. 1.1). The start or front-end of the gene is termed the *5' end* and the finish or back-end of the gene is referred to as the *3' end*. The start of the transcribed region (transcription start site) of the gene usually begins several hundred to thousands of nucleotides (bases) into the gene from the 5' end, analogous to an indentation at the start of a new paragraph. Transcription proceeds from that point toward the 3' end of the gene where transcription stops at a specified point which is short of the 3' end of the gene. The transcribed region is further divided into a region that contains the nucleotides that are "read" in triplets (each triplet or codon represents an amino acid in that gene's protein). These nucleotides are referred to as the *protein coding region*. However, in most mammalian genes this region is not contiguous but rather is separated by variable stretches of nucleotides that do not "print" for amino acids belonging to that protein, thus resulting in the division of the protein coding region into a number of discontinuous segments (each of which is called an *exon*). The noncoding regions separating the exons are transcribed along with the exons into mRNA and are known as *introns*. The exact function of these regions is still unknown, but nevertheless introns must be removed (edited) from the mRNA before it can be decoded and translated into a protein. Introns are literally "cut" from mRNA and the exons "spliced" together just as words that are not desired may be removed from a sentence and the remaining words connected together to form a sentence (protein's RNA code). The 3' end of the gene also contains a region that is transcribed into the 3' end of the mRNA. The 3' end of the mRNA is known as the *3' untranslated region* since it is not translated into amino acids. At the start of this 3' untranslated region is the nucleotide triplet sequence (UAA, UAG, or UGA) that designates the end of the protein coding region of the mRNA (translation termination codon). Protein synthesis (translation) of the mRNA stops when the codon is "read" by the protein assembling machinery (ribosome). Another important sequence is located in the DNA (gene). Most eucaryotic mRNAs contain a stretch of adenosine nucleotides at the 3' end of its transcribed region (poly-A tail). This "tail" is added to the mRNA after transcription is complete and occurs as part of the "editing" of the precurser mRNA. The nucleotide sequence that signals the addition of this tail is termed the poly-adenylation site and can be found within the 3' untranslated region of the gene and its mRNA. The second major portion of the gene, the nontranscribed regions, includes the nucleotide sequences from the very start (5' end) of the gene to the start of the protein coding region (called the *5' untranscribed region*) and from the termination site of transcription to the very end (3' end) of the gene (designated the *3' untranscribed region*). Although not copied into the mRNA molecules, the 5' untranscribed region is known to contain distinct nucleotide sequences important in regulating several aspects of gene function. The *promoter region* of the 5' untranscribed region is the site where an enzyme can initiate transcription. The *enhancer regions* in the 5' untranscribed region are sites where proteins interact with the DNA with a resultant increase in transcription rate. Enhancer regions are on the same DNA strands containing the gene's coding and are called the *cis* regulatory regions. The proteins which interact with the enhancer are known as *trans factors*. Returning to the mRNA transcript, when the mRNA is finally copied and "edited," it is now ready to be decoded and translated into a protein.

The mRNA functions analogously to Federal Express in the transport business. The mRNA "transports" a copy of the genes coded "sentence" to the protein manufacturing site where the blueprint is "read" by the cells protein synthetic machinery (ribosomes) which decodes (translates) the nucleotide alphabetic code sequence of the mRNA into "words" (amino acids) and assembles them into meaningful "sentences" (proteins). These sentences are further transported to other locales in the cell where they are structured into "paragraphs" (protein–protein or protein–lipid or protein–carbohydrate interactions), "chapters" (cells), and "books" (organisms) whose story is just now unfolding through the powerful techniques and tools developed and being used in the field of molecular biology.

Most of the techniques used in molecular biology are aimed at (*a*) isolating DNA sequences belonging to particular protein genes, (*b*) determining the exact "spelling" (nucleotide sequence) of a specific protein's gene or its mRNA, (*c*) identifying cis-acting regulatory sequences within the gene (5′ untranscribed region) that are important for regulating how much protein is made, (*d*) identifying trans-acting proteins that interact with a portion of a gene's cis regulatory sequence to govern the gene's expression, and (*e*) measuring mRNA quantity. The following reviews some of the tools and techniques currently used to study the gene and its regulation.

Enzymes (called *restriction endonucleases*) will cut DNA at specific DNA sequences. For example, the restriction endonuclease *Pst* I cuts at the sequence spelled:

$$dCdTdGdCdAdG$$
$$| \quad | \quad | \quad | \quad | \quad |$$
$$dGdAdCdGdTdC$$

Note that the top strand of DNA has a spelling the inverse order of the bottom strand (that is, the 1st letter of the top strand is the 6th letter in the bottom strand, etc.). This inversion of spelling occurs at all sites where restriction endonucleases cut DNA.

Restriction endonucleases are very powerful tools employed by molecular biologists as components of procedures to identify gene fragments and to multiply (clone) specific DNA words. Examples are given next. A string of DNA in mammalian cells can be 10^9 contiguous letters (nucleotides) long, which makes it very difficult to study specific sequences. Restriction endonucleases can cut long DNA strings into shorter DNA lengths (fragments). Having shorter lengths of DNA (hundreds to thousands of letters long) facilitates the identification of individual genes or portions of an individual gene. Restriction endonucleases can also be used to add or insert mammalian DNA fragments into the DNA of a virus that will infect (i.e., transfect) a bacteria. The virus in the bacteria is multiplied in number by growing it in a bacterial medium. Thus a particular DNA fragment of interest can be placed into a virus and multiplied (cloned) within the bacteria. The purpose is to obtain many copies of the DNA sequence so that this segment may be more completely and easily studied. However, the DNA or mRNA sequences for a particular protein's gene must first be isolated and identified by procedures called *screening a genomic library* (for DNA) or *screening a cDNA library* (for mRNA). The genomic library is made by fragmenting long strings of DNA into shorter lengths with a restriction endonuclease (as described above) and placing each fragment into its own microorganism. The cDNA library is made by taking all the cellular mRNA, copying it to its complementary DNA spelling, and inserting the DNA with restriction endonucleases into a microorganism (as described above). The term *library* implies that all genes from a mammalian cell or that all mRNA existing within a cell type are available to be checked out (isolated) by browsing (screening) the catalog of listings (the DNA or mRNA fragments) in the microorganism (library). Potentially any gene for any protein may be studied in this way. The principle underlying one type of screening utilizes the fact that DNA nucleotides (letters) must bond in specific pairs, as discussed earlier.

Two nucleotides that are able to bind one another are said to be complementary. For example, adenosine (A) and uridine (U) are *complementary nucleotides*. Likewise, DNA is a double-stranded molecule in which the nucleotides (letters) in one strand matches exactly with their bonding-mate nucleotides in the opposite strand. Thus, the two DNA strands are referred to as *complementary strands*. Since the strands of DNA are bound together by hydrogen bonding, the ability to form these bonds can be modulated experimentally by altering conditions (stringency) which effect hydrogen bond formation such as temperature and salt concentration. For example, under very high temperature and very low salt conditions no hydrogen bonding occurs; therefore, complementary strands of DNA cannot bond together, but remain single stranded or *denatured*. If temperature is slightly lowered and the salt concentration is slightly raised (high stringency), hydrogen bonding occurs only between two perfectly matched complementary strands. The two perfectly matched DNA strands anneal to one another or *hybridize* together. When two denatured strands of DNA do not share complementary sequences or are not a perfect match (*noncomplementary strands*), then not enough bonding occurs between them to hold them together and they remain single stranded under high stringency conditions. Thus under carefully modulated conditions, complementary strands can be allowed to hybridize together while noncomplementary strands are left single stranded. This principle is used as a tool to screen genomic and cDNA libraries. If a small segment of nucleotides (>20 bases long) has been identified to be the partial nucleotide sequence of a gene and if this DNA segment is labeled with a radioactive label (such as phorphorus 32), then it can be used as a "probe" to find its complementary strand among the many fragments of DNA or mRNA stored in the libraries. The use of radio-labeled nucleic acid (hybridization) probes is analogous to employing a small magnet to locate a needle in a haystack. A radiolabeled nucleic acid probe (analogous to the magnet) will find a specific complementary DNA sequence (analogous to the needle) among many nonmatching (noncomplementary) DNA sequences (analogous to the hay) and will hybridize (analogous to the magnetic force) to the complementary DNA sequence. This process of the matching and binding (hybridization) of complementary DNA strings serves to identify and quantify specific genes (DNA) or specific messenger RNAs in libraries, cell cultures, or tissue. Molecular biologists routinely employ hybridization procedures to identify and quantitate a string of DNA or mRNA by using a radiolabeled probe to search for the needle (complementary spelling) in an excess of noncomplementary words (hay). Often the probe locates a DNA fragment that is longer than the probe. If this is repeated enough, DNA words (5' and 3' untranscribed regions) before and after the DNA protein coding region can be located. This is important to the study of genetic regulation since many of the DNA sequences that determine how much messenger RNA is transcribed are nucleotide sequences 5' to the coding region of the gene. They are called the 5' untranscribed region of the gene, or cis-regulatory regions of genes.

The spelling of cis-acting regulatory regions for gene transcription can be determined by techniques categorized as DNA sequencing. *Sequencing* refers to obtaining the exact nucleotide "spelling" of a DNA. The DNA sequences (spellings) can then be compared to a stored list of DNA spellings contained in a computerized bank of gene (DNA) sequences. Such comparisons have netted common DNA sequences known to control DNA transcription of multiple messenger RNAs.

If the stringency conditions are lowered so that the match of a hybridization probe to a complementary (second) string of DNA is not 100% perfect, but is only 80% correct (low stringency), then relatives to a protein can be found. From the DNA spellings of other family members, available computer programs can be employed to predict the amino acid sequence for the protein which could be made from the DNA sequence and to predict the secondary and tertiary structure of the protein.

Knowledge of the spelling of DNA words can be used to synthesize artificially short segments of the DNA words, called oligonucleotides. Synthesized oligonucleotides can be hybridized to a complementary nucleotide sequence, just as natural DNA strings can be hybridized. When synthesized oligonucleotides are hybridized to a longer string of DNA, they can act as synthetic promoters (synthetic primers) for the lengthening of the second strand with nucleotides to form two long strings of DNA. This technique is used to determine such information as the length of a gene transcript and the location of the 3′ and 5′ ends of a gene.

This brief introduction of terms should indicate the potential power of molecular biology to answer many questions in the biological sciences. Techniques in molecular biology now provide the ability to determine the spelling of the entire human genome and map the location of specific genes or chromosomes, to add significant new insight to the process of evolution of animals, to provide gene transfer to cure diseases caused by mutated genes, to describe at the level of the molecule how animals develop after fertilization, and to provide information as to how genes are turned on and off as an animal adapts to new environments, such as exercise training or detraining. The remainder of this review will attempt to show how molecular biological techniques have been applied to exercise physiology and then will attempt to speculate how molecular biology might be applied to exercise physiology research in the future.

CURRENT APPLICATION OF MOLECULAR BIOLOGY TO EXERCISE SCIENCES

Major research in molecular biology of interest to the field of exercise sciences to date has been in the determination of the levels of specific mRNAs in muscle undergoing a change in contractile activity and in the identification of multigene families in skeletal muscle. Each of these will be discussed in turn.

Messenger RNA in Chronic Exercise

A major application of molecular biology to the field of exercise physiology has been to employ messenger RNA hybridization probes to estimate changes in the levels of mRNAs in skeletal muscle during training or detraining. By correlating the time course of the changes in mRNA level, protein concentration, and/or protein synthesis rate it is possible to indicate whether pretranslational and/or translational control mechanisms may be altering the protein synthesis rates during the training period. Pretranslational control means that mRNA quantity is rate limiting and that some factor (such as gene transcription or mRNA stability) alters the mRNA concentration. Translational control implies that mRNA quantity is in excess and that some factor alters the efficiency of the usage of the mRNA on the polyribosome to make a nascent polypeptide. Thus protein synthesis rate is limited by the ability of the ribosome and the translational cofactors to utilize an overabundance of mRNA. Posttranslational control of protein quantity implies that many events happen to a protein after it is synthesized on the ribosome, like transport or

TABLE 1.1
Contractile Activities[a]

Increased contractile activity
　Physiological model (exercise)
　　1. Run
　　2. Weight lift
　　3. Bicycling
　Nonphysiological model
　　1. Chronic electrical stimulation (24 hours/day)
　　2. Ablation
Decreased contractile activity
　Physiological model
　　1. Bed rest
　　2. Limb immobilization
　　3. Weightlessness
　　4. Detraining from running, etc. training
　Nonphysiological model
　　1. Hindlimb suspension

[a]Contractile activity = quantity or quality of muscle contraction.

assembly. In order to distinguish between translational control and post-translational control, the rate of protein synthesis on polyribosomes must be compared to the rate that the protein is assembled into its functional site in the cell. If the rate of cytochrome-c transport across the outer mitochondrial membrane or the rate of heme incorporation into cytochrome c were shown to be less than its protein synthesis rate, then posttranslational control would be rate limiting for this protein.

The predominance of pretranslational, translational, and posttranslational controls varies depending on the stage of the training and the type of muscle. As an early response to a change in contractile activity, a translational or posttranslational control appears to alter protein synthesis rates for mitochondrial and contractile proteins in fast-twitch muscle. Little is known about the relative importance of pretranslational, translational, or posttranslational controls in slow-twitch muscle to account for the early changes in protein synthesis to alterations in contractile activity. On the other hand, during more prolonged training or detraining (designated as long-term responses to altered contractile activity) pretranslational control of protein synthesis rate in both slow- and fast-twitch skeletal muscle becomes more predominant. Evidence for these statements is given after the next paragraph in which exercise terms are defined.

In Table 1.1 the term "contractile activity" is equated with the quantity and quality of muscle contraction. As shown in Table 1.1, contractile activity can be separated into two major subdivisions: increased contractile activity and decreased contractile activity. Increased contractile activity is further subdivided into the categories of physiological models of contractile activity and nonphysiological models of contractile activity. The distinction between these two categories is that contractile activities such as chronic electrical stimulation for 24 hours per day and ablation of muscles to produce overload hypertrophy of remaining muscles are types of contractile activities rarely experienced by humans. Thus they are categorized as nonphysiological models because there is no guarantee at this time that all biochemical events occurring in nonphysiological models mimic physiological models. For example, skeletal muscle that undergoes chronic electrical stimulation for 24 hours per day has increased mitochondrial density and muscle atrophy [36]. On the other hand, 2 hours of daily running doubles mitochondrial density but does not alter muscle size [10]. Obviously the biochemical events for control of contractile protein quantity differ between continuous electrical stimulation and treadmill running. Thus it is possible that other biochemical control mechanisms also differ between these two types of contractile activity since mitochondrial density increases 1-fold after repeated daily bouts of 2 hours of treadmill running [10] but increases 5-fold after weeks of continuous electrical stimulation [36].

The conclusion that translational or posttranslational control plays an important role in altering protein synthesis rates as an early response to a change in contractile activity comes from inferential reasoning rather than a direct measurement of translation rate on polyribosomes in vivo. As shown in Figure 1.2, a rapid 67% decrease in the synthesis rate of actin protein without any concomitant change in α actin mRNA quantity implies a decreased translation of the α actin mRNA into newly synthesized actin protein in fast-twitch muscle during the first 5 hours of hindlimb immobilization [34]. The reasoning is that cellular levels of α actin mRNA did not decrease significantly in these 5 hours and thus α actin mRNA could not be rate limiting. That is, actin protein synthesis fell even though α actin mRNA did not fall.

A second example which implies a role for an increase in translation of existing mRNA as an early response to a change in contractile activity is shown in Figure 1.2. These data illustrate an increase in the activity of citrate synthase without any change in the level of its mRNA [25]. The reasoning which leads to a conclusion that an increased translation is responsible for the early increase in citrate synthase activity during the first 6 days of 12-hour daily stimulation of fast-twitch muscle is as follows: (*a*) The synthesis rate of citrate synthase is inferred to be increased from data of others showing that another mitochondrial protein, cytochrome-c protein, has an increased synthesis rate during an exercise program which increases mitochondrial content [5, 21], and (*b*) the increase in citrate synthase synthesis rate without any change in its mRNA implies that citrate synthase mRNA quantity was not rate limiting in the control condition. Thus the deduction can be made that translation of

FIGURE 1.2

Dissociation between the lack of an acute change in mRNA quantity and either the amount of protein or the synthesis rate of this protein. **Top**, *After 5 hours of immobilization of the gastrocnemius muscle. (Reproduced with permission from Watson PA, Stein JP, Booth FW: Changes in actin synthesis and α-actin-mRNA content in rat muscle during immobilization.* Am J Physiol 247:C39–C44, 1984.) **Bottom**, *During the first 6 days of electrically induced contraction (12 hours day) of the extensor digitorum longus muscle (Reproduced with permission from Seedorf UE, Leberer E, Kirschbaum BJ, Pette D: Neural control of gene expression in skeletal muscle. Effects of chronic stimulation on lactate dehydrogenase isoenzymes and citrate synthase.* Biochem J 239:115–120, 1986.)

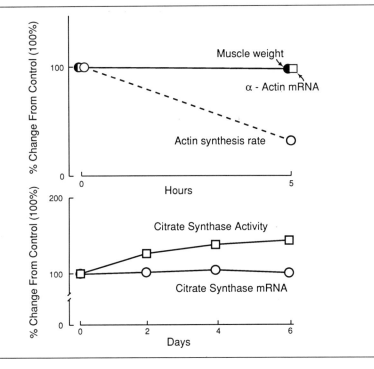

citrate synthase must be rate limiting if pretranslational control, that is, mRNA level, is not rate limiting and if posttranslational control is not playing a role. Little is known about the potential modification of posttranslational control by exercise. For example, citrate synthase is synthesized by cytoplasmic ribosomes and transported into the mitochondria. Could acute exercise alter posttranslational processing of citrate synthase or other proteins?

TABLE 1.2
Correlations among mRNA Quantity, Protein Quantity, and Protein Synthesis Rates for Specific Proteins during Muscle Atrophy or Increased Contractile Activity

1	2	3	4	5	6	7	8
Altered Contractile Activity	Days of Altered Contractile Activity	mRNA and/or Protein Measured in Columns 4, 5, and 6	Change in Concentration of mRNA in Column 3 (% of Control)	Change in Whole Muscle Content of Protein in Column 3 (% of Control)	Change in Synthesis Rate of Protein in Column 3 (% of Control)	Muscle	Reference
Hindlimb immobilization (ankle extensors are fixed in a shortened position)	7	Cytochrome c	60	60	81	Red quadriceps	21
		Actin	53	73	34	Gastrocnemius	22
Hindlimb unweighting (muscles can contract without bearing weight)	7	Cytochrome c	80–83	—	—	Gastrocnemius and soleus	3
		Actin	67–71	—	—		
		Myofibrillar	—	79	41	Soleus	29
		Slow myosin	—	60	—	Soleus	
Hindlimb denervation (muscles cannot contract or bear weight)	7	Cytochrome c	60–61	—	—	Gastrocnemius and soleus	3
		Actin	44–53	—	—		
Chronic electrical stimulation (12 hr/day) of hindlimb fast-twitch muscle	28	Citrate synthase	700	400	—	Extensor digitorum longus	25
		Heart isoform of lactate dehydrogenase	170	200	—		
		Muscle isoform of lactate dehydrogenase	50	60	—		

Condition	Protein					Muscle	Ref
	Parvalbumin	28	13	5	—	Extensor digitorum longus	17
	Sarcoplasmic reticular Ca++ATPase	52	80	80	—	Extensor digitorium longus	25
Chronic electrical stimulation (24 hr/day) of hindlimb fast-twitch muscle	Citrate synthase	10	200	—	—	Tibialis anterior	35
	Citrate synthase	10	—	213	—	Tibialis anterior	6
	Cytochrome oxidase		—	215	—		—
	VIC subunit of cytochrome oxidase		112	—	—		—
	βsubunit of F1 ATPase		197	—	—		—
	Cytochrome b		252	—	—		—
	Citrate synthase	21	—	500	—	Tibialis anterior or extensor digitorum longus	37
	Cytochrome b		500	—	—		—
	Aldolase		24	30	—		—
	Citrate synthase	21	—	557	—	Tibialis anterior	36
	Cytochrome oxidase		—	412	—		—
	VIC subunit of cytochrome oxidase		220	—	—		—
	βsubunit of F1 ATPase		265	—	—		—
	Cytochrome b		654	—	—		—
	Aldolase A		32	—	—		—
	Myoglobin	21	1540	—	—	Tibialis anterior	31

The conclusion that as a later response to altered contractile activity pretranslational control plays an important role in altering protein synthesis rates is derived from data shown in Table 1.2 The correlations among directional changes in mRNA amount, protein quantity, and protein synthesis rate imply that the altered quantity of mRNA played some role in changing the synthesis rate of its protein, and thus the protein quantity. For example, decreases in actin and cytochrome-c protein synthesis rates are associated with decreases in their mRNAs after 7 days of limb immobilization that cause a 25% loss of skeletal muscle mass [21, 22]. Likewise, after 28 days of electrical stimulation (12 hours per day), the quantities of the protein and mRNA for the muscle isoform of lactate dehydrogenase are proportionally decreased in skeletal muscle [25]. In contrast, the percentage increases in the quantities of the protein and mRNA for either citrate synthase or the heart isoform of lactate dehydrogenase are roughly equivalent after 28 days of chronic stimulation of skeletal muscle [25]. Since the amount of a mRNA can be altered by multiple factors (such as altered transcription rate by a gene to form the immature mRNA, altered processing of the immature to mature mRNA in the nucleus, or altered stability [degradation] of the mRNA), future research will be required to delineate which of the above are responsible for altered mRNA quantities which appear as a late change to an alteration in contractile activity.

Gene Families
In addition to detecting changes in specific mRNAs with exercise, studies have noted isoform switching with changes in contractile activity. A protein which exists in multiple isoforms may be derived from a multigene family. For example, the actin protein family has at least six different proteins whose sequences vary only at a few amino acid residues but are encoded by six separate actin genes identified as α skeletal, α cardiac, α smooth, γ smooth, β nonmuscle, and γ nonmuscle [32]. While each actin isoform likely has a different function based on different structures resulting from the various amino acid sequences, this speculation has not yet been proved. The expression of α skeletal actin and α cardiac actin in muscle is tissue and age dependent. The age-dependent expression of actin isoforms in skeletal muscle is as follows. The percentage of the total actin that is α cardiac actin is 80% in the 11-day-old chick embryonic leg muscle, 50% in the same muscle just prior to birth, and 5% in the adult muscle [32]. The remaining percentage of actin at each developmental stage is composed of α skeletal actin. In contrast, the effect of age on isoform expression in the heart is the inverse of that described for skeletal muscle. Thus the actin isoform is expressed in pairs in striated muscle. From these data it is now considered that α cardiac actin is the embryonic isoform of actin in skeletal muscle while

the embryonic form in the heart is α skeletal actin. This information may be of importance to research on the effects of exercise because of the possibility that certain types of exercise cause muscle remodeling [16] and may result in the induction of satellite cell division [6]. It is thought that these newly formed cells could initially express embryonic isoforms such as α cardiac actin in the regenerating fibers of adult skeletal muscle following exercise that damages muscle fibers. This puts forth the possibility of gaining novel information on the appearance of embryonic isoforms of proteins and offers an additional marker of skeletal muscle injury and its initiation process.

An example of another multigene family is the myosin heavy chain protein. Although multiforms of myosin heavy chain protein were known to exist prior to molecular biology, the use of recombinant DNA technology has furthered comprehension in this area. The laboratory of Nadel-Ginard [19] has screened cDNA and genomic libraries to identify seven members of the myosin heavy chain multigene family. Some of the new insight from this work was the conclusive proof that (*a*) the same gene produces cardiac ventricular β-myosin heavy chain protein and slow-twitch skeletal muscle myosin heavy chain protein, (*b*) that there are two different fast-twitch skeletal myosin heavy chain genes (types IIA and IIB), and (*c*) that there are two developmental genes (embryonic and neonatal myosin heavy chain).

The application of these findings to exercise physiology would be the use of radiolabeled nucleic acid probes for detecting mRNA levels to answer questions such as, Does the concentration of slow myosin heavy chain mRNA decrease in the soleus muscle during hindlimb suspension? (It is known that slow myosin protein content decreases in the suspended soleus muscle [29].) Does endurance training cause a down-regulation of the type IIB myosin heavy chain and the up-regulation of type IIA in fast-twitch skeletal muscle? Does sprinting training cause the reverse effect? Measurements of specific mRNA levels with various hybridization probes will help answer these and related questions. For example, it is now feasible to place fast-twitch myosin heavy chain cDNA sequences into a bacterial expression vector which will result in an overproduction of a fragment of the protein encoded by the cDNA. The produced protein is used to form an antibody to one of the fast-twitch myosin heavy chains and the antibody used to localize the particular fast-twitch myosin heavy chain using immunohistochemical techniques. Another question which can be posed, with the availability of probes for embryonic and neonatal myosin heavy chains, is when and to what degree these mRNAs are expressed after exhaustive exercise. The occurrence of muscle fiber regeneration 2 days after eccentric contraction during downhill running by rats has been reported by Armstrong et al. [2]. In addition, Everett and Sparrow [7] observed a transient up-regulation of either a fast-twitch or an embryonic myosin heavy chain in slow-twitch muscle during stretch hypertrophy. (The antibody employed did not distinguish between the two aforementioned myosin isoforms.) They suggested that either regeneration followed injury to muscle because of the stretch or focal embryonic events occurred where satellite cells fused into hyper-trophying muscle fibers [7]. The above suggestions illustrate a few of the questions which might be posed in exercise physiology and that can now be answered with the use of detection probes not only for all of the myosin heavy chains but for potentially any protein. A future challenge for exercise physiologists could be to delineate the functional or phys-iological significance to athletic performance of isoform switching in response to exercise.

POTENTIAL APPLICATIONS OF MOLECULAR BIOLOGY TO EXERCISE SCIENCES IN FUTURE RESEARCH

As stated in the initial paragraph of this review, previous application of existing scientific methods to exercise sciences has resulted in an im-proved athletic performance. Thus the foresight to incorporate new methods and research findings into practical application is not novel. However, since the area of molecular biology is a relatively unexplored aspect of exercise, it may be beneficial to outline some specific avenues through which these two disciplines may be integrated. Therefore the purpose of the third part of this review is to suggest future applications of molecular biological techniques to the exercise sciences. It is hoped that some of the suggested approaches will provide a more in-depth look into acute and chronic mechanisms that regulate the human body during exercise. These applications are presented in the form of responses to research questions in exercise.

How does endurance training coregulate the gene expression of most mito-chondrial proteins in the trained skeletal muscle? It is well known that quan-titatively similar increases of many mitochondrial proteins occur in par-allel [9, 11]. Techniques in molecular biology permit the determination of whether a common DNA sequence (spelling) occurs in the 5′ untran-scribed region of mitochondrial genes. Once the complete DNA se-quence of, for example, a mitochondrial gene is found (including the sequences 5′ to the gene [untranscribed region], the coding region with any introns, and sequences 3′ to the gene [untranslated region]), then the sequence of this mitochondrial gene can be compared to the DNA sequences of other known mitochondrial genes by computer analysis to identify particular segments of base sequences with a high percentage of homology or similarity. The rationale underlying this strategy is as follows. If a subset of genes are expressed in unison, then it is likely that a common DNA-binding regulatory factor interacts with a common DNA sequence to all the mitochondrial genes up-regulated by endurance exercise. Thus comparison of DNA sequences among mitochondrial proteins which are coexpressed in endurance training should yield a common DNA sequence in each of these which is a common regulatory region. (If this speculation is not true, then a separate DNA regulating factor for each mitochondrial protein must each exist and be coregulated so that exercise elicits proportional increases in all factors and mitochondrial proteins.) Although the above methodology is possible and the question vital, very little data currently exist to verify this speculative hypothesis as the molecular regulatory mechanism involved in the endurance-training-induced coexpression of mitochondrial genes.

Which enzymes are responsible for the shift in metabolic fuels that occur with endurance training? An important concept in exercise physiology is to understand the identity of the rate-limiting enzyme in a metabolic pathway in untrained and trained muscles or tissue [24]. Some techniques in molecular biology might be able to add to our present understanding of rate-limiting enzymes. Experiments can now be performed in vitro in which the tissue concentrations of a single enzyme can be studied by isolation of specific genes and observing expression under varied conditions following transfer into a bacterial host. For example, Walsh and Koshland [33] studied the role of different activities of citrate synthase on the utilization of carbon chains either from glucose or from acetate. Using recombinant DNA techniques, the citrate synthase gene was put under control of a synthetic promoter which permitted adjustable expression of the enzyme's gene so that citrate synthase activities were varied from 10% to 5000% of normal. This recombinant (gene and promoter) was transfected into *Escherichia coli*. Walsh and Koshland [33] indicated the following premises. If the level of citrate synthase activity is increased and is the rate-limiting enzyme in its metabolic pathway, then flux of substrate through its pathway should increase. However if citrate synthase is not a rate-controlling enzyme, its increase would not alter metabolic flux. The results of Walsh and Koshland's study [33] are given next. When citrate synthase activity in the bacteria was increased, carbon flow from acetate increased. Moreover, when citrate synthase enzyme protein was underproduced, carbon flux through the Krebs cycle was decreased if acetate was the sole carbon source, but carbon flux through the Krebs cycle was unaffected if glucose was the main nutrient. They interpreted the results to mean that citrate synthase activity was rate limiting when acetate was the sole carbon source but was not rate limiting if glucose was a main nutrient. These in vivo results in bacteria cannot be extrapolated to mammalian metabolism. However, they do illustrate that a similar experimental design could be employed in animals when gene transfer techniques into adult mammalian skeletal muscle becomes a reality in the future. Questions such as what the rate-limiting step is in β-oxidation of fatty acids or in glycolytic flux during physical exercise could be further examined.

What chemical signal(s) induced by weight-lifting cause skeletal muscle hypertrophy? The rationale for the next discussion is that knowledge of factors inducing uncontrolled growth in tumors could provide insight into mechanisms by which weight-lifting training causes the regulated enlargement of skeletal muscle. Some of the genetic factors in retroviruses which induce uncontrolled DNA proliferation after retroviral integration into the host genome have been identified and are designated as oncogenes [14]. It is also known that many of these oncogenes are truncated or slightly mutated DNA segments that were originally derived from normal eukaryotic DNA. It is speculated that a retrovirus "stole" a normal eukaryotic growth signal and placed it into its retroviral genome. (The progenitor eukaryotic DNA sequences have been named cellular oncogenes or proto-oncogenes.) When a retrovirus infects a cell and the retroviral DNA is integrated into the host DNA, the oncogene DNA from the retrovirus can be continuously expressed. The resultant increase in growth factor protein from an expressed oncogene in the host could cause the cell to have unregulated DNA proliferation. Since the viral oncogenes initiate uncontrolled cellular growth, it has been speculated that cellular oncogenes could play a role in normal controlled growth. An obvious extension of these ideas is that weight-lifting exercise induces some of the eukaryotic cellular oncogenes through an unknown sequence of steps. The activated cellular oncogene could then increase its mRNA, which would translate more of the cellular oncogene protein causing muscle enlargement by an enhancement of growth. It is known that many viral oncogenes induce uncontrolled growth, and it is speculated that cellular oncogenes could play a signaling role in the induction of physiological growth.

Presently, many researchers are attempting to determine the mechanism by which oncogene proteins induce their actions. For example, it is believed that the proteins from oncogenes c-*myc* and c-*fos* may interact with DNA or with proteins interacting with DNA while other cellular oncogenes have different sites of action in cellular metabolism [14]. A simple first step toward testing the hypothesis that weight-lifting induces muscle hypertrophy through the activation of some of the cellular oncogenes is to measure oncogene mRNA quantities. Commercial sources of cDNA probes for some cellular oncogene mRNAs are available. Antibodies to some of the oncogene proteins are also available commercially.

Speculation as to how cellular oncogenes might act in exercise might be the following. Laurent et al. [16] observed a proliferation of DNA in skeletal muscle during stretch-induced hypertrophy. Marshall [20] has argued that the proteins from c-*myc* mRNA and c-*fos* mRNA are effectors that link events at the cell surface to nuclear events, such as changes in gene transcription and the initiation of DNA synthesis. It is generally accepted that the oncogenes c-*myc* and c-*fos* proteins are localized in the nucleus and their mRNAs have a peak expression within 30–120 minutes of treatment. Using the hypothesis of Marshall [20] it can be speculated that stretch of the sarcolemma could trigger the transient induction of c-*myc* and c-*fos* in satellite cells resulting in proliferation of satellite cells, which play some role in the increase in DNA per muscle fiber which occurs in stretch-induced hypertrophy.

If satellite cells were to migrate to existing muscle fibers to become new nuclei on the sarcolemma of hypertrophying fibers because of weight-lifting, an additional question employing another mechanism can be posed. How does the enlarging sarcolemma sense an increased distance among its nuclei and then signal satellite cells to be recruited so to return intranuclear distances on the sarcolemma to distances found in control sarcolemma? Is there an exercise signal from weight-lifting to cause the oncogenes c-*myc* and c-*fos* to increase in satellite cells, and does this increase induce satellite cell proliferation? Research into oncogenes and satellite cells should engage more interest by exercise physiologists in the future.

The possibility remains, although untested, that the study of a potential role of cellular oncogenes as a signal in the pathway leading from weight bearing to muscular enlargement will have to be done in vivo rather than in muscle culture. Previously many of the investigators employed tissue culture to determine how viral oncogenes transformed cells to tumors. Now, according to Marshall [20], it seems as if such systems clearly represent a gross oversimplification of the neoplastic process. Marshall [20] indicates that a number of researchers have now turned to more complex living systems with the hope that they may more closely mimic the situation in vivo. One of many recent examples is the report of Sinn et al. [27] in which transgenic animals are genetically engineered so that the organism expresses an exogenous oncogene implanted into fertilized eggs. We interpret the progression of cancer research from tissue culture to whole animals as a research template for exercise physiology. Just as oncology has learned that a tissue culture can provide misinformation about the whole animal, we believe the same will be true for the field of exercise physiology where the complex integration of organ systems under stress cannot be reproduced by a culture of homogeneous embryonic cells.

Another potential family of growth factors that could be involved in the signal pathway from weight-lifting to increased protein expression is the polypeptide growth factors. For example, Turner et al. [30] have reported an increased quantity of insulin-like growth factor I and insulin-like growth factor II mRNAs in skeletal muscles of rats having an overproduction of growth hormone. Insulin-like growth factor I is a mitogenic polypeptide with growth-promoting effects [8]. The regenerating soleus muscle has increased insulin-like growth factor I immunoreactivity in its satellite cells, myoblasts, and myotubes [13]. Thus any type of exercise that could cause muscle regeneration such as weightlifting or eccentric exercise might have increased insulin-like growth factor I associated with muscle fiber remodeling. Darr and Schultz [6] have reported an activation of satellite cells in skeletal muscles which underwent eccentric contractions during a single bout of downhill running by rats. It would be interesting to determine whether insulin-like growth factor I gene expression is increased in skeletal muscles undergoing an initial bout of eccentric-type of exercise or weight lifting. Probes for insulin-like growth factor I mRNA would be used in this quantification.

What DNA regulatory sequences are important for altering transcription of an mRNA? It is now possible to identify in muscle cultures the DNA sequences of transcriptional regulatory regions for specific genes. An example of one such study will be described in order to indicate one approach that was used to obtain information about control of the transcription of the human α skeletal actin gene.

Previous work has isolated and sequenced the human α skeletal actin gene and the 2000 bases preceding the mRNA coding region. Muscat and Kedes [23] took the 2000 bases of DNA consisting of the putative regulatory region preceding the human α skeletal actin gene and placed them upstream before the coding region for the bacterial chloramphenicol acetyltransferase (CAT) gene. Since the CAT gene is not in mammalian cells, the appearance of CAT protein from the CAT gene serves to report how much the putative regulatory region driving the human α skeletal actin gene is turned on in the muscle cells. Thus, assay of the kinetics of bacterial CAT activity in the muscle serves as a reporter for the amount of cellular control of candidate regulatory regions from the actin gene. For example, if the 2000-base sequence preceding the mRNA coding region of the human α skeletal actin gene is important for transcription, factors inducing actin gene expression and produced by weight-bearing exercise will interact with the region and cause increased activity in the muscle. If not, CAT activity will be unchanged from control. To further localize specific control sequences within the 5' end regulatory region, various portions of the DNA sequence in the 2000 bases upstream from the coding region for the human α skeletal actin gene were deleted by Muscat and Kedes [23]. Each of these shortened fragments with the attached CAT gene was placed into separate aliquots of cultured muscle cells, and the level of the resultant CAT activity was assayed. The strategy of the deletions was that when a regulatory DNA sequence which was necessary for human α skeletal actin gene transcription was deleted, then CAT activity made would be decreased. Using the above reasoning, Muscat and Kedes [23] transfected (placed) the various deletion constructs of the human α skeletal actin with the CAT gene into two immortalized or transformed lines of skeletal muscle cells (L8 and C2C12 cell lines).

The results of the above experiment indicated that the particular DNA sequence(s) as well as any interacting factor required to regulate the human α skeletal actin gene were dependent on the type of muscle cell line employed [23]. Muscat and Kedes observed that whereas deletion of DNA sequences 2000 to 626 bases before the start of the human α skeletal actin gene reduced the expression of the marker gene CAT by 93% in C2C12 muscle cultures, the same deletion only decreased marker gene expression by 35% in L8 muscle cultures (Fig. 1.3). The major reduction in CAT expression in L8 cells occurred upon removal of additional bases that were 626 to 87 bases before the coding region for actin. The conclusion drawn by Muscat and Kedes [23] from these observations was that a DNA-binding factor that was present in the C2C12 muscle culture was absent in the L8 culture of transformed muscle cells. The significance of this interpretation to future research in exercise physiology is given in the next paragraph.

If muscle cultures were to be stretched for the purpose of determining which DNA sequence or sequences were necessary as a regulatory region to increase the transcription of the actin gene, so as to produce more actin mRNA and more actin protein, then it is possible that the results could be dependent on the type of muscle cells stretched in the tissue culture. Thus two different muscle culture lines might give two different answers for the identity of the DNA-base sequence utilized for increased transcription of the actin gene and thus could imply two different DNA-binding factors induced from the stretching of the muscle cells. If this speculation were to be confirmed, then the selection of which, if either, muscle cell line mimicked the in vivo state in a whole animal would have to be done in vivo. Thus it is likely that future research into the identity of DNA-binding sequences and factors which are affected by exercise will have to be performed in whole animals rather than in tissue culture systems. Transfer of deletion constructs of genes into adult skeletal muscles for the purpose of identifying DNA sequences and binding factors required for altered gene expression during exercise will be a possible area of research in years to come.

What are the proteins that regulate skeletal muscle function? Some of the methodologies of molecular biology have been employed to identify new proteins in skeletal muscle that are important for modulation of cellular function. Knowing a partial or entire nucleotide sequence of a gene of known importance provides an extremely powerful tool for additional information. The nucleotide sequence of the Duchenne muscular dystrophy gene by the laboratory of Kunkel will be employed to illustrate

FIGURE 1.3

The DNA sequence for the 2000 bases before the human α skeletal actin coding region is attached to the chloramphenicol acetyltransferase (CAT) coding region. If bases −2000 to −626 are deleted and the remaining DNA sequence is placed into C2C12 cells, CAT activity is reduced by 93% [23]. Placing the same construct (without bases −2000 to −626) into L8 cells decreases CAT activity by only 35%. This demonstrates that the DNA region deleted contains different information for the control of human α skeletal actin expression in each specific cell line. (Reproduced with permission from Muscat GEO, Kedes L: Multiple 5′-flanking regions of human α-skeletal actin gene synergistically modulate muscle-specific expression. Mole Cell Biol 7:4089–4099, 1987.)

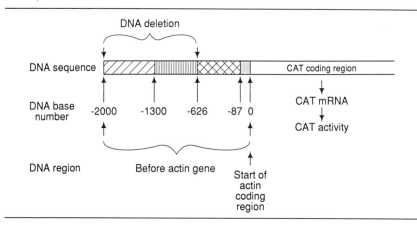

the potency of knowing a gene's nucleotide sequence [15]. Fragments of the Duchenne muscular dystrophy gene were fused to the 3′ terminus of the *E. coli trpE* gene and the resultant protein from the fused gene was made by an expression vector. The protein, containing the amino acid sequence of a part of the protein product of Duchenne muscular dystrophy gene was used to produce a polyclonal antibody. With this antibody, the size of dystrophin (427 kilodaltons), the cellular content (about 0.002% of striated muscle protein is dystrophin), and the cellular distribution (associated with the sarcolemma) were determined [15]. Using the complete nucleotide sequence of the Duchenne muscular dystrophy gene, Kunkel's laboratory has been able to predict the amino acid sequence of dystrophin. Having dystrophin's amino acid sequence permitted them to use computer programs to predict the structure of dystrophin (rod shaped) and to discover that certain amino acid sequences for the protein dystrophin were similar to the amino acid sequences of the cytoskeletal proteins spectrin and α-actinin.

The similarity of functional domains in protein families is a fact that can be applied to identify previously unrecognized proteins using the following experimental strategy. Members of a protein family often have a conserved or similar amino acid sequence within their structure that is important for their functional activity. For example, the catalytic site of the members within a family of protein kinases can have very similar, if not identical, nucleotide sequences. Using a molecular probe, which has the nucleotide sequence of the catalytic site of a known protein kinase, under conditions of low hybridization stringency can detect new or previously unknown protein kinases with similar catalytic sites [12].

Protein kinases will be used next in this review as an example of the potential application of new proteins to answer questions in exercise physiology.

Protein kinases play a role in the transduction of many signals within the cell. Their role has been likened to off/on switches and amplifiers (up to 20-fold) [12]. Since the finding of the first protein kinase, muscle phosphorylase b kinase, nearly two decades ago, nearly 100 different protein kinases have been discovered [12]. Many of these protein kinases span the plasma membrane or are associated with its inner surface, and are thus in a position to transduce a signal across the membrane [12]. At least 15 protein kinases are oncogenic and could play a role in mitogenic response pathways. Many protein kinases have been found to be in families; for example, protein kinase C has five different isoforms from four different genes [12]. One consequence of the existence of at least 100 different protein kinases to the field of exercise physiology is that the coordination of various intracellular pathways in the contracting muscle cell is likely very complex. However, the techniques of molecular biology used to form this multifactorial regulatory scheme have also presented exercise scientists with new candidate proteins, such as additional protein kinases, which may play a role in explaining an exercise response or adaptation. For example, Shepherd et al. [26] recently suggested that another protein kinase, acting independently of cAMP and cAMP-dependent protein kinase may operate in the regulation of hormone-sensitive lipase in fat cells after endurance training. Hunter [12] indicates that many new protein kinases are now being identified with the cloning strategy of screening cDNA libraries with a catalytic domain probe at a lowered stringency so as to identify other membranes of a protein family. Maybe this approach could be employed to test the suggestion of Shepherd et al. [26] that another protein kinase in fat cells is responsible for the increased sensitivity to catecholamines of fat cells from endurance-trained animals.

What are the factors important for the study of the differential gene expression occurring in response to different and similar changes in contractile activity?

Many models altering contractile activity are available. It is well known that differential gene expression occurs in adult skeletal muscle and is dependent on the kind of exercise training performed. For example, running daily for weeks increases mitochondrial density without altering muscle size, while weight-lifting training increases muscle size without changing mitochondrial density [10]. Thus the choice of the type of exercise must be appropriate for the specific gene to be studied.

The next question to be discussed is the factors to consider for the application of molecular biological techniques to investigate how different or even similar alterations in contractile activity result in differential gene expression in skeletal muscle.

In an elegant recent publication, Alford et al. [1] demonstrated the importance of loading skeletal muscle in the maintenance of muscle mass. They observed the loss of mass in skeletal muscle which had normal electromyographic activity but which did not have to support the body weight. This demonstrated that any experiment studying the role of exercise on contractile proteins gene expression must be able to employ loading of muscle. At present tissue culture systems cannot load cells in culture. Although cells can be stretched in culture, the phenotypic response of stretch in vivo differs from loading in vivo. Spector et al. [28] observed that skeletal muscle which was stretched without loading in vivo had longer fibers with diameters equal to control. Diameters of muscle fibers increase because of weight-lifting [18]. So the response of muscle fiber diameter differs between stretch in vivo and weight-lifting. Thus there is no conclusive proof, at present, that molecular mechanisms occurring in stretched muscle cells in culture and in weight-lifting are identical.

Previously in this review, certain results from a study by Muscat and Kedes [23] were cited to show that the regulatory factors for transcription of a gene varied in two types of muscle culture systems. These data suggested that the portion of a gene shown to be a regulatory region in transformed muscle cells in culture was dependent on the selection of the type of muscle culture. Thus transformed muscle cells may not respond to contractile activity through identical mechanisms as those occurring in human exercise training.

From the above description it seems likely that many, if not all, experiments which employ molecular biological techniques to delineate mechanisms responsible for the altered gene expression in humans after exercise training will need to employ whole animals. Procedures to transfer genes into adult skeletal muscles will be developed in the future for gene therapy, and these techniques will be able to be used by exercise scientists in their studies of molecular biology.

In summary, the factors to consider in studying exercise-induced differential gene expression include (*a*) the selection of an appropriate exercise model to study the protein of interest, and (*b*) the differential effects between muscle cultures and intact adult skeletal muscle in whole animals on the protein gene.

Recent Advances to Simplify the Application of Molecular Biology:
The Synthetic Oligonucleotide
By far, one of the more labor-intensive aspects of molecular biology is, and will continue to be, the screening or searching of cDNA or genomic libraries for the clone sequence of interest. However, if one can obtain or infer nucleotide sequence information, considerable time savings can be realized by synthesizing a short oligomer (25 or more bases) of the desired sequence. Cost-effective custom synthesis is now offered, sometimes for as little as five or ten dollars per base. In addition, custom oligonucleotides synthesized that are biotinylated or fluorescently labeled offer additional savings in some cases by circumventing the need for radioisotopes. Thus, for some experimenters, the advent of an "off the shelf" technology offers distinct advantages to obtain pilot information to justify the intensive effort to obtain a purified gene or mRNA for cloning of molecular probes. Further information concerning the application of introductory methods in molecular biology to exercise was presented in a recent review [4].

SUMMARY

Past progress in exercise biochemical research has often depended on the use of knowledge and techniques which were originally reported from other disciplines. With the advent of newer methodologies in molecular biology, the purpose of this review has been to document the status of information gained from the application of molecular biological techniques to questions in exercise physiology. Furthermore, this review has speculated how new methods in molecular biology might be employed to answer classic questions in exercise physiology. A powerful revolution in science, that is, molecular biology, will provide new information about exercise mechanisms, which ideally will improve the training programs for elite athletes as well as continue to be associated with the public's interest in exercise training.

ACKNOWLEDGMENTS

The author thanks Don Thomason, Ph.D., and Ted Wong for their idea-generating critical discussions and their encouraging support. Mr. Wong also contributed through his extensive editing of the review, particularly his assistance in writing the section on molecular biology terms. The author thanks Ms. Stefanie Duhon for excellent typing. This review was supported by National Institutes of Health Grant AR 19393.

REFERENCES

1. Alford EK, Roy RR, Hodgson JA, Edgerton VR: Electromyography of rat soleus, medial gastrocnemius, and tibialis anterior during hindlimb suspension. *Exp Neurol* 96:635–649, 1987.
2. Armstrong RB, Ogilvie RW, Schwane JA: Eccentric exercise-induced injury to rat sketal muscle. *J Appl Physiol* 54:80–93, 1983.
3. Babij P, Booth FW: α-Actin and cytochrome c mRNAs in atrophied adult rat skeletal muscle. *Am J Physiol* 254:C651–C656, 1988.
4. Babij P, Booth FW: Biochemistry of exercise: advances in molecular biology relevant to adaptation of muscle to exercise. *Sports Med* 5:137–143, 1988.
5. Booth FW, Holloszy JO: Cytochrome c turnover in skeletal muscle. *J Biol Chem* 252:416–419, 1977.
6. Darr KC, Schultz E: Exercise-induced satellite cell activation in growing and mature skeletal muscle. *J Appl Physiol* 63:1816–1821, 1987.
7. Everett AW, Sparrow MP: Transient appearance of a fast myosin heavy chain epitope in slow-type muscle fibres during stretch hypertrophy of the anterior latissimus dorsi muscle in the adult chicken. *J Musc Res Cell Mot* 8:220–228, 1987.
8. Florini JR: Hormonal control of muscle growth. *Muscle and Nerv* 10:577–598, 1987.
9. Green HJ, Reichmann H, Pette D: Fibre type specific transformations in the enzyme activity pattern of rat vastus lateralis muscle by prolonged endurance training. *Pflugers Arch* 399:216–222, 1983.
10. Holloszy JO, Booth FW: Biochemical adaptations to exercise in muscle. *Ann Rev Physiol* 38:273–291, 1976.
11. Holloszy JO, Oscai LB, Don IJ, Mole PA: Mitochondrial citric acid cycle and related enzymes: adaptive response to exercise. *Biochem Biophys Res Comm* 40:1368–1373, 1970.
12. Hunter T: A thousand and one protein kinases. *Cell* 50:823–829, 1987.
13. Jennische E, Hannsson HA: Regenerating skeletal muscle cells express insulin-like growth factor I. *Acta Physiol Scand* 130:327–332, 1987.
14. Kahn P, Graf T: *Oncogenes and Growth Control.* New York, Springer-Verlag, 1986.
15. Koenig M, Monaco AP, Kunkel LM: The complete sequence of dystrophin predicts a rod-shaped cytoskeletal protein. *Cell* 53:219–228, 1988.
16. Laurent GJ, Sparrow MP, Millward DJ: Turnover of muscle protein in the fowl. *Biochem J* 176:407–417, 1978.
17. Leberer E, Seedorf U, Pette D: Neural control of gene expression in skeletal muscle. Calcium-sequestering proteins in developing and chronically stimulated rabbit skeletal muscles. *Biochem J* 239:295–300, 1986.
18. Luthi JM, Howald H, Claassen H, Rosler K, Vock P, Hoppeler H: Structural changes in skeletal muscle tissue with heavy-resistance exercise. *Int J Sports Med* 7:123–127, 1986.
19. Mahdavi V, Strehler EE, Periasamy M, Wieczorek DF, Izumo S, Nadal-Ginard B: Sarcomeric myosin heavy chain gene family: organization and pattern of expression. *Med Sci Sports Exerc* 18:299–308, 1985.
20. Marshall CJ: Oncogenes and growth control 1987. *Cell* 49:723–725, 1987.
21. Morrison PR, Montgomery JA, Wong TS, Booth FW: Cytochrome c protein-synthesis rates and mRNA contents during atrophy and recovery in skeletal muscle. *Biochem J* 241:257–263, 1987.
22. Morrison PR, Muller GW, Booth FW: Actin synthesis rate and mRNA level increase during early recovery of atrophied muscle. *Am J Physiol* 253:C205–C209, 1987.
23. Muscat GEO, Kedes L: Multiple 5'-flanking regions of human α-skeletal actin gene synergistically modulate muscle-specific expression. *Mole Cell Biol* 7:4089–4099, 1987.

24. Newsholme EA: Use of enzyme activity measurements in studies on the biochemistry of exercise. *Int J Sports Med* 1:100–102, 1980.
25. Seedorf UE, Leberer E, Kirschbaum BJ, Pette D: Neural control of gene expression in skeletal muscle. Effects of chronic stimulation on lactate dehydrogenase isoenzymes and citrate synthase. *Biochem J* 239:115–120, 1986.
26. Shepherd RE, Bah MD, Nelson KM: Enhanced lipolysis is not evident in adipocytes from exercise-trained SHR. *J Appl Physiol* 61:1301–1308, 1986.
27. Sinn E, Muller W, Pattengale P, Tepler I, Wallace R, Leder P: Coexpression of MMTV/ v-Ha-*ras* and MMTV/c-*myc* genes in transgenic mice: synergistic action of oncogenes in vivo. *Cell* 49:465–475, 1987.
28. Spector SA, Simard CP, Fournier M, Sternlicht E, Edgerton VR: Architectural alterations of rat hind-limb skeletal muscles immobilized at different lengths. *Exp Neurol* 76:94–110, 1982.
29. Thomason DB, Herrick RE, Surdyka D, Baldwin KM: Time course of soleus muscle myosin expression during hindlimb suspension and recovery. *J Appl Physiol* 63:130– 137, 1987.
30. Turner J, Rotwein P, Novakofski J, Bechtel P: Induction of mRNA for IGF-I and -II during growth hormone stimulated muscle hypertrophy. *Am J Physiol* 255:E513– E517, 1988.
31. Underwood LE, Williams RS: Pretranslational regulation of myoglobin gene expression. *Am J Physiol* 252:C450–C453, 1987.
32. Vanderkerckhove J, Bugaisky G, Buckingham M: Simultaneous expression of skeletal muscle and heart actin proteins in various striated muscle tissues and cells. *J Biol Chem* 261:1838–1843, 1986.
33. Walsh K, and Koshland DE Jr: Characterization of rate-controlling steps in vivo by use of an adjustable expression vector. *Proc Natl Acad Sci* 82:3577–3581, 1985.
34. Watson PA, Stein JP, Booth FW: Changes in actin synthesis and α-actin-mRNA content in rat muscle during immobilization. *Am J Physiol* 247:C39–C44, 1984.
35. Williams RS: Mitochondrial gene expression in mammalian striated muscle. *J Biol Chem* 261:12390–12394, 1986.
36. Williams RS, Garcia-Moll M, Mellor J, Salmons S, Harlan W: Adaptation of skeletal muscle to increased contractile activity. *J Biol Chem* 262:2764–2767, 1987.
37. Williams RS, Salmons S, Newsholme EA, Kaufman RE, Mellor J: Regulation of nuclear and mitochondrial gene expression by contractile activity in skeletal muscle. *J Biol Chem* 261:376–380, 1986.

2
A Review of Metabolic and Physiological Factors in Fatigue

DON P. M. MACLAREN, M.Sc.
HENRY GIBSON, Ph.D.
MARK PARRY-BILLINGS, B.Sc.
RICHARD H. T. EDWARDS, M.D.

INTRODUCTION

This review examines and discusses the many studies reported in the literature on the factors contributing to human skeletal muscle fatigue. The exact nature as to the cause of fatigue still remains unclear and thus it is not intended here to provide a simple answer to what is a complex phenomenon. General agreement exists as to what constitutes fatigue during muscular contractions [10, 75, 210]. We have taken as our definition of fatigue that proposed by Gibson and Edwards [95], who stated that fatigue is a failure to maintain the required or expected force or power output.

Whether fatigue is central or peripheral in origin was the source of early controversy. Because there is more literature concerned with peripheral fatigue, we are therefore giving greater emphasis to it. The modes of investigation of peripheral human muscular fatigue have followed from two general schools of thought: metabolic and electrophysiological. Many metabolic studies have been made on dynamically active muscle, whereas electrophysiological studies have generally been made on isometrically contracting muscle. The integration and interpolation of data from the different protocols used in the literature are made with caution, since the mechanism of fatigue is likely to depend on the type of activity and the contractile history of the muscle.

CENTRAL FATIGUE

The command chain for voluntary muscular activity involves many steps from the brain to the formation of actin–myosin cross bridges within the muscle (Fig. 2.1), and fatigue may occur as a result of a failure at any one link in this chain [75]. The first classification is whether fatigue is either central or peripheral on a structural basis [10], or whether central fatigue is caused by a failure in neural drive and peripheral fatigue by an impairment of force generation by the muscle [95].

Early studies considered fatigue to be central in origin [171, 234]. By employing a finger ergograph, Mosso [171] showed in a colleague that more work could be performed and less fatigue exhibited following presentation of a lecture. This was attributed to nervous arousal. More recent work has involved supramaximally stimulating muscle (via motor nerves or motor end points) and comparing forces developed to that with maximum voluntary contractions (MVC). Merton [163], who found no differences between the two forces for the adductor pollicis muscle, concluded that fatigue was peripheral in origin, but Ikai et al. [123] demonstrated in the same muscle an enhancement of contractile force with tetanic stimulation, implying fatigue was central. In experiments on the quadriceps muscle, five out of nine subjects consistently showed central fatigue while the remainder did not, suggesting that this may explain individual motor performance [33]. Motivation clearly influences fatigue: Schwab [205] observed that exercise was prolonged in subjects promised a reward or in those running to catch a train. Further laboratory experiments support the idea that a central component in fatigue exists [10].

Central fatigue may occur because of malfunction of nerve cells or inhibition of voluntary effort; the action of sensory pathways on the reticular formation has been suggested to be critical [10]. Setchenov [208] demonstrated that the recovery of an exhausted limb could be accelerated if the opposite, previously rested, limb was exercised. This was attributed to a "recharging with energy" the fatigued motor centers as a result of afferent impulses from the active, nonfatigued limb. Weber [236] opposed this explanation, claiming that the enhanced recovery was due to an increase in blood flow which removed harmful metabolites. This "circulatory" theory was disputed by the findings of Asmussen and Mazin [11, 12], who showed that small, static movements and mental activity during rest periods aided recovery of the fatigued muscles and as expected found that these "diverting activities" did not increase blood flow. A mechanism was proposed in which the feedback of nerve impulses from fatigued muscles to the reticular formation caused the inhibition of voluntary effort. Diverting activity produced an increased inflow of impulses from nonfatigued muscle to the facilitatory part of the reticular formation and this shifted the balance from inhibition toward facilitation [10].

Further evidence for the concept of central fatigue was put forward by Rojtbak and Dedabrishvili [193], who recorded the electroencephalogram (EEG) from exercising subjects. The alpha rhythm of the EEG, which is characteristic of lowered arousal, appeared in fatigue and disappeared during diverting activity. The alpha rhythm was also evident when subjects closed their eyes, but not present when they opened them. Hence it was assumed that central inhibition resulted when subjects closed their eyes and that reduced inhibition and facilitation occurred on opening them [12]. Exercise studies supported this theory, with subjects who worked to "exhaustion" with closed eyes able to continue to exercise immediately upon opening them.

Central fatigue may be caused by an inhibition of motor areas elicited by nervous impulses from receptors (probably a form of chemoreceptor) in the fatigued muscle [10]. A psychological component in fatigue is obviously a possibility, for example, in the case of athletes who learn to ignore painful or inhibitory sensory inputs and approach performance limits set by the motor pathways and muscle fibers; however, its presence should not be considered to diminish the importance of clear evidence of peripheral fatigue. The idea of a neural rather than a metabolic cause for changes in brain function during exercise was supported by the suggestion that acidosis within the brain occurs only in pathological conditions and that exercise lactacidosis has a negligible effect on brain function [209]. However, recently it has been hypothesized that central fatigue during sustained exercise may occur because of an increase in the plasma tryptophan:branched chain amino acid ratio, which in turn results in an increase in synthesis of the neurotransmitter 5-hydroxytryptamine in the brain [184].

Exercise is also associated with an increase in ammonia production by skeletal muscle, and the extramuscular action of ammonia is directed mainly toward the central nervous system, particularly the brain. In the brain NH_3 accumulation may alter the concentration of vital neurotransmitters [152] and reduce the level of ATP [3]. Central fatigue has also been attributed to the "overexcitation" of neural tissue by ammonia, caused by a reduction in postsynaptic inhibition [124]. In addition, it has been demonstrated that an elevated ammonia level stimulates ventilation [206]. Hyperpnea is a possible contributor toward central perceptions of fatigue [14, 39].

PERIPHERAL FATIGUE

Peripheral fatigue occurs at three possible sites: the neuromuscular junction and muscle cell membrane (excitation), the calcium release mechanism (activation), and the sliding filaments (contractile processes) (Fig. 2.1). Early work by Asmussen [9] demonstrated the existence of these sites in an experiment on an isolated preparation of lizard intercostal muscle. He stimulated the fibers indirectly (via the motor nerve) until

FIGURE 2.1

The command chain for muscular contraction and the major causes of fatigue.
(Modified from Edwards RHT: Biochemical basis of fatigue. In Knuttgen HG
(ed): Biochemistry of Exercise. *Champaign, IL, Human Kinetics, 1983, pp*
3–28.)

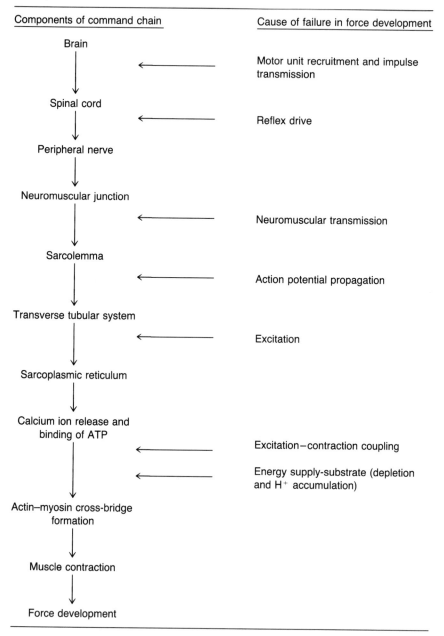

Components of command chain	Cause of failure in force development
Brain	Motor unit recruitment and impulse transmission
Spinal cord	Reflex drive
Peripheral nerve	
Neuromuscular junction	Neuromuscular transmission
Sarcolemma	Action potential propagation
Transverse tubular system	Excitation
Sarcoplasmic reticulum	
Calcium ion release and binding of ATP	Excitation–contraction coupling
	Energy supply-substrate (depletion and H⁺ accumulation)
Actin–myosin cross-bridge formation	
Muscle contraction	
Force development	

force declined, which indicated failure of the "transmission mechanism" (i.e., excitation). Direct stimulation resulted in an increase in force before fatigue occurred again. The second decrease was attributed to impairment in the contractile mechanism. These findings were supported by similar experiments on the tibialis muscle of decerebrate cats [43]. The distinction between excitation and activation mechanisms was shown by the work of Merton [163], who demonstrated a decline in contractile force without loss of excitation in the indirectly stimulated adductor pollicis muscle. Peripheral fatigue may obviously be affected by metabolic factors in muscle.

Simonson [210] proposed two hypotheses for the cause of fatigue within muscle—the "accumulation hypothesis" and the "exhaustion hypothesis." The former was considered to be related to the accumulation of metabolites which may result in impaired force generation, whereas the latter was deemed to arise as a result of depletion of metabolites.

Accumulation Hypothesis

The accumulation hypothesis relates to the accumulation of a number of metabolites, namely hydrogen ions (H^+), ammonia (NH_3), and inorganic phosphate (P_i), which have been shown to result in an impairment of force generation by the muscle fibers. The earliest reported work which claimed that accumulation of a substance did in fact limit performance was that of Weichardt [237], who labeled this substance "kenotoxin." In 1935, Muller [174] demonstrated a faster onset of fatigue in occluded limbs and suggested that the occlusion resulted in an accumulation of some unidentified products of metabolism which caused the fatigue. Hill [114] claimed that lactic acid was the "fatigue substance."

HYDROGEN ION ACCUMULATION. Exercise of short duration and high intensity recruits predominantly fast glycolytic (FG) fibers and draws on anaerobic glycolysis for the synthesis of the majority of the ATP necessary for muscle contraction [200], with accumulation of lactic acid in both muscle and blood. At a pH of 6.5, 99.8% of lactic acid exists in its ionized form [198] and therefore there is a concomitant increase in hydrogen ion concentration.

Evidence to support the theory that H^+ accumulation results in failure to maintain force during muscular contraction has been provided by studies employing a wide range of techniques including iodoacetate poisoned muscle preparations [195], skinned mammalian muscle fibers [67], nuclear magnetic resonance (NMR) [59], and muscle biopsy analysis [196]. Further evidence has been provided by studies which induced a state of alkalosis or acidosis in subjects prior to exercise. Sodium bicarbonate and sodium citrate ingestion have been shown to elevate preexercise blood pH and increase speed and endurance [157, 222] while ingestion of ammonium chloride has resulted in a reduction in preexercise pH and a decrease in time to exhaustion [122, 132, 222]. H^+ accumulation may impair muscle performance through its effect on glycolysis, on the contractile process itself, or on certain physiologically important equilibrium reactions.

Hydrogen Ions and Glycolysis. Ronzoni and Kerly [194] noted that inhibition of the conversion of hexomonophosphates to lactate occurred in acidic conditions. Reduced enzyme activity is associated with a decrease in the rate of glycolysis and a decline in ATP resynthesis [108]. Phosphofructokinase (PFK) is almost completely inhibited at pH 6.5 [53, 230]. H^+ ions may affect PFK activity by increasing the level of $HATP^{3-}$ [53], which has been found to be a potent inhibitor of the enzyme [154]. PFK inhibition has been found to lead to an elevated glucose-6-phosphate concentration resulting from high levels of fructose-6-phosphate [228]. The latter has been shown to be a powerful inhibitor of both hexokinase and phosphorylase [186]. Inhibition of glycolysis may thus occur at sites remote from the initial inhibition of PFK.

Although PFK is probably the key limiting enzyme in glycolysis, the effect of acidosis on phosphorylase activity may also be a possible fatigue mechanism. The transformation of phosphorylase b to active phosphorylase a is slowed, and the maximum level of phosphorylase a has been found to be reduced as a consequence of acidosis [53, 195]. The reduction in activity of phosphorylase is brought about by an inhibition of phosphorylase b kinase at low pH [74, 144]. Danforth [53] has linked substrate depletion and glycolytic enzyme activity, demonstrating that low muscle glycogen resulted in a low level of phosphorylase a.

Hydrogen ion accumulation may adversely affect the activity of enzymes other than PFK and phosphorylase [131]. Lactate dehydrogenase (LDH) activity is inhibited by physiological concentrations of lactate, and therefore variations in individual LDH levels may affect peak lactic acid production [212, 224]. The influence of pH changes on nonglycolytic enzymes may also constitute a mechanism for impaired tension development. A reduction in myosin-ATPase activity in acidic conditions has been shown to result in the early onset of fatigue [202]. The rate at which ATP is synthesized from anaerobic glycogenolysis is therefore limited by the inhibition of key enzymes as a consequence of the accumulation of H^+.

Hydrogen Ions and the Contractile Process. The introduction of the in vitro "skinned fiber" technique was a significant development in the investigation of the effect of changes in pH on the contractile machinery because it allowed the control of substrate and Ca^{2+} concentrations [66]. A decrease in muscle pH was found to reduce tension development and increase the Ca^{2+} requirement to develop the same tension [67, 88, 192]. Ca^{2+} release by the sarcoplasmic reticulum at a lower pH has been found to be reduced [178]. Competition of H^+ for activating Ca^{2+} sites in cross-bridge formation can also reduce force generation [138], as can reduced muscle filament binding capacity for Ca^{2+} through inactivation of the myofibrillar protein troponin [94, 139]. Experiments using the skinned fiber technique have cast doubt on the concept of H^+ competition for the Ca^{2+} sites but not for the enhanced binding of Ca^{2+} in the sarcoplasmic reticulum at low pH [66]. Furthermore, the results from skinned fiber work have established that the most likely explanation of reduced force generation as a consequence of increases in H^+ concentration is due to product inhibition of actomyosin ATPase [67, 107, 227]. The linear relationship observed between the decline of force and the increase in H^+ concentration in fatiguing frog muscle fibers and the decline in utilization of ATP that occurs during fatigue appear to be consistent with product inhibition of myofibrillar ATPase.

It has been suggested that H^+ accumulation inhibits generation of action potentials in excitable membranes [62] by causing physical changes in the arrangement of membrane proteins or as a result of the electric field generated by their charge [16]. Experimental evidence for this suggestion has been provided by Orchardson [187], who demonstrated that membrane excitability decreased when intracellular pH decreased. Since conduction velocity is directly related to membrane excitability, an increase in acidity in the membrane environment would be expected to cause a decrease in membrane conduction velocity. The interaction between pH and conduction velocity is not firmly established, but it is significant that Mills and Edwards [169] showed that the power spectral shift in electromyography (EMG) with fatigue also occurs in patients with myophosphorylase deficiency.

Hydrogen Ions and Equilibrium Reactions. The accumulation of H^+ affects the position of reactions which involve the consumption or production of H^+. These include three important equilibria which are altered in such a way as to enhance the onset of fatigue:

1. The creatine kinase reaction:

$$PCr + ADP + H^+ \rightleftharpoons Cr + ATP$$

   At low pH the forward reaction is more rapid, because of the increase in H^+ resulting in a faster depletion of PCr, an important short-term energy substrate [167].
2. The hydrolysis and resynthesis of ATP:

$$ATP \rightleftharpoons ADP + P_i + H^+$$
$$ATPase$$

   The decrease in the ATP:ADP ratio during exercise-induced acidosis was attributed partly to the altered distribution between ionic forms due to the increase in H^+ concentration [102]. Both ATP and ADP are composed of different ionic species, including Mg^{2+}, K^+, and H^+, and in most enzymatic reactions involving ATP and ADP the active species are magnesium ion complexes. Sahlin [195] reported that the Mg^{2+}-complex concentrations declined in acidosis and suggested that this caused inhibition of reactions involving the adenosine nucleotides.

3. A number of glycolytic reactions are linked to the $NAD^+/NADH$ or $NADP^+/NADP$ couples, including the lactate/pyruvate equilibrium:

$$\text{Pyruvate} + NADH + H^+ \rightleftharpoons \text{LACTATE} + NAD^+$$
$$\text{LDH}$$

An increase in H^+ concentration increases lactate production. Indeed the lactate:pyruvate ratio increases more than 10-fold at exhaustion [197], and this reaction has been stated as the main controller of the cellular level of NAD^+ [73]. The importance of the availability of NAD^+ for glycolysis has been stressed by a number of workers, who claimed that a high glycolytic rate depended on a high $NAD^+:NADH$ ratio [40, 238]. It is therefore significant that H^+ accumulation may reduce the level of the hydrogen acceptor NAD^+ and so reduce glycolysis.

Other Effects of Hydrogen Ion Accumulation. The adverse effects of H^+ accumulation have been outlined above in connection with predominantly anaerobic exercise. In long-term, low-intensity exercise the lactic acid production and concomitant decrease in pH are comparatively small. It is important to remember that lactic acid is formed whenever FG motor units are activated, even when the supply of oxygen is adequate. In addition to the effects previously described, a decrease in pH has been shown to inhibit the mobilization of free fatty acids (FFA) from adipose tissue [207] and result in a faster glycogen depletion and earlier onset of fatigue.

Although there appear to be profound effects of H^+ accumulation, some evidence suggests that fatigue in certain muscles cannot be explained by the concomitant decline in pH. When cat gastrocnemius and soleus muscles were made to contract, the lactate output was the same from both muscles and yet the gastrocnemius fatigued to a greater extent than the soleus [117]. Moreover, patients with McArdle's syndrome (a congenital lack of myophosphorylase) produce no lactic acid and yet their muscles fatigue even more rapidly than normal muscle [85, 242]. PFK-deficient patients have also been studied using NMR [80] and results show that virtually no change in pH occurs (i.e., pH 7.24–7.18) whereas a significant fall could be realized in normal subjects (i.e., pH

7.18–7.05) during periods of exercise and ischemia. Hence, other possible mechanisms to account for muscular fatigue must be considered.

AMMONIA ACCUMULATION. The accumulation of ammonia (NH_3) and the ammonium ion (NH_4^+) in muscle and blood cannot be overlooked as a possible inhibitory metabolite contributing to fatigue [175]. Intense or prolonged exercise is accompanied by release of large amounts of ammonia from muscle [6]. This is as a result of an increase in the myokinase reaction (Equation 1) and the enhancement of the purine–nucleotide cycle [153], converting AMP to inosine monophosphate (IMP) with the formation of ammonia (Equation 2):

$$2\ ADP \xrightarrow{\text{myokinase}} ATP + AMP \qquad 1$$

$$AMP + H_2O \xrightarrow{\text{adenylate deaminase}} IMP + NH_3 \qquad 2$$

Ammonia production was first linked to fatigue by Tashiro [223], and since then it has been confirmed that during exercise the formation of ammonia is increased [6, 42] and is positively related to work intensity [244]. Muscle is the major source of ammonia in an active subject [153], but it may exert its effects both intracellularly and extracellularly. The accumulation of ammonia may cause central fatigue, as discussed earlier, but it may also adversely affect muscle metabolism. Greater ammonia accumulation has been observed in predominantly FG than in slow oxidative (SO) muscles [70, 165] and may partially explain the separate fatigue characteristics of the muscles. A possible site of influence of the NH_4^+ ion is at the surface membrane of the muscle, where it may reduce overall muscle tension as a result of a progressive loss of electrically excitable fibers [106]. In addition, ammonia has been found to stimulate PFK activity [153], inhibit the Krebs cycle [137] and gluconeogenesis [45], and reduce mitochondrial oxidation [249]. Overall this will result in a larger lactic acid production and faster glycogen depletion. It is possible that ammonia might initiate the decline in pH associated with the onset of fatigue [143].

In contrast, it has been suggested that ammonia may help to delay the onset of fatigue [106] since it is a base which will buffer H^+ ions and at low levels potentiate twitch tension. However, the beneficial effects of ammonia appear to be negligible and its main effects are harmful, for example, hepatic coma and epileptic seizures. It still remains to be shown what role ammonia accumulation plays in the development of fatigue [148].

The ingestion of aspartic acid salts or sodium glutamate in order to reduce the exercise-induced increases in blood ammonia have resulted in equivocal findings. Recent studies in humans [156, 161], however, have failed to show beneficial effects of such administration in terms of promoting performance during cycle ergometry. For a more detailed account of ammonia and exercise stress, Banister et al. [15] should be consulted.

IORGANIC PHOSPHATE ACCUMULATION. Using topical magnetic resonance spectroscopy, it has been shown that inorganic phosphate (P_i) is present in muscle cells at a concentration of 4.4 mmol·kg^{-1} [246]. Maximal voluntary isometric contractions in humans may result in a 4-fold increase of P_i (i.e., 15–16 mmol·kg^{-1} wet weight) [58], and similar results have been obtained for isometrically contracting isolated frog sartorius muscle [59]. Accumulation of P_i has also been found to occur during ischemic rest [80] and muscular activity [81]. This accumulation of P_i may further contribute to force loss.

Direct evidence of P_i-induced force reduction has been obtained from skinned muscle fibers [41, 112]. It has been suggested that P_i may bind to myosin in such a way so as to increase the forward rate of cross-bridge cycling and thereby to reduce force output [50, 140]. Furthermore as H^+ accumulates during intense exercise, the acid form of P_i ($H_2PO_4^-$) may be produced which may result in force reduction [245]. Moreover, patients with McArdle's syndrome demonstrate greater fatiguability than normal individuals [85] and a concomitantly larger increase in P_i accumulation [149]. The evidence supports a plausible role for P_i in fatigue. Most studies have employed a model of isometric muscle contraction and the little evidence available on the role of P_i in fatigue during dynamic is indirect [38, 103].

"Exhaustion" Hypothesis

Simonson [210] claimed that fatigue may result from the depletion of certain metabolites, in particular the energy substrates ATP, PCr, and glycogen. The contribution of this mechanism to fatigue in anaerobic and aerobic exercise will be reviewed as well as the role of phosphate depletion in the impairment of muscle contraction.

ATP, PCR, AND GLYCOGEN DEPLETION DURING ANAEROBIC EXERCISE. During work which is predominantly anaerobic, muscle contraction may be impaired by the depletion of the short-term energy substrates ATP and PCr, and also by reduced levels of glycogen [98, 225]. Metabolite depletion may be localized and may not be reflected in altered whole-muscle metabolite levels, for example, ATP depletion at the heads of the myosin cross-bridges or glycogen depletion in highly recruited fibers.

Low levels of ATP have been recorded at exhaustion after dynamic exercise [37, 190], yet the role of ATP depletion in fatigue remains equivocal. Use of NMR has shown only small changes in total ATP, ADP, and AMP levels after exercise [59], indicating that fatigue is unlikely to be accounted for by ATP depletion. In contrast, after 1–2 minutes of maximal work the level of PCr is practically zero or is severely depleted [120, 136]. Indeed, PCr concentration has been positively correlated to tension development [125, 214] and so it appeared that PCr depletion was a major cause of fatigue. However, Dawson et al. [59] observed no proportional relationship between PCr and force development. Furthermore, it has been claimed there was no obvious biochemical basis for postulating that PCr depletion was directly responsible for force reduction [108]. Successive isometric contractions each held to fatigue with continuous ischemia, (i.e., no aerobic recovery possible), resulted in two further contractions [76]. This experiment indicates the difficulty in distinguishing muscle pain from fatigue and further illustrates that both pain and fatigue may simply reflect "hard times" in the muscle, which limit performance by influencing central factors, including motivation.

The depletion of glycogen may also limit muscle performance. A large and rapid breakdown of glycogen occurs during brief, intense exercise but only about one-half of the total muscle stores are depleted [111]. Consequently, it may be concluded that a lack of muscle glycogen could not account for fatigue in this type of exercise [108], although the early depletion of glycogen in highly recruited FG fibers may result in a decline in tension development [72, 99].

The available evidence shows that no simple relationship exists between concentrations of the energy substrates ATP, PCr, and glycogen and the development of force. It has been suggested that fatigue may be due not to the absolute level of any one substrate, but to the relative kinetics of supply and demand, as determined by a few key enzymes [119].

FAT, GLYCOGEN, AND GLUCOSE AVAILABILITY DURING AEROBIC EXERCISE. During submaximal work slow oxidative fibers are primarily recruited and the energy required is provided predominantly by two fuels, glucose and FFA which are stored in the form of glycogen and triglycerides, respectively [182]. No evidence has been found to indicate that fat deposits are depleted during submaximal work [87]. Indeed fatty acids could theoretically support 5 days of continuous running, and therefore it is obvious that the total body fat stores are more than sufficient to provide fuel for long-term exercise [182].

The major source of glucose for muscle metabolism is the glycogen stored within the muscle fibers [183]. A number of studies which have employed muscle biopsy techniques and subsequent histochemical analysis have found that muscle glycogen stores were depleted during sustained exercise at 65–75% of the maximum oxygen uptake ($\dot{V}O_2$max) and that this depletion was closely associated with fatigue [21, 110].

Furthermore, some data suggest that glycogen stores do not influence fatigue until depleted; perhaps an "all or none" response exists [199, 200]. Glycogen is first depleted in SO fibers, and if exercise is continued glycogen stores in FG fibers may also become depleted [99]. Earlier studies indicate that exhaustion after exercise at moderate and low intensity (i.e., 55% $\dot{V}O_2$max or less) may not coincide with muscle glycogen depletion. These findings must be reconsidered in view of more recent work [232, 233] which demonstrates that even at low exercise intensities glycogen depletion may be important in fatigue.

Once the primary source of glucose—muscle glycogen—is exhausted, blood glucose becomes more important as a fuel for aerobic metabolism. However, it has been found that the oxidation of the blood-borne fuels, glucose and FFA, cannot provide energy at a sufficient rate to satisfy muscle demands [182, 183]. Therefore in response to the lower availability of ATP, exercise intensity must be decreased, constituting fatigue when this is defined in terms of power output. The continued utilization of blood glucose in oxidative metabolism may lead to a condition of hypoglycemia, which has been shown to affect the central nervous system, because of its dependence on blood glucose as a fuel. Hypoglycemia is not a problem in marathon runners [229], although Ahlborg and Felig [4] observed hypoglycemia in subjects exercising for long periods (2.5–3.5 hours). Low blood glucose concentration will stimulate glycogenolysis with resulting depletion of hepatic glycogen stores seen with prolonged exercise [13, 118]. Glucose for muscle metabolism may also be provided by gluconeogenesis in the liver. Felig and Wahren [89] estimated that conversion of amino acids to glucose provided 30% of the carbohydrate utilized by skeletal muscle during exercise of low intensity (30% $\dot{V}O_2$max). However, in elite marathon runners, who utilize 70–80% $\dot{V}O_2$max, its quantitative importance is questionable [182].

Further support for the concept that the availability of muscle glycogen limits performance has been provided by studies which employed high- and low-carbohydrate diets prior to exercise. A low-carbohydrate diet has been found to reduce endurance time compared to that achieved after a normal diet [49]. Moreover, a high-carbohydrate diet consumed for 3 days has been shown to increase muscle glycogen levels and to offset fatigue in long-term exercise [21]. Conversely, the administration of beta-blockers, which depress the mobilization of FFA from adipose tissue, leads to earlier exhaustion as a result of earlier muscle glycogen depletion [211]. Studies involving ingestion of caffeine prior to exercise have shown a delay in the onset of fatigue [52], due to a stimulation of FFA mobilization [96], leading to a glycogen-sparing effect [113]. A combination of carbohydrate loading and caffeine ingestion has recently been reported as prolonging endurance activities [158].

The oxidation of FFA during long-term exercise is important since it has a sparing effect on the limited glycogen reserves and so helps in delaying the onset of fatigue due to glycogen depletion. A number of underlying mechanisms for this effect have been suggested. An increase in the β-oxidation of FFA to acetyl coenzyme A leads to an increase in the acetyl coenzyme A:coenzyme A ratio, which has been shown to inhibit pyruvate oxidation and so reduce the glycolytic rate [186]. In addition, a high rate of fat oxidation elevates citrate concentration via the Krebs cycle, which in turn has been found to inhibit PFK activity [127].

The concept that the turnover of FFA becomes increasingly important when exercise is prolonged, as a result of the depletion of carbohydrate stores, has been challenged by the findings of Hermansen et al. [110]. They found that the respiratory exchange ratio (R) remained above 0.9 during 1.5 hours of exercise, indicating that carbohydrates were being predominantly oxidized. In contrast, during more prolonged exercise (24 hours) a steady decline in R, implying an increased dependence on fat as a fuel, has been observed [54]. Therefore it appears that glycogen depletion may not occur in some subjects during long-term exercise (1.5–2.5 hours duration), while glycogen stores may limit performance in more prolonged exercise and during more intense exercise of a similar duration.

PHOSPHATE DEPLETION. Traditionally the depletion hypothesis refers to the exhaustion of energy subtrates; however, the depletion or loss of ionic phosphate (P_i) from muscle may also be considered of importance. In dynamic exercise, the release of phosphate ions from muscle is increased; this is in contrast to the findings of P_i accumulation during isometric exercise (described earlier). Stella [218] was the first to report a higher rate of P_i diffusion from fatigued muscle. Furthermore, experiments on fast- and slow-twitch muscles of rats showed that phosphate release was significantly elevated and force declined by 50% in the gastrocnemius, while the soleus showed no change in either phosphate release or force development [117]. These findings are in agreement with the fact that the muscle membrane is permeable to P_i when depolarized during activation [1, 116].

A number of mechanisms by which P_i depletion may result in fatigue have been proposed. Lack of intracellular phosphate may reduce PCr resynthesis and lead to faster depletion of this immediate energy store [117]. Low concentrations of P_i may also reduce ATP resynthesis as a result of inadequate stimulation of ATPase activity [44]. In addition, the activity of phosphorylase is critically dependent on P_i concentration: Low intramuscular concentrations have been associated with a decline in activity [48], while Ca^{2+} release from the vesicles of the sarcoplasmic reticulum is impaired after phosphate depletion [159].

After 3–4 minutes of maximal exercise the loss of ionic phosphate from the contracting muscles may impair force generation [117]. Phosphate depletion in fatigue during submaximal exercise appears doubtful, and its effect on intense exercise of less than 1 minute duration remains unresolved.

Interaction between the Accumulation and Exhaustion Hypotheses
The accumulation of metabolites and the depletion of energy substrates and phosphate do not occur independently. A large degree of interaction exists between these two fatigue mechanisms. Thorstensson [226] claimed that during predominantly anaerobic exercise the fatigue characteristics of FG fibers were due to both a significant glycogen depletion and a large H^+ accumulation. Furthermore Bergstrom et al. [20] suggested that phosphagen depletion was limiting and was caused by a low glycolytic rate due to a H^+ inhibition of PFK, followed by the effect of elevated glucose-6-phosphate levels on phosphorylase activity. During prolonged aerobic exercise a degree of interaction is also evident. As mentioned earlier, fatigue may be caused by a pH-induced inhibition of FFA mobilization which leads to a more rapid depletion of glycogen stores [238].

Oxygen as a Limiting Factor
Optimal performance in long-term exercise relies on the body's utilizing as large a proportion of the $\dot{V}O_2max$ as possible without stimulating a significant lactic acid production. The question as to whether it is the oxidative capacity of muscle or the oxygen transport capacity of the cardiovascular system that limits $\dot{V}O_2max$ and hence affects endurance performance remains unresolved. A full discussion of this issue is beyond the scope of this review, although the two opposing arguments are briefly highlighted.

During exhausting exercise the oxygen content of venous blood from the active muscle groups remains elevated above 10 mm Hg [65, 134]. The critical level of oxygen below which normal oxidative reactions are limited by oxygen availability is believed to be 10 mm Hg [216, 217]. Therefore, even during maximal exercise there is an adequate supply of oxygen to the muscle, and it is the capacity of the oxidative reactions themselves that limits oxygen uptake. However, Wenger and Reed [238] stated that a high venous oxygen level could not be taken to indicate adequate oxygen delivery to the muscle because of the interfiber variation in oxygen utilization. The oxygen extraction by FG fibers may be negligible, while SO fibers may empty the blood of all available oxygen and therefore aerobic metabolism in these fibers would be impaired by an inadequate oxygen supply.

In contrast, it has been claimed that mitochondrial respiratory capacity exceeds that which could be achieved with a maximal oxygen delivery and therefore oxygen supply does indeed limit the aerobic metabolism of contracting muscle. Evidence includes the observation that muscle oxidative capacity is greater than whole body maximal oxygen consumption [97] and greater than the calculated upper limit of the heart to deliver oxygen [7, 201]. Furthermore, the enhancement of $\dot{V}O_2$max following red blood cell reinfusion [247] also suggests that it is oxygen transport capacity and not the oxidative capacity of the muscle which is limiting.

It would appear that the mitochondrial respiratory capacity is adequate to meet the demands of maximal exercise and yet the oxygen available in the circulation is not fully compromised. However, since the oxygen is required in the mitochondria and studies have not clearly established the mitochondrial oxygen tension, this topic remains equivocal.

Other Metabolic Factors
Several additional metabolic mechanisms by which aerobic exercise may be limited have been proposed and these will be reviewed briefly.

During long-term exercise fatty acids constitute an important energy substrate, as discussed previously in this review. FFA must bind to proteins in the muscle cytosol and then be esterified with a carrier, carnitine, to permit transport into the mitochondria. Therefore the availability of FFA-binding proteins [231] and the concentration of carnitine may limit FFA utilization within the muscle fiber [186].

In aerobic metabolism the majority of ATP is generated via the respiratory chain, which entails a series of exchange reactions involving H^+ (and their electrons) within the mitochondrial matrix. H^+ produced by glycolysis and the Krebs cycle are transported to the site of the respiratory chain reactions bound to the coenzyme nicotinamide adenine dinucleotide (NAD). Both the sarcolemma and particularly the inner mitochondrial membrane are resistant to the diffusion of NADH. Consequently hydrogen is transferred across the two membranes by a number of shuttle mechanisms (glycerophosphate-dihydroxyacetone phosphate, β-hydroxybutyrate-acetoacetate, and malate-oxaloacetate). Therefore the concentration of the shuttle mechanism components and also the activity of the dehydrogenase enzymes in glycolysis and Krebs cycle may limit ATP synthesis via the respiratory chain. Edington et al. [74] reported that the postexercise NAD:NADH ratio following prolonged stimulation was higher in untrained rats indicating a comparatively low level of NADH in the mitochondria of animals. Hence they suggested that the delivery of NADH to the respiratory chain may be a limiting factor in long-term exercise. Even when the supply of NADH to the respiratory chain is adequate the transfer of hydrogen to the cytochrome components of the chain may be limited by the concentration and activity of the NADH diaphorases which catalyze the reaction [238].

More recently, investigations into the enzyme levels of the NADH shuttle systems comparing SO and FG muscle fibers and comparing untrained versus endurance trained individuals have highlighted the importance of malate-aspartate shuttle enzymes [203, 204]. Approximately 50% higher activities were found in the endurance-trained athletes, whereas there was no change in the α-glycerophosphate shuttle. Human skeletal muscle adapts to endurance training through increased activities of the malate-aspartate shuttle enzymes whereas the α-glycerophosphate shuttle enzyme activities do not change. These changes would play an important role in the reduced lactate response at submaximal exercise intensities exhibited by endurance-trained athletes, although the validity of the quantitative assumptions in these experiments may be questionable in view of the nature of the reactions studied [185].

A further fatigue mechanism relating to the transport of metabolites across membranes was proposed by Wenger and Reed [238]. They suggested that the transfer of ATP from the mitochondrion matrix, where it is synthesized, to the contractile proteins of the fiber may be limited by the concentration of ATP translocases at the inner mitochondrial membrane, but this has not been tested experimentally. Furthermore, the diffusion of ATP between its site of production and site of utilization could be a limiting factor for the contractile process. It has been proposed that the ADP–ATP diffusion limitation is overcome by the transfer of high-energy phosphate by means of a PCr shuttle system [23]. It has been reported that there is an increase in the relative amount of creatine kinase bound to the mitochondria as a result of endurance training [8]. This would result in enhancement of ATP transfer from the mitochondria and the facilitation of translocation of ADP into the mitochondria. Reviews on this topic may be found by consulting Meyer et al. [166], Bessman and Carpenter [22], and Jacobus [126].

Other metabolic events which may cause fatigue include a decrease in mitochondrial respiratory control and loss of structural integrity of the sarcoplasmic reticulum due to the liberation of free radicals. During prolonged exercise, the rate of oxygen consumption is increased and so it is likely that more superoxide and hydrogen peroxide are formed. Free radical linked muscle damage as a result of exercise has been observed in rats [57] and in marathon runners [235]. The accumulation of calcium ions within the mitochondria may also result in the cessation of work. A proportion of the calcium ions released from the sarcoplasmic reticulum during contraction are sequestered by the mitochondria [47]. This process consumes oxygen and so reduces that which is available for the synthesis of ATP which may eventually result in complete uncoupling of oxidative phosphorylation. Furthermore, continual recycling of calcium ions between mitochondria and sarcoplasm could result in high rates of respiration [64], thereby ensuring that energy turnover was excessive in relation to the needs of the muscle and possibly contributing to fatigue.

TRANSMISSION (EXCITATION AND ACTIVATION) FATIGUE

Energy metabolism is undoubtedly of considerable interest. However, there are possibly more important alterations in the excitation and activation of muscle contraction which may override it in determining the onset of fatigue [75]. Much physiological evidence is available suggesting that a failure of a part of the excitation and activation processes, in both anaerobic and aerobic activity, results in impairment of muscle contraction. Failure of propagation of sarcolemmal excitation prevents energy resource utilization in the muscle cell, while defective excitation–contraction coupling (activation) results in less force generation [77, 86].

Electrophysiological Studies of Fatigue
The use of electrical stimulation of muscle, as well as surface and intramuscular EMG recording of myoelectrical activity, has been widely employed in the study of fatigue. Such techniques have allowed the investigation of the electrical aspects of fatigue following isometric/dynamic exercise under either ischemic or oxidative conditions as a result of stimulated and voluntary contractions. Coupled with the measurement of other physiological variables, e.g., relaxation rate [240] and metabolic heat production [241], a greater understanding of the electrical and metabolic factors underlying human muscle fatigue has been attained.

ELECTRICAL STIMULATION. Tetanic electrical stimulation of muscle via the motor nerve trunk [163] or via intramuscular motor end nerves by percutaneous stimulation [86] has been used to fatigue muscles as well as to provide a means of documenting the frequency–force characteristics of fresh and fatigued muscle [33, 51, 86, 123]. Direct stimulation of human muscle in vivo has also been employed in the investigation of fatigue, involving stimulation voltages of 1000 volts or more [115]. Unlike indirect stimulation, which is safe and not particularly painful, direct stimulation of muscle is dramatically painful [75].

In a small hand muscle, the adductor pollicis, application of a series of frequency trains, that is, the programmed stimulation EMG, allows documentation of the frequency–force relationships together with the evoked action potential and relaxation rate [51, 75]. In large muscles of the leg the validity of percutaneous stimulation to obtain this has been questioned since it has been suggested the curve obtained in this way is voltage dependent [56]. Further work on the quadriceps muscle has shown this is not the case except at low voltages [78].

Two types of peripheral fatigue have been defined as a response to electrical stimulation: high-frequency fatigue (HFF), a reduction of force with high-frequency tetanic stimulation, and low-frequency fatigue (LFF), a reduction of force with low-frequency tetanic stimulation [75, 84, 129].

High-Frequency Fatigue. The establishment of frequency–force curves in humans [86] has indicated that after fatiguing activity, supramaximal stimulation with high-frequency trains of impulses (80–100 Hz) results in a reduction in force, while force generation may be maintained at low frequencies [75]. A concomitant decline in the peak-to-peak surface recorded synchronous evoked action potential also occurs, indicating a failure of electrical excitement along the sarcolemmal membrane. Similarly, continuous high-frequency stimulation (80–100 Hz) leads to a rapid decline in force with a concomitant decline in surface evoked action potential amplitude which may be reversed by reducing the frequency of stimulation [30, 130]. This rapid reversal is important in differentiating the influences of excitatory and metabolic factors on force reduction, since it is suggestive of redistribution of ionic fluxes across the sarcolemmal membrane, whereas PCr recovery (half-time about 30 seconds; 105) is too slow to account for the rapid recovery of excitation or force. Accompanying the decline in action potential amplitude is a broadening in shape suggestive of a slowing in conduction velocity [30, 46]. Fatigue of directly stimulated isolated muscle can be overcome by increasing stimulus intensity or duration indicating that a change in excitation threshold occurs [128, 145], further supporting the suggestion that membrane properties are altered in HFF.

Calculations by Adrian and Peachey [2] indicate that in frog sartorius muscle, for each muscle action potential the Na^+ concentration in the T-tubules may decline by 0.5 mM and K^+ concentration increase by 0.28 mM. Such changes may dramatically alter both resting membrane potentials and Na^+/K^+ conductances, hence affecting amplitude and propagation of the action potential. The accumulation of K^+ or depletion of Na^+ has been suggested to occur in the interfiber space [24] and in the extracellular fluid of the transverse tubular system [33] during muscle contraction. Indeed, K^+ loss from muscle cells is well established [91, 220] and has been related to glycogen breakdown [18].

An increase in K^+ conductance is thought to explain the reports of low membrane resistance observed in metabolically fatigued single muscle fibers [100]. This observation has been further confirmed in subsequent studies [92], and more recently an ATP-dependent K^+ channel has been identified in skeletal muscle [215] further suggesting that K^+ conductance may be altered by metabolic factors. In addition, 1–2 nM caffeine added to the bathing medium of normal frog sartorius muscle fibers (thereby elevating free internal Ca^{2+}) also results in a reduction in membrane resistance, indicating a role for Ca^{2+} in the activation of K^+ channels [92]. Indeed, Ca^{2+}-sensitive K^+ channels have recently been identified in rat muscle [188] which may be influenced by accumulation of Ca^{2+} in the T-tubular space with high-frequency activity [25].

The accumulation of extracellular K^+ has been suggested to be greatest in the T-tubules where diffusion is restricted because of the high surface-to-volume ratio [2, 33]. This may additionally account for the failure of contractile elements within the fiber where loss of the sarcolemmal action potential is not observed [24]. However, recent studies involving the measurement of T-tubule action potentials in amphibia muscle (penetrating the surface membrane) indicate this may not necessarily occur [63]. It is a distinct disadvantage that no direct information about T-tubular function is possible by EMG in human muscle.

Alterations in extracellular K^+ concentration may not be the sole determinant of HFF. Accumulation of K^+ in the extracellular space would result in an expected alteration in resting membrane potential. Investigations in amphibia and mammalian muscle seem to indicate little change in the resting membrane potential [100, 145, 164], suggesting that an alternative mechanism may be responsible for excitation failure.

The hypothesis that HFF results from electrical pertubations of the action potential has also recently been challenged. Metzger and Fitts [164] have postulated that events distal to the sarcolemma are responsible for fatigue at both high and low frequencies of stimulation. This conclusion was based on rat phrenic nerve–diaphragm preparations stimulated at 5 and 75 Hz which showed a marked difference in the tetanic response during recovery (more fatigue at high frequency) despite identical changes in recovery of the action potential. Further evidence to suggest that changes in sarcolemmal properties are not responsible for fatigue has been obtained from observations of the length dependency of muscle to fatigue [93]. Shortened muscle fatigues to a lesser degree than optimum length muscle indicating a possible energy-dependent phenomenon related to the number of cross-bridge interactions. Shortened muscle length may result in deformation of T-tubules, preventing the propagation of excitation to all parts of the cell and thereby resulting in some parts of the contractile apparatus not being equally fatigued. This means that studies of fatigue with muscles contracting at short length are difficult to interpret.

The physiological significance of HFF during voluntary muscular contraction is unclear since it is unlikely high-tetanic rates of motoneuron discharge rates are ever achieved except briefly during the initial stages of a contraction. Nevertheless, the accommodation of muscle motoneuron discharge rates and concomitant slowing of relaxation during maximal voluntary contractions (see section entitled Slowing of Relaxation) would seem to minimize this form of fatigue.

Low-Frequency Force Fatigue. Despite the changes in electrical function of the sarcolemmal membrane reported during high-frequency stimulation thought to result in fatigue, it is still not clear as to what causes fatigue at lower stimulation frequencies. Low-frequency fatigue is characterized by a selective long-term loss of force at low-stimulation frequency (of several hours), although following fatiguing activity force generation at high frequency appears to rapidly return to normal [84]. This form of fatigue can be demonstrated following a series of contractions made under anaerobic conditions [84] and also following specific forms of voluntary dynamic contractions [55, 56, 84]. The mean firing frequency of a sustained maximal contraction may be 10–30 Hz [17], although this may be greater at the start of a contraction. Therefore it is likely that this type of fatigue may result in significant force reduction unless a compensatory increase in firing frequency can be achieved or there is a concomitant recruitment of further motor units in parallel.

The cause of this type of fatigue is probably located further down the command chain, in a failure of excitation–contraction coupling (Fig. 2.1). This may be in part due to a reduction in Ca^{2+} release or impaired transmission in the transverse tubular system [75]. This conclusion is further supported by work carried out on rats which, in addition, appear to suggest that type II fibers are more likely to demonstrate LFF than type I fibers [147]. Low-frequency fatigue is not simply due to lactic acid accumulation as a consequence of activity, since it may be demonstrated in conditions in which there is no lactate (and hence H^+) production with exercise, for example, in patients who lack myophosphorylase or phosphofructokinase [242].

The comparatively slow recovery of force postexercise (a day or more; [84, 180]) indicates structural damage to the sarcoplasmic reticulum or tubular system, but this has not been demonstrated microscopically. Low-frequency fatigue is more pronounced following eccentric contractions, in which the muscle is stretched during activity (resulting in greater force per unit fiber cross-sectional area than that obtained in concentric contractions) which does produce sarcomere disruption, further supporting the suggestion that some form of cellular damage may contribute to LFF [181]. In addition, plasma creatine kinase levels (an indicator of muscle damage) are markedly elevated in some individuals several days after eccentric exercise [179].

That energetic factors may be responsible in development of LFF is unlikely. The energetic cost of eccentric contractions is about one-sixth less than of concentric contractions as indicated by oxygen uptake measurements during cycle ergometry [27]. The slow recovery rate also dismisses regeneration of high-energy phosphates as the cause since rates of recovery are markedly faster. The time course of glycogen recovery following depletion does follow a similar time scale to long-term LFF [19, 189]. It is unlikely, however, that a state of glycogen depletion has occurred following short-term intermittent ischemic exercise [76] or following eccentric exercise where a similarly worked concentrically contracting muscle shows less LFF [79].

VOLUNTARY CONTRACTIONS. The loss of force from sustained maximal voluntary ischemic isometric contractions is accompanied by a similar decrement in the smooth rectified (integrated) EMG from surface and intramuscular recordings [31, 130, 141, 219]. These studies appear to indicate force loss is a consequence of excitation failure.

Failure of Neuromuscular Transmission. An obvious candidate for consideration was the neuromuscular junction (NMJ), which was initially thought to be the cause of excitation failure [177]. Considered in more detail, the possible sites of failure include inhibition of presynaptic nerve terminals, depletion of transmitter or decreased postsynaptic end-plate excitability [145].

The involvement of the NMJ in peripheral fatigue was disputed by the work of Merton [163], who found no decline in the surface-measured evoked potential amplitude when applied during a sustained MVC of the adductor pollicis at a time when force could no longer be generated. Later studies by Bigland-Ritchie et al. [34], using both surface and intramuscular recordings of EMG, similarly showed no decline in amplitude or area of the evoked signal for up to 60 seconds in a sustained MVC, even though the smooth rectified EMG signal declined. However, these observations were not consistent with reports by Stephens and Taylor [219] of a reduction in the evoked EMG signal from the first dorsal interosseous muscle and by Marsden et al. [160] of reduced evoked EMG signal in the adductor pollicis. The reason for these differences remains unclear since similar changes were observed using paired impulses (to remove the effects of interference from voluntary motor impulses) and single impulses [34]. Bigland-Ritchie et al. [34] attributed these differences to the methods employed to analyze the EMG signal.

Direct high-frequency stimulation of curarized mouse muscle, by-passing the NMJ, has been shown to produce a force loss similar to that of indirect high-frequency stimulation of the human adductor pollicis [130]. This most important observation suggests that certain postsynaptic factors lead to a decline in EMG and force. However, no means of in vivo measurement of NMJ function during fatigue is as yet possible.

Changes in Motor Unit Firing Frequency. During sustained voluntary contractions, motor units discharge asynchronously at different rates with a mean discharge rate of up to 30 Hz, depending on the muscle group contracting and the force held [17, 26]. The asynchronous discharge of motor units allows full tetanic tension to be achieved at a lower rate than would be required if the units discharged synchronously as demonstrated by multielectrode stimulation techniques in cat muscle [191]. Intramuscular EMG recordings have demonstrated a decline in mean firing frequency of motor units and of single units during sustained contraction [31, 32, 101], and peak frequencies as high as 190 Hz have been recorded [160]. Interestingly, force failure during a MVC can be simulated during stimulated contractions by gradually reducing the stimulation frequency [130, 160]; this has been termed "artificial wisdom" [160]. This observation has an important role in the study of fatigue, since it permits investigation of the whole muscle as if it were a single cell. However, such a model has been considered too simple, since single-unit EMG recordings indicate optimal frequencies differ between motor units [160].

It can be argued that a decline in motor neuron firing rate would cause a loss of force (viz., frequency–force curve; 86). However, accompanying this is a slowing of relaxation of the muscle [32]. It is thought that this slowing is probably sufficient to allow full activation of the muscle despite a reduction in discharge rate, and furthermore it has been suggested that during a fatiguing MVC the decline of the discharge rate may alter in response to the slowing of relaxation with fatigue [35]. This might be advantageous to motor control and may further explain a matching of motor neuron discharge rates and the contractile properties of human muscle with different fiber composition (biceps brachii and soleus; 17). A reduction in motor unit discharge rates during a sustained voluntary contraction would also minimize the tendency to fatigue at high frequencies, thus possibly protecting against action potential failure at the peripheral nerve, NMJ, and/or the sarcolemmal membrane itself [160].

The origin of the decline in motor neuron firing rate is thought (although controversy has surrounded its origin) to be a fatigue-induced reflex in the central nervous system or the muscle [28]. A lack of recovery of motor unit discharge rates during ischemia of the quadriceps muscle observed by Woods et al. [248] suggests a peripheral inhibitory reflex may act to reduce motoneuron firing rate without impairment of neuromuscular transmission or subject effort.

Synchronization of Discharge Rates. Synchronization of motor unit discharge rates (defined as the tendency of motor units to discharge regularly at or near a time that other motor units discharge [61]) during prolonged contractions has been reported to occur during fatigue [151], but this is unlikely to be an important contributor to fatigue for reasons given below.

Slowing of Relaxation. Slowing of relaxation of muscle with fatigue has long been recognized [90, 171]. Slowing of relaxation will potentiate force at low frequencies, as can be demonstrated by cooling of fresh muscle [85]. It has been proposed that slowing of relaxation may protect against force loss at low stimulation frequencies such as would occur with synchronization of discharge rates by increasing fusion of tetani and subsequently increasing mean force generated [32, 129]. Such a mechanism could be advantageous in view of the mean low-frequency discharge of motor units encountered during a sustained or intermittent ischemic contraction.

The mechanisms leading to slowing of muscle relaxation are still elusive. Following an isometric contraction, the recovery rate of relaxation follows an approximately exponential curve [239], and relaxation rate appears dependent on muscle fiber composition [243] and intramuscular temperature of the muscle [240]. A Q_{10} of 1.8 [241] correlates favorably with Q_{10} values of 2–3 found for the velocity of many enzyme-catalyzed reactions and appears therefore to be consistent with some metabolic process being the principle determinant of relaxation rate.

The mechanisms determining relaxation of muscle are likely to be reuptake of Ca^{2+} by the sarcoplasmic reticulum or the requirement of cross-bridges for ATP necessary for detachment [82, 227]. Since both mechanisms require energy it has been suggested relaxation rate should be an indirect measure of the energy status of the muscle [85, 121]. Questions thus arise as to which metabolic process or metabolite is related to relaxation rate and what mechanism is involved. Recovery of relaxation rate appears to correlate with PCr [213]. The failure of recovery of slowing of relaxation rate or PCr following fatiguing contractions under anaerobic conditions [104] further supports a possible link, though this may be indirect, both being dependent on a third, as yet unmeasured factor.

It is unlikely that lactate accumulation or pH changes are responsible [109] since rapid normalization of relaxation is observed for small changes in pH [105]. Further, iodoacetate-poisoned muscle [82] and patients with myophosphorylase deficiency [242] still show slowing of relaxation, despite the lack of H^+ accumulation. That H^+ is not involved at all, however, is unlikely considering its affect on membrane function. ATP content of human muscle does not systematically decline during fatiguing contractions in which relaxation is slowed [83], but it has been proposed that a decrease in cross-bridge dissociation would be reflected in a reduced turnover of cross-bridges, implying a reduced ATP turnover rate. Intramuscular heat production measurements during voluntary and stimulated contractions, which depend on the sum of enthalpy changes or metabolic reactions (principally PCr splitting and glycolysis) appeared to support this concept. Toward the end of a contraction when relaxation is slowed, heat production per unit force declines [83, 239]. However, how much ATP hydrolysis during contraction is actually associated with cross-bridge cycling is unknown, as is the force in relation to cross-bridge number during relaxation.

Dawson et al. [60], using NMR techniques to follow metabolite changes in fatiguing frog muscle, found no change in the rate of ATP turnover per unit force when relaxation was slowed. A close relationship between relaxation and affinity for ATP hydrolysis was shown, expressed as the free energy change per mole of ATP hydrolyzed. Together with evidence from aequorin studies of Ca^{2+} movement in frog muscle fibers [36], it was concluded relaxation may be related to the rate of Ca^{2+} uptake into the sarcoplasmic reticulum, which may depend on the free-energy change for ATP hydrolysis. However, cross-bridge dissociation is also energy dependent, and both mechanisms may be involved in slowing by this process.

Other EMG Techniques Used to Elucidate Fatigue
The use of measurement of surface evoked potentials and detection of the integrated and smooth rectified EMG signal in the investigation of fatigue mechanisms have already been reviewed above in detail. The analysis of the frequency power spectrum of the EMG signal is yet another tool that has been more recently applied as technological advances in signal analysis progress [133, 135, 168, 173]. The interest in use of this technique has become more widespread in the last decade since a greater understanding of fatigue problems are required in industry as well as in the laboratory. Advantage has also been taken of the development of portable apparatus such as a "muscle fatigue monitor" for "in the field" use [221].

The power spectrum of the EMG demonstrates a shift from high to low frequencies during muscular activity [142]. The relationship between these changes and fatigue is unclear, however. Moxham et al. [172] studied the high:low frequency ratio of power spectra during exercise and found the largest shift in frequency occurred earlier than the loss of force. DeLuca [62] has similarly observed a more rapid decline in the median frequency of the power spectrum before force loss when a 50% MVC of the first dorsal interosseous muscle was held to fatigue. The rate of decline of the mean power frequency (MPF) has also been shown to be dependent on the contraction strength held [146], a more rapid decline occurring with higher contraction forces. To explain the changes observed, the MPF has been demonstrated to be related to the conduction velocity of excitation propagation along the sarcolemmal membranes [29, 71, 170]. Although disputed by Naeije and Zorn [176] using cross-correlation techniques to measure conduction velocity, further studies [162] have confirmed this relationship.

Lindstrom et al. [150] presented an elegant mathematical description to provide evidence that the changes in MPF observed were due to metabolic factors, particularly lactate accumulation (see section entitled "Hydrogen Ion Accumulation"). This is further evidenced by cooling the muscle [29, 162]. However, it is likely the observed changes are the result of the change in shape of the action potential, which may well be a consequence of the ionic alterations in the extracellular fluid, but then these factors too may be related. That lactate may contribute to the change of the power spectrum is also disputed since similar findings occur in individuals deficient in myophosphorylase activity [169, 242]. Alternatively, fatigue-induced changes in MPF may be the result of synchronization of motor units [29]. However, such activity occurs later than the shift in MPF [62].

The use of MPF as an indicator of fatigue [221] has also been questioned [75]. It does not reveal any information about excitation–contraction coupling: No shift in the frequency spectrum occurs with low-frequency fatigue [173]. However, measurement of MPF does appear to give an indication of the changes in the electrical characteristics of motor units during fatigue and has shown indirectly altered conduction velocities as a consequence of the fatiguing contraction.

INTERACTION BETWEEN CONTRACTILE FATIGUE AND TRANSMISSION FATIGUE

Undoubtedly there is a close relationship between energy metabolism and excitation processes: Failure of one will affect the extent of the other. Changes in the evoked action potential shape are further enhanced during ischemic conditions than during intermittent nonischemic contractions [68], highlighting a possible dependency on energy supply for membrane function or removal of metabolites and ions. Of significance is the study by Luttgau [155] in which iodoacetate/cyanide-poisoned amphibian muscle (inhibiting glycolysis and oxidative phosphorylation) could still conduct action potentials without a reduction in amplitude, whereas muscle still able to contract showed a declining amplitude when stimulated at 100 Hz. He concluded from this that action potential failure was the consequence of products produced by the contractile process itself. Accumulation of lactate and hence hydrogen ions may have important effects on membrane function, inhibiting generation of action potentials in excitable membranes [62] as pH decreases [187], possibly by causing physical changes in the arrangement of membrane proteins or due to the electric field generated by their charge [16]. However, recent studies indicate little correlation between lactate concentrations and excitation recovery following sustained and intermittent contractions of the human flexor carpi ulnaris [69].

Much has been learned from patients with selected enzyme defects of metabolism in muscle, providing alternative models for the investigation of fatigue and the indication of possible interactions of excitation processes and energy metabolism. Already discussed are patients who are unable to utilize glycogen because of phosphorylase deficiency. An important observation in these patients is the rapid decline in the surface recorded evoked action potential amplitude [85] and the failure of recovery during local ischemia following an ischemic-stimulated contraction at 20 Hz [239], which in normal subjects recovers rapidly. Conversely, hypothyroid patients are unable to sustain force for longer periods than normal subjects at less ATP cost [243]. In these individuals an improved preservation of excitation is also noted, possibly accounting for the improved endurance. Clearly, energy plays an important role influencing excitation and electrolyte balance within the cell.

To highlight the possible interaction between "energy" and "electricity," Edwards [75] proposed a three-dimensional model, based on the "catastrophe theory" [250] to illustrate the interaction between the two principal factors involved in the onset of fatigue. The theory, applied to many biological and sociological phenomena [250], describes the sudden discontinuities that occur in what would otherwise be a continuous system as a consequence of the interaction of one or more factors. Two controlling axes, "energy" and "excitation/activation," together affect the third axis, "force" (Fig. 2.2). Failure of excitation/activation clearly leads to a fall in force without energy loss, whereas a reduction in energy supply without failure of activation would also prove to limit force production. That rigor does not arise with the depletion of ATP, and hence irreparable damage to the muscle cell is prevented by excitation/activation loss as illustrated by the fold of the cusp, whereupon the stability of the system is maintained only with a sudden decline in force generation, thus reducing contractile activity and hence ATP demand.

The catastrophe theory has also been applied to muscle contraction by Alesso [5] in which tension (resulting from external neighboring contractile mechanisms exerting counterforces was used as a determinant of calcium ion release, the two interacting to cause a change in fibril length when the cusp was reached. Such a model describes changes within the cell and may help to predict the changes resulting in LFF, where a decline in force may occur as a consequence of reduced calcium ion release.

The actual decline of force observed is gradual, whereas the catastrophe model predicts a sudden fall in force. However, the muscle cell is complex, and the events occurring at one site of the cell may not necessarily occur at another. In a whole muscle, the more gradual appearance of fatigue as a slow decline in force may be explained by the "catastrophe" occurring at different times in different cell populations.

The models of fatigue put forward emphasize that when a muscle fatigues, there may be a predominant influence of one or both principal mechanisms. The importance of this interplay between "energy" and "electricity" has also been stressed by other workers [219].

FIGURE 2.2

The catastrophe theory of muscular fatigue: the interaction between energy loss and excitation/activation loss in the development of fatigue. Pathway 1 shows a "pure" loss of energy and the attendant risk of rigor (ATP depletion). Pathway 4 shows a "pure" loss of excitation/activation. Pathway 3 shows a possible route to fatigue during exercise. Pathway 2 represents a "safety mechanism" preventing rigor or muscular damage. (Reproduced with permission from Edwards RHT: Biochemical basis of fatigue. In Knuttgen HG (ed): Biochemistry of Exercise. Champaign, IL, Human Kinetics, 1983, pp 3–28.)

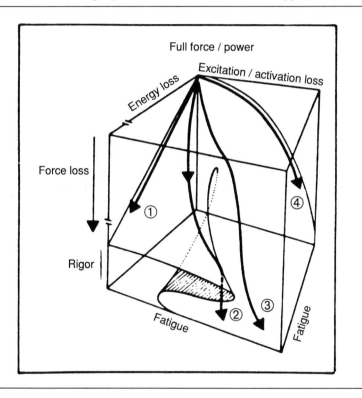

ACKNOWLEDGMENTS

Support from the Muscular Dystrophy Group of Great Britain and Northern Ireland, ICI Pharmaceuticals, and Mersey Region Health Authority is gratefully acknowledged. H. Gibson was a holder of a University of Liverpool Research Studentship during the preparation of this review.

REFERENCES

1. Abood LG, Koketsu K, Miyamoto S: Outflux of various phosphates during membrane depolarization of excitable tissues. *Am J Physiol* 202:469–474, 1962.
2. Adrian RH, Peachey LD: Reconstruction of the action potential of frog sartorius muscle. *J Physiol* 235:103–131, 1973.
3. Agrest A, Debercovich C, Navon S: Ammonia and ATP in the central nervous system of rats with dyspnoea and chronic hypercapnia. *Clin Sci* 28:401–405, 1965.
4. Ahlborg G, Felig P: Lactate and glucose exchange across the forearm, legs, and splanchnic bed during and after prolonged leg exercise. *J Clin Invest* 69:45–54, 1982.
5. Alesso HP: Reliability analysis of the elementary catastrophe theory model of muscle contraction. *Eng Med* 7:21–30, 1978.
6. Allen SI, Conn HO: Observations on the effect of exercise on blood ammonia concentrations in man. *Yale J Biol Med* 33:133–144, 1960.
7. Anderson P, Saltin B: Maximal perfusion of skeletal muscle in man. *J Physiol* 366:233–249, 1985.
8. Apple FS, Rogers A, Casal DC, Sherman WM, Ivy JL: Creatine kinase-MB isoenzyme adaptations in stressed human skeletal muscle of marathon runners. *J Appl Physiol* 59:149–153, 1985.
9. Asmussen E: Untersuchungen uber die mechanische Reaktion der Skelettmuskelfuser. *Skand Arch Physiol* 70:233–272, 1934.
10. Asmussen E: Muscle fatigue. *Med Sci Sports Exerc* 11:313–321, 1979.
11. Asmussen E, Mazin B: Recuperation after muscular fatigue by diverting activities. *Eur J Appl Physiol* 38:1–8, 1978a.
12. Asmussen E, Mazin B: A central nervous component in local muscular fatigue. *Eur J Appl Physiol* 38:9–15, 1978b.
13. Baldwin KM, Reitman JS, Terjung RL, Winder WW, Holloszy JO: Substrate depletion in different types of muscle and in liver during prolonged running. *Am J Physiol* 225:1034–1050, 1973.
14. Banister EW: The perception of effort: an inductive approach. *Eur J Appl Physiol* 41:141–150, 1979.
15. Banister EW, Rajendra W, Mutch BJC: Ammonia as an indicator of exercise stress: implications of recent findings to sports medicine. *Sports Med* 2:34–46, 1985.
16. Bass L, Moore WJ: The role of protons in nerve conduction. *Prog Biophys Mol Biol* 27:143–151, 1973.
17. Bellemare F, Woods JJ, Johansson R, Bigland-Ritchie B: Motor-unit discharge rates in maximal voluntary contractions of three human muscles. *J Neurophysiol* 50:1380–1392, 1983.
18. Bergstrom J, Beroniade V, Hultman E, Roch-Norland AE: Relation between glycogen and electrolyte metabolism in human muscle. In Kruck F (ed): *Symposium uber Transport und Function Intracellularer Elektrolyte.* Munchen-Berlin-Wein, Schuren und Schwarzenberg, 1967, pp 108–117.
19. Bergstrom J, Hultman E: Muscle glycogen synthesis after exercise: an enhancing factor localized to the muscle cell in man. *Nature* 210:309–310, 1966.
20. Bergstrom J, Harris RC, Hultman E, Nordesjo LO: Energy rich phosphagens in dynamic and static work. In Pernow B, Saltin B (eds): *Muscle Metabolism during Exercise.* London, Plenum Press, 1971, pp 342–356.
21. Bergstrom J, Hermansen L, Hultman E, Saltin B: Diet, muscle glycogen and physical performance. *Acta Physiol Scand* 71:140–150, 1967.
22. Bessman SP, Carpenter CL: The creatine–creatine phosphate energy shuttle. *Annu Rev Biochem* 54:831–862, 1985.
23. Bessman SP, Geiger PJ: Transport of energy in muscle: the phosphorylcreatine shuttle. *Science* 211:448–452, 1981.

24. Bezanilla F, Caputo C, Gonzalez-Serratos H, Venosa RA: Sodium dependence of the inward spread of activation in isolated twitch muscle fibers of the frog. *J Physiol* 223:507–523, 1972.
25. Bianchi CP, Narayan S: Muscle fatigue and the role of transverse tubules. *Science* 215:295–296, 1982.
26. Bigland B, Lippold OCJ: Motor unit activity in the voluntary contraction of human muscle. *J Physiol* 125:322–335, 1954.
27. Bigland-Ritchie B, Woods JJ: Integrated electromyogram and oxygen uptake during positive and negative work. *J Physiol* 260:267–277, 1976.
28. Bigland-Ritchie B, Dawson NJ, Johansson R, Lippold OCJ: Reflex control of motor neuron firing rates during fatigue in man. *J Physiol* 365:23P, 1985.
29. Bigland-Ritchie B, Donovan EF, Roussos CS: Conduction velocity and EMG power spectrum changes in fatigue of sustained maximal efforts. *J Appl Physiol: Respir Environ Exerc Physiol* 51:1300–1305, 1981.
30. Bigland-Ritchie B, Jones DA, Woods JA: Excitation frequency and muscle fatigue: electrical responses during human voluntary and stimulated contractions. *Exp Neurol* 64:414–427, 1979.
31. Bigland-Ritchie B, Johansson R, Lippold OLJ, Smith S, Woods JJ: Changes in motorneuron firing rates during sustained maximal voluntary contractions. *J Physiol* 340:335–346, 1983a.
32. Bigland-Ritchie B, Johansson R, Lippold OCJ, Woods JJ: Contractile speed and EMG changes during fatigue of sustained maximal voluntary contractions. *J Neurophysiol* 50:313–324, 1983b.
33. Bigland-Ritchie B, Jones DA, Hosking GP, Edwards RHT: Central and peripheral fatigue in sustained maximum voluntary contractions of human quadriceps muscle. *Clin Mol Med* 54:609–614, 1978.
34. Bigland-Ritchie B, Kakula CB, Lippold OLJ, Woods JJ: The absence of neuromuscular transmission failure in sustained maximal voluntary contractions. *J Physiol* 330:265–278, 1982.
35. Bigland-Ritchie B, Woods JJ: Changes in muscle contractile properties and neural control during human muscle fatigue. *Muscle Nerve* 7:691–699, 1984.
36. Blinks JR, Rudel R, Taylor SR: Calcium transients in isolated amphibian skeletal muscle fibers: detection with aequorin. *J Physiol* 277:291–323, 1978.
37. Boobis LH: Metabolic aspects of fatigue during sprinting. In Macleod D, Maughan R, Nimmo M, Reilly T, Williams C (eds): *Exercise: Benefits, Limits and Adaptations.* London, E & FN Spon, 1987, pp 116–143.
38. Boobis LH, Williams C, Wootton SA: Human muscle metabolism during brief maximal exercise. *J Physiol* 338:21–22P, 1982.
39. Borg GAV: *Physical Performance and Perceived Exertion.* Lund, Sweden, Gleerups, 1962, pp 1–63.
40. Boxer GE, Devlin TM: Pathways of intracellular hydrogen transport. *Science* 134:1495–1501, 1961.
41. Brandt PW, Cox RN, Kawai M, Robinson T: Regulation of tension in skinned muscle fibers. *J Gen Physiol* 79:997–1016, 1982.
42. Brodan V, Kuhn E, Pechar J, Placer Z, Slabochova Z: Effects of sodium glutamate infusion on ammonia formation during intense physical exercise in man. *Nutr Rep Int* 9:223–232, 1974.
43. Brown GL, Burns BD: Fatigue and neuromuscular block in mammalian skeletal muscle. *Proc R Soc Lond (Biol)* 136:182–195, 1949.
44. Bruell W, Ruegg JC, Steiger GJ, Ulbrich M: Cross-bridge properties derived from mechano-enzymic experiments on fibrillar muscle. Proceedings of the IUPS Vol. IX, XXV Int. Congress. Munich, German Physiological Society, 1971; 82.

46. Buchthal F, Engbaek L: Refractory period and conduction velocity of the striated muscle fiber. *Acta Physiol Scand* 59:199–220, 1963.
47. Carafoli E, Lehninger AL: A survey of the interaction of calcium ions with mitochondria from different tissues and species. *Biochem J* 122:681–690, 1971.
48. Chasiotis D, Sahlin K, Hultman E: Regulation of glycogenolysis in human muscle at rest and during exercise. *J Appl Physiol: Respir Environ Exerc Physiol* 53:708–715, 1982.
49. Christensen EH, Hanson O: Arbeitsfahigkeit und Ernahrung. *Skand Arch Physiol* 81:160–175, 1939.
50. Cooke R, Pate E: Inhibition of muscle contraction by the products of ATP hydrolysis: ADP and phosphate. *Biophys J* 47:25a, 1985.
51. Cooper RG, Edwards RHT, Gibson H, Stokes M: Human muscle fatigue: frequency dependence of excitation and force generation. *J Physiol* 397:585–599, 1988.
52. Costill DL, Dalsky GP, Fink WJ: Effects of caffeine ingestion on metabolism and exercise performance. *Med Sci Sports Exerc* 10:155–158, 1978.
53. Danforth WH: Activation of the glycolytic pathway in muscle. In Chance B, Estabrook RW (eds): *Control of Energy Metabolism.* New York, Academic Press, 1965, pp 287–298.
54. Davies CTM, Thompson MW: Aerobic performance of female marathon and male ultramarathon athletes. *Eur J Appl Physiol* 41:233–245, 1979.
55. Davies CTM, White MJ: Muscle weakness following eccentric work in man. *Pflugers Arch* 392:168–171, 1981.
56. Davies CTM, White J: Muscle weakness following dynamic exercise in humans. *J Appl Physiol: Respir Environ Exerc Physiol* 53:236–241, 1982.
57. Davies KJA, Quintanilha AT, Brooks GA, Packer L: Free radicals and tissue damage produced by exercise. *Biochem Biophys Res Commun* 107:1198–1205, 1982.
58. Dawson MJ: Phosphorus metabolism and the control of glycolysis studies by nuclear magnetic resonance. In Knuttgen HG (ed): *Biochemistry of Exercise.* Champaign IL, Human Kinetics, 1983, pp 116–125.
59. Dawson MJ, Gadian DG, Wilkie DR: Muscular fatigue investigated by phosphorus nuclear magnetic resonance. *Nature* 274:861–866, 1978.
60. Dawson MJ, Gadian DG, Wilkie DR: Mechanical relaxation rate and metabolism studied in fatiguing muscle by phosphorus nuclear magnetic resonance. *J Physiol* 299:365–484, 1980.
61. De Luca CJ, LeFever RS, McCue MP, Xenakis AP: Control scheme governing concurrently active human motor units during voluntary contractions. *J Physiol* 329:129–142, 1982.
62. De Luca CJ: Myoelectrical manifestations of localized muscular fatigue in humans. *CRC Crit Rev Biomed Eng* 11:251–279, 1984.
63. Deleze J, Lazrak A, Rakotonirina VS: Isolation of the tubular action potential in the frog skeletal muscle fiber. *J Physiol* 371:149P, 1986.
64. Di Mauro S, Bonilla E, Lee CP, Schotland DL, Scarpa A, Conn H, Chance B: Luft's disease: further biochemical and ultrastructural studies of skeletal muscle in the second case. *J Neurol Sci* 27:217–232, 1976.
65. Doll E, Keul J, Maiwald C: Oxygen tension and acid-base equilibria in venous blood of working muscle. *Am J Physiol* 215:23–29, 1968.
66. Donaldson SKB: Effect of acidosis on maximum force generation of peeled mammalian skeletal muscle fibers. In Knuttgen HG (ed): *Biochemistry of Exercise.* Champaign IL, Human Kinetics, 1983, pp 126–133.
67. Donaldson SK, Hermansen L, Bolles L: Differential direct effects of H^+ and Ca^{2+}-activated force of skinned fibers from the soleus, cardiac and adductor magnus muscles of rabbits. *Pflugers Arch* 376:55–65, 1978.
68. Duchateau J, Hainault K: Electrical and mechanical failures during sustained and intermittent contractions in humans. *J Appl Physiol: Respir Environ Exerc Physiol* 58:942–947, 1985.

69. Duchateau J, Montigny L, Hainaut K: Electro-mechanical failures and lactate production during fatigue. *Eur J Appl Physiol* 56:287–291, 1987.

70. Dudley GA, Staron RS, Murray TF, Hagerman FC, Luginbuhl A: Muscle fiber composition and blood ammonia levels after intense exercise in humans. *J Appl Physiol: Respir Environ Exerc Physiol* 54:582–586, 1983.

71. Eberstein A, Beattie B: Simultaneous measurement of muscle conduction velocity and EMG power spectrum changes during fatigue. *Muscle Nerve* 8:786–773, 1985.

72. Edgerton RV, Saltin B, Esen B, Simpson DR: Glycogen depletion in specific types of human skeletal muscle fibers after various work routines. Presented at the Second International Symposium in Biochemistry of Exercise, Magglingen, 1973.

73. Edington DW: Pyridine nucleotide oxidized to reduced ratio as a regulator of muscular performance. *Experientia* 26:601–602, 1970.

74. Edington DW, Ward GR, Saville WA: Energy metabolism of working muscle: concentration profiles of selected metabolites. *Am J Physiol* 244:1375–1380, 1971.

75. Edwards RHT: Human muscle function and fatigue. In Porter R, Whelan J (eds): *Human Muscle Fatigue: Physiological Mechanisms* (Ciba Foundation Symposium No. 82). London, Pitman Medical, 1981, pp 1–18.

76. Edwards RHT: Biochemical basis of fatigue. In Knuttgen HG (ed): *Biochemistry of Exercise*. Champaign IL, Human Kinetics, 1983, pp 3–28.

77. Edwards RHT: Interaction of chemical with electromechanical factors in human skeletal muscle fatigue. *Acta Physiol Scand* 128 (Suppl 556):149–155, 1986.

78. Edwards RHT, Newham DJ: Force:frequency relationship determined by percutaneous stimulation of the quadriceps muscle. *J Physiol* 353:129P, 1984.

79. Edwards RHT, Mills KR, Newham DJ: Greater low frequency fatigue produced by eccentric than concentric muscle contractions. *J Physiol* 317:17P, 1981.

80. Edwards RHT, Dawson MJ, Wilkie DR, Gordon RE, Shaw D: Clinical use of nuclear magnetic resonance in the investigation of myopathy. *Lancet* 1:725–731, 1982a.

81. Edwards RHT, Griffiths RG, Cady EB: Topical magnetic resonance for the study of muscle metabolism in human myopathy. *Clin Physiol* 5:93–109, 1985.

82. Edwards RHT, Hill DK, Jones DA: Metabolic changes associated with the slowing of relaxation in fatigued mouse muscle. *J Physiol* 251:287–301, 1975a.

83. Edwards RHT, Hill DK, Jones DA: Heat production and chemical changes during isometric contractions of human quadriceps muscle. *J Physiol* 251:303–315, 1975b.

84. Edwards RHT, Hill DK, Jones DA, Merton PA: Fatigue of long duration in human skeletal muscle after exercise. *J Physiol* 272:769–778, 1977b.

85. Edwards RHT, Wiles CM: Energy exchange in human skeletal muscle during isometric contraction. *Circ Res* 48:I11-I17 (Suppl 1), 1981.

86. Edwards RHT, Young A, Hosking GP, Jones DA: Human skeletal muscle function: description of tests and normal values. *Clin Sci Mol Med* 52:283–290, 1977.

87. Essen B, Hagenfeldt L, Kaijser L: Utilization of blood-borne and intramuscular substrates during continuous and intermittent exercise in man. *J Physiol* 265:489–506, 1977.

88. Fabiato A, Fabiato F: Effect of pH on the myofilaments and the sarcoplasmic reticulum of skinned cells from cardiac and skeletal muscles. *J Physiol* 276:233–255, 1978.

89. Felig P, Wahren J: Fuel homeostatis in exercise. *N Engl J Med* 293:1078–1084, 1975.

90. Feng TP: The heat-tension ratio in prolonged tetanic contractions. *Proc R Soc Lond (Biol)* 108:522–537, 1931.

91. Fenn WO: Electrolytes in muscle. *Physiol Rev* 16:450–487, 1936.

92. Fink R, Luttgau HC: An evaluation of the membrane constants and the potassium conductance in metabolically exhausted muscle fibers. *J Physiol* 263:215–238, 1976.

93. Fitch S, McComas A: Influence of human muscle length on fatigue. *J Physiol* 362:205–213, 1985.

94. Fuchs F, Reddy Y, Briggs FN: The interaction of cations with the calcium binding site of troponin. *Biochim Biophys Acta* 221:407–409, 1970.

95. Gibson H, Edwards RHT: Muscular exercise and fatigue. *Sports Med* 2:120–132, 1985.
96. Giles D, MacLaren DPM: Effects of caffeine and glucose ingestion on metabolic and respiratory functions during prolonged exercise. *J Sports Sci* 2:35–46, 1984.
97. Gollnick PD, Armstrong RB, Saubertiv CW, Piehl K, Saltin B: Enzyme activity and fiber composition in skeletal muscle of untrained and trained men. *J Appl Physiol* 33:312–319, 1972.
98. Gollnick PD, Armstrong RD, Sembrowich WL, Shepherd RE, Saltin B: Glycogen depletion pattern in human skeletal muscle fibers after heavy exercise. *J Appl Physiol* 34:615–618, 1973.
99. Gollnick PD, Karlsson J, Piehl K, Saltin B: Selective glycogen depletion in skeletal muscle fibers in man following sustained contractions. *J Physiol* 241:59–67, 1974.
100. Grabowski W, Lobsiger EA, Luttgau H: The effect of repetitive stimulation at low frequencies upon the electrical and mechanical activity of single muscle fibers. *Pflugers Arch* 334:222–239, 1972.
101. Grimby L, Hannerz J, Hedman B: The fatigue and voluntary discharge properties of single motor units in man. *J Physiol* 316:545–554, 1981.
102. Harris RC, Sahlin K, Hultman E: Phosphagen and lactate contents of m. quadriceps femoris of man after exercise. *J Appl Physiol* 43:852–857, 1977.
103. Harris RC, Hultman E: Adenine nucleotide depletion in human muscle in response to intermittent stimulation in situ. *J Physiol* 365:73P, 1985.
104. Harris RC, Hultman E, Kaijser L, Nordesjo L-O: The effect of circulatory occlusion on isometric exercise capacity and energy metabolism of the quadriceps muscle in man. *Scand J Clin Lab Invest* 35:87–95, 1975.
105. Harris RC, Edwards RHT, Hultman E, Nordesjo L-O: The time course of phosphorylcreatine resynthesis during recovery of the quadriceps in man. *Eur J Physiol* 367:137–142, 1976.
106. Heald DE: Influence of ammonium ions on mechanical and electro-physiological responses of skeletal muscle. *Am J Physiol* 229:1174–1179, 1975.
107. Hermansen L: Effect of acidosis on skeletal muscle performance during maximal exercise in man. *Bull Eur Physiopathol Respir* 15:229–238, 1979.
108. Hermansen L: Effect of metabolic changes on force generation in skeletal muscle during maximal exercise In Porter R, Whelan J (eds): *Human Muscle Fatigue: Physiological Mechanisms* (Ciba Foundation Symposium No. 82). London, Pitman Medical, 1981, pp 75–78.
109. Hermansen L, Osnes JB: Blood and muscle pH after maximal exercise in man. *J Appl Physiol* 32:304–308, 1972.
110. Hermansen L, Hultman E, Saltin B: Muscle glycogen during prolonged severe exercise. *Acta Physiol Scand* 71:129–139, 1976.
111. Hermansen L, Vaage O: Lactate disappearance and glycogen synthesis in humans after maximal exercise. *Am J Physiol* 233:E422-E429, 1977.
112. Hibberd MG, Dantzig JA, Trentham DR, Goldman YE: Phosphate release and force generation in skeletal muscle fibers. *Science* 228:1317–1319, 1985.
113. Hickson RC, Rennie MJ, Conlee RK, Winder WW, Holloszy JO: Effects of increased plasma free fatty acids on glycogen utilization and endurance. *J Appl Physiol* 43:829–833, 1977.
114. Hill AV: *Muscular Activity*. Baltimore, Williams & Wilkins, 1925.
115. Hill DK, McDonnell MJ, Merton PA: Direct stimulation of the adductor pollicis in man. *J Physiol* 300:2P–3P, 1979.
116. Hilton SM, Vrbova G: Inorganic phosphate—a new candidate for mediator of functional vasodilation in skeletal muscle. *J Physiol* 206:29P, 1970.
117. Hudlicka O: Differences in development of fatigue in slow and fast muscles In Keul J (ed): *Limiting Factors of Physical Performance*. Stuttgart, G. Thieme, 1971, pp 36–41.
118. Hultman E: Regulation of carbohydrate metabolism in the liver during rest and exercise with special reference to diet In Landry F, Orban WAR (eds): *3rd International*

Symposium of the Biochemistry of Exercise. Miami, FL, Symposia Specialists, 1978, pp 99–126.

119. Hultman E, Bergstrom J: Local energy-supplying substrates as limiting factors in different types of leg muscle work in normal man. In Keul J (ed): *Limiting Factors of Physical Performance.* Stuttgart, G. Thieme, 1971, pp 113–125.

120. Hultman E, Bergstrom J, McLennan Anderson N: Breakdown and resynthesis of adenosine triphosphate in connection with muscular work in man. *Scand J Clin Lab Invest* 19:56–66, 1967.

121. Hultman E, Sjoholm H, Sahlin K, Edstrom L: Glycolytic and oxidative energy metabolism and contraction characteristics in intact human muscle. In Porter R, Whelan J (eds): *Human Muscle Fatigue: Physiological Mechanisms* (Ciba Foundation Symposium No. 82). London, Pitman Medical, 1981, pp 19–40.

122. Hultman E, Del Canale S, Sjoholm: Effect of induced metabolic acidosis on intracellular pH, buffer capacity and contraction force of human skeletal muscle. *Clin Sci* 69:505–510, 1985.

123. Ikai M, Yabe K, Ishu K: Muskelkraft und muskulare Ermudung bein willkurlicher Anspannung und elektrischer Reizung des Muskels. *Sportartz Sportmed* 5:197–211, 1967.

124. Iles JF, Jack JJB: Ammonia: assessment of ion action on postsynaptic inhibition as a cause of convulsions. *Brain* 103:555–578, 1980.

125. Infante AA, Klaupiks D, Davies RE: Phosphorylcreatine consumption during single working contraction of isolated muscle. *Biochim Biophys Acta* 94:504–515, 1965.

126. Jacobus WE: Respiratory control and the integration of the heart high-energy phosphate by mitochondria. Coupling of creatine kinase. *Annu Rev Physiol* 47:707–712, 1985.

127. Jansson E: Diet and muscle metabolism in man with reference to fat and carbohydrate utilization and its regulation. *Acta Physiol Scand* (Suppl) 487, 1980.

128. Jones DA: Change in excitation threshold as a cause of muscular fatigue. *J Physiol* 295:90P–91P, 1979.

129. Jones DA: Muscle fatigue due to changes beyond the neuromuscular junction. In Porter R, Whelan J (eds): *Human Muscle Fatigue: Physiological Mechanisms* (Ciba Foundation Symposium No. 82). London, Pitman Medical, 1981, pp 178–196.

130. Jones DA, Bigland-Ritchie B, Edwards RHT: Excitation frequency and muscle fatigue: mechanical responses during voluntary and stimulated contractions. *Exp Neurol* 64:401–413, 1979.

131. Jones NL: Hydrogen ion balance during exercise. *Clin Sci* 59:85–96, 1980.

132. Jones NL, Sutton JR, Taylor R, Toews CJ: Effect of pH on cardiorespiratory and metabolic responses to exercise. *J Appl Physiol* 43:959–964, 1977.

133. Kadefors R, Kaiser E, Petersen I: Dynamic spectrum analysis of myopotentials with special reference to muscle fatigue. *Electromyography* 8:39–74, 1968.

134. Kaijser L: Limiting factors for aerobic muscle performance. The influence of varying oxygen pressure and temperature. *Acta Physiol Scand* (Suppl) 346:1–96, 1970.

135. Kaiser E, Petersen I: Frequency analysis of muscle action potentials during tetanic contraction. *Electromyography* 3:5–17, 1963.

136. Karlsson J: Muscle ATP, CP and lactate in submaximal and maximal exercise In Pernow B, Saltin B (eds): *Muscle Metabolism During Exercise.* London, Plenum Press, 1971, pp 383–394.

137. Katanuma N, Okada M, Nishii Y: Regulation of the urea cycle and TCA cycle by ammonia. In Weaver G (ed): *Advances in Enzyme Regulation* New York, Pergamon Press, 1966, Vol 4, pp 317–335.

138. Katz A: Contractile proteins of the heart. *Physiol Rev* 50:63–158, 1970.

139. Katz A, Hecht H: The early "pump" failure of the ischemic heart. *Am J Med* 47:497–502, 1969.

140. Kawai M, Wolen C, Cornaccia T: The effect of phosphate (P_i) on crossbridge kinetics in psoas fibres indicates that the forward cycling rate increases with P_i. *Biophys J* 47:24a, 1985.

141. Komi PV, Rusko H: Quantitative evaluation of mechanical and electrical changes

during fatigue loadings of eccentric and concentric work. *Scand J Rehabil Med* 3:121–126, 1974.

142. Komi PV, Tesch P: EMG frequency spectrum, muscle structure and fatigue during dynamic contractions in man. *Eur J Appl Physiol* 42:41–50, 1979.

143. Koyuncuoclu H, Keyer M, Simsek S, Sagduyu H: Ammonia intoxication: changes of brain levels of putative neurotransmitter and related compounds and its relevance to hepatic coma. *Pharmacol Res Commun* 10:787–807, 1978.

144. Krebs EG, Love DS, Bratvold GE, Trayser KA, Meyer WL, Fischer EH: Purification and properties of rabbit skeletal muscle phosphorylase b kinase. *Biochemistry* 3:1022–1033, 1964.

145. Krnjevik K, Miledi R: Failure of neuromuscular propagation in rats. *J Physiol* 140:440–461, 1958.

146. Kroon GW, Naeije M: Electromyographical power spectrum changes during fatigue of the human masseter muscle at different contraction levels. *J Physiol* 366:99P, 1985.

147. Kugelberg E, Lindegren B: Transmission and contraction fatigue of rat motor units in relation to succinate dehydrogenase activity of motor unit fibers. *J Physiol* 288:285–300, 1979.

148. Kvamme E: Ammonia metabolism in the CNS. *Prog Neurobiol* 20:109–132, 1983.

149. Lewis SF, Haller RG, Cook JD, Nunnally RL: Muscle fatigue in McArdle's disease studied by ^{31}P-NMR: effect of glucose infusion. *J Appl Physiol* 59:1991–1994, 1985.

150. Lindstrom L, Magnusson R, Petersen I: Muscular fatigue and action potential conduction velocity changes studied with frequency analysis of EMG signals. *Electroencephalogr Clin Neurophysiol* 10:341–356, 1970.

151. Lippold OCJ, Redfearn JWT, Vuco J: The electromyography of fatigue. *Ergonomics* 3:121–131, 1960.

152. Lockwood AH, McDonald JM, Reiman RE: The dynamics of ammonia metabolism in man: effects of liver disease and hyper-ammonemia. *J Clin Invest* 63:449–460, 1979.

153. Lowenstein JM: Ammonia production in muscle and other tissues: the purine nucleotide cycle. *Physiol Rev* 52:382–414, 1972.

154. Lowry OH, Passonneau JV: Kinetic evidence for multiple binding sites on phosphofructokinase. *J Biol Chem* 241:2268–2279, 1966.

155. Luttgau HC: The effect of metabolic inhibitors on the fatigue of the action potential in single muscle fibers. *J Physiol* 178:45–67, 1965.

156. MacLaren DPM, Jackson K: The effect of monosodium glutamate and aspartic acid ingestion on blood ammonia levels during exhaustive exercise. *J Sports Sci* 3:222, 1985.

157. MacLaren DPM, Morgan GM: Effects of sodium bicarbonate ingestion on maximal exercise. *Proc Nutr Soc* 44:26A, 1985.

158. MacLaren DPM, Ricketts S: Effect of glycogen loading and caffeine on endurance performance. *J Sports Sci* 1:141–142, 1983.

159. Makinose M: ATP synthesis by the sarcoplasmic reticulum pump. *Proc IUPS*, Vol. IX, XXV Int. Congress Munich. 1971: 362.

160. Marsden CD, Meadows, Merton PA: "Muscular wisdom" that minimizes fatigue during prolonged effort in man: peak rates of motoneuron discharge and slowing of discharge during fatigue. In Desmedt JE (ed): *Motor Control Mechanisms in Health and Disease*. New York, Raven Press, 1983, pp 169–211.

161. Maughan RJ, Saddler DJ: The effect of oral administration of salts of aspartic acid on the metabolic response to prolonged exhausting exercise in man. *Int J Sports Med* 4:119–123, 1983.

162. Merletti R, Sabbahi MA, De Luca CJ: Median frequency of the myoelectric signal. Effects of muscle ischemia and cooling. *Eur J Appl Physiol* 52:258–265, 1984.

163. Merton PA: Voluntary strength and fatigue. *J Physiol* 123:553–564, 1954.

164. Metzger JM, Fitts RH: Fatigue from high- and low-frequency muscle stimulation: role of sarcolemma action potentials. *Exp Neurol* 93:320–333, 1986.

165. Meyer RA, Dudley GA, Terjung RL: Ammonia and IMP in different skeletal muscle fibers after exercise in rats. *J Appl Physiol* 49:1037–1041, 1980.
166. Meyer RA, Sweeney HL, Kushmerick MJ: A simple analysis of the "creatine shuttle." *Am J Physiol* 246:C365–377, 1984.
167. Meyerhof O, Lohmann K: Uber Atmung und Kohlenhydratumsatz tierischer Gewebe I. Mitteilung: Milchsaurebildung und Milchsaure-schwund in tierischen Geweben. *Biochim Z* 171:381–402, 1926.
168. Mills KR: Power spectral analysis of electromyogram and compound muscle action potential during muscle fatigue and recovery. *J Physiol* 326:401–409, 1982.
169. Mills KR, Edwards RHT: Muscle fatigue in myophosphorylase deficiency: power spectral analysis of the electromyogram. *Electroencephalogr Clin Neurophysiol* 57:330–335, 1984.
170. Mortimer JT, Magnussen RI, Petersen I: Conduction velocity in ischemic muscle: effect on EMG frequency spectrum. *Am J Physiol* 219:1324–1329, 1970.
171. Mosso A: *Fatigue* (Drummond M, Drummond WG, trans). London, Allen and Unwin, 1915.
172. Moxham J, De Troyer A, Farkas G, Macklem PT, Edward RHT, Roussos C: Relationship of EMG power spectrum with low and high frequency fatigue in human muscle. *Physiologist* 22:91, 1979.
173. Moxham J, Edwards RHT, Aubier M, De Troyer G, Farkas G, Macklem PT, Roussos C: Changes in EMG power spectrum (high to low ratio) with force fatigue in humans. *J Appl Physiol: Respir Environ Exerc Physiol* 53:1094–1099, 1982.
174. Muller EA: Die Erholung nach statischer Haltearbeit. *Arlbeitsphysiol* 8:72, 1935.
175. Mutch BJC, Banister EW: Ammonia metabolism in exercise and fatigue: a review. *Med Sci Sports Exerc* 15:41–40, 1983.
176. Naeije M, Zorn H: Relation between EMG power spectrum shifts and muscle fiber action potential conduction velocity changes during local muscular fatigue in man. *Eur J Physiol* 50:23–33, 1982.
177. Naess K, Storm-Mathisen A: Fatigue and sustained tetanic contractions. *Acta Physiol Scand* 34:351–366, 1955.
178. Nakamura Y, Schwartz A: Possible control of intracellular calcium metabolism by [H^+]: sarcoplasmic reticulum of skeletal and cardiac muscle. *Biochem Biophys Res Commun* 41:330–386, 1970.
179. Newham DJ, Edwards RHT. Plasma creatine kinase changes after eccentric and concentric contractions. *Muscle Nerve* 9:59–63, 1986.
180. Newham DJ, Mills KR, Quigley BM, Edwards RHT: Pain and fatigue after concentric and eccentric muscle contractions. *Clin Sci* 64:55–62, 1983a.
181. Newham DJ, McPhail G, Mills KR, Edwards RHT: Ultrastructural changes after concentric and eccentric contractions of human muscle. *J Neurol Sci* 61:102–122, 1983b.
182. Newsholme EA: The glucose/fatty acid cycle and physical exhaustion. In Porter R, Whelan J (eds): *Human Muscle Fatigue: Physiological Mechanisms* (Ciba Foundation Symposium No. 82). London, Pitman Medical, 1981, pp 89–96.
183. Newsholme EA: Metabolic control and its importance in sprinting and endurance running. In Marconnet P, Poortmans J, Hermanson L (eds): *Medicine and Sport Science*. Karger, Basel, 1982, vol 17, pp 1–8.
184. Newsholme EA, Acworth IN, Blomstrand E: Amino acids, brain neurotransmitters and a functional link between muscle and brain that is important in sustained exercise. In Benzi G (ed): *Advances in Myochemistry*. London, John Libbey, 1987, pp 127–133.
185. Newsholme EA, Crabtree B: Theoretical principles in the approaches to control of metabolic pathways and their application to glycolysis in muscle. *J Mol Cell Cardiol* 11:839–856, 1979.
186. Newsholme EA, Start C: *Regulation in Metabolism*. London, John Wiley, 1973.

187. Orchardson R: The generation of nerve impulses in mammalian axons by changing the concentrations of the normal constituents of extracellular fluid. *J Physiol* 275:177–189, 1978.

188. Pallotta BS: Calcium activated potassium channels in rat muscle inactivated from a short duration open state. *J Physiol* 363:501–516, 1985.

189. Piehl K: Time course for refilling of glycogen stores in human muscle fibers following exercise induced glycogen depletion. *Acta Physiol Scand* 90:297–302, 1974.

190. Piper J, di Prampero PE, Certelli P: Oxygen debt and high-energy phosphate in gastrocnemius muscle of the dog. *Am J Physiol* 215:523–531, 1968.

191. Rack PMH, Westbury DR: The effects of length and stimulus rate on tension in the isometric cat soleus muscle. *J Physiol* 204:443–460, 1969.

192. Robertson S, Kerrick W: The effect of pH on submaximal calcium ion-activated tension in skinned frog skeletal fibers. *Biophys J* 16:73A, 1976.

193. Rojtbak AJ, Dedabrishvili CM: On the mechanism of active rest. *Dik Akad Nauk U.S.S.R.* 124:957–960, 1959.

194. Ronzoni E, Kerly M: The effect of pH on carbohydrate changes in isolated anaerobic frog muscle. *J Biol Chem* 103:175–181, 1933.

195. Sahlin K: Effects of acidosis on energy metabolism and force generation in skeletal muscle. In Knuttgen HG, Vogel H (eds): *Biochemistry of Exercise.* Champaign, IL, Human Kinetics, 1983, pp 151–160.

196. Sahlin K, Harris RC, Hultman E: Creatine kinase equilibrium and lactate content compared with muscle pH in tissue samples obtained after isometric contraction. *Biochem J* 152:173–180, 1975.

197. Sahlin K, Harris RC, Nylind B, Hultman E: Lactate content and pH in muscle samples obtained after dynamic exercise. *Pflugers Arch* 367:143–149, 1976.

198. Sahlin K, Henriksonn J: Buffer capacity and lactate accumulation in skeletal muscle of trained and untrained men. *Acta Physiol Scand* 122:331–339, 1984.

199. Saltin B, Hermansen L: Glycogen stores and prolonged severe exercise. In Blix (ed): *Symposia of the Swedish Nutrition Foundation.* Uppsala, Almoqvist and Wiksell, 1967, Vol 5, pp 32–46.

200. Saltin B, Karlsson J: Muscle glycogen utilization during work of different intensities. In Pernow B, Saltin B (eds): *Muscle Metabolism During Exercise.* New York, Plenum Press, 1971, pp 289–299.

201. Savard G, Kiens B, Saltin B: Central cardiovascular factors as limits to endurance; with a note on the distinction between maximal oxygen uptake and endurance fitness. In Macleod D, Maughan R, Nimmo M, Reilly T, Williams C (eds): *Exercise: Benefits, Limits and Adaptations.* London, E & FN Spon, 1987, pp 162–180.

202. Schadler M: Proportionale Aktivierung von ATPase—Aktivitat und kontraktionss-pannung durch Caliumionen in isolierten contractilen Strukturenn verschiedener Muskelaten. *Pflugers Arch* 296:70–90, 1967.

203. Schantz PG, Henriksson J: Enzyme levels of the NADH shuttle systems: measurements in isolated muscle fibers from humans of differing physical capacity. *Acta Physiol Scand* 129:505–515, 1987.

204. Schantz PG Sjoberg B, Svedenhag J: Malate-aspartate and alpha-glycerophosphate shuttle enzyme levels in human skeletal muscle: methodological considerations and effect of endurance training. *Acta Physiol Scand* 128:397–407, 1986.

205. Schwab RS: Motivation and measurement of fatigue. In Floyd WF, Welford HT (eds): *Fatigue.* London, Lewis, 1953, pp 193–248.

206. Schwartz AE, Lawrence W Jr, Roberts KE: Elevation of peripheral blood ammonia following muscular exercise. *Proc Soc Exp Biol Med* 98:548–550, 1958.

207. Sembrovich WL, Shepherd RE, Gollnick PD: Regulation of lipolysis in norepineph-rine stimulated isolated fat cells. Presented at the annual meeting of the American College of Sports Medicine, Seattle, 1973.

208. Setchenov IM: Zur Frage nach der Einwirkung sensitiver Reize auf die Muskelarbeit

des Menchen. In *Selected Works*. Moscow, USSR Academy of Sciences, 1935, pp 246–260.

209. Siesjo BK: Lactic acidosis in the brain: occurrence, triggering mechanisms and pathophysiological importance. *Ciba Found Symp* 87:77–88, 1982.

210. Simonson E: *Physiology of Work Capacity and Fatigue*. Springfield, IL, Charles C. Thomas, 1971.

211. Simpson WT: Nature and effects of unwanted effects with atenolol. *Postgrad Med J* 53 (Suppl. 3):162–167, 1977.

212. Sjodin B: Lactate dehydrogenase in human skeletal muscle. *Acta Physiol Scand (Suppl)* 436:5–32, 1976.

213. Sjoholm H, Sahlin K, Edstrom L, Hultman E: Quantitative estimation of anaerobic and oxidative energy metabolism and contraction characteristics in intact human skeletal muscle in response to electrical stimulation. *Clin Physiol* 3:227–239, 1983.

214. Spande JI, Schottelius BA: Chemical basis of fatigue in isolated mouse soleus. *Am J Physiol* 219:1490–1496, 1970.

215. Spruce AE, Standen NB, Stanfield PR: Voltage-dependent ATP sensitive potassium channels of skeletal muscle membrane. *Nature* 316:736–738, 1985.

216. Stainsby WN: Some critical oxygen tensions and their physiological significance. In Hatcher JB, Jennings DB (eds): *International Symposium on the Cardiovascular and Respiratory Effects of Hypoxia*. Basel, Karger, 1966, pp 29–40.

217. Stainsby WN, Otis AB: Blood flow, blood oxygen tension, oxygen uptake and oxygen transport in skeletal muscle. *Am J Physiol* 206:858–866, 1964.

218. Stella G: The concentration and diffusion of inorganic phophate in living muscle. *J Physiol* 66:19, 1928.

219. Stephens JA, Taylor A: Fatigue of maintained voluntary muscle contraction in man. *J Physiol* 220:1–18, 1972.

220. Streter FA: Distribution of water, sodium and potassium in resting and stimulated mammalian muscle. *Can J Biochem* 41:1035–1045, 1963.

221. Stulen FB, De Luca CJ: Muscle fatigue monitor: a non-invasive device for observing localized muscular fatigue. *IEEE Trans Biomed Eng* 29:760–768, 1982.

222. Sutton JR, Jones NL, Toews CJ: Effect of pH on muscle glycolysis during exercise. *Clin Sci* 61:331–338, 1981.

223. Tashiro S: Ammonia production in the nerve fiber during excitation. *Am J Physiol* 60:519–543, 1922.

224. Tesch P: Muscle fatigue and muscle lactate concentration. In Asmussen E, Jorgensen K (eds): *Biomechanics VI-A: International Series on Biomechanics*. Baltimore, University Park Press, 1978, pp 68–72.

225. Tesch P: Muscle fatigue in man with special reference to lactate accumulation during short term intense exercise. *Acta Physiol Scand (Suppl)* 480, 1980.

226. Thorstensson A: Muscle strength, fiber types and enzyme activities in man. *Acta Physiol Scand (Suppl)* 443, 1976.

227. Trentham DR, Eccleston JF, Bagshaw CR: Kinetic analysis of ATPase mechanisms. *Quart Rev Biophys* 9:217–281, 1976.

228. Trividi B, Danforth WH: Effect of pH on the kinetics of frog muscle phosphofructokinase. *J Biol Chem* 241:4110–4114, 1966.

229. Tunstall-Pedoe DS: Exercise and the heart. Lecture given at the Medical Institute, Liverpool, February 14, 1985.

230. Ui M: A role of phosphofructokinase in pH dependent regulation of glycolysis. *Biocheim Biophys Acta* 124:310–322, 1966.

231. Veerkamp JH, Paulussen RJA: Fatty acid transport in muscle: the role of fatty acid binding proteins. *Biochem Soc Trans* 15:331–336, 1987.

232. Vollestad NK, Blom PCS: Effect of varying exercise intensity on glycogen depletion in human muscle fibers. *Acta Physiol Scand* 125:395–405, 1985.

233. Vollestad NK, Vaage O, Hermansen L: Muscle glycogen depletion patterns in type

I and subgroups of type II fibers during prolonged severe exercise in man. *Acta Physiol Scand* 122:433–441, 1984.

234. Waller AD: The sense of effort: an objective study. *Brain* 14:179–249, 1891.
235. Warhol MJ, Seigel AJ, Evans WJ, Silverman LM: Skeletal muscle injury and repair in marathon runners after competition. *Am J Pathol* 118:331–339, 1985.
236. Weber E: Eine Physiologische Methode, die Leistungsfahigkeit ermudeter Muskeln zu erhohen. *Arch Physiol (Leipzig)* 385–420, 1914.
237. Weichardt W: Uber das Ermudungtoxin und—Autitoxin. *Muench Med Wochenschr* 51:2121, 1904.
238. Wenger HA, Reed AT: Metabolic factors associated with muscular fatigue during aerobic and anaerobic work. *Can J Appl Sports Sci* 1:43–48, 1976.
239. Wiles CM: The determinants of relaxation rate of human muscle in vivo. Ph.D. Thesis, University of London, 1980.
240. Wiles CM, Edwards RHT: The effect of temperature, ischemia and contractile activity on the relaxation rate of human muscle. *Clin Physiol* 2:485–497, 1982a.
241. Wiles CM, Edwards RHT: Metabolic heat production in isometric ischemic contractions of human adductor pollicis. *Clin Physiol* 2:449–512, 1982b.
242. Wiles CM, Jones DA, Edwards RHT: Fatigue in human muscle myopathy. In Porter R, Whelan J (eds): *Human Muscle Fatigue: Physiological Mechanisms* (Ciba Foundation Symposium No. 82). London, Pitman Medical, 1981, pp 120–129.
243. Wiles CM, Young A, Jones DA, Edwards RHT: Muscle relaxation rate, fiber-type composition and energy turnover in hyper- and hypothyroid patients. *Clin Sci* 57:375–384, 1979.
244. Wilkerson JE, Batterton DL, Horvath SM: Exercise induced changes in blood ammonia levels in humans. *Eur J Appl Physiol* 37:255–263, 1977.
245. Wilkie DR: Muscular fatigue: effects of hydrogen ions and inorganic phosphate. *Fed Proc* 45:2921–2923, 1986.
246. Wilkie DR, Dawson MJ, Edwards RHT, Gordon RE, Shaw D: ^{31}P NMR studies of resting muscle in normal human subjects. In Pollack G, Sugi H (eds): *Cross-Bridge Mechanisms in Muscle Contraction: Proceedings of the 2nd International Symposium*. Seattle, 1983.
247. Williams MH, Wesseldine S, Somma T, Schuster R: The effects of induced erythrocythemia upon 5-mile treadmill run time. *Med Sci Sports Exerc* 13:169–175, 1981.
248. Woods JJ, Furbish F, Bigland-Ritchie BR: Evidence for a fatigue-induced reflex inhibition of motoneuron firing rates. *J Neurophys* 58:125–137, 1987.
249. Worcel A, Erecinska M: Mechanism of inhibitory action of ammonia on the respiration of rat-liver mitochondria. *Biochim Biophys Acta* 67:27–33, 1964.
250. Zeeman EC: *Catastrophe Theory. Selected Papers 1972–1977*. London: Addison-Wesley, 1977, pp 1–64.

3
Skeletal Muscle Disorders and Associated Factors That Limit Exercise Performance

STEVEN F. LEWIS, Ph.D.
RONALD G. HALLER, M.D.

INTRODUCTION

The many factors which, in humans, limit the performance of various types of exercise have been studied extensively [cf. 105, 157] but in general are poorly understood. The problem is of immense complexity, encompassing virtually all relevant physiological systems: for example, cardiovascular, respiratory, neuromuscular, metabolic, and hormonal. Much of the difficulty lies in isolating the most critical factor(s) limiting each type of in vivo exercise performance from one or more of these systems. An approach traditional to medical science, that is, learning about normal physiology through study of the associated pathophysiology, may provide a framework appropriate for this task. In the past two decades major increases in knowledge of exercise pathophysiology have been made in a number of clinical fields [25] including cardiology [3, 113, 155], pulmonology [49, 100, 199], and endocrinology [76, 195]. This information has proved valuable for diagnostic and treatment purposes and also for the understanding of normal human exercise physiology and the limitations to performance. In contrast, systematic research on exercise in human muscle disease has received only minor emphasis partly because of the rarity of many muscle diseases and associated limitations to their recognition and diagnosis. Available technology was for many years a diagnostic barrier. For example, in 1951 the first disorder of muscle energy metabolism was described as a defect in glycogen breakdown [134], but it took 8 additional years for the specific deficiency of glycogen phosphorylase in this disorder to be identified by direct assay [141, 178]. The emergence of new clinically applicable noninvasive techniques such as magnetic resonance spectroscopy [41, 61, 160] and imaging [137, 145] and advances in the field of molecular biology are likely to make it feasible to characterize with minimal discomfort the precise nature of many metabolic and structural muscle defects and to facilitate the assessment of clinical and experimental interventions related to exercise performance.

There is increasing recognition that research on skeletal muscle disease can provide unique insights into a number of the mechanisms by which humans adjust to exercise and ultimately become fatigued [cf. 42, 66, 79, 121, 122, 158, 201]. These insights have been derived largely, but not entirely, from the emerging field of studying muscle metabolic disorders [cf. 6, 35, 55, 65, 67, 87 88, 92, 114, 129, 163]. Research on human metabolic defects has provided valuable information on various aspects of normal physiology, but until recently this approach has largely been neglected in the study of regulatory mechanisms during exercise. Nevertheless, the consequences of certain specific defects of muscle energy metabolism for exercise performance are often so striking as to permit definitive conclusions.

The physiological limitations to exercise performance may be considered in two broad categories. This review primarily deals with the more general metabolic and physiologic factors which set an upper limit to performance in patients with a variety of specific disorders affecting the metabolism or structure of skeletal muscle. We have placed less emphasis on the factors more directly responsible for an inability to continue exercise, that is, the end points or fatigue factors, in patients with muscle disorders. Recent reviews or monographs [61, 121, 157, 201] have more specifically considered the problem of fatigue in certain muscle disorders and the reader is referred to these sources for additional detail.

BACKGROUND

Sources of Energy for Exercise Performance in Healthy Subjects
Adenosine triphosphate (ATP) is the immediate source of energy for muscle contraction and relaxation. Skeletal muscle ATP is stored in very limited quantity, sufficient to supply energy for only a few seconds of maximal exercise if it is not resynthesized. Virtually all ATP is resynthesized by four metabolic processes: Oxidative phosphorylation, glycolysis, and the creatine kinase and adenylate kinase reactions (Table 3.1). Oxidative metabolism is the major quantitative source of energy for ATP resynthesis whereas anaerobic glycolysis and creatine kinase play much more limited quantitative roles (Tables 3.1 and 3.2). The adenylate kinase reaction has a negligible capacity for ATP resynthesis and is coupled to that of adenosine monophosphate (AMP) deaminase. The major function of the coupled adenylate kinase/AMP deaminase reactions appears to be to buffer transient increases in the ATP hydrolysis product adenosine diphosphate (ADP).

Variables Affecting Exercise Performance in Healthy Subjects
For any individual the specific metabolic requirements of a given exercise depend on a number of variables. One important variable is the *mode of contraction*, that is, whether exercise is *dynamic* (brief contractions repeated rhythmically and involving a change in muscle length) or *static*

TABLE 3.1
Adenosine Triphosphate (ATP) Resynthesis/Adenosine Diphosphate (ADP) Utilization in Skeletal Muscle

Oxidative phosphorylation

A. $glycogen_{(n)} + 6O_2 + 37P_i + 37ADP \rightarrow glycogen_{(n-1)} + 6CO_2 + 42H_2O + 37ATP$

B. $glucose + 6O_2 + 36P_i + 36ADP \rightarrow 6CO_2 + 42H_2O + 36ATP$

C. $palmitate + 23O_2 + 129P_i + 129ADP \rightarrow 16CO_2 + 145H_2O + 129ATP$

Anaerobic glycolysis

A. $glycogen_{(n)} + 3P_i + 3ADP \rightarrow glycogen_{(n-1)} + 2 \text{ lactate} + 2H_2O + 3ATP$

B. $glucose + 2P_i + 2ADP \rightarrow 2 \text{ lactate} + 2H_2O + 2ATP$

Creatine kinase reaction

$ADP + PCr + H^+ \leftrightarrow ATP + Cr$

Adenylate kinase/AMP deaminase reactions

$2ADP \leftrightarrow ATP + AMP/AMP + H_2O \rightarrow NH_3 + IMP + 2P_i$

P_i = inorganic phosphate; PCr = phosphocreatine; Cr = creatine; AMP = adenosine monophosphate; IMP = inosine monophosphate.

(a sustained isometric contraction). Walking, running, swimming, and cycling are examples of dynamic exercise. Lifting, pushing or pulling heavy objects, and downhill or water skiing largely involve static muscle contractions. The degree to which active muscle is ischemic is an important metabolic consideration in static exercise. A large increase in intramuscular pressure during high-intensity static exercise [181] lowers effective perfusion pressure and limits muscle blood flow and O_2 delivery, thereby increasing the dependency on anaerobic glycogenolysis. During isometric contraction under conditions of total ischemia, lactate production accounts for approximately 60% of the ATP turnover [104] with the remainder attributable to the other anaerobic sources including the local ATP stores.

In the context of muscle disease, dynamic exercise testing performed under conditions of externally induced ischemia is commonly employed to screen for disorders of muscle glycogen metabolism. The test involves repeated maximal effort handgrip contractions performed to fatigue during total ischemia of the active forearm muscles produced by inflation of a pressure cuff around the upper arm [144]. The pressure cuff is deflated immediately following exercise, and samples of venous blood draining the active muscles are obtained at specified times during recovery for measurement of lactate. Dynamic exercise is, however, normally performed under nonischemic conditions and is largely supported by oxidative metabolism. In dynamic exercise at approximately 70% of maximal oxygen uptake ($\dot{V}O_2max$) lactate production has been calculated to account approximately 2% of total ATP resynthesis [171]. During dynamic exercise at 100% of $\dot{V}O_2max$ the entire contribution from the anaerobic processes can account for only about 16% of the total ATP turnover [171].

The *active muscle mass* also is critical. In general, the larger the mass of active muscle the greater will be the responses of the cardiovascular, pulmonary, and neuroendocrine systems for transport of oxygen and mobilization of extramuscular oxidizable substrate to meet a greater demand for oxidative metabolism [127]. Overall assessment of oxidative metabolism consists of measuring $\dot{V}O_2$max and its components, maximal cardiac output, and arteriovenous oxygen difference (a-v O_2 difference) in large-muscle exercise on a bicycle ergometer or treadmill. Figure 3.1 strikingly illustrates how major pathologic restriction of either a-v O_2 difference or cardiac output can diminish the upper limits of oxidative metabolism to a similar extent. In patients with severe limitations of O_2 utilization due to primary defects in skeletal muscle oxidative metabolism, maximal cardiac output is essentially normal but maximal systemic a-v O_2 difference, indicative of muscle O_2 extraction, and $\dot{V}O_2$max are markedly depressed. In contrast, in patients with a markedly subnormal oxygen transport capacity resulting from chronic heart failure, maximal systemic a-v O_2 diff, and muscle O_2 extraction are within normal limits but there is a dramatically attenuated maximal cardiac output and a subnormal level of $\dot{V}O_2$max [202] very similar to that of the muscle disease patients.

The factors limiting $\dot{V}O_2$max in healthy humans have been controversial. Andersen and Saltin [4] recently provided strong evidence implying that maximal cardiac output is a limiting factor. They demonstrated that maximal perfusion and oxygen uptake of a relatively small active muscle mass (i.e., the quadriceps muscle of one leg) are sufficiently high that the rate of delivery of oxygenated blood necessary to achieve a maximal metabolic rate of a large muscle mass would greatly exceed the maximal cardiac pump capacity. Consistent with this are findings of a reduced vascular conductance (i.e., an increased vascular resistance) in working limbs as cardiac output approaches maximum in large-muscle exercise [108, 179]. The diminished local vascular conductance provides a means for maintaining systemic arterial perfusion pressure when cardiac output is near maximal [164] but may contribute to fatigue by compromising blood flow to working muscle [108, 179]. Comprehensive assessment of the factors limiting exercise performance in muscular disorders should therefore include large- and small-group effort.

Other critical variables include the *intensity* and *duration* of exercise. Exercise intensity is generally expressed in *absolute* terms, that is, in terms of an individual's power output (in watts of external work accomplished or liters of oxygen consumed) in dynamic exercise or force generated (in newtons or kilograms) in static exercise, or in *relative* terms, that is, as a percentage of an individual's maximal oxygen uptake in dynamic

FIGURE 3.1

A comparison of oxygen uptake, cardiac output, and systemic arteriovenous oxygen difference (a-v O_2 Diff.) during maximal cycle exercise in patients with defects in skeletal muscle oxidative metabolism, patients with chronic heart failure, and healthy control subjects. The muscle disease group consists of a total of 15 patients with defects in the availability (6 with McArdle's syndrome, 5 with phosphofructokinase deficiency) or utilization (4 with defects of mitochondrial electron transport) of oxidizable substrate. Data for the individual patient groups (88, 120, 128; Haller and Lewis, unpublished data) are given in Table 3.4, and the pathophysiology of these defects is described in text. Values for the eight heart failure patients were calculated from the data of Wilson et al. (202). Means and standard deviations for the controls (nine men, eight women) were obtained from Haller et al. (87, 88) and Lewis and Haller (unpublished data) and are given separately for each sex in Table 3.4.

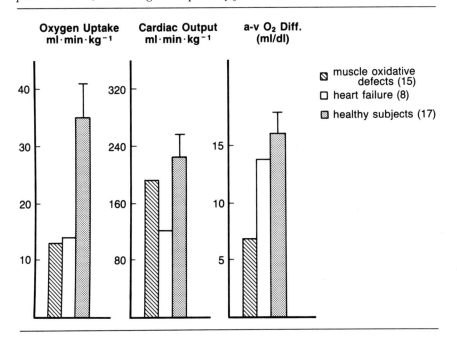

exercise or maximal force generated in static exercise. The maximum power output achievable correlates positively with the maximal rate of ATP turnover. A rapid acceleration to a high maximal rate of ATP turnover can be provided by anaerobic energy sources, but these sources are rapidly depletable (Table 3.2) resulting in a marked attenuation of maximal power output if exercise is continued. In maximal large-muscle effort of sufficiently high intensity as to lead to exhaustion within 1 minute, the majority of energy for ATP resynthesis is derived from intramuscular anaerobic sources—local stores of phosphocreatine and breakdown of glycogen to lactic acid—and the ability to perform this type of exercise depends critically on the availability of these anaerobic fuels. In contrast, oxidative metabolism can provide a maximal ATP turnover rate approximately one-third that from anaerobic sources with a much slower rate of acceleration (Table 3.2). Consequently, oxidative metabolism is associated with a more limited maximal power output. If carbohydrate is exclusively combusted, oxidative metabolism requires approximately 3 minutes to reach a maximal level of ATP turnover (Table 3.2). This delay is primarily due to the time needed for the cardiovascular and pulmonary adjustments necessary to increase O_2 delivery. For free fatty acid (FFA) oxidation the maximal ATP turnover rate is about 50% that of carbohydrate and about 30 minutes normally are needed to reach a maximal FFA oxidation rate. The delay in FFA oxidation is attributable to the time required for FFA mobilization from adipose tissue. Thus in comparison with carbohydrate oxidation, the acceleration in FFA oxidation is slow and FFA is able to support exercise of lower power output.

The upper limit to maximal oxidative metabolism and large-muscle exercise performance in effort of between 3 and 10 minutes' duration normally is established by the capacity for systemic oxygen delivery, that is, cardiac output [4, 172], and normally requires carbohydrate in the form of muscle glycogen as a virtually exclusive oxidizable substrate [173]. In more prolonged *sub*maximal effort, the duration of performance is markedly affected by the relation between exercise intensity and selection of metabolic fuel. At exercise intensities below 50% of $\dot{V}O_2$max, plasma FFA and blood glucose are the primary oxidative substrates [2]. The fraction of total oxygen uptake by active muscle attributable to FFA gradually increases over the duration of mild exercise [2], and because the supply of FFA available from adipose tissue depots is virtually unlimited (Table 3.2) healthy subjects can potentially perform mild to moderate intensity dynamic exercise for many hours [203]. With increasing exercise intensity there is, however, a progressive increase in carbohydrate relative to lipid oxidation, and muscle glycogen has been identified as the dominant fuel for work above 50% of $\dot{V}O_2$max [173]. The duration of exercise performance at exercise intensities requiring 70–80% of $\dot{V}O_2$max was shown to be directly related to the initial glycogen content of active muscle [1], the point of fatigue corresponding to virtually complete glycogen depletion [93]. Fatigue related to glycogen depletion in the muscles of healthy subjects usually occurs between 1 and 2 hours of exercise at this intensity [93].

The *dietary conditions* on the days preceding exercise and more immediately before exercise can modify the availability of carbohydrate,

TABLE 3.2
Metaboblic Characteristics of Fuels for Human Muscle Contraction[a]

Fuels	Available Energy (mol ATP[b])	Endurance Time at 70% $\dot{V}o_2$max (minutes)	Maximum ATP Turnover Rate (mmol ATP/kg dm/s)	Time to Maximum ATP Turnover Rate	O_2 Requirement (mmol O_2/ATP)
Anaerobic					
ATP	0.02	0.03	11.2	<1 s	0
PCr[c]	0.34	0.5	8.6	<1 s	0
CHO[d] → Lactate	0.7–5.2	0.9–6.9	5.2	<5 s	0
Aerobic					
CHO → CO_2 + H_2O	70	93	2.7	3 min	0.162[f]
FFA[e] → CO_2 + H_2O	8,000	10,600	1.4	30 min	0.177

The available energy was calculated from 20 kg muscle with a glycogen content of 70 mmol/kg wet weight, from a liver glycogen store of 500 mmol, and from a fat depot of 15 kg. The endurance time was calculated from a $\dot{V}o_2$max of 4.0 l/minute and with the hypothetical assumption that the specific energy process is the sole source of ATP.

The maximal ATP turnover rate of the anaerobic energy sources was calculated from Hultman and Sjoholm [96]. The maximal aerobic power was calculated from an assumed $\dot{V}o_2$max of 4.0 l/minute of which 72% is utilized by the working legs and working muscle mass of 20 kg (= 4.7 kg dm). The maximal ATP turnover rate of FFA oxidation was assumed to correspond to 50% of the total aerobic power, which seems to be the upper limit [48, 121]. A relatively long time for acceleration to the maximal ATP turnover rate for FFA oxidation is expected due to the necessity of mobilizing FFA from the fat depots into the blood.

[a] Modified from Sahlin K: Metabolic changes limiting muscle performance. In Saltin B (ed): *Biochemistry of Exercise VI*. Champaign, IL, Human Kinetics, 1986, pp 323–343.
[b] Adenosine triphosphate.
[c] Phosphocreatine.
[d] Carbohydrate.
[e] Free fatty acid.
[f] Assumes muscle glycogen is sole CHO oxidized.

the degree to which it is oxidized relative to lipid, and the duration of exercise performance. A high-carbohydrate diet on the days prior to exercise can ensure optimal filling of the muscle glycogen stores, thereby enhancing endurance in heavy submaximal exercise [18]. However, carbohydrate intake shortly before exercise has been shown to inhibit lipolysis [44], thereby increasing the dependency of active muscle on glycogen as a fuel. This is associated with an accelerated muscle glycogen depletion [44] and a diminished endurance [73]. Increases in the rate of glycogen depletion and reduced endurance also have been demonstrated after the administration of the antilipolytic agent nicotinic acid [19, 153]. In contrast, interventions which increase the availability of plasma FFA, such as consumption of a fatty meal plus heparin administration, have been demonstrated to attenuate the rate of muscle glycogen depletion [44] and may improve endurance when administered prior to exercise.

An individual's level of *physical conditioning* can modify the upper limits to maximal oxidative metabolism and endurance in heavy exercise. $\dot{V}O_2$max is the most commonly used single indicator of degree of physical conditioning. The relative increases in $\dot{V}O_2$max resulting from 2–3 months of physical conditioning in initially sedentary healthy individuals represent the sum of approximately equal percentagewise increases in cardiac output and a-v O_2 difference [174]. In contrast, the large increase in $\dot{V}O_2$max observed when physical conditioning is sustained for several years is primarily due to a markedly larger maximal cardiac output and stroke volume [22]. The increased endurance in heavy submaximal exercise observed after physical conditioning in healthy subjects is related to an increased oxidation of fat and a sparing of muscle glycogen at a given power output [94]. Patients with muscle glycogen unavailability due to phosphorylase or phosphofructokinase deficiency (see below) are highly dependent on fat oxidation for exercise performance [119] but typically are deconditioned due to exercise intolerance. Physical conditioning which leads to an increased capacity for fat oxidation may therefore be of potential benefit to these patients.

The *oxygen cost* of exercise is another determinant of performance in dynamic exercise. In healthy human subjects there are reasonably constant and predictable relationships between the rate of oxygen consumed in moving the body and the speed of walking and running [13, 133] and between the rate of oxygen consumption and the external power output, as in stationary cycling [45]. In general, the less "skill" or neuromuscular coordination involved in performing a given task the more accurately the oxygen cost of the task can be predicted. For a simple task such as pedaling a cycle ergometer the O_2 cost can be predicted from an equation based on the power output and the individual's body weight (a factor accounting for the greater energy requirement of moving heavier legs) with a remarkably low standard deviation of ± 90 ml [45]. In comparison with stationary cycling, the O_2 cost of walking and running is somewhat more variable due in part to interindividual differences in vertical displacement of the center of gravity and acceleration and deceleration of the trunk with each step [40, 46]. Another factor which can affect the O_2 cost of exercise is the relative proportion of lipid to carbohydrate oxidized. Approximately 10% less O_2 is necessary to resynthesize a mole of ATP from glycogen than from FFA (Table 3.2). Fuel selection ordinarily plays a relatively minor role in determining the O_2 cost of exercise in healthy individuals able to oxidize both fat and carbohydrate but could assume greater importance in patients with impairments in carbohydrate or fatty acid metabolism in skeletal muscle. In general, for individuals with subnormal $\dot{V}O_2$max, such as most patients with skeletal muscle disorders, a given deviation from the normal oxygen cost of exercise would have a relatively larger effect on maximal work capacity.

Regulation of Cardiac Output
In healthy human subjects cardiac output normally increases 5–6 l for each liter of increase in total body oxygen uptake from rest to exercise [57, 69, 127]. Factors that affect resting cardiac output such as age, sex, body weight, level of physical fitness, or posture [196] have little influence on the slope of the cardiac output–oxygen uptake relation in exercise. The link between cardiac output and oxygen uptake is indicative of a tight, approximately 1:1 coupling of O_2 transport and utilization. One liter of arterial blood contains approximately 200 ml of O_2. Thus in order to *transport* 1 l of O_2, cardiac output must increase by approximately 5 l. The mechanisms responsible for the close coupling of O_2 transport and utilization are poorly defined, but patients with disordered availability or utilization of oxidizable substrate by skeletal muscle are providing important clues [26, 80, 87, 89, 112, 114, 119–122, 129]. In these patients hemoglobin levels are normal and cardiac output is normal at rest but increases 10–15 l per liter of increase in oxygen uptake during exercise.

Patients whose muscle oxidative metabolism is dependent on the circulatory delivery of extramuscular oxidative substrate due to an impaired intramuscular substrate availability, for example, those with phosphorylase or phosphofructokinase deficiency (see section entitled "Disorders of Glycogenolysis/Glycolysis"), have a 2- to 3-fold greater than normal slope of increase in cardiac output in relation to oxygen uptake [26, 87, 88, 112, 123, 128] implying their $\dot{V}O_2$max is not limited by O_2 delivery. In these patients $\dot{V}O_2$max is a function of maximal cardiac output and blood levels of oxidizable substrate (primarily FFA) as determined by substrate mobilization rate(s).

The large number of factors which can limit exercise performance enhances the significance of studying human skeletal muscle disorders and, in particular, defects of muscle energy metabolism. Specific human metabolic defects have been identified which have critical implications for the metabolic requirements of exercise of a certain type, intensity, or duration under specific dietary conditions. In contrast, animals with similar in-born metabolic defects are unavailable or not physiologically comparable [27, 194, 198].

CLASSIFICATION OF SKELETAL MUSCLE DISORDERS

From the standpoint of exercise performance, skeletal muscle diseases can be classified into three major groups. One group consists of *primary disorders of muscle energy metabolism* (Table 3.3). This group includes enzymatic defects in metabolic pathways for ATP resynthesis from its hydrolysis products, ADP and inorganic phosphate (P_i) (Table 3.1). Intolerance to sustained exercise and premature fatigability are characteristic features of these metabolic muscle defects. Muscle weakness and atrophy are less common. *Consistent with the concept that oxidative metabolism is the major source of energy for contracting muscle, patients with disordered muscle oxidative metabolism—that is, patients with defects in the availability or utilization of oxidizable substrate—typically demonstrate severely impaired exercise performance.*

A second major group includes *disorders in which there is a decreased muscle mass due to muscle necrosis, atrophy, and the replacement of muscle by fat or connective tissue.* These disorders are exemplified by the various muscular dystrophies in which the capacity for exercise is severely impaired due to muscle wasting and weakness in spite of largely normal pathways for muscle ATP resynthesis.

A third group includes *disorders in which there is impaired activation of muscle contraction* or *impaired muscle relaxation.* These disorders may be considered in two subcategories. In the first, impaired activation or relaxation of contractile activity is due to intrinsic dysfunction of sarcolemma, sarcoplasmic reticulum, or excitation–contraction coupling, including diseases associated with myotonia [200] or periodic paralysis [116]. Published information on the exercise responses of patients with these disorders is extremely limited [cf. 38, 118, 190]. In the second subcategory, there is a primary abnormality in the "chain of command" of neural excitation of muscle originating in the motor cortex. These disorders involve impaired muscle activation related to diseases of the central nervous system, motor nerves, or neuromuscular junction. Diseases of this type typically are associated with muscle atrophy secondary to disuse or denervation. An example is the motor neuron disease amy-

TABLE 3.3
Classification of Selected Skeletal Muscle Diseases and Implications for Exercise Performance

Disorder	Primary Defect	Exercise Limitation
Metabolic myopathies	Impaired ATP resynthesis/ADP utilization	Premature muscle fatigue (likely related to accumulation of ATP hydrolysis products, i.e., ADP, P_i, H^+)
Glycogen storage diseases		
1. Phosphorylase deficiency (McArdle's disease)	Impaired utilization of muscle glycogen	Low $\dot{V}O_2$max/muscle pain, contracture in strenuous or ischemic exercise
2. Phosphofructokinase deficiency	Impaired utilization of muscle glycogen and blood glucose	Low $\dot{V}O_2$max/muscle pain, contracture in strenuous or ischemic exercise
3. Debranching enzyme deficiency	Attenuated muscle and liver glycogenolysis	Low $\dot{V}O_2$max, weakness may or may not be present
Disorders of lipid metabolism		
1. Carnitine palmitoyl transferase deficiency	Defective long-chain fatty acid oxidation	Intolerance to prolonged exercise aggravated by fasting or low carbohydrate diet
2. Acyl-CoA dehydrogenase deficiencies	Defect in short-, medium-, or long-chain fatty acid oxidation associated with secondary carnitine deficiency	Low $\dot{V}O_2$max/weakness
Electron transport defects	Impaired oxidation of NADH and/or flavin-linked substrates	Low $\dot{V}O_2$max/easy fatigue/weakness
AMP deaminase deficiency	Impaired purine nucleotide metabolism	? Premature fatigue in moderately strenuous exercise
Dystrophies		
Duchenne's dystrophy	Absence of dystrophin[a]	Marked and rapidly progressive weakness/severe muscle atrophy
Becker's dystrophy	Absence of dystrophin[a]	Progressive weakness/muscle atrophy
Facioscapulohumeral dystrophy	Unknown	Slowly progressive weakness/muscle atrophy
Limb-girdle dystrophy	Unknown	Slowly progressive weakness/muscle atrophy
Myotonic dystrophy	Unknown	Weakness/atrophy; myotonia

ATP = adenosine triphosphate; ADP = adenosine diphosphate; P_i = inorganic phosphate; NADH = nicotinamide adenine dinucleotide; AMP = adenosine monophosphate.
[a]Dystrophin is a protein coded on the X chromosome apparently associated with muscle triads, the intracellular junctions of the muscle membrane, and sarcoplasmic reticulum where electrical excitation of the muscle triggers contraction.

otrophic lateral sclerosis which has recently been studied from the standpoint of exercise by Sanjak et al. [175, 176].

The remaining discussion will focus on the effects of impaired muscle energy metabolism and muscular dystrophy on exercise performance. This scope primarily relates to difficulties in interpreting the extremely limited and unsystematic published information regarding exercise in the disorders of muscle activation mentioned above. For example, in many previous reports, exercise data from a variety of disorders each comprised of a very small number of patients have been lumped together under the category "neuromuscular diseases" [cf. 24, 72, 132, 139]. Another example involves myasthenia gravis, a defect of neuromuscular transmission which exhibits major variation in the anatomical distribution and severity of muscle weakness [182]. In myasthenia gravis, most [98, 111, 124, 199] but not all [148, 180] published reports on voluntary exercise involve diverse protocols each performed by a single patient with little or no mention of the location or degree of muscle weakness. The scarcity of systematic information for muscle diseases in general is particularly apparent in the literature relating to muscular strength [cf. 74, 95, 135, 139, 190, 193]. For this reason, we also have placed limited emphasis on the topic of muscular strength.

DISORDERS OF MUSCLE ENERGY METABOLISM

The known disorders of muscle energy metabolism include specific defects in muscle carbohydrate and lipid metabolism, disorders of the mitochondrial respiratory chain, and abnormalities of purine nucleotide metabolism (Figs. 3.2 and 3.3). Several recent reviews [32, 50, 54, 65, 68, 70, 78, 154, 166, 187] have covered the clinical aspects of these defects in detail, and only the principal features will be discussed here.

Disorders of Glycogenolysis/Glycolysis

CLINICAL FEATURES. These are genetic defects consisting of an absent or, less frequently, a catalytically inactive enzyme protein in the metabolism of skeletal muscle glycogen [Fig. 3.2]. The exercise pathophysiology of patients with glycogen phosphorylase deficiency (McArdle's disease) and phosphofructokinase (PFK) deficiency has been studied in some detail [7, 8, 20, 26, 31, 42, 63, 79, 83, 88, 92, 109, 112, 119, 121, 123, 125, 134, 140, 150, 152, 156, 163, 165, 197, 201]. In contrast, limited data are available for the other defects of glycogen metabolism [6, 55, 82, 91, 107, 162]. Patients with PFK deficiency and McArdle's disease demonstrate a lack of elevation of blood lactate following fatiguing ischemic exercise, the biochemical hallmark of absent glycolysis. The clinical hallmark of these defects is the occurrence of an electrically silent muscle contracture resulting from intense or ischemic exercise. The onset of symptoms is usually in childhood or early adult life and consists of complaints of

FIGURE 3.2

A schematic of the major known defects in the pathways of energy supply in human skeletal muscle. The individual enzymatic defects are highlighted in **bold print** *and* underlined. *The specific location of each defect is shown by the* thick lines *crossing the* thinner lines, *denoting the known sequence of reactions in the relevant metabolic pathways.*

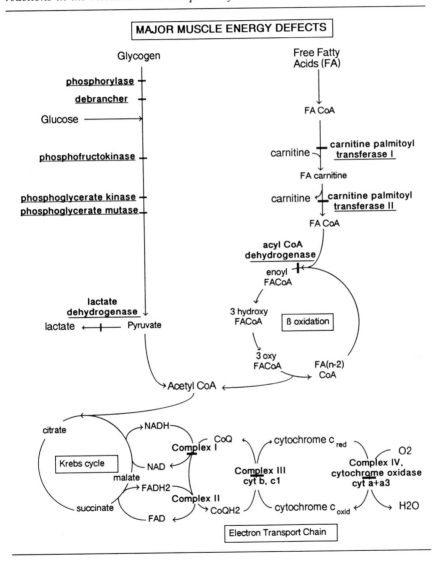

FIGURE 3.3

Relations between the adenylate kinase reaction, the adenosine monophosphate (AMP) deaminase reaction, the purine nucleotide cycle, and the production of inosine monophosphate (IMP) degradation products and fumarate in skeletal muscle.

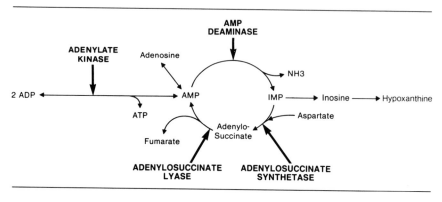

exercise intolerance with muscle fatigue, pain, or cramps during strenuous or ischemic muscle activity. Mild exercise usually can be performed without difficulty but heavy or ischemic exercise can lead to muscle pain, muscle swelling, soreness, and rhabdomyolysis (widespread necrosis of active muscle) with elevated serum creatine kinase and sometimes myoglobinuria. Extreme muscle fatigue, cramps, and/or painful contractures may impair maximal exercise performance in patients with McArdle's disease and PFK deficiency.

ANAEROBIC MUSCLE PERFORMANCE. The unavailability of muscle glycogen severely limits the ability to perform exercise in which active muscle is subjected to anaerobic conditions. In McArdle's disease and PFK deficiency the available anaerobic energy sources are virtually restricted to phosphocreatine (PCr) and ATP stored in muscle. Repeated maximal handgrip contractions performed under ischemic conditions by these patients typically lead to complete muscle exhaustion within 1 minute. In contrast, healthy subjects usually can tolerate this type of exercise for at least 2–3 minutes. The observations for McArdle and PFK-deficient patients are consistent with calculations indicating that without other sources of ATP resynthesis, local stores of ATP and PCr would theoretically be exhausted within 1 minute (Table 3.2). It is intriguing that despite a rapid, marked depletion of muscle PCr during maximal ischemic exercise in McArdle's disease [163], muscle ATP levels usually show no change or only a modest decline [66, 163, 165]. Maximal ischemic exercise also has little effect on total muscle ATP levels in PFK deficiency [63]. Factors other than gross muscle ATP depletion therefore appear responsible for the greatly diminished capacity to exercise under anaerobic conditions in these disorders.

MAXIMAL OXYGEN UPTAKE. Because of the striking failure of lactate to accumulate and the presence of muscle contractures during ischemic or high-intensity nonischemic exercise, it is conventionally believed that glycogenolytic and glycolytic disorders are primarily defects of anaerobic energy supply. Oxidative metabolism, however, is the major quantitative mode of ATP resynthesis in skeletal muscle. The complete aerobic oxidation of glycogen and glucose to CO_2 and water provides net gains of 37 and 36 ATPs, respectively (Table 3.1). By comparison, the anaerobic oxidation of glycogen and glucose to lactate provides net gains of only 3 and 2 ATPs, respectively (Table 3.1). Recent evidence from patients with McArdle's disease and PFK deficiency supports the hypothesis that the unavailability of muscle glycogen as a fuel for oxidative metabolism is a major reason for the greatly diminished work capacity [88, 119, 121].

In the American patients thus far studied with McArdle's disease and PFK deficiency $\dot{V}O_2$max measured during cycle exercise typically is 35–50% of normal (Table 3.4). This level of $\dot{V}O_2$max represents a 4-to-6-fold increase over resting oxygen uptake in comparison with 10-to-12-fold increases in oxygen uptake from rest to maximal exercise typical for healthy subjects. A higher $\dot{V}O_2$max reported in a single McArdle patient from Norway also was considered by the authors [112] approximately 50% of normal in comparison with physically fit Scandinavian subjects [12]. The low $\dot{V}O_2$max in PFK deficiency and McArdle's disease appears largely to be the result of markedly subnormal muscle oxygen extraction. This is reflected by a 25–50% increase in systemic a-v O_2 difference from rest to maximal exercise in contrast to the 3- to 4-fold elevation normally observed [88, 119, 128]. Impaired myocardial pump performance does not appear responsible for the low $\dot{V}O_2$max in PFK deficiency and McArdle disease. Cardiac muscle is spared and maximal cardiac output is within the normal range (Table 3.4) apparently related to the presence of tissue-specific isozymes of phosphorylase [51] and PFK [166]. In contrast, $\dot{V}O_2$max and systemic a-v O_2 difference are essentially normal in patients with a selective defect in muscle long-chain fatty acid oxidation due to carnitine palmitoyltransferase deficiency [35, 87]. These findings are in agreement with evidence that the availability of muscle glycogen as an oxidizable substrate is critical for normal muscle O_2 extraction and the expression of $\dot{V}O_2$max [88, 119, 121]. In both PFK deficiency and McArdle's disease there is a lack of access to muscle glycogen as a metabolic fuel while glucose oxidation by muscle is blocked in PFK deficiency but not in McArdle's disease (Fig. 3.2) The similarity of $\dot{V}O_2$max in PFK deficiency and McArdle's disease (Table 3.4) is there-

TABLE 3.4
Maximal Exercise Data (Mean ± Standard Deviation) in Skeletal Muscle Disorders

Subjects	Exercise	Reference[a]	N	Age (yr)	Sex	Weight (kg)	Workload (Watts)	$\dot{Q}$ (ml/min/kg)	HR (beats/min)	SV (ml)	$a\text{-}vO_2D$ (ml/dl)	$\dot{V}O_2$ (ml/min/kg)	$\Delta\dot{Q}$[b]$/\Delta\dot{V}O_2$	$\dot{V}E$ (l/min)	$\dot{V}E/\dot{V}O_2$	RER
McArdle's disease	Cycle	88, 123	6	30 ±14	4M 2F	82 ±13	58 ±20	168 ±23	152 ±20	92 ±14	7.7 ±2.0	13 ±3	11.0 ±2.7	50 ±10	43 ±6	0.95 ±0.08
		79, 92	8	29 ±7	4M 4F	68 ±9	73 ±30	—[c]	187	—	—	16 ±4	—	46	43 ±12	1.05[d] ±0.14
	Treadmill	112	1	26	M	60	100	338	192 ±8	106	9.0	30	11.0	42	23	1.04
		107	2	—	M	59	—	—	184	—	—	27	—	60	32	0.86
Glycogen debrancher disease	Cycle	82	1	46	F	74	50	142	142	74	12.6	18	5.4	55	42	0.83
		91	1	36	M	—	125	—	136	—	—	1.62	—	—	—	—
Phosphofructokinase deficiency	Cycle	128	5	22 ±14	3M 2F	55 ±16	16 ±5	203 ±28	154 ±7	73 ±8	6.4 ±1.0	13 ±2	12.3 ±3.1	30 ±7	43 ±7	1.04 ±0.13
Carnitine palmitoyl-transferase deficiency	Cycle	87	2	20	2M	74	215	254	183	102	16.1	41	4.3	132	43	1.14
		35	1	23	M	79	230	—	200	—	—	41	—	—	—	—
Electron transport defects	Cycle	89, 120	4	22 ±10	2M 2F	38 ±11	22 ±19	208 ±60	176 ±5	45 ±18	6.0 ±0.1	13 ±4	14.4 ±0.4	41 ±21	85 ±25	1.29 ±0.28
		23	2	14	M,F	60	90	—	198	—	—	22	—	54	42	1.20
		67	1	20	M	—	65	—	183	—	—	0.54[e]	—	102	188	3.33
Dystrophies																
Duchenne	Cycle	185	13	8 ±1	M	26 ±5	—	202[f]	136 ±13	41 ±13	7.7 ±5.0	14 ±5	7.0[f]	8 ±4	22[f]	—
		38	1	11	M	37	—	—	—	—	—	13	—	—	—	—
Other	Cycle	87	8	32 ±12	M	72 ±18	59 ±25	163 ±26	164 ±24	66 ±19	13.1 ±1.9	21 ±5	6.2 ±1.7	62 ±16	45 ±7	1.08 ±0.11
		38	6	24 ±14	M	72 ±27	102 ±71	—	—	—	—	20 ±10	—	—	—	—
		72	3	33 ±11	M	81 ±4	—	—	—	—	—	21 ±1	—	—	—	—

TABLE 3.4
Continued

Group	Mode	Source	Ref.	n	Sex												
Myalgia	Cycle	Haller	87	11	M	33 ±9	82 ±18	153 ±35	190 ±44	165 ±14	94 ±15	14.2 ±1.8	27 ±5	5.3 ±0.8	86 ±17	40 ±7	1.08 ±0.07
		unpublished		6	F	33 ±5	55 ±7	83 ±29	107 ±87	168 ±16	53 ±8	12.5 ±0.5	22 ±5	5.6 ±0.9	55 ±8	47 ±3	1.10 ±0.08
			38	8	M	29 ±13	82 ±15	163 ±64	—	—	—	—	31 ±9	—	—	—	—
Healthy controls	Cycle	Lewis	127	9	M	26 ±3	78 ±10	229 ±32	237 ±36	190 ±10	96 ±14	16.7 ±2.1	39 ±5	4.7 ±0.6	135 ±26	45 ±6	1.15 ±0.07
		unpublished		8	F	26 ±4	60 ±7	136 ±22	207 ±13	186 ±5	65 ±10	15.0 ±1.2	31 ±3	5.0 ±0.8	77 ±14	42 ±6	1.14 ±0.06
			38	7	M	33 ±5	76 ±7	193 ±47	—	—	—	—	36 ±5	—	—	—	—
			38	8	F	26 ±2	56 ±7	182 ±24	—	—	—	—	37 ±6	—	—	—	—
			185	13	M	8 ±1	27 ±5	—	378[f]	190 ±8	49 ±15	11.8 ±3.1	40 ±4	7.0[f]	32 ±8	29	—

$\dot{Q}$ = cardiac output; HR = heart rate; SV = stroke volume; a-vO$_2$D = systemic arteriovenous oxygen difference; $\dot{V}O_2$ = oxygen uptake, STPD; $\Delta\dot{Q}/\Delta\dot{V}O_2$ = slope of cardiac output (l/min) in relation to oxygen uptake (l/min, BTPS) to oxygen uptake (l/min, STPD); $\dot{V}E$ = pulmonary ventilation, BTPS; $\dot{V}E/\dot{V}O_2$ = ratio of pulmonary ventilation (l/min, BTPS) to oxygen uptake (l/min, STPD); RER = respiratory exchange ratio: carbon dioxide production (l/min, STPD)/oxygen uptake (l/min, STPD).

[a] The references cited in some cases do not contain all data presented in this table. Supplementary unpublished data (Lewis and Haller; Hagberg and co-workers) were made available in these instances.

[b] Calculated as the mean ± standard deviation slope of the cardiac output on oxygen uptake based on separate linear regression equations for each individual in each group. Cardiac output was measured by the acetylene rebreathing technique [82, 87–89, 120, 123, 128] described by Blomqvist et al. [191], by the dye-dilution technique [112] or by an electrical impedance method [185].

[c] Unavailable data.

[d] Mean and standard deviation for four subjects only.

[e] Patient body weight not published; units for $\dot{V}O_2$ = l/min.

[f] Calculated or estimated from original data.

fore consistent with the concept that blood glucose normally makes a very minor contribution as a fuel for brief intense dynamic exercise [101].

In McArdle's disease and PFK deficiency, cardiac output typically increases 200–300% more than normally for a given increase in oxygen uptake from rest to exercise (Table 3.4). Muscle blood flow data are lacking in PFK deficiency, but in McArdle's disease blood flow to active muscle is exaggerated relative to muscle oxygen demand [126; Jorfeldt Pernow, Havel, Saltin, and Wahren, unpublished observations]. The possible mechanisms responsible for the abnormally large increase in oxygen delivery to muscle have been discussed elsewhere [121] and likely involve the fact that in McArdle's disease and PFK deficiency oxidative metabolism is limited by the delivery of extramuscular oxidizable fuels rather than the delivery of O_2 [119]. Delivery of a given substrate is a function of blood flow to active muscle and the substrate concentration in the blood. Thus, as in healthy subjects, maximal cardiac output probably sets an upper limit to $\dot{V}O_2max$ in PFK deficiency and McArdle's disease. However, a salient difference is that *oxidative metabolism in McArdle or PFK-deficient patients also is limited by the rate of mobilization of extramuscular fuels*, that is, FFA from adipose tissue (in both disorders) and glucose from liver (in McArdle's disease only). Normalization of the exaggerated cardiac output and muscle blood flow during interventions that increase blood levels of oxidative substrate [81, 88, 123, 126, 128] links the steeper than normal rise in cardiac output in PFK deficiency and McArdle's disease with a rate of extramuscular fuel mobilization insufficient to satisfy muscle oxidative demands. Fuel mobilization insufficient to meet muscle oxidative requirements may therefore be associated with attainment of maximal cardiac output at a subnormal oxygen uptake. A reduction in local vascular conductance in large active muscle groups normally is observed as maximal cardiac output is reached [164]. Whether this occurs in McArdle's disease and PFK deficiency is unknown. Reduced local conductance could represent an additional restriction to substrate delivery and thereby contribute to the markedly subnormal capacity for large-muscle exercise performance in glycolytic disorders. Increased maximal cardiac output such as that observed in healthy individuals after physical conditioning [174] might improve large-muscle exercise performance in patients with McArdle's disease or PFK deficiency by increasing the overall capacity for substrate delivery to muscle. However, data specifically addressing this issue are lacking.

A markedly subnormal $\dot{V}O_2max$ and impaired muscle oxygen extraction in PFK deficiency and McArdle's disease reflects the virtual absence of muscle pyruvate [197], the preferred substrate for oxidative metabolism [77]. It has been postulated [121] that a diminished supply of muscle pyruvate limits the rate of production of acetyl CoA for incorporation into the citric acid cycle. This, in turn, will attenuate maximal rates of formation of citrate and production of reducing potentials, chiefly nicotinamide adenine dinucleotide (NADH), thus limiting the rate of oxygen uptake by the mitochondrial respiratory chain. Measurements of muscle NADH during exercise in patients with McArdle's disease [56; Sahlin, Haller, Henriksson, Areskog, Lewis, and Jorfeldt, unpublished data] support this postulate. Also consistent are observations that $\dot{V}O_2$max in PFK deficiency and McArdle's diseases varies with the availability of oxidizable substrates. In McArdle's disease increasing the availability to active muscle of glucose (by intravenous infusion) or FFA (by prolonged fasting or overnight fasting plus 45 minutes of moderate intensity exercise) increases $\dot{V}O_2$max by approximately 20% [37, 88, 121]. Similarly, in PFK deficiency increasing the availability of lactate (by intravenous infusion) or FFA, substrates which can bypass the defect in PFK [Fig. 3.2], increased $\dot{V}O_2$max by more than 30% [81, 128]. Conversely, interventions that reduce the supply of FFA to working muscle—oral administration of the antilipolytic agent nicotinic acid in McArdle's disease [123] and intravenous glucose infusion in PFK deficiency [81]—are associated with a reduced $\dot{V}O_2$max.

Limited observations indicate that $\dot{V}O_2$max also is abnormally low in glycogen debranching enzyme (amylo 1,6 glucosidase) deficiency, but is not reduced to the same extent as in McArdle's disease (Table 3.4;) [82, 91]. Because glycogen phosphorylase is normal in debranching enzyme deficiency [52], this likely is due in part to the debrancher patient's ability to metabolize a limited number of glucosyl units from the outer branches of the glycogen molecule through the action of phosphorylase. In contrast to McArdle's disease and PFK deficiency, in debrancher deficiency there is a partial but subnormal elevation of venous effluent lactate to approximately one-fourth the level observed in normal subjects [82] after maximal ischemic forearm exercise. Correspondingly, when glycogen is incubated with purified phosphorylase in the absence of debranching enzyme, about 30–35% of the molecule is converted to glucose-1-phosphate [33]. In contrast to the very depressed $\dot{V}O_2$max in McArdle's disease, PFK deficiency, and debrancher disease, a $\dot{V}O_2$max of 80–90% of normal and an essentially normal blood lactate increase with maximal treadmill exercise have been reported in a patient with phosphoglycerate mutase deficiency [107]. This may be related to a residual phosphoglycerate mutase activity of approximately 5% of normal residing in the BB isozyme [107]. ^{31}P nuclear magnetic resonance (NMR) findings in another phosphoglycerate-mutase-deficient patient [6] are in general agreement. In this patient phosphoglycerate mutase was approximately 6% of normal and muscle pH fell, although less than normally, with ischemic forearm exercise [6]. In contrast, muscle pH typically increases slightly with exercise in McArdle's disease [55, 125, 162] and remains unchanged in PFK deficiency [20, 55, 162]. Phosphoglycerate mutase activity normally is more than 10-fold that of phosphorylase or PFK [29]. Thus, a residual activity of 5–6% is consistent with a substantial capacity of glycolytic flux and formation of pyruvate and may explain a less severe limitation to exercise performance in phosphoglycerate mutase deficiency.

OXYGEN COST OF EXERCISE. At a given power output, total body oxygen uptake is, in some cases, slightly greater than normal in McArdle's disease [112, 121, 156] and PFK deficiency (Fig. 3.4**A**). This may be explained in part by an increased oxidative metabolism of the cardiac and respiratory muscles due to an excessive tachycardia [112, 123, 134] and systolic blood pressure [121] and a greater than normal pulmonary ventilation [83]. Based on the respiratory exchange ratio there is also, at a given exercise intensity in McArdle patients, a greater than normal utilization of fat relative to carbohydrate as an oxidative fuel [88]. A larger O_2 consumption is required to generate the same quantity of ATP from fat than from carbohydrate (Table 3.2). In PFK deficiency a virtually total absence of carbohydrate oxidation due to the lack of access to glycogen and glucose as fuels is consistent with and may contribute importantly to the tendency toward an augmented O_2 cost of exercise. The normal relation between oxygen uptake and exercise intensity in patients with exertional myalgia but no physical or laboratory evidence for neuromuscular disease (Fig. 3.4**F**) implies that the tendency for an increased O_2 cost of exercise in McArdle's disease or PFK deficiency is unrelated to muscle pain which may occur with exercise in these disorders.

In contrast to the tendency for an increased total body O_2 cost of exercise in McArdle's disease and PFK deficiency, patients with McArdle's disease have been reported to have a decreased rate of muscle energy turnover during fatiguing submaximal static contractions performed under ischemic conditions [201]. The reduced energy turnover rate has been postulated to relate to compensatory mechanisms for conserving the limited energy resources of phosphorylase-deficient muscle as fatigue ensues [201].

SUBMAXIMAL EXERCISE PERFORMANCE AND THE SECOND-WIND PHENOMENON. Because muscle glycogen normally is the critical fuel for strenuous submaximal exercise, reduced endurance also is a prominent feature in muscle glycogenoses. During moderately strenuous exertion in patients with McArdle's disease and PFK deficiency there is a premature onset of muscle fatigue, discomfort, cramping, and/or pain. Depending on the relative exercise intensity and dietary conditions, the patients may have to quit entirely or slow down or rest for a few minutes before continuing. Sometimes the same or higher exercise rate can be sustained or resumed with a dramatic reduction of fatigue or other symptoms. The spontaneous increase in the capacity for exercise and attenuation or abolition of symptoms was termed the "second wind" [150] and appears attributable largely to increased delivery of blood-borne oxidizable substrate, principally FFA, to active muscle [152]. A second-wind response associated with increased FFA availability can result from an increased FFA mobilization from adipose tissue stores and/or increased blood flow to active muscle [152]. The reduced dependency on muscle glycogen as an oxidative fuel related to the increased capacity to oxidize FFA normally observed after physical conditioning [94] would be particularly beneficial in PFK deficiency and McArdle's disease. Preliminary data are consistent with an increased exercise tolerance associated with augmented capacities for muscle O_2 extraction and FFA oxidation after physical conditioning in PFK deficiency [86]. Limited observations [91; Haller and Lewis, unpublished data] suggest that the second-wind phenomenon is not as prominent or not present in glycogen debrancher deficiency. The partial availability of muscle glycogen as a fuel in debrancher deficiency [32] may facilitate the transition from rest to strenuous exercise.

METABOLIC FACTORS INVOLVED IN MCARDLE'S DISEASE AND PFK DEFICIENCY. A precise explanation for the premature fatigue in these defects is presently unavailable. However, the similarity of the clinically observed features of fatigue in both disorders and recent findings, including data obtained by ^{31}P NMR [20, 42, 63, 125, 158, 163], suggest that fatigue related to accumulation of muscle ADP may be a common denominator. The metabolic factors commonly studied in relation to human muscle fatigue are shown in Table 3.5. These factors include muscle ATP and PCr depletion and H^+, P_i, and ADP accumulation. As mentioned earlier in this review, fatigue appears unrelated to gross muscle ATP depletion because muscle ATP falls at most only modestly during exhaustive exercise in PFK deficiency [20, 63] or McArdle's disease [66, 125, 165]. This does not, however, eliminate the possibility of fatigue due to depletion of a critical subcellular compartment of ATP in these defects. Depletion of PCr is not consistently related to fatigue in muscle glycogenoses. There is a marked decline of PCr in active muscle in McArdle's disease [125, 163], but the drop in muscle PCr is attenuated in PFK deficiency [20].

Accumulation in muscle of the products of ATP hydrolysis—H^+, P_i, or ADP—could result in muscle fatigue due to product inhibition of the ATPase participating in the interaction of actin and myosin or the ATPases involved in ion pumping across muscle membranes in muscle activation or relaxation [43]. In PFK deficiency and McArdle's disease muscle fatigue is not caused by H^+ accumulation. There is no decline in pH of active muscle in these defects [20, 42, 63, 125, 162, 163]. Findings to date imply that P_i accumulation could play an important role in fatigue in McArdle's disease, but not in PFK deficiency. The increase of muscle

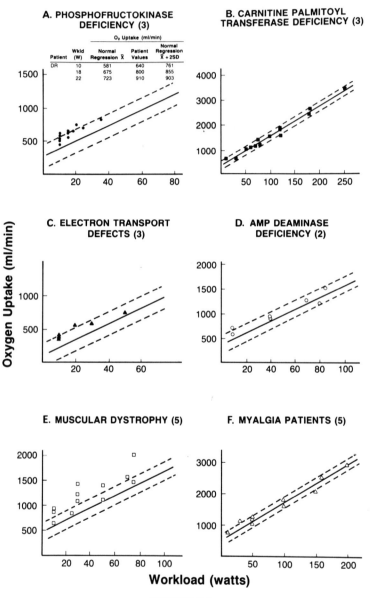

FIGURE 3.4

FIGURE 3.4

A–F, *O_2 uptake in relation to external workload during cycle exercise in several skeletal muscle disorders (Lewis and Haller, unpublished data). For each disorder, individual points from selected patients with similar body weight are plotted relative to the regression line* (solid line) *and ± 2 standard deviation limits (± 180 ml O_2) from the regression line* (dashed lines) *derived from the equation of Cotes (45): $\dot{V}O_2$ (ml/minute) = 11.8W + 6.84wt − 94, where W = power output in watts and* wt = *body weight in kg, based on healthy subjects with the same average body weight as the patients. For each disorder, the relation of O_2 uptake to external workload was very similar in patients whose data are shown and patients whose data are not shown because their body weight differed from the majority of the group. This is demonstrated in* **A**, *which gives O_2 cost of cycling in a patient with phosphofructokinase (PFK) deficiency whose body weight (81 kg) was considerably higher than the mean weight of the other PFK-deficient patients (53 kg). In agreement with the plotted data for O_2 uptake in PFK deficiency,* **A** *shows that O_2 uptake in the heavier patient is higher than the regression mean or the regression line ± 2 standard deviations for healthy subjects weighing 81 kg.*

TABLE 3.5
Metabolic Correlates of Muscle Fatigue

	McArdle's Disease	Phosphofructokinase Deficiency
Depletion		
Adenosine triphosphate	−	−
Phosphocreatine	+	−
Accumulation		
H$^+$	−	−
Inorganic phosphate	+	−
Adenosine diphosphate	+	+

− = no; + = yes.

P_i with respect to exercise intensity is exaggerated in McArdle's disease [125, 163] and relates to the lack of glycogen as a substrate to support oxidative phosphorylation and anaerobic glycolysis. There is a shift in ATP resynthesis/ADP utilization from oxidative phosphorylation and glycolysis to the metabolic reactions leading to net accumulations of P_i, that is, the creatine kinase reaction and the coupled adenylate kinase/AMP deaminase reactions [121]. Increased PCr breakdown [125, 163] and ammonia production [90, 140, 167] are associated with fatigue of phosphorylase deficient muscle [121]. In contrast, despite larger than normal elevations of ammonia in muscle venous effluent [109, 140], elevations of P_i in active muscle are markedly attenuated during fatiguing exercise in PFK deficiency [20, 42, 63]. The limited rise in muscle P_i in PFK deficiency is attributable to incorporation of P_i into phosphorylated glycolytic intermediates proximal to PFK [42, 188] and attenuated PCr breakdown [20]. Increased production of ammonia and the inosine monophosphate degradation products inosine and hypoxanthine by active muscle in the absence of an decline in muscle pH in PFK deficiency [109, 140] and McArdle's disease [31, 90, 140, 167], is consistent with activation of AMP deaminase by elevations of muscle ADP [170, 189] in both defects. Based on ^{31}P NMR findings and the equilibrium characteristics of the creatine kinase reaction, Radda has calculated that in McArdle's disease ADP accumulates to a level which can be inhibitory to myosin ATPase [158]. Cooke et al. [43] suggest that accumulation of ADP, per se, is more likely to cause fatigue by inhibition of the Na^+-K^+ ATPase of the sarcolemma involved in muscle activation or the Ca^{++} ATPase of the sarcoplasmic reticulum involved in muscle relaxation than by inhibition of the myosin ATPase responsible for actin–myosin interaction. Inhibition of the ATPases involved in ion pumping could cause a failure of electrical activation of the muscle or of muscle excitation–contraction coupling. The finding of a close temporal association between the decline in force production and the fall in the muscle action potential in PFK deficiency and McArdle disease [201] is consistent with a role for impaired muscle excitation in fatigue in these disorders.

Carnitine Palmitoyltransferase Deficiency

CLINICAL FEATURES. In this disorder there is a genetic deficiency of carnitine palmitoyltransferase (CPT), a translocation enzyme that enables long-chain fatty acids, the principal lipid fuel of muscle, to pass through the inner mitochondrial membrane and reach the inner mitochondrial space where they are oxidized to CO_2 and water. Demonstrations of a markedly subnormal oxidation of ^{14}C-palmitate in muscle homogenate [35, 53] and a diminished oxidation of ^{14}C-palmitate intravenously infused in an exercising patient [117] are consistent with the enzymatic defect. Symptoms usually begin in late childhood or early adult life and consist of recurrent muscle pain, tenderness, and swelling and myoglobinuria triggered by metabolic circumstances which normally would require fatty acid oxidation as the major source of muscle energy production, including prolonged exercise, fasting, a low-carbohydrate, high-fat diet, or cold exposure [54]. Most patients appear normal on routine clinical examination and muscle mass and strength are usually normal [54].

MAXIMAL OXYGEN UPTAKE. In CPT deficiency, $\dot{V}O_2$max and short-term exercise tolerance are fully normal as long as carbohydrate availability is maintained. Under normal dietary conditions, in which muscle glycogen is readily available as a source of oxidizable substrate, $\dot{V}O_2$max in bicycle exercise was 41 ± 7 ml/minute/kg in three men with CPT deficiency and 41 ± 5 ml/minute/kg in healthy men (Table 3.4). A high respiratory exchange ratio at rest and during submaximal exercise in CPT deficiency [35, 117] is consistent with an increased dependency on the oxidation of carbohydrate. Prolonged fasting can be extremely deleterious to exercise performance likely related to depletion of muscle glycogen. A CPT-deficient patient was unable to exercise after fasting for 38 hours [37]. In contrast, 30–45 minutes of exercise at approximately 50% of $\dot{V}o_2$max can be performed without apparent complications after a 12-hour fast [Haller and Lewis, unpublished observations].

OXYGEN COST OF EXERCISE. Less O_2 is required to generate the same quantity of ATP from carbohydrate than from fat (Table 3.2) However, despite greater than normal carbohydrate utilization as suggested by a high respiratory exchange ratio [35, 117], the relation between total body O_2 uptake and exercise intensity appears normal in CPT deficiency (Fig. 4**B**).

ANAEROBIC MUSCLE PERFORMANCE. There is very limited published information on anaerobic exercise performance in CPT deficiency. In one study, a patient with CPT deficiency performed maximal ischemic forearm exercise under two conditions: after eating and after fasting for 48 hours [21]. Measurement of the plasma purine compounds hypoxanthine and inosine, indicators of AMP deamination (Fig. 3.3) and net ATP catabolism, were made under each condition. Total plasma purine compounds in the venous effluent from active ischemic muscle were markedly higher after fasting than postprandially, suggesting an increased net degradation of ATP after fasting. The exaggerated levels of purine compounds found in muscle venous effluent of patients with PFK deficiency and McArdle's disease [31, 109, 140], who lack access to muscle glycogen, imply that glycogen normally is a critically important source of fuel for ATP resynthesis in ischemic exercise. In CPT deficiency, glycogen depletion during fasting may be accelerated because of the impairment in fatty acid oxidation. This hypothesis would predict a diminished capacity for anaerobic muscle performance after fasting in CPT deficiency.

Mitochondrial Defects

LUFT'S SYNDROME. *Clinical/Biochemical Features.* The clinical presentation in the two reported cases of this disorder was one of hypermetabolism characterized by elevated basal metabolic rate, tachycardia, and excessive sweating in the presence of normal thyroid function. Normally the oxygen consumption of isolated mitochondria is closely coupled to the formation of ATP from ADP and P_i and reflects the fact the cellular respiration is regulated according to energy demand.

The primary defect in Luft's syndrome is a "loose coupling" of the phosphorylation of ADP to oxygen consumption in mitochondria isolated from skeletal muscle. That is, O_2 consumption of mitochondria from affected patients proceeds at a nearly maximal rate even in the absence of a continuous supply of ADP to the mitochondrial incubation medium. As a consequence, resting metabolic rate is 2- to 3-fold greater than normal [58, 131]. Affected patients have been markedly underweight despite an increased caloric intake and exhibit exercise intolerance, premature fatigue, and weakness commensurate with a poorly developed musculature.

Responses to Exercise. Published data on a single patient studied by Edelman et al. [58] suggest a normal O_2 cost of exercise. Despite a 3-fold higher than normal resting oxygen consumption, there was an approximately normal increase from rest to exercise in the absolute level of total body O_2 uptake during submaximal and maximal treadmill walking. Maximal treadmill walking speed was 4 miles per hour (mph), a speed that normally requires a 4- to 6-fold increase over resting O_2 uptake [45]. Because of the elevated resting O_2 uptake there was, however, only a 2-fold increase in O_2 uptake from rest to walking at 4 mph. The patient's ability to walk may have been limited by alveolar ventilation because arterial hypoxia and hypercapnia were observed in maximal exercise. This likely was related to respiratory muscle weakness or fatigue because the pulmonary ventilation achieved during walking at 4 mph was similar to the markedly diminished value obtained in a test of maximal voluntary ventilation [58].

It is difficult to reconcile the above findings with the report of Luft et al. [131] in which the patient performed cycle ergometer exercise. Maximal cycle ergometer work capacity was approximately 35% of normal with respect to body size, and cardiac output increased more steeply than normally during exercise. Luft et al. [131] do not report the primary data but state that there was an "unchanged arteriovenous oxygen difference" during exercise. Because resting a-v O_2 difference values were not reported, the relative contributions of cardiac output and a-v O_2 difference to the elevated resting O_2 uptake cannot be determined.

ELECTRON TRANSPORT DEFECTS. *Clinical/Biochemical Features.* In the last decade a number of distinct abnormalities involving the composition or function of the human electron transport chain have been identified. Defects involving skeletal muscle electron transport at the levels of complex I, III, and IV (Fig. 3.2) have been described [50, 89, 142, 143, 154, 161]. Traditional biochemical techniques used to define these defects include (*a*) measurement of oxygen uptake in isolated mitochondria using substrates linked with NAD and flavin cofactors, (*b*) determination of cytochrome content in isolated mitochondria, and (*c*) measurement of enzyme activities in isolated mitochondria or crude muscle homogenates. In some cases the defect is present in the central nervous system and other tissues in addition to skeletal muscle. However, in most patients in whom exercise responses have been reported the disorder affected primarily skeletal muscle. In general, the primary impairment affecting exercise performance is a markedly diminished ability of active muscle to oxidize NADH and/or flavin-linked substrates derived from lipids or carbohydrates. As a consequence of the oxidative defect there is an increased anaerobic glycogenolysis and a striking blood lactic acidosis [23, 67, 89, 142, 143, 161]. Exercise intolerance is severe; trivial exertion leads to premature muscle fatigue, dyspnea, and palpitations. A dramatic tachycardia in relation to exercise intensity has been documented [23, 67, 89, 142, 143, 161]. A chronic adaptation to electron transport defects appears to be an increase in the synthesis of oxidative metabolic machinery; that is, mitochondrial volume increases [50] and there are increases in the levels of mitochondrial oxidative enzymes [67, 84].

Maximal Oxygen Uptake. $\dot{V}O_2$max is approximately 3–5 times resting oxygen uptake, which is dramatically lower than normal (Table 3.4). Maximal cardiac output is similar to that of normal sedentary subjects (Table 3.4) [89, 120], consistent with a probable sparing of the heart from the metabolic defects in patients studied to date and with a lack of cardiac limitation to $\dot{V}O_2$max. The very low $\dot{V}O_2$max appears primarily attributable to a markedly attenuated muscle oxygen extraction. Systemic a-v O_2 difference increases by approximately 25% from rest to maximal exercise in comparison with the >300% increase observed for healthy subjects [89, 120]. A greatly exaggerated increase in pulmonary ventilation in relation to oxygen uptake (Table 3.4) may contribute to the markedly depressed work capacity in some affected patients. The excessive ventilatory response is associated with the breathlessness which is a prominent symptom of exercise intolerance in patients with mitochondrial myopathies [85]. Resting cardiac output is normal, but during exercise the slope of increase in cardiac output in relation to oxygen uptake is approximately 300% of normal [89, 120].

In contrast to patients with McArdle's disease and PFK deficiency, there is no direct evidence that $\dot{V}O_2$max in electron transport defects can be altered by changes in dietary composition or intravenous substrate infusions. However, case reports have indicated that exercise tolerance in some patients may be improved by treatment with vitamins or cofactors. For example, in one patient with a deficiency in the NADH-coenzyme Q reductase complex, 100 mg of oral riboflavin taken daily for 3 months resulted in a 33% increase in $\dot{V}O_2$max [11]. The mechanism of benefit is unclear but flavin nucleotide compounds, the physiologically active forms of riboflavin, serve as cofactors in several electron transport flavoproteins.

Oxygen Cost of Exercise. The available data, although limited, appear consistent with a somewhat higher than normal total body oxygen uptake at a given exercise intensity in patients with respiratory chain defects (Fig. 3.4C). This may be explained in part by marked increases in cardiac and respiratory muscle work resulting from an exaggerated tachycardia [23, 67, 89, 142, 143, 161] and systolic blood pressure response [Lewis and Haller, unpublished data] and a greatly augmented ventilatory drive (Table 3.4).

Anaerobic Muscle Performance. Limited data suggest that patients with defects of electron transport have a relatively normal capacity for ischemic or high-intensity static exercise [67] and do not display increased muscle fatigue or discomfort in this mode of exertion. The rate of muscle ATP turnover in ischemic isometric contraction also appears to be virtually normal [67]. A likely explanation is that the capacity for ischemic or high-intensity static exercise depends largely on anaerobic glycogenolysis and PCr breakdown as sources for ATP resynthesis/ADP removal, and neither of these processes are abnormal in patients with electron transport defects.

Muscle Fatigue. The cause of the premature muscle fatigue in patients with electron transport defects has not been systematically investigated. In spite of the severe impairment in the capacity for oxidative ATP resynthesis in respiratory chain defects, there is little or no decline in the levels of muscle ATP as measured by ^{31}P NMR [10, 64] or conventional assay of muscle biopsy specimens [67]. On the basis of the very low levels of $\dot{V}O_2$max and disproportionate elevations in systemic venous blood lactate in relation to exercise intensity [23, 67, 89, 142, 143, 161] it is reasonable to postulate that the impairment in oxidative metabolism would result in an abnormally rapid and pronounced activation of anaerobic glycolysis and a commensurate decline in muscle pH. However, several ^{31}P NMR studies [10, 64, 75, 159] have failed to document an exaggerated decline in muscle pH, and in a few patients the fall in muscle pH was even slightly attenuated relative to controls [9]. Why pH in active muscle does not fall excessively while blood lactate rises precipitously is presently unknown, as is the precise cause of premature muscle fatigue in these patients.

OTHER OXIDATIVE DEFECTS. *Patients of Linderholm et al. and Larsson et al.* Larsson et al. [114] and Linderholm et al. [129] performed detailed physiological studies in patients with a hereditary myopathy characterized by premature fatigue, palpitations, and dyspnea with trivial exertion and recurrent myoglobinuria indicative of rhabdomyolysis. The pathophysiology was largely restricted to exercise and consisted of easy fatigability but not weakness. Muscle strength was within normal limits. Resting cardiac output and ventilation were normal as were maximal voluntary ventilation and lung function. Arterial O_2 saturation and hemoglobin levels and heart and blood volume also were normal. Normal blood pressures, including ventricular filling pressures measured during cardiac catheterization and a normal stroke volume in relation to heart volume suggested a lack of myocardial involvement in the disease. During exercise there were excessive increases in heart rate, cardiac output, and ventilation in relation to oxygen uptake. Estimated blood flow to active muscle was disproportionately elevated and there was a greater than normal release of lactate from the exercising legs related to a subnormal O_2 extraction. A low lactate/pyruvate ratio in the venous effluent from the exercising legs suggested an underlying disorder of pyruvate oxidation, but the precise metabolic lesion has not been identified to date.

$\dot{V}O_2$max was dramatically low in these patients, averaging approximately 10 ml/minute/kg [114, 129]. Maximal cardiac output was normal but systemic a-v O_2 difference failed to rise normally with exercise, implying that a restricted capacity for muscle oxygen utilization limited $\dot{V}O_2$max. The slope of increase in cardiac output in relation to oxygen uptake was approximately 15–20 in comparison with the normal value of 5, indicative of a fundamental disturbance in O_2 transport during exercise.

Total body oxygen uptake was within the normal range or slightly higher than normal in relation to external workload [129]. As in the oxidative defects of muscle discussed earlier in this review, an elevated oxygen uptake may partly relate to an abnormally high heart rate, systolic blood pressure, and pulmonary ventilation, that is, an increased oxygen demand of the myocardium and ventilatory muscles.

Acyl-CoA Dehydrogenase Deficiency/Carnitine Deficiency. Fatty acid β-oxidation defects at the level of long-, medium-, and short-chain acyl-CoA dehydrogenases and multiple acyl-CoA dehydrogenase deficiency related to a riboflavin-dependent reaction common to straight and branched chain acyl-CoA moieties have been described [68, 78, 192]. Organic aciduria related to the excretion of unmetabolized fatty acids typically is associated. Secondary depletion of carnitine, a cofactor involved in the transport of long-chain fatty acyl-CoA units into mitochondria, typically occurs as a consequence of the action of carnitine acyl transferases on accumulated acyl-CoA esters with the formation of acylcarnitine compounds. Many patients described with carnitine deficiency prior to recognition of these enzyme defects likely had acyl-CoA dehydrogenase deficiency with secondary carnitine deficiency. The clinical presentation of these disorders includes weakness, exercise intolerance, and metabolic crises triggered by increased plasma FFA levels. Accumulation of triglyceride is prominent in skeletal muscle. Dramatic impairment of exercise performance associated with abnormal skeletal muscle weakness and fatigability has been observed in some patients with short-chain or multiple acyl-CoA dehydrogenase deficiency and/or carnitine deficiency [39, 80, 192].

$\dot{V}O_2$max in some patients is markedly reduced (approximately one-third normal) [39, 80]. We studied a patient with a lipid myopathy, carnitine deficiency, and ethyl malonic aciduria compatible with multiple acyl-CoA dehydrogenase deficiency in whom $\dot{V}O_2$max and maximal a-v O_2 difference were both markedly low [80] consistent with impaired O_2 extraction by working muscle. The presence of a severe oxidative defect in this type of lipid myopathy contrasts with normal oxidative capacity in CPT deficiency. Its mechanism is unclear. Interventions which modify or bypass the metabolic defect have increased $\dot{V}O_2$max in similar patients [39; Haller, Cook, and Lewis, unpublished data] likely by improving the capacity for muscle O_2 extraction. Carroll et al. [39] found that $\dot{V}O_2$max approximately doubled after 3 months of treatment with riboflavin, increasing from 9 to 20 ml/minute/kg. Supplemental carnitine had no effect on $\dot{V}O_2$max or exercise performance in patient studied by Carroll et al. [36]. In our patient [80], treatment with medium-chain triglycerides and supplementary vitamins was associated with an increase in $\dot{V}O_2$max from 12 to 24 ml/minute/kg and an increase in maximal systemic a-v O_2 difference from 6.2 to 12.3 ml/dl. Maximal cardiac output and heart rate did not change after triglyceride and vitamin therapy.

Very limited observations [177; Lewis and Haller, unpublished data] indicate that oxygen uptake during cycle exercise largely falls within the expected range for a given exercise intensity and body weight.

Cardiac output measurements are available from only one patient [80]. The slope of increase in cardiac output in relation to that for oxygen uptake ranged between 10 and 15 in comparison with the normal slope of approximately 5–6. This is indicative of an uncoupling of the normal approximately 1:1 relation between oxygen transport and utilization during exercise similar to that observed in patients with severe defects in muscle oxidative metabolism, that is, patients with McArdle's disease, PFK deficiency, or electron transport disorders, and those studied by Linderholm et al. and Larsson et al. (see above).

Anaerobic muscle performance has not been studied in detail, but systemic lactate levels during cycle exercise were markedly elevated for a given power output in comparison with those of healthy controls [39, 80, 177, 192] and resemble the levels observed during exercise in patients with established disorders of mitochondrial electron transport [23, 67, 89, 142, 143, 161].

AMP Deaminase Deficiency

CLINICAL FEATURES AND SIGNIFICANCE OF THE DEFECT. This deficiency was discovered accidentally when a large number of muscle biopsy specimens were stained histochemically for AMP deaminase activity [71]. About half of the patients in whom muscle AMP deaminase activity has been found deficient have exercise intolerance, myalgia, and/or muscle cramps, but others are asymptomatic or have other well-defined neuromuscular diseases [70]. The relationship between the enzyme defect and the symptoms has not been convincingly demonstrated [136], though theoretical considerations suggest a possible role in exercise intolerance.

AMP deaminase catalyzes the first of the three reactions of the purine nucleotide cycle [Fig. 3.3], resulting in AMP deamination to inosine monophosphate (IMP) and ammonia [130]. The significance of AMP deaminase deficiency for muscle energy metabolism has two major aspects. The first involves AMP deamination, per se, as a means of ADP utilization. The second concerns the reamination of IMP and conversion of aspartate to fumarate by the combination of the two remaining purine nucleotide cycle reactions catalyzed by adenylosuccinate synthetase and adenylosuccinate lyase. An increased production of fumarate provides a potential means for expansion of the pool of citric acid cycle intermediates which may be important under conditions of increased energy demand, that is, exercise. An increased pool of citric acid cycle intermediates could increase the rate of acetyl-CoA oxidation and production of NADH thereby enhancing muscle oxidative capacity. The significance of the AMP deaminase reaction and purine nucleotide cycle for energy metabolism and exercise performance has been covered in detail in a recent review [170]. The present discussion will largely be limited to the possible significance of the absence of these processes for exercise performance in affected patients.

ADP/AMP Removal. Accumulation of muscle ADP can result from imbalances between the rates of ATP production/ADP utilization during exercise. The adenylate kinase ($2ADP \leftrightarrow ATP + AMP$) reaction is in a near equilibrium state [115] and is coupled with the AMP deaminase ($AMP + H_2O \rightarrow IMP + NH_3$) reaction such that deamination of a molecule of AMP is associated with utilization of two molecules of ADP (Table 3.1, Fig. 3.3). The major function of the coupled adenylate kinase/ AMP deaminase reactions appears to be to buffer increases in ADP in active skeletal muscle when the rates of energy demand and ATP hydrolysis exceed the rates of ADP removal via oxidative phosphorylation, anaerobic glycolysis, and the creatine kinase reaction. Patients with AMP deaminase deficiency would theoretically have a reduced capacity for buffering ADP accumulation and on this basis may have an increased susceptibility to muscle fatigue.

The Purine Nucleotide Cycle and Citric Acid Expansion. There is evidence from studies performed *in vitro* and *in situ* in experimental animals both in favor of [5, 34] and against [138] the hypothesis that the deamination of aspartate to fumarate accompanying IMP reamination in the remainder of the purine nucleotide cycle (Fig. 3.3) contributes to an expansion of the pool of citric acid cycle intermediates during exercise. The discrepancy relates in part to conflicting findings about whether or not AMP deamination to IMP and IMP reamination occur simultaneously during exercise [5, 138]. Findings concerning purine nucleotide cycle function in healthy humans [102, 103, 170] appear less controversial. During exercise at 50% of $\dot{V}O_2$max, there is virtually no muscle IMP or NH_3 production, and hence no evidence for AMP deaminase activity [102]. In maximal dynamic or static exercise there is IMP and NH_3 formation but the findings do not suggest IMP reamination [102, 103]. There are, however, data suggesting AMP deamination and IMP reamination during exercise at 70% of $\dot{V}O_2$max [170]. However, pathways other than the purine nucleotide cycle also can serve to expand the pool of citric acid cycle intermediates during exercise [170]. Because previous studies of AMP-deaminase-deficient patients have not included direct measurements of citric acid cycle intermediates in active muscle, it is difficult to evaluate the anaplerotic significance of AMP deaminase deficiency.

EXERCISE PERFORMANCE. The precise limitations to exercise performance in patients with AMP deaminase deficiency are unknown. Sabina et al. [168] found a subnormal endurance time and total work performance during cycle exercise of progressively increasing intensity in AMP-deaminase-deficient patients compared to patients with myalgia but no physical or laboratory evidence of neuromuscular disease. The reduction in the concentration of total muscle phosphagen (PCr + ATP) was several-fold greater in the AMP-deaminase-deficient patients than in those with myalgia, suggesting to the authors that AMP deaminase deficient skeletal muscle has a diminished capacity for aerobic energy production [168].

Sinkeler et al. [183] found no difference in the endurance time or the force-time integral between AMP-deaminase-deficient patients and healthy subjects performing exhaustive static exercise at 50% of maximal voluntary contraction under ischemic conditions. The muscles of AMP-deaminase-deficient patients and healthy controls had similar resting levels of PCr and levels of lactate after ischemic exercise [183]. This suggests that AMP-deaminase-deficient muscle has a normal capacity for heavy anaerobic exercise and could be at variance with the hypothesis that ADP accumulation is important in the development of muscle fatigue. A similar conclusion could be drawn from the very similar capacities for maximal exercise reported for patients with McArdle's disease and two patients with combined AMP deaminase deficiency and phosphorylase deficiency (McArdle's disease) [92; Haller and Lewis, unpublished data].

OXYGEN COST OF EXERCISE. On the basis of limited observations, the O_2 cost of exercise appears normal in AMP deaminase deficiency (Fig. 3.4D).

MUSCULAR DYSTROPHIES

Clinical Features
In the major types of muscular dystrophy, including Duchenne's dystrophy, Becker's dystrophy, facioscapulohumeral (FSH) dystrophy, limb girdle (LG) dystrophy, and myotonic dystrophy, there is skeletal muscle weakness related to muscle fiber atrophy and/or necrosis, with replacement of muscle fibers with fat or connective tissue. The severity of the muscle weakness varies considerably relative to the type of muscular dystrophy and the stage of progression of the disease. Profound weakness relative to normal age-matched control subjects often is observed in Duchenne's dystrophy. In comparison with the approximately linear increase in strength of limb and trunk muscles in healthy boys from 5 to 15 years of age, there is virtually no increase or even a loss in strength of these muscles in Duchenne's dystrophy boys over this age span [30, 62, 74]. Cardiac and respiratory involvement in the muscular dystrophies generally is most severe and common in Duchenne's dystrophy, particularly in its advanced stage [97, 146]. Echocardiographic studies performed under resting conditions comparing a group of myotonic, FSH, LG, and Duchenne's dystrophy patients with cardiovascularly normal orthopedic patients bedridden for 21–71 days suggest that muscular dystrophy is associated with an abnormality in myocardial relaxation unrelated to physical deconditioning [110]. Subnormal ventilation in advanced Duchenne's dystrophy, in spite of peripheral and central chemoreceptors which are adequately sensitive to hypercapnia and hypoxia [17], appears primarily due to respiratory muscle weakness [184].

Maximal Oxygen Uptake
$\dot{V}O_2$max is abnormally low in patients with muscular dystrophy (Table 3.4) largely because of weakness and muscle atrophy. Most published values for cycle $\dot{V}O_2$max in FSH and LG dystrophy patients 14–47 years of age fall between 15–30 ml/minute/kg [38, 72, 87]. In comparison, $\dot{V}O_2$max is approximately 25–35 ml/minute/kg and 35–40 ml/minute/kg for similar-aged patients with exertional muscle pain but no evidence for muscle disease and healthy subjects, respectively [38, 87]. In 13 boys with Duchenne's dystrophy $\dot{V}O_2$max averaged 14 ml/minute/kg compared with 40 ml/minute/kg in age- and weight-matched boys (Table 3.4; 185). The relation between the severity of dystrophy or degree of

muscle wasting and $\dot{V}O_2$max has not been systematically evaluated, but limited observations suggest an inverse correlation. For example, patients with Duchenne's dystrophy, in whom leg weakness is severe, have a lower $\dot{V}O_2$max (14 ± 5 ml/minute/kg) than patients with FSH dystrophy (22 ± 5 ml/minute/kg) in whom leg muscles are less affected [38, 87, 185].

In the absence of significant associated cardiac disease, $\dot{V}O_2$max of patients with muscular dystrophy is not likely to be limited by impaired cardiovascular O_2 delivery. Normal increases in cardiac output relative to increasing oxygen uptake have been observed during exercise in patients with LG, FSH [87], and Duchenne's dystrophy [185] (Table 3.4). In Duchenne's dystrophy the extent of muscle capillarization is essentially normal [99], and the capacity to increase blood flow to active muscle does not appear diminished in Duchenne's, LG, or FSH dystrophy [28, 149]. Pulmonary O_2 intake probably does not limit $\dot{V}O_2$max. Limited data indicate that ventilation relative to oxygen uptake during maximal exercise in patients with Becker's, LG, FSH, and myotonic dystrophy is within the normal range (Table 3.4; Haller and Lewis, unpublished data). In patients with Duchenne's dystrophy maximal ventilation relative to oxygen uptake tends to be subnormal (Table 3.4; 185) but probably insufficiently to limit $\dot{V}O_2$max. Decreased oxygen extraction per unit of active muscle also does not appear to explain the markedly diminished $\dot{V}O_2$max. Primary abnormalities of muscle energy metabolism that could lead to a impaired oxygen extraction are unlikely [60]. Muscle mitochondria isolated from Duchenne's dystrophy patients appear to have a normal capacity for oxidative phosphorylation, unless the disease is very advanced [147, 151]. The markedly depressed $\dot{V}O_2$max in muscular dystrophy is at least partly attributable to a reduced total systemic metabolic demand due to the loss of functional muscle mass [85]. In eight men with moderate muscle atrophy and weakness due to LG, FSH, Becker's, and myotonic dystrophy studied in our laboratory, maximal systemic a-v O_2 difference and maximal heart rate were slightly lower than normal, that is, 13.1 ± 1.9 ml/dl and 164 ± 24 beats/minute compared with 16.7 ± 2.1 ml/dl and 190 ± 10 beats/minute, respectively, in nine healthy men (Table 3.4). In contrast, in boys with more pronounced muscle atrophy and weakness due to Duchenne's dystrophy, maximal a-v O_2 difference (7.7 ± 5 ml/dl) and heart rate (136 ± 13 beats/minute) were more strikingly attenuated in comparison with healthy boys (11.8 ± 31 ml/dl and 190 ± 8 beats/minute, respectively). (Table 3.4; [185]). In healthy individuals, maximal heart rate, cardiac output, and systemic a-v O_2 difference are, within limits, functions of the active muscle mass and total metabolic demand [127]. These findings suggest that reductions in maximal heart rate and a-v O_2 difference in muscular dystrophies may be due to reductions in active muscle mass.

Values for $\dot{V}O_2$max relative to body weight in muscular dystrophy likely are diminished not only by muscle atrophy but also by muscle fiber necrosis and replacement of affected muscle by fat or connective tissue. A normal or more nearly normal $\dot{V}O_2$max expressed in relation to body weight, lean body mass, or limb volume has been reported in malnourished children with reduced muscle mass [47, 186]. Also the magnitude of reduction in $\dot{V}O_2$max relative to body weight, in adults with subnormal body weight and muscle mass due to severe malnutrition [14] or semi-starvation [106], tends to be less marked than in Duchenne's dystrophy. The quantitative contribution of physical deconditioning to the subnormal $\dot{V}O_2$max of muscular dystrophy is unknown. Limited observations on two patients, one with congenital muscular dystrophy and one with LG dystrophy, indicate that $\dot{V}O_2$max can be increased by approximately 25% by endurance-type physical conditioning [72]. Whether endurance-type conditioning can be clinically beneficial in muscular dystrophy is unclear [193]. Resting levels of plasma creatine kinase and myoglobin, markers of muscle damage, were approximately 30% higher after conditioning in these two patients [72].

Oxygen Cost of Exercise
Figure 3.4**E** depicts a higher than normal and, in some cases, a very exaggerated total body oxygen uptake for a given exercise workload in patients with Becker's, LG, FSH, and myotonic dystrophy. Weaker patients tended to have higher values for O_2 cost. This may relate to augmented activation of ancillary muscle groups to support leg muscles responsible for the external work and trunk and arm muscles involved in postural stabilization during cycling.

Anaerobic Muscle Performance
In Duchenne's dystrophy patients there is a greatly depressed capacity for high-power-output anaerobic exercise as indicated by a markedly subnormal peak power and mean power output expressed in absolute units or corrected for body weight in the 30-second Wingate anaerobic leg cycling or arm cranking test [15, 16]. In well-motivated healthy subjects, performance in the Wingate test of anaerobic power depends primarily on the active muscle mass and the maximal rates and capacities for ATP resynthesis/ADP utilization via anaerobic glycogenolysis and PCr breakdown in active muscle. It is likely that the vast majority of the decrement in anaerobic muscle performance in Duchennes's dystrophy is due to a severely reduced muscle mass, but reports of a subnormal ratio of PCr to ATP in muscle from Duchenne's patients [59] suggest that a small portion of the impaired performance might be attributable to a limited energy availability. An intriguing finding in Duchenne's dystrophy patients is a reduction in the intrinsic fatigability of active

muscle as determined from recordings of force in response to electrical activation of muscle [62]. The diminished fatigability of Duchenne's muscle was observed under both ischemic and nonischemic conditions [62]. The mechanisms involved are presently unknown.

SUMMARY

The study of skeletal muscle disorders is providing potentially important insights into regulatory mechanisms in human exercise and fatigue and information useful for diagnostic and treatment purposes. This review primarily concerned the general metabolic and physiological factors which set upper limits to performance of various types of exercise in patients with a variety of muscle disorders. From the standpoint of exercise performance, skeletal muscle diseases can be classified into three major groups. One group consists of primary disorders of muscle energy metabolism, including defects in muscle carbohydrate and lipid metabolism, disorders of mitochondrial electron transport, and abnormalities of purine nucleotide metabolism. Exercise performance largely reflects the capacity for ATP resynthesis. Oxidative phosphorylation is the dominant quantitative source of energy for ATP resynthesis under most exercise conditions. Consequently, patients with disordered oxidative metabolism (i.e., patients with defects in the availability or utilization of oxidizable substrate, such as those with phosphorylase or PFK deficiency or those with defects in mitochondrial electron transport) typically demonstrate severely impaired exercise performance. Intolerance to sustained exercise and premature fatigability are salient features of muscle oxidative disorders. Maximal oxygen uptake and maximal a-v O_2 difference are markedly subnormal related to an attenuated muscle oxygen extraction. Muscle weakness and atrophy are less common. Anaerobic muscle performance is dramatically limited in patients with virtually complete defects of glycogenolysis/glycolysis but appears relatively normal in those with electron transport defects. A second major group of disorders includes patients with decreased muscle mass due to muscle necrosis, atrophy, and replacement of muscle by fat and connective tissue. These disorders are exemplified by the various muscular dystrophies (Duchenne's dystrophy, Becker's dystrophy, LG dystrophy, FSH dystrophy, and myotonic dystrophy) in which exercise performance is severely impaired due to muscle wasting and weakness in spite of largely normal pathways for muscle ATP resynthesis. In muscular dystrophy patients, the degree to which maximal oxygen uptake and anaerobic muscle performance are impaired appears to be a function of the severity of muscle weakness and atrophy. A third group of disorders includes patients with impaired activation of muscle contraction or relaxation. These disorders may be considered in two subcategories. In the first, impaired activation or relaxation of contractile activity is due to intrinsic muscle dysfunction (e.g., diseases associated with myotonia or periodic paralysis). In the second subcategory, there is impaired muscle activation due to a primary abnormality in the central nervous system, motor nerves, or neuromuscular junction. Diseases of this type (e.g., the motor neuron disease, amyotrophic lateral sclerosis) typically are associated with muscle atrophy secondary to disuse or denervation. Research on exercise performance in patients with impaired muscle activation or relaxation has received little or no systematic attention. The emergence of new clinically applicable noninvasive techniques such as magnetic resonance spectroscopy and imaging is allowing a better understanding of the pathophysiology of many skeletal muscle disorders and is helping to facilitate the assessment of clinical and experimental interventions related to exercise performance.

ACKNOWLEDGMENTS

Invaluable general support for work related to this review was provided by Dr. C. G. Blomqvist. The expert secretarial assistance of Ms. Gladys Carter is gratefully appreciated.

Research funds for this work were provided by National Heart, Lung and Blood Institute Grant HL-06296, the Muscular Dystrophy Association, the Veterans Administration, and the Harry S. Moss Heart Center. S. F. Lewis is the recipient of Research Career Development Award HL-01581.

REFERENCES

1. Ahlborg B, Bergstrom J, Ekelund L-G, Hultman E: Relationship between muscle glycogen concentration and exercise endurance time. *Acta Physiol Scand* 70:129–142, 1967.
2. Ahlborg G, Felig P, Hagenfeldt L, Hendler R, Wahren R: Substrate turnover during prolonged exercise in man. Splanchnic and leg metabolism of glucose, free fatty acids and amino acids. *J Clin Invest* 53:1080–1090, 1974.
3. Amsterdam EA, Wilmore JH, DeMaria AN (eds): *Exercise in Cardiovascular Health and Disease.* New York, Yorke Medical Books, 1977.
4. Andersen P, Saltin B: Maximal perfusion of skeletal muscle in man. *J Physiol* 366:233–249, 1985.
5. Aragon JJ, Lowenstein JM: The purine nucleotide cycle. Comparison of the levels of citric acid cycle intermediates with the operation of the purine nucleotide cycle in rat skeletal muscle during exercise and recovery from exercise. *Eur J Biochem* 110:371–377, 1980.
6. Argov Z, Bank WJ, Boden B, RO Y-I, Chance B: Phosphorus magnetic resonance spectroscopy of partially blocked muscle glycolysis. An in vivo study of phosphoglycerate mutase deficiency. *Arch Neurol* 44:614–617, 1987.
7. Argov Z, Bank WJ, Leigh JS Jr, Chance B: Muscle energy metabolism in human phosphofructokinase deficiency as recorded by ^{31}P NMR. *Ann Neurol* 22:46–51, 1986.

8. Argov Z, Bank WJ, Maris J, Chance B: Muscle energy metabolism in McArdle's syndrome by in vivo phosphorus magnetic resonance spectroscopy. *Neurology* 37:1720–1724, 1987.
9. Argov Z, Bank WJ, Maris J, Peterson P, Chance B: Bioenergetic heterogeneity of human mitochondrial myopathies as demonstrated by in vivo phosphorus magnetic resonance spectroscopy (^{31}P-NMR). *Neurology* 37:257–262, 1987.
10. Arnold DL, Taylor DJ, Radda GK: Investigation of human mitochondrial myopathies by phosphorus nuclear magnetic resonance spectroscopy. *Ann Neurol* 18:189–195, 1985.
11. Arts WFM, Scholte HR, Bogaard JM, Kerrebijn KF, Luyt-Houwen IEM: NADH-CoQ reductase deficient myopathy: successful treatment with riboflavin. *Lancet* 2:581–582, 1983.
12. Åstrand I: Aerobic work capacity in men and women with special reference to age. *Acta Physiol Scand* 49(Suppl 169):1–92 1960.
13. Åstrand P-O: *Experimental Studies of Physical Working Capacity in Relation to Age and Sex.* Munksgaard, Copenhagen, 1952.
14. Barac-Nieto M, Spurr GB, Maksud M, Lotero H: Aerobic work capacity in chronically undernourished adult males. *J Appl Physiol* 44:209–215, 1978.
15. Bar-Or O: Pathophysiological factors which limit the exercise capacity of the sick child. *Med Sci Sports Exerc* 18:276–282, 1986.
16. Bar-Or O: *Pediatric Sports Medicine for the Practitioner.* New York, Springer-Verlag, 1983.
17. Begin R, Bureau M-A, Lupien L, Lemieux B: Control of breathing in Duchenne's muscular dystrophy. *Am J Med* 69:227–234, 1980.
18. Bergstrom J, Hermansen L, Hultman E, Saltin B: Diet, muscle glycogen and physical performance. *Acta Physiol Scand* 71:140–150, 1967.
19. Bergstrom J, Hultman E, Jorfeldt L, Pernow B, Wahren J: Effect of nicotinic acid on physical working capacity and on metabolism of muscle glycogen in man. *J Appl Physiol* 26:170–176, 1969.
20. Bertocci LA, Nunnall RL, Lewis SF, Haller RG: Attenuated depletion of phosphocreatine in human muscle PFK deficiency during handgrip exercise. *Proc Soc Magn Res Med* 1:192, 1988.
21. Bertorini TE, Shively V, Taylor B, Palmieri GMA, Fox IH: ATP degradation products after ischemic exercise: hereditary lack of phosphorylase or carnitine palmityl-transferase. *Neurology* 35:1355–1357, 1985.
22. Blomqvist CG, Saltin B: Cardiovascular adaptations to physical training. *Annu Rev Physiol* 45:169–184, 1983.
23. Bogaard JM, Busch HFM, Arts WFM, Heijsteeg M, Stam H, Versprille A: Metabolic and ventilatory responses to exercise in patients with a deficient O_2 utilization by a mitochondrial myopathy. *Adv Exp Med Biol* 191:409–417, 1984.
24. Bohannon RW: Relative dynamic muscular endurance of patients with neuromuscular disorders and of healthy matched control subjects. *Phys Ther* 67:18–23, 1987.
25. Bove AA, Lowenthal DT (eds): *Exercise Medicine: Physiological Principles and Clinical Applications.* New York, Academic Press, 1983.
26. Braaakhekke JP, deBruin MI, Stegeman DF, Wevers, Binkhorst RA, Joosten EMG: The second wind phenomenon in McArdle's disease. *Brain* 109:1087–1101, 1986.
27. Bradley R, Fell BF: Myopathies in animals. In J Walton (ed): *Disorders of Voluntary Muscle.* New York, Churchill-Livingstone, 1981, pp 824–872.
28. Bradley WG, O'Brien MD, Walder DN, Murchison D, Johnson M, Newell DJ: Failure to confirm a vascular cause of muscular dystrophy. *Arch Neurol* 32:466–473, 1975.
29. Bresolin N, RoY-I, Reyes M, Miranda AF, DiMauro S: Muscle phosphoglycerate mutase (PGAM) deficiency: a second case. *Neurology* 33:1049–1053, 1983.

30. Brooke MH, Fenichel GM, Griggs RC, Mendell JR, Moxley R, Miller PJ, Province MA, CIDD Group: Clinical investigation in Duchenne dystrophy: 2. Determination of the "power" of theraputic trials based on the natural history. *Muscle Nerve* 6:91–103, 1983.

31. Brooke MH, Patterson VH, Kaiser KK: Hypoxanthine and McArdle's disease: a clue to metabolic stress in the working forearm. *Muscle Nerve* 6:204–206, 1983.

32. Brown BI: Debranching and branching enzyme deficiencies. In Engel AG, Banker BQ (eds): *Myology*, New York, McGraw-Hill, 1986, vol 2, pp 1653–1661.

33. Brown DH: Glycogen metabolism and glycolysis in muscle. In Engel AG, Banker BQ (eds): *Myology*, New York, McGraw-Hill, 1986, vol 1, pp 673–695.

34. Canela EI, Ginesta I, Franco R: Simulation of the purine nueleotide cycle as an anaplerotic process in skeletal muscle. *Arch Biochem Biophys* 254:142–155, 1987.

35. Carroll JE, Brooke MH, DeVivo DC, Kaiser KK, Hagberg JM: Biochemical and physiologic consequences of carnitine palmityltransferase deficiency. *Muscle Nerve* 1:103–110, 1978.

36. Carroll JE, Brooke MH, DeVivo DC, Shumate MD, Kratz R, Ringel SP, Hagberg JM: Carnitine "deficiency": lack of response to carnitine therapy. *Neurology* 30:618–121, 1980.

37. Carroll JE, DeVivo DC, Brooke MH, Planer GJ, Hagberg JH: Fasting as a provocative test in neuromuscular diseases. *Metabolism* 28:683–687, 1979.

38. Carroll JE, Hagberg JM, Brooke MH, Shumate JB: Bicycle ergometry and gas exchange measurements in neuromuscular diseases. *Arch Neurol* 36:457–461, 1979.

39. Carroll JE, Shumate JB, Brooke MG, Hagberg JM: Riboflavin-responsive lipid myopathy and carnitine deficiency. *Neurology* 31:1557–1559, 1981.

40. Cavagna GA, Saibene FP, Margaria R: External work in walking. *J Appl Physiol* 18:1–9, 1963.

41. Chance B: Applications of ^{31}P NMR to clinical biochemistry. *Ann NY Acad Sci* 428:318–332, 1984.

42. Chance B, Eleff S, Bank W, Leigh JS Jr, Warnell R: ^{31}P NMR studies of control of mitochondrial function in phosphofructokinase-deficient human skeletal muscle. *Proc Natl Acad Sci USA* 79:7714–7718, 1982.

43. Cooke R: The inhibition of muscle contraction by the products of ATP hydrolysis. In Taylor AW (ed): *Proceedings of the 7th International Biochemistry of Exercise Conference.* Champaign, IL, Human Kinetics, In press.

44. Costill DL, Coyle E, Dalsky G, Evans B, Fink W, Hoopes D: Effects of elevated plasma FFA and insulin on muscle glycogen usage during exercise. *J Appl Physiol* 43:695–699, 1977.

45. Cotes JE: *Lung Function*, ed 4. Oxford, England, Blackweh, 1979, pp 299–304.

46. Cotes JE, Mead F: The energy expenditure and mechanical energy demand in walking. *Ergonomics* 3:97–119, 1960.

47. Davies CTM: The relationship of leg volume (muscle plus bone) to maximal aerobic power output on a bicycle ergometer: The effects of anemia, malnutrition and physical activity. *Ann Hum Biol* 1:47–55, 1974.

48. Davies CTM, Thompson MW: Aerobic performance of female and male ultramarathon athletes. *Eur J Appl Physiol* 41:233–245, 1979.

49. Dempsey JA, Reed CE (eds): *Muscular Exercise and the Lung.* Madison, WI, University of Wisconsin Press, 1977.

50. DiMauro S, Bonilla E, Zeviani M, Nakagawa M, DeVivo DC: Mitochondrial myopathies. *Ann Neurol* 17:521–528, 1985.

51. DiMauro S, Bresolin N: Phosphorylase deficiency. In Engel AG, Banker BQ (eds). *Myology.* New York, McGraw-Hill, 1986, pp 1585–1601.

52. DiMauro S, Hartwig GB, Hays A, Eastwood AB, Franco R, Olarte M, Chang M, Roses AD, Fetell M, Schoenfeldt RS, Stern LZ: Debrancher deficiency: neuromuscular disorder in 5 adults. *Ann Neurol* 5:422–436, 1979.
53. DiMauro S, Melis-DiMauro PM: Muscle carnitine palmityltransferase deficiency and myoglobinuria. *Science* 182:929–930, 1973.
54. DiMauro S, Papadimitriou A: Carnitine palmitoyltransferease deficiency. In Engle AG, Banker BQ (eds): *Myology*. New York, McGraw-Hill, 1986, pp 1697–1708.
55. Duboc D, Jehenson P, Tran Dinh S, Marsac C, Seota A, Fardeau M: Phosphorus NMR spectroscopy study of muscular enzyme deficiencies involving glycogenolysis and glycolysis. *Neurology* 37:663–671, 1987.
56. Duboc D, Renault G, Polianski J, Muffat-Joly M, Toussaint M, Guerin F, Pocidalo J-J, Fardeau M: NADH measured by laser fluorimetry in McArdle's disease. *N Engl J Med* 316:1664–1665, 1987.
57. Durand J, Mensch-Dechene J: Physiological meaning of the slope and intercept of the cardiac output-oxygen uptake relationship during exercise. *Bull Eur Physiopathol Respir* 15:977–998, 1979.
58. Edelman NH, Santiago TV, Conn HL: Luft's syndrome: O_2 cost of exercise and chemical control of breathing. *J Appl Physiol* 39:857–859, 1975.
59. Edwards RHT: Energy metabolism in dystrophic muscle. In Serratrice G, Desnuell C, Pellissier JF, Cros D, Gastruat JL, Pouget J, Schiano A (eds): *Neuromuscular Diseases*. New York, Raven Press, 1984, pp 105–109.
60. Edwards RHT: Energy metabolism in normal and dystrophic human muscle. In Rowland LP (ed): *Pathogenesis of Human Muscular Dystrophies*. Amsterdam, Excerpta Medica, 1977, pp 415–428.
61. Edwards RHT: New techniques for studying human muscle function, metabolism and fatigue. *Muscle Nerve* 7:599–609, 1984.
62. Edwards RHT, Chapman SJ, Newham DJ, Jones DA: Practical analysis of variability of muscle function measurements in Duchenne muscular dystrophy. *Muscle Nerve* 10:6–14, 1987.
63. Edwards RHT, Dawson MJ, Wilkie DR, Gordon RE, Shaw D: Clinical use of nuclear magnetic resonance in the investigation of myopathy. *Lancet* 1:725–731, 1982.
64. Edwards RHT, Griffiths RD, Cady EB: Topical magnetic resonance for the study of muscle metabolism in human myopathy. *Clin Physiol* 5:93–109, 1985.
65. Edwards RHT, Jones DA: Diseases of skeletal muscle. In Peachey LD, Adrian RH, Geiger SR (eds): *Handbook of Physiology. Section 10: Skeletal muscle*. Bethesda, MD, American Physiological Society, 1983, pp 633–672.
66. Edwards RHT, Wiles CM: Energy exchange in human skeletal muscle during isometric contraction. *Circ Res* 48(Suppl I):11–17, 1981.
67. Edwards RHT, Wiles CM, Gohil K, Krywawych S, Jones DA: Energy metabolism in human myopathy. In Schotland DL (ed): *Disorders of the Motor Unit*. New York, John Wiley, 1982, pp 715–735.
68. Engel AG: Carnitine deficiency syndromes and lipid storage myopathies. In Engel AG, Banker BQ (eds): *Myology*. New York, McGraw-Hill, 1986, pp 1663–1696.
69. Faulkner JA, Heigenhauser GF, Schork MA: The cardiac output–oxygen uptake relationship of men during graded bicycle ergometry. *Med Sci Sports Exerc* 9:148–154, 1977.
70. Fishbein WN: Myoadenylate deaminase deficiency: inherited and acquired forms. *Biochem Med* 33:158–169, 1985.
71. Fishbein WN, Armbrustmacher VW, Griffin JL: Myoadenylate deaminase deficiency: a new disease of muscle. *Science* 200:545–548, 1978.

72. Florence JM, Hagberg JM: Effect of training on the exercise responses of neuromuscular disease patients. *Med Sci Sports Exerc* 16:460–465, 1984.
73. Foster C, Costill DL, Fink WJ: Effects of pre-exercise feedings on endurance performance. *Med Sci Sports Exerc* 11:1–5, 1979.
74. Fowler WM Jr, Gardner GW: Quantitative strength measurements in muscular dystrophy. *Arch Phys Med Rehabil* 48:629–644, 1967.
75. Gadian D, Radda G, Ross B, Hockaday J, Bore P, Taylor D, Styles P: Examination of a myopathy by phosphorus nuclear magnetic resonance. *Lancet* 2:774–775, 1981.
76. Galbo H: *Hormonal and Metabolic Adaptation to Exercise*. Stuttgart, Georg Thieme Verlag, 1983.
77. Gollnick PD: Metabolism of substrates. Energy substrate metabolism during exercise and as modified by training. *Fed Proc* 44:353–357, 1985.
78. Gregersen N: Riboflavin-responsive defects of β-oxidation. *J Inherited Metab Dis* 8(Suppl 1):65–69, 1985.
79. Hagberg JM, Coyle EF, Carroll JE, Miller JM, Martin WH, Brooke MH: Exercise hyperventilation in patients with McArdle's disease. *J Appl Physiol:Respir Environ Exerc Physiol* 52:991–994, 1982.
80. Haller RG, Cook JD, Lewis S, Blomqvist CG: A "lipid myopathy" associated with a hyperkinetic circulatory response to exercise. *Trans Am Neurol Assoc* 104:117–119, 1979.
81. Haller RG, DiMauro S, Vora S, Lewis SF: Glucose impairs exercise performance in muscle phosphofructokinase deficiency: the "out of wind" effect. *Neurology* 39(Suppl 1): 270, 1988.
82. Haller RG, Gunder M, Combes B, Lewis SF: Debrancher versus myophosphorylase deficiency: effects on muscle energy metabolism in exercise. *Muscle Nerve* 9(Suppl 5):187, 1986.
83. Haller RG, Lewis SF: Abnormal ventilatory response to exercise in McArdle's disease: modulation by availability of substrate. *Neurology* 36:716–719, 1986.
84. Haller RG, Lewis SF:Human muscle respiratory chain defects: metabolic and physiologic implications. In Taylor AW (ed): *Biochemistry of Exercise VII*. Champaign, IL, Human Kinetics, in press.
85. Haller RG, Lewis SF: Pathophysiology of exercise performance in muscle disease. *Med Sci Sports Exerc* 16:456–459, 1984.
86. Haller RG, Lewis SF: Physical conditioning: a rational treatment of muscle phosphofructokinase deficiency. *Neurology* 38(Suppl 1):341, 1988.
87. Haller RG, Lewis SF, Cook JD, Blomqvist CG: Hyperkinetic circulation during exercise in neuromuscular disease. *Neurology* 33:1283–1287, 1983.
88. Haller RG, Lewis SF, Cook JD, Blomqvist CG: Myophosphorylase deficiency impairs muscle oxidative metabolism. *Ann Neurol* 17:196–199, 1985.
89. Haller RG, Lewis SF, Estabrook RW, Nunnally R, Foster DW: A skeletal muscle disorder of electron transport associated with deficiency of cytochromes aa3 and b and abnormal cardiovascular regulation in exercise. *Clin Physiol* 5(Suppl 7):34, 1985.
90. Haller, RG, Lewis SF, Gunder M, Dennis M: Ammonia production during exercise in McArdle's syndrome—an index of muscle energy supply and demand. *Neurology* 35:207, 1985.
91. Hartwig GB, Leatherman NE, McNeil WP, Kylstra J: Exercise performance in debrancher deficiency myopathy. *Trans Am Neurol Assoc* 104:248–252, 1979.
92. Heller SL, Kaiser KK, Planer GJ, Hagberg JM, Brooke MH: McArdle's disease with myoadenylate deaminase deficiency: observations in a combined enzyme deficiency. *Neurology* 37:1039–1042, 1987.
93. Hermansen L, Hultman E, Saltin B: Muscle glycogen during prolonged severe exercise. *Acta Physiol Scand* 71:129–139, 1967.

94. Holloszy JO, Coyle EG: Adaptations of skeletal muscle to endurance exercise and their metabolic consequences. *J Appl Physiol* 56:831–838, 1984.

95. Hosking GP, Bhat US, Dubowitz V, Edwards RHT: Measurements of muscle strength and performance in children with normal and diseased muscle. *Arch Dis Child* 51:957–963, 1976.

96. Hultman E, Sjoholm H: Substrate availability. In Knuttgen HG, Vogel JA, Poortmans J (eds): *Biochemistry of Exercise.* Champaign, IL, Human Kinetics, 1983, pp 63–75.

97. Hunter S: The heart in muscular dystrophy. *Br Med Bull* 36:133–134, 1980.

98. Ionasescu I, Luca N: Studies of carbohydrate metabolism in myasthenia gravis in conditions of ischemic exercise. *Acta Neurol Scand* 42:244–254, 1966.

99. Jerusalem F, Engel AG, Gomez MR: Duchene dystrophy. I. Morphometric study of the muscle microvasculature. *Brain* 97:115–132, 1974.

100. Johnson RL Jr: Oxygen transport. In Willerson JT, Saunders CA (eds): *Clinical Cardiology, The Science and Practice of Clinical Medicine*, New York, Grune and Stratton, vol 3, 1977.

101. Katz A, Broberg S, Sahlin K, Wahren J: Leg glucose uptake during maximal dynamic exercise in humans. *Am J Physiol* 251:E65-E70, 1986.

102. Katz A, Broberg S, Sahlin K, Wahren J: Muscle ammonia and amino acid metabolism during dynamic exercise in man. *Clin Physiol* 6:365–379, 1986.

103. Katz A, Sahlin K, Henriksson J: Muscle ammonia metabolism during isometric contraction in humans. *Am J Physiol* 250:C834-C840, 1986.

104. Katz A, Sahlin K, Henriksson J: Muscle ATP turnover rate during isometric contraction in humans. *J Appl Physiol* 60:1839–1842, 1986.

105. Keul J (ed): *Limiting Factors of Physical Performance.* Stuttgart, Georg Thieme, 1973.

106. Keys A, Brozek J, Henschel A, Mickelsen O, Taylor HL: *The Biology of Human Starvation.* Minneapolis, MN, University of Minnesota Press, 1950, pp 735–742.

107. Kissel JT, Beam W, Bresolin N, Gibbons G, DiMauro S, Mendell JR: Physiologic assessment of phosphoglycerate mutase deficiency: incremental exercise tests. *Neurology* 36:106–108, 1986.

108. Klausen K, Secher NH, Clausen JP, Hartling O, Trap-Jensen J: Central and regional circulatory adaptations to one-leg training. *J Appl Physiol* 52:976–983, 1982.

109. Kono N, Mineo I, Shimizu T, Hara N, Yamada Y, Nonaka K, Tarui S: Increased plasma uric acid after exercise in muscle phosphofructokinase deficiency. *Neurology* 36:106–108, 1986.

110. Kovick RB, Fogelman AM, Abbasi AS, Peter JB, Pearce ML: Echocardiographic study of posterior left ventricular wall motion in muscular dystrophy. *Circulation* 52:447–454, 1975.

111. Kozlowski S, Brzezinska Z, Nazar K, Kowalski W, Franczyk M: Plasma catecholamines during sustained isometric exercise. *Clin Sci Mol Med* 45:723–731, 1973.

112. Lange Andersen K, Lund-Johansen P, Clausen G: Metabolic and circulatory responses to muscular exercise in a subject with glycogen storage disease (McArdle's disease). *Scand J Clin Lab Invest* 24:105–113, 1969.

113. Larsen OA, Malmborg RO (eds): *Coronary Heart Disease and Physical Fitness.* Copenhagen, Munksgaard, 1971.

114. Larsson L-E, Linderholm H, Muller R, Ringqvist T, Sornas R: Hereditary metabolic myopathy with paroxysmal myoglobinuria due to abnormal glycolysis. *J Neurol Neurosurg Psychiatry* 27:361–380, 1964.

115. Lawson JW, Veech RL: Effects of pH and free Mg^+ on the Keq of the creatine kinase reaction and other phosphate transfer reactions. *J Biol Chem* 254:6528–6537, 1979.

116. Layzer RB: Pathophysiology of the periodic paralyses: overview and theoretical aspects. In Serratrice G, Desnuell C, Pellissier JF, Cros D, Gastruat JL, Pouget J, Schiano A (eds): *Neuromuscular Diseases*. New York, Raven Press, 1984, pp 173–177.

117. Layzer RB, Havel RJ, McIlroy MB: Partial deficiency of carnitine palmityltransferase: physiologic and biochemical consequences. *Neurology* 30:627–633, 1980.

118. Lehmann-Horn F, Hopfel D, Rudel R, Ricker K, Kuther G: In vivo P-NMR spectroscopy: muscle energy exchange in paramyotonia patients. *Muscle Nerve* 8:606–610, 1985.

119. Lewis SF, Haller RG: Disorders of muscle glycogenolysis/glycolysis: the consequences of substrate-limited oxidative metabolism in humans. In Taylor AW (ed): *Biochemistry of Exercise VII*. Champaign, IL, Human Kinetics, in press.

120. Lewis SF, Haller RG: Human disorders of muscle oxidative metabolism: significance for metabolic and cardiovascular regulation during exercise. In Barnes C, Gollnick PD (eds): *Limiting Factors in Muscular Exercise*. New York, Academic Press, in press.

121. Lewis SF, Haller RG: The pathophysiology of McArdle's disease: clues to regulation in exercise and fatigue. *J Appl Physiol* 61:391–401, 1986.

122. Lewis SF, Haller RG, Blomqvist CG: Neuromuscular diseases as models of cardiovascular regulation during exercise. *Med Sci Sports Exerc* 16:466–471, 1984.

123. Lewis SF, Haller RG, Cook JD, Blomqvist CG: Metabolic control of cardiac output response to exercise in McArdle's disease. *J Appl Physiol* 57:1749–1753, 1984.

124. Lewis SF, Haller RG, Cook JD, Blomqvist CG: Neuromuscular diseases: models for studying oxygen transport to skeletal muscle. In Loeppky JA, Riedesel ML (eds): *Oxygen Transport to Human Tissue*. New York, Elsevier North Holland, 1982, pp 366–367.

125. Lewis SF, Haller RG, Cook JD, Nunnally RL: Muscle fatigue in McArdle's disease studied by ^{31}P NMR: effect of glucose infusion. *J Appl Physiol* 59:1991–1994, 1985.

126. Lewis SF, Haller RG, Henriksson KG, Areskog N-H, Jorfeldt L: Availability of oxidative substrate and leg blood flow during exercise in McArdle's disease. *Fed Proc* 45:783, 1986.

127. Lewis SF, Taylor WF, Graham RM, Pettinger WA, Schutte JE, Blomqvist CG: Cardiovascular responses to exercise as functions of absolute and relative workload. *J Appl Physiol* 54:1314–1323, 1983.

128. Lewis SF, Vora S, DiMauro S, Haller RG: Disordered oxidative metabolism in muscle phosphofructokinase deficiency. *Neurology* 38(Suppl 1):269, 1988.

129. Linderholm H, Muller R, Ringqvist T, Sornas R: Hereditary abnormal muscle metabolism with hyperkinetic circulation during exercise. *Acta Med Scand* 185:153–166, 1969.

130. Lowenstein JM: Ammonia production in muscle and other tissues: the purine nucleotide cycle. *Physiol Rev* 52:382–414, 1972.

131. Luft R, Ikkos D, Palmieri G, Ernster L, Afzelius B: A case of severe hypermetabolism of nonthyroid origin with a defect in the maintenance of mitochondrial respiratory control: a correlated clinical, biochemical, and morphological study. *J Clin Invest* 41:1776–1801, 1962.

132. Lyager S, Naeraa N, Pedersen OF: Cardiopulmonary responses to exercise in patients with neuromuscular diseases. *Respiration* 45:89–99, 1984.

133. Margaria R, Cerretelli P, Aghemo P, Sassi G: Energy cost of running. *J Appl Physiol* 18:367–370, 1963.

134. McArdle B: Myopathy due to a defect in muscle glycogen breakdown. *Clin Sci* 10:13–33, 1951.

135. McCartney N, Moroz D, Garner SH, McComas AJ: The effects of strength training in patients with selected neuromuscular disorders. *Med Sci Sports Exerc* 20:362–368, 1988.
136. Mercelis R, Martin J-J, de Barsy T, Van den Berghe G: Myoadenylate deaminase deficiency: absence of correlation with exercise intolerance in 452 muscle biopsies. *J Neurol* 234:385–389, 1987.
137. Mettler FA Jr, Muroff LR, Kularni MV (eds): *Magnetic Resonance Imaging and Spectroscopy.* New York, Churchill Livingstone, 1986.
138. Meyer RA, Terjung RL: AMP deamination and IMP reamination in working skeletal muscle. *Am J Physiol* 239:C32-C38, 1980.
139. Milner-Brown HS, Miller RG: Muscle strengthening through high-resistance weight-training in patients with neuromuscular disorders. *Arch Phys Med Rehabil* 69:14–19, 1988.
140. Mineo I, Kono N, Hara N, Shimizu T, Yamada Y, Kawachi M, Kiyokawa H, Wang YL, Tarui S: Myogenic hyperuricemia: a common physiologic feature of glycogenosis types III, V and VII. *N Engl J Med* 317:75–80, 1987.
141. Mommaerts WFHM, Illingworth B, Pearson CM, Guillory RJ, Seradorian K: A functional disorder of muscle associated with the absence of phosphorylase. *Proc Natl Acad Sci USA* 45:791–797, 1959.
142. Morgan-Hughes JA, Darveniza P, Kahn SN, Landon DN, Sheratt RM, Land JM, Clark JB: A mitochondrial myopathy characterized by a deficiency in reducible cyctochrome b. *Brain* 100:617–640, 1977.
143. Morgan-Hughes JA, Darveniza P, Landon DN, Land JM, Clark JB: A mitochondrial myopathy with a deficiency of respiratory chain NADH-CoQ reductase activity. *J Neurol Sci* 43:27–46, 1979.
144. Munsat TL: A standardized forearm ischemic exercise test. *Neurology* 20:1171–1178, 1970.
145. Murphy WA, Totty WG, Carroll JE: MRI of normal and pathologic skeletal muscle. *Am J Physiol* 146:565–574, 1986.
146. Newsom-Davis J: The respiratory system in muscular dystrophy. *Br Med Bull* 36:135–138, 1980.
147. Olson E, Vignos PJ, Woodlock J, Perry T: Oxidative phosphorylation of skeletal muscle in human muscular dystrophy. *J Lab Clin Med* 71:220–231, 1968.
148. Patten BM, Oliver KL, Engel WK: Effect of lactate infusions on patients with myasthenia gravis. *Neurology* 986–990, 1974.
149. Paulson OB, Engel AG, Gomez MR: Muscle blood-flow in Duchenne type muscular dystrophy, limb-girdle dystrophy, polymyositis, and in normal controls. *J Neurol Neurosurg Psychiatry* 37:685–690, 1974.
150. Pearson CM, Rimer DG, Mommaerts WFHM: A metabolic myopathy due to absence of muscle phosphorylase. *Am J Med* 30:502–517, 1961.
151. Pennington RFT: Biochemical aspects of muscle disease. In Walton Sir J (ed): *Disorders of Voluntary Muscle.* New York, Churchill Livingstone, 1981, pp 417–447.
152. Pernow BB, Havel RJ, Jennings DB: The second wind phenomenon in McArdle's syndrome. *Acta Med Scand (Suppl)* 472:294–307, 1967.
153. Pernow B, Saltin B: Availability of substrates and capacity for prolonged exercise in man. *J Appl Physiol* 31:416–422, 1971.
154. Petty RKH, Harding AE, Morgan-Hughes JA: The clinical features of mitochondrial myopathy. *Brain* 109:915–938, 1986.
155. Pollock ML, Schmidt DH (eds): *Heart Disease and Rehabilitation* ed 2, New York, John Wiley and Sons, 1986.

156. Porte D Jr, Crawford DW, Jennings JB, Aber C, McIlroy MB: Cardiovascular and metabolic responses to exercise in a patient with McArdle's syndrome. *N Engl J Med* 275:406–412, 1966.

157. Porter R, Whelan J (eds): *Human Muscle Fatigue: Physiological Mechanisms* (Ciba Foundation Symposium No. 82). London, Pitman Medical, 1981.

158. Radda GK: Control of bioenergetics: from cells to man by phosphorus nuclear magnetic resonance spectroscopy. *Biochem Soc Trans* 14:517–525, 1986.

159. Radda GK, Bore PJ, Gadian DG, Ross BD, Styles P, Taylor DJ, Morgan-Hughes J: ^{31}P NMR examination of two patients with NADH-CoQ reductase deficiency. *Nature* 295:608–609, 1982.

160. Radda GK, Taylor DJ: Applications of nuclear magnetic resonance spectroscopy in pathology. *Int Rev Exp Pathol* 27:285–287, 1985.

161. Reichmann H, Rohkamm R, Zeviani M, Servidei S, Ricker K, DiMauro S: Mitochondrial myopathy due to complex III deficiency with normal reducible cytochrome *b* concentration. *Arch Neurol* 49:957–961, 1986.

162. Ross BD, Radda GK: Application of ^{31}P NMR to inborn errors of metabolism. *Biochem Soc Trans* 11:627–630, 1983.

163. Ross BD, Radda GK, Gadian DG, Rocker G, Esiri M, Falconer-Smith J: Examination of a case of suspected McArdle's syndrome by ^{31}P nuclear magnetic resonance. *N Engl J Med* 304:1338–1342, 1981.

164. Rowell LB: *Human Circulation During Physical Stress*. New York, Oxford University Press, 1986.

165. Rowland LP, Araki S, Carmel P: Contracture in McArdle's disease. *Arch Neurol* 13:541–544, 1965.

166. Rowland LP, DiMauro S, Layzer R: Phosphofructokinase deficiency. In Engel AG, Banker BQ (eds): *Myology*. New York, McGraw-Hill, 1986, pp 1603–1617.

167. Rumpf KW, Wagner H, Kaiser H, Meinck HM, Goebel HH, Scheler F: Increased ammonia production during forearm ischemic work test in McArdle's disease. *Klin Wochenschr* 59:1319–1320, 1981.

168. Sabina RL, Swain JL, Olanow CW, Bradley WG, Fishbein WN, DiMauro S, Holmes EW: Myoadenylate deaminase deficiency. Functional and metabolic abnormalities associated with disruption of the purine nucleotide cycle. *J Clin Invest* 73:720–730, 1984.

169. Sahlin K: Metabolic changes limiting muscle performance. In Saltin B (ed): *Biochemistry of Exercise VI*. Champaign, IL, Human Kinetics, 1986, pp 323–343.

170. Sahlin K, Katz A: Purine nucleotide metabolism during muscle contraction. In Poortmans J (ed): *Principles of Exercise Biochemistry*. Basel, Karger, 1988.

171. Sahlin K, Katz A, Henriksson J: Redox state and lactate accumulation in human skeletal muscle during dynamic exercise. *Biochem J* 245:551–556, 1987.

172. Saltin B: Oxygen transport by the circulatory system in man. In Keul J (ed): *Limiting Factors of Physical Performance*. Stuttgart, Georg Thieme, 1971, pp 235–252.

173. Saltin B, Karlsson J: Muscle glycogen utilization during work of different intensities. In Pernow B, Bengt Saltin (eds): *Advances in Experimental Medicine and Biology: Vol. 11. Muscle Metabolism During Exercise*. New York, Plenum Press, 1971, pp 289–299.

174. Saltin B, Rowell LB: Functional adaptations to physical activity and inactivity. *Fed Proc* 39:1506–1513, 1980.

175. Sanjak M, Paulson D, Sufir R, Reddan W, Beaulieu D, Erickson L, Shug A, Brooks BR: Physiologic and metabolic responses to progressive and prolonged exercise in amyotrophic lateral sclerosis. *Neurology* 37:1217–1220, 1987.

176. Sanjak M, Reddan W, Brooks BR: Role of muscular exercise in amyotrophic lateral sclerosis. *Neurol Clin* 5:251–268, 1987.
177. Scarlato G, Pellegrini G, Cerri C, Meola G, Veicsteinas A: The syndrome of carnitine deficiency: morphological and metabolic correlations. *J Can Sci Neurol* 5:205–213, 1978.
178. Schmid R, Mahler R: Chronic progressive myopathy with myoglobinuria: demonstration of a glycogenolytic defect in the muscle. *J Clin Invest* 38:2044–2058, 1959.
179. Secher NH, Clausen JP, Klausen K, Noer I, Trap-Jensen J: Central and regional circulatory effects of adding arm exercise to leg exercise. *Acta Physiol Scand* 100:288–297, 1977.
180. Secher NH, Petersen S: Fatigue of voluntary contractions in normal and myasthenic human subjects. *Acta Physiol Scand* 122:243–248, 1984.
181. Sejersted OM, Hargens AR, Kardel AR, Blom P, Jensen O, Hermansen L: Intramuscular fluid pressure during contraction of human skeletal muscle. *J Appl Physiol* 56:287–295, 1984.
182. Simpson JA: Myasthenia gravis and myasthenic syndromes. In Walton Sir J (ed): *Disorders of Voluntary Muscle*, ed 4, New York, Churchill Livingstone, 1981, pp 585–624.
183. Sinkeler SPT, Binkhorst RA, Joosten EMG, Wevers RA, Coerwinkel MM, Oei TL: AMP deaminase deficiency: study of the human skeletal muscle purine metabolism during ischemic isometric exercise. *Clin Sci* 72:475–482, 1987.
184. Smith PEM, Calverley PMA, Edwards RHT, Evans GA, Campbell EJM: Practical problems in the respiratory care of patients with muscular dystrophy. *N Engl J Med* 316:1197–1205, 1987.
185. Sockolov R, Irwin B, Dressendorfer RH, Bernauer EM: Exercise performance in 6- to 11-year old boys with Duchenne muscular dystrophy. *Arch Phys Med Rehabil* 58:195–201, 1977.
186. Spurr GB, Barac-Nieto M, Maksud MG: Childhood undernutrition: implications for adult work capacity and productivity. In Folinsnsbee LJ (ed): *Environmental Stress: Individual Human Adaptations*. New York, Academic Press, 1978, pp 165–182.
187. Swain JL, Sabina RL, Holmes EW: Myoadenylate deaminase deficiency. In Stanburg JB, Wyngaarden JB, Frederickson DS, Goldstein JL, Brown MS (eds): *The Metabolic Basis of Inherited Disease*, ed 5. New York, McGraw-Hill, 1983, pp 1184–1191.
188. Tarui S, Mineo I. Shimizu T, Sumi S, Kono N: Muscle phosphofructokinase deficiency and related disorders. In Serratrice G, Desnuell C, Pellissier JF, Cros D, Gastruat JL, Pouget J, Schiano A (eds): *Neuromuscular Diseases*. New York, Raven Press, 1984, pp 71–77.
189. Terjung RL, Dudley GA, Meyer RA: Metabolic and circulatory limitations to muscular performance at the organ level. *J Exp Biol* 115:307–318, 1985.
190. Torres C, Moxley RT, Griggs RC: Quantitative testing of handgrip strength, myotonia, and fatigue in myotonic dystrophy. *J Neurol Sci* 60:157–168, 1983.
191. Triebwasser JH, Johnson RL Jr, Burpo RP, Campbell JC, Reardon WC, Blomqvist CG: Noninvasive determination of cardiac output by a modified acetylene rebreathing procedure utilizing mass spectrometer measurements. *Aviat Space Environ Med* 48:203–209, 1977.
192. Turnbull DM, Bartlett K, Stevens DL, Alberti KGMM, Gibson GJ, Johnson MA, McCulloch AJ, Sherratt HSA: Short-chain acyl-CoA dehydrogenase deficiency associated with a lipid-storage myopathy and secondary carnitine deficiency. *N Engl J Med* 311:1232–1236, 1984.
193. Vignos PJ Jr: Physical models of rehabilitation in neuromuscular disease. *Muscle Nerve* 6:323–338, 1983.

194. Vora S, Giger U, Turchen S, Harvey JW: Characterization of the enzymatic lesion in inherited phosphofructokinase deficiency in the dog: an animal analogue of human glycogen storage disease type VII. *Proc Natl Acad Sci USA* 82:8109–8113, 1985.

195. Vranic M, Horvath S, Wahren J (eds): Proceedings of a conference on diabetes and exercise. *Diabetes* 28(Suppl 1):1–113, 1979.

196. Wade OL, Bishop JM: *Cardiac Output and Regional Blood Flow.* Oxford, Blackwell, 1962.

197. Wahren J, Felig P, Havel RJ, Jorfeldt L, Pernow B, Saltin B: Amino acid metabolism in McArdle's syndrome. *N Engl J Med* 288:774–777, 1973.

198. Walvoort HC: Glycogen storage diseases in animals and their potential value as models of human disease. *J Inherited Metab Dis* 6:3–16, 1983.

199. Wasserman K, Hansen JE, Sue D, Whipp BJ: *Principles of Exercise Testing and Interpretation.* Philadelphia, Lea & Febiger, 1987, p 218.

200. Wiles CM, Edwards RHT: Weakness in myotonic syndromes. *Lancet* 2:598–601, 1977.

201. Wiles CM, Jones DA, Edwards RHT: Fatigue in human metabolic myopathy. In Porter R, Whelan J (eds): *Human Muscle Fatigue: Physiological Mechanisms.* London, Pitman Press, 1981, pp 264–276.

202. Wilson JR, Martin JL, Schwartz D, Ferraro N: Exercise intolerance in patients with chronic heart failure: role of impaired nutritive flow to skeletal muscle. *Circulation* 69:1079–1087, 1984.

203. Young DR, Pelligra R, Adachi RR: Serum glucose and free fatty acids in man during prolonged exercise. *J Appl Physiol* 21:1047–1052, 1966.

4
Lactate Uptake by Skeletal Muscle
L. BRUCE GLADDEN, Ph.D.

INTRODUCTION

Lactic acidosis is a typical response to strenuous muscular exercise [72]. It is important because of the metabolic role of lactate as well as the effect of lactic acidosis on the performance of both cardiac [155, 199] and skeletal muscle [70, 84, 122, 136, 203]. Lactic acidosis is also observed clinically [32, 144] as a result of circulatory insufficiency [10, 31]; systemic disorders such as diabetes, liver, and renal failure [31, 118, 144]; and drugs or toxins such as phenformin and methanol [32, 118, 144]. The overall mortality from clinical lactic acidosis is greater than 50% [144] and is worsened with increased blood lactate concentration and more severe acidosis [11, 31].

Blood lactate concentration is a balance between production and utilization. In this scheme, skeletal muscle has usually been viewed as a producer of lactate. However, during sodium lactate infusion or an elevation in blood lactate concentration due to exercise, skeletal muscle actually takes up lactate, acting as both a passive sink and a utilizer [1, 2, 51, 65, 131, 148, 178]. The fact that skeletal muscle may play an important role in lactate uptake under certain conditions has not been widely appreciated. In addition, the significance of a possible specific transport mechanism for lactate in skeletal muscle, in either exercise or clinical disease states, remains unknown.

Before discussing the factors which might control lactate uptake by muscle, it is appropriate to explain the terminology that will be used.

Terminology
Lactic acid is properly referred to as lactate in body fluids. As illustrated in Figure 4.1, lactic acid has a pK on the order of 3.7 [71], which means that it is more than 99.5% dissociated at pH values of 6.4–7.4, the range likely to be encountered from inside fatigued muscle to normal arterial blood. Whether the uptake of lactate is more appropriately called "lactate uptake" or "lactic acid uptake" is a more difficult question. Several lines of evidence suggest that a significant component of lactate translocation (either uptake or output) involves the membrane transfer of the undissociated lactic acid molecule either by simple or facilitated diffusion. This lactic acid component of total lactate movement has been described variously as a "fraction" of the total flux, a "large fraction" of the total

FIGURE 4.1

Dissociation curve for lactic acid at 38°C. (Redrawn with permission from Gladden LB, Yates JW: Lactic acid infusion in dogs: effects of varying infusate pH. J Appl Physiol 54:1254–1260, 1983.)

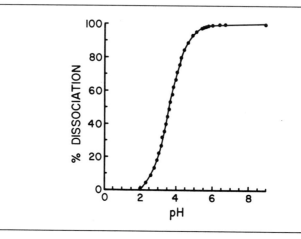

flux, the "predominant" component of lactate entry, or "of similar magnitude" to the ionic flux [124, 129, 130, 153, 163]. Once inside cells, whether lactate is converted to glucose/glycogen or oxidized, protons are consumed with lactate in an equimolar fashion [71, 144, 147, 162]. In other words, the net effect is the same as if lactic acid is metabolized.

It can be argued that the most accurate terminology is "lactate concentration," "lactic acid uptake [or output]," and "lactic acid utilization [or oxidation or production]." However, there are also several reasons for using the terms "lactate uptake" and "lactate output": (*a*) There is still uncertainty, especially under varying physiological conditions, concerning the relative amounts of membrane transport of lactic acid versus lactate; (*b*) both net uptake and net output are typically determined by measuring changes in lactate concentration in the blood or extracellular medium; and (*c*) less importantly, "lactate uptake" has been the more widely used term. Therefore, for simplicity and consistency, this review will refer to lactate uptake, utilization, etc., with only occasional exceptions.

Factors Affecting Lactate Uptake

In this review, lactate uptake will be discussed from the viewpoint presented in Figure 4.2, that is, that lactate uptake may be limited by either (*a*) the rate of lactate utilization or (*b*) membrane characteristics relating to lactate uptake. During transient periods of rapid change in the transmembrane lactate gradient, membrane characteristics are more likely to

FIGURE 4.2

Graph depicting hypothetical response of muscle lactate uptake (L̇) to sudden increase in blood lactate concentration to 10 mM at time zero. Note small lactate output at time zero before sudden increase in lactate concentration. Key concept is that lactate uptake may be limited by membrane transport factors during initial transient period (0–5 minutes?) whereas lactate uptake is most likely limited by utilization in the steady state (20+ minutes ?).

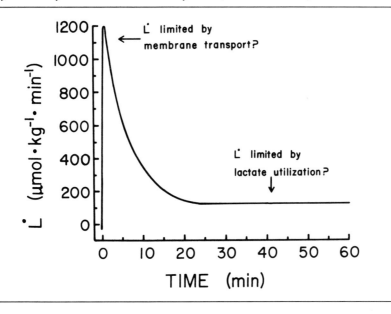

represent the limiting factor in lactate translocation. In the steady state, however, net lactate uptake cannot be greater than the rate of lactate utilization. Factors affecting the rate of lactate utilization will be divided into metabolic control, hormonal control, and metabolic rate. In addition, four other factors which might interact with both utilization and membrane transport of lactate will be discussed: hydrogen ion concentration, perfusion, muscle fiber type, and endurance training.

RATE OF LACTATE UTILIZATION

Lactate utilization refers to the metabolism of lactate to form pyruvate which can (*a*) accumulate, (*b*) be released from the muscle, (*c*) be converted to alanine, (*d*) be used to synthesize glycogen, and (*e*) be oxidized as a fuel for energy metabolism. Figure 4.3 indicates the important pathways for lactate utilization and suggests that lactate utilization would

FIGURE 4.3

Pathways for lactate utilization. In a steady state, the rate of accumulation of lactate and pyruvate will be zero. NAD = nicotinamide adenine dinucleotide; TCA = tricarboxylic acid.

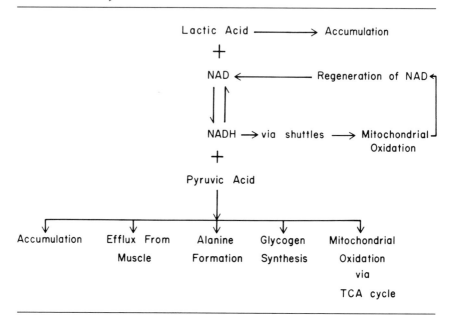

be maximized by conditions which favor rapid pyruvate formation from lactate followed by rapid metabolism of pyruvate and oxidation of the reduced form of nicotinamide adenine dinucleotide (NADH) to replenish NAD. Lactate utilization in the presence of an already elevated lactate concentration should also be enhanced if the glycolytic rate is depressed to decrease the formation of pyruvate and NADH from sources other than the lactate that is already present.

Factors determining the rate of lactate utilization by skeletal muscle can be broadly divided into metabolic control, hormonal control, and metabolic rate.

Metabolic Control of Lactate Utilization

While it is clear that if lactate utilization is to proceed rapidly there must be rapid conversion of lactate to pyruvate, adequate catabolism of pyruvate, and a constant replenishment of NAD, there is relatively little information concerning the metabolic control of lactate utilization. On the other hand, the metabolic changes that stimulate lactate production have been widely investigated and reviewed [17–19, 69, 92, 172]. A brief listing of stimulants of lactate production follows:

1. Lactate production appears to increase any time the glycolytic rate increases.
2. The glycolytic rate is increased by factors that stimulate the controlling enzymes of the glycolytic pathway, particularly phosphorylase and phosphofructokinase.
3. Phosphorylase is activated directly by muscle contractions, apparently by way of the increase in cytosolic calcium concentration. Phosphorylase is also activated by the catecholamines, especially epinephrine.
4. Increases in metabolic rate such as occur during exercise decrease the concentration of adenosine triphosphate (ATP) while increasing the concentrations of adenosine diphosphate (ADP), adenosine monophosphate (AMP), inorganic phosphate (Pi), and ammonia. All of these changes tend to activate phosphofructokinase and thereby glycolysis. There may also be a slight rise in cytosolic pyruvate and NADH concentrations.
5. Oxidative phosphorylation may be more slowly activated than glycolysis, thus resulting in an increase in cytosolic NADH concentration.
6. Lactic acid production at any glycolytic rate depends on the balance of competition for pyruvate and NADH between lactic dehydrogenase (LDH) on the one hand, and alanine transaminase, the NADH shuttles, and the tricarboxylic acid cycle on the other. With even small increases in pyruvate and NADH such as may occur with an increase in metabolic rate, the formation of lactate is likely due to the extremely high catalytic activity and low Michaelis-Menten constant (K_m) of LDH.

As a first approximation, it seems likely that any circumstance which decreases the glycolytic rate while activating pyruvate dehydrogenase and oxidative phosphorylation in the presence of elevated lactate concentration would hasten lactate utilization. However, there are no data with which to evaluate these possibilities.

Although there is considerable debate concerning the role of an inadequate oxygen supply in lactate production during exercise in normoxia [17, 18, 34, 35, 43, 69, 92, 110, 172, 190, 191], it is well known that hypoxia stimulates an increase in lactate production [21, 34, 89–91, 111, 113, 193]. It seems reasonable that hypoxia would therefore inhibit lactate utilization, whereas hyperoxia might enhance lactate utilization. I am not aware of any study concerning the effect of hypoxia on lactate uptake. However, the effect of hyperoxia during exercising recovery in humans has been tested in two studies [178, 197] and found to cause no change in the rate of blood lactate decline. This finding is in accord with reports that hyperoxia does not significantly decrease lactate production and release by active in situ muscle, either in humans [194] or in dogs [200], despite the fact that it depresses lactate concentration in intact humans during exercise [89, 90, 193, 194]. Nevertheless, there has been no direct investigation of the effect of hyperoxia on skeletal muscle lactate uptake and utilization during elevated blood lactate concentration.

Another factor which apparently does affect lactate uptake and utilization is muscle glycogen concentration. Essen et al. [59] had subjects perform an exercise protocol designed to reduce muscle glycogen 1 day prior to experimentation. This regimen was performed with only one leg so that during the actual experiments, the subjects had one leg which had a "normal" glycogen content and one leg which had only about half as much glycogen. The subjects then performed two-legged cycle exercise while blood was periodically collected from arterial and right and left femoral venous catheters. Even though both legs did the same amount of work at the same intensity, the leg with the lower glycogen content took up lactate while the "normal" leg released lactate.

This could be due to an increased glycogen synthesis from lactate in the low-glycogen leg or, more likely, a decreased glycolytic rate due to the low glycogen [99]. A lower glycolytic rate in the low-glycogen leg would decrease endogenous pyruvate and lactate production, thereby promoting utilization of exogenous lactate perfusing the leg. I am unaware of any other reports on the role of glycogen concentration in muscle lactate utilization.

As noted earlier, pyruvate metabolism must proceed quickly if lactate utilization is to occur rapidly. In this context, a well-known stimulant of pyruvate dehydrogenase is dichloroacetate [38, 61, 198]. Dichloroacetate has been shown to lower blood lactate concentration during submaximal exercise in dogs (135; by as much as 60%) and humans [22]. Blood and muscle lactate concentrations were found to be lower with dichloroacetate in rats following nonexhaustive swimming [161]. There is additional evidence that dichloroacetate inhibits muscle lactate production at rest [28], during hypoxia [75], and during contractions [119, 120]. Finally, Goodman et al. [74] observed that dichloroacetate caused lactate output to reverse to lactate uptake in the resting, perfused rat hindquarter. Apparently no other measurements of lactate uptake during dichloroacetate administration have been reported.

Brevetti et al. [16] speculated that L-carnitine can indirectly activate pyruvate dehydrogenase to reduce lactate formation. However, neither this hypothesis, nor the possibility that carnitine might promote lactate utilization has been tested.

The availability of alternative substrates could also exert metabolic control over lactate utilization by muscle. Dunn and Critz [54] infused sodium lactate into anesthetized dogs to increase the arterial blood lactate concentration to about 2 mM. At the same time nicotinic acid was infused to depress arterial free fatty acid levels. Under these conditions, the dog hindlimb extracted lactate from the blood. However, in a separate group of dogs, 2 mM lactate accompanied by infusion of a heparin-fat emulsion to elevate free fatty acids resulted in a hindlimb arteriovenous lactate difference of zero. In other words, an increase in free fatty acid availability apparently reduced lactate utilization by hindlimb muscle. This notion deserves further study.

In summary, it seems reasonable that any factor which (*a*) decreases endogenous lactate production, (*b*) increases pyruvate and NADH oxidation, or (*c*) accomplishes both a and b at the same time will increase lactate utilization:

1. Low muscle glycogen levels appear to decrease muscle lactate production and increase lactate utilization as a result.
2. Dichloroacetate stimulates pyruvate dehydrogenase and seems to promote lactate utilization. It is speculated that L-carnitine might also enhance lactate utilization by indirectly stimulating pyruvate dehydrogenase.
3. Elevated free fatty acids serve as an alternative substrate to lactate, and may reduce lactate utilization.
4. Indirect evidence suggests that hyperoxia does not affect lactate utilization.
5. There appear to be no studies concerning the effects of hypoxia on lactate uptake and utilization. However, lactate utilization would probably be overridden by the high endogenous lactate production accompanying hypoxia.

Hormonal Control Of Lactate Utilization
In addition to the effects of metabolites and other chemical agents, it seems likely that the hormonal milieu, particularly epinephrine concentration, could play a prominent role in determining the rate of lactate utilization. Epinephrine has been shown to activate phosphorylase, hastening glycogenolysis and increasing muscle lactate concentration and output in rat hindlimb [150, 152] and intact humans [26, 171]. Epinephrine may also activate phosphofructokinase [126]. In addition, Stainsby et al. [174, 175] have observed an increased lactate output by the contracting, in situ dog gastrocnemius during infusion of either epinephrine or norepinephrine, with epinephrine being the more potent of the two. In another study, Stainsby et al. [176] reported that lactate output by contracting in situ dog muscle was increased by epinephrine and isoproterenol (a relatively pure β-receptor agonist) infusion. The epinephrine response was inhibited by propranolol (a general β-blocker) but enhanced by phenoxybenzamine (a general α-receptor blocker). From

these data, they [176] suggested that β-activation increases, whereas α-activation decreases, lactate output by contracting muscle. A lower lactate output from muscles during β-blockade has also been shown in human studies [106]. In intact humans, the effects of catecholamines on muscle may be confounded by the systemic effects of catecholamines on cardiac output, blood flow, and other organs [106, 112]. None of these studies deals directly with lactate utilization. Nevertheless, they do raise the possibility that muscle lactate utilization might be enhanced by β-receptor blockade and α-receptor activation.

Metabolic Rate

Typically, an elevated metabolic rate is associated with an elevated glycolytic rate and concomitant lactate production. However, if the metabolic rate is elevated without a large increment in glycolysis (such as during low-intensity submaximal exercise), then net lactate utilization might be increased as a result of a faster rate of pyruvate and NADH oxidation.

There are four types of studies in the literature that relate to the effect of metabolic rate on lactate utilization: studies of lactate uptake by resting human muscle, studies of lactate decline during exercising recovery in humans, isotopic tracer studies, and in situ muscle studies. These four types of studies are discussed in the following sections.

LACTATE UPTAKE BY HUMAN MUSCLE. There is little doubt that resting muscle can act as a large sink for lactate during both exercise and lactate infusion. For example, Karlsson et al. [107] found that leg exercise caused a large increase in arm muscle lactate concentration from approximately 1.0 to 9.7 millimoles per kilogram of wet weight (mmol·kg^{-1}). Similarly, arm exercise caused leg muscle lactate concentration to rise from about 1.0 to 7.8 mmol·kg^{-1}. As early as 1923, Barr and Himwich [8] noted that venous blood draining an inactive arm had a lower lactate concentration than arterial blood during exercise with the legs. More recently, Harris et al. [83] studied lactate uptake and output in the resting arm during rest and exercise with the legs in patients with rheumatic heart disease. Under resting conditions, the arms and legs released lactate and the liver took up lactate. During exercise with the legs, lactate was released from the legs while there was considerable lactate uptake in the resting arm which continued well into recovery. These investigators [83] speculated that the lactate was actively metabolized by the arm muscles since there was no evidence of increased lactate release from the arm following leg exercise. However, their [83] results were only qualitative in nature since their findings were based only on arteriovenous lactate concentration differences without any blood flow measurements. Similarly, Poortmans et al. [148] measured arteriovenous lactate difference across the resting forearm during progressive leg exercise in healthy subjects. They surmised that resting muscle lactate uptake was directly correlated with the arterial lactate concentration, once again without the benefit of blood flow measurements. On the basis of arteriovenous lactate differences in resting limbs during exercise of other limbs, Freyschuss and Strandell [65] suggested that 5–12% of the lactate produced in the exercising muscles might be removed by resting muscles.

Ahlborg et al. [1] determined blood flow by dye dilution and observed increases in lactate uptake by a nonexercising leg during exercise with the contralateral leg and during exercise with the arms. This uptake amounted to 0.3–1.0 mmol·min^{-1}. Since oxygen uptake ($\dot{V}O_2$) by the inactive leg rose by as much as 45% during exercise, a significant percentage of the lactate taken up could have been oxidized. In a subsequent study, Ahlborg et al. [2] infused sodium lactate into healthy subjects and measured the exchange of lactate in the leg and in forearm muscle. They estimated that skeletal muscle metabolized 35% of the infused lactate. Woll and Record [202] also infused sodium lactate into healthy subjects and estimated skeletal muscle uptake on the basis of forearm blood flow (strain gauge plethysmography), arterialized venous blood samples (dorsal vein of hand heated to 55–60°C), and venous blood samples from the contralateral antecubital vein. Extrapolating to the entire muscle mass, they [202] estimated that about 26% of the administered lactate was removed by skeletal muscle.

As a group, these studies clearly indicate that resting skeletal muscle can take up significant amounts of lactate during periods of elevated blood lactate concentration.

LACTATE DECLINE DURING EXERCISING RECOVERY. While it seems clear that resting muscle can metabolize lactate, especially when the arterial lactate concentration is increased, what is the effect of an increase in metabolic rate? As early as 1928, Jervell [100] observed that blood lactate concentration fell more rapidly in recovery when moderate exercise was performed instead of a passive resting recovery. (This observation was made in two experiments performed on one subject.) Jervell's work was extended by Newman et al. [141] in 1937 who found that the rate of blood lactate decline during recovery increased with the intensity of exercise during recovery up to a critical level of activity. It was speculated that the increased rate of lactate decline during an exercising recovery might be due to an increased blood flow with more rapid transport of lactate to removal centers and to increased utilization of lactate as a fuel for the exercise. Numerous similar studies [7, 9, 12, 15, 42, 51, 66, 68, 85, 133, 149, 157, 178, 179, 196, 197] have been done since 1937, but the interpretations of Newman et al. [141] have been altered only slightly. Typical data for blood lactate decline during recovery at rest and with exercise are shown in Figure 4.4.

FIGURE 4.4

Typical data for blood lactate decline during recovery while resting as compared to performing moderate exercise. Line with solid circles *indicates passive recovery.* Dashed line with Xes *indicates exercise at 35% of* $\dot{V}O_2max$ *during recovery. Exercise was performed on a cycle ergometer.* (*Redrawn with permission from Dodd S, Powers SK, Callender T, Brooks E: Blood lactate disappearance at various intensities of recovery exercise.* J Appl Physiol 57:1462–1465, 1984.)

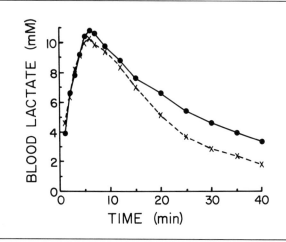

A number of studies have been directed toward determining the optimal exercise intensity for blood lactate decline during recovery. In other words, at what exercise intensity does lactate concentration in the blood decline most rapidly? Apparently the first of these studies was done by Davies et al. [42]. Following heavy exercise, they [42] observed lactate decline at rest and during exercise at approximately 15, 30, 45, and 60% of maximal $\dot{V}O_2$ ($\dot{V}O_2max$). Their results suggested that the rate of lactate decline would be greatest at approximately 40% of $\dot{V}O_2max$, an exercise intensity which was just below the lactate threshold of their subjects. (For the purposes of this review, lactate threshold can be defined as that exercise intensity above which blood lactate concentration is significantly greater than the resting level.) During treadmill exercise, Hermansen and Stensvold [85] found that lactate decline following maximal intermittent exercise was most rapid at an exercise intensity of 60–80% of $\dot{V}O_2max$. Once again, the recovery exercise intensity producing the fastest rate of lactate decline corresponded to the lactate threshold of the subjects, that is, 60–80% of $\dot{V}O_2max$.

Ryan et al. [157] took a different approach to the question of lactate metabolism during exercise. They [157] infused sodium L(+)-lactate at a constant rate of 0.05 mmol·kg^{-1}·min^{-1} during rest and exercise at 25, 50, and 66% of $\dot{V}O_2$max. At rest, the lactate infusion resulted in an increase of 3.5 mM in plasma lactate. An increase in lactate uptake during exercise was strikingly illustrated by the fact that blood lactate concentration fell when the subjects began exercising at 25% of $\dot{V}O_2$max, even though the lactate infusion continued. Plasma lactate during the different exercise intensities was only 1.2 mM higher during the lactate infusion than during the same power output with saline infusion. No evidence of an impaired ability to metabolize infused lactate was evident in these subjects up to an exercise intensity of 66% of $\dot{V}O_2$max.

In another interesting study, McGrail et al. [133] studied the effect of increasing the mass of exercising muscle during recovery on the rate of lactate decline. Following an intense exercise bout to elevate blood lactate, subjects exercised during recovery with arms only, legs only, or both arms and legs. In all three cases, the exercise intensity was 27% of $\dot{V}O_2$max for the particular exercise regimen employed. However, the absolute $\dot{V}O_2$ ranged from 0.73 l per minutes (l·min^{-1}) for the arm recovery exercise to 1.23 l·min^{-1} for the legs-plus-arms exercise. There was a significant correlation ($r = 0.92$) between the rate of lactate decline and the absolute $\dot{V}O_2$ of the recovery exercise. This suggests that lactate uptake is enhanced by increasing the active muscle mass, provided that the metabolic rate remains below the lactate threshold for the particular exercise being performed.

On the basis of the experiments discussed above [42, 85, 133, 157] and many others [9, 12, 51, 68, 156, 178, 179, 196, 197], the 1937 speculations of Newman et al. [141] can be refined as follows: (*a*) Recovery exercise performed with the greatest muscle mass at the highest intensity which elicits little or no increase in blood lactate concentration when started from rest should be the optimal recovery pattern for blood lactate decline. In other words, exercise with a large muscle mass at an intensity just below the lactate threshold should produce the greatest rate of lactate decline. (*b*) The primary fate of lactate during exercising recovery is probably oxidative metabolism by skeletal muscle. (This notion has been consistently supported by isotopic tracer studies which will be discussed next.) (*c*) The high rate of lactate decline during exercise recovery is probably related to the increased skeletal muscle blood flow. (*d*) The beneficial effects of increased muscle blood flow are probably reduced at higher exercise intensities by increased lactate production within the muscles and reduced splanchnic blood flow to remove the lactate from the blood.

Isotopic Tracer Studies. Several studies have used isotopically labeled lactate to study lactate metabolism during exercise in intact rats

[20, 52], dogs [47, 57, 98], and men [94, 131, 181], and across exercising muscle groups in rats [164], dogs [37, 80, 143] and men [103, 182]. Tracer studies of lactate metabolism have been reviewed extensively elsewhere [17–19], and their results will only be summarized briefly here:

1. Oxidation is a major route of lactate disposal during both rest (40–50% of lactate produced) and exercise (55–87% of lactate produced during light exercise).
2. The rate of lactate production increases during exercise, but so does the rate of lactate removal.
3. Lactate removal occurs to a large extent in exercising muscles, most likely by way of oxidation. Lactate oxidation is linearly related to metabolic rate (oxygen uptake). Tracer studies have provided strong support for the notion that most of the lactate removal during exercising recovery is by way of oxidation.
4. Perhaps the most interesting suggestion of lactate tracer studies [19, 20, 98, 103, 182] is that muscle produces, removes, and oxidizes lactate, all at the same time. This idea will be discussed later in the context of muscle fiber type and lactate uptake.

All of these tracer studies as well as those cited elsewhere in this review must be interpreted with caution. In 1966, Krebs et al. [117] incubated slices of kidney cortex with lactate and acetoacetate. In this system, lactate was largely converted to glucose whereas acetoacetate was the major fuel of respiration. Nevertheless, a large portion of uniformly labeled [^{14}C]lactate appeared in CO_2. Krebs et al. [117] suggested that there was a "crossing over" of carbons and that the fate of the label did not allow predictions to be made about the *net* fate of the labeled metabolites.

Several investigators have suggested that labeled lactate can rapidly equilibrate with pyruvate. This would allow any metabolism of pyruvate to contribute to the calculated lactate turnover, and cause an overestimate of lactate production and oxidation. On this basis, Cohen and Iles [30] state that convincing resolution of the problem of measuring lactate production and removal "will only be achieved by careful measurement of arteriovenous concentration differences of lactate and flow rates across the critical organs." Similarly, Sahlin [158] argues that net lactate production (defined as the net release of lactate by a cell or organ) and net lactate removal (defined as the net uptake of lactate by a cell or organ) cannot be determined by tracer techniques.

Recently, Wolfe et al. [201] provided experimental evidence that lactate kinetics as usually determined more closely reflect pyruvate kinetics rather than lactate kinetics. They [201] infused [$3 - ^{13}$C]lactate into six anesthetized dogs and subsequently determined the percentages of lactate and pyruvate which were labeled. Pyruvate was labeled to almost the same extent as lactate, indicating rapid isotopic equilibration between lactate and pyruvate. These results raise serious questions concerning the conclusions reached from typical isotopic lactate tracer studies.

Despite the criticisms of isotopic tracer studies, it should be noted that some of the conclusions from these studies are in agreement with the circumstantial evidence provided by the studies of lactate decline during exercise recovery. Specifically, the following are points of agreement among the isotopic studies and the recovery exercise studies as well as the in situ muscle studies which are discussed next: (*a*) Resting muscle takes up and oxidizes lactate, and (*b*) Lactate uptake and oxidation by exercising muscle is greater than lactate uptake and oxidation by resting muscle.

IN SITU MUSCLE STUDIES. Although lactate output by in situ skeletal muscle has been studied extensively [6, 24, 27, 35, 76, 77, 87, 88, 104, 168–170, 173–177, 183, 195, 200], there has been considerably less investigation of lactate uptake [59, 71, 134, 145, 177, 192, 195]. Stainsby and Welch [177, 195] were among the first investigators to emphasize the ability of skeletal muscle to take up lactate even during contractions. More recently, a few studies [71, 134, 192] have reported lactate uptake by resting muscle exposed to an elevated blood or perfusate lactate concentration. For example, Gladden and Yates [71] followed lactate uptake by the resting, in situ dog gastrocnemius muscle at an arterial lactate concentration of about 10 mM. The arteriovenous blood lactate difference across the muscle was small, ranging between 0.1 and 0.6 mM. Before lactic acid infusion, lactate output was prevalent, averaging 51.5 micromoles per kg of wet muscle per minute (μmol·kg^{-1}·min^{-1}). Output changed to uptake during lactic acid infusion. Lactate uptake during 1 hour of infusion varied from 9.7 to 99.0 μmol·kg^{-1}·min^{-1}.

Recently, Gladden (unpublished data) investigated the effect of increasing metabolic rate due to muscle contractions on lactate uptake by the in situ dog gastrocnemius. In 11 experiments, control measures of resting $\dot{V}O_2$ and lactate output were followed by infusion of a lactic acid/lactate solution at a pH of 3.6 (to maintain control acid–base status as described by Gladden and Yates [71]). Infusion raised the arterial lactate concentration to an average of 8.7 mM, which was maintained for 90 minutes. During the first 30 minutes of infusion, the muscles remained at rest; from 30 to 60 minutes the muscles were stimulated to contract with twitches at 1.0 Hz; and from 60 to 90 minutes the stimulation frequency was increased to 4.0 Hz.

At the elevated lactate concentration, resting $\dot{V}O_2$ was almost 12 ml·kg^{-1}·min^{-1}; $\dot{V}O_2$ increased to 38 ml·kg^{-1}·min^{-1} at 1.0 Hz contractions and then to about 125 ml·kg^{-1}·min^{-1} at 4.0 Hz. Figure 4.5 shows that lactate uptake by resting muscle was quite high only 1 minute after

FIGURE 4.5

Lactate uptake ($\dot{L}$) by in situ dog gastrocnemius muscle with blood lactate concentration elevated to 8.7 mM during rest, twitch contractions at 1.0 Hz, and twitch contractions at 4.0 Hz (Gladden, unpublished data). N = 11.

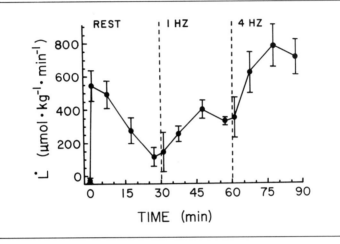

the infusion was begun, then declined over the remainder of the 30-minute resting period. Although the value at the first minute is a non-steady-state value and must be interpreted with caution, the high initial uptake followed by a decline most likely reflects a rapid wash-in of lactate in response to the sudden increase in the transmembrane lactate gradient at the onset of infusion. After 27 minutes of infusion, the lactate uptake is 113 μmol·kg^{-1}·min^{-1}, and probably reflects the steady-state uptake (lactate utilization) of the resting muscle since this value compares favorably with our previously published data for lactate uptake by resting muscle during 20–60 minutes of infusion [71].

At the onset of 1.0 Hz twitch contractions, lactate uptake changes very little, but then rises to a steady-state value which is almost three times greater than the steady-state resting lactate uptake. Again, at the onset of 4.0 Hz contractions, the lactate uptake changes very little, but then rises to a steady-state level which is approximately twice that at 1.0 Hz. The lack of an initial increase in lactate uptake at the onset of contractions or an increase in contraction frequency presumably reflects the absence of an increase in lactate utilization by the muscle. This could occur because of a transient increase in lactate production by the muscle in spite of the exogenous lactate perfusing it. This fits the known response of lactate output by dog muscle at the onset of contractions with normal, resting blood lactate concentrations [24, 87, 88, 174, 177, 195]. The dog gastrocnemius releases lactate for the first 5–15 minutes of contractions, and the rate of release is greater at higher contraction frequencies.

The explanation for a transient increase in lactate production and release, and a lag in the increase in lactate utilization, at the onset of contractions or an increase in contraction frequency may be the same. As noted earlier, phosphorylase is activated by the elevated cytosolic calcium which accompanies muscle contractions. This activation is due to the stimulatory effect of calcium on phosphorylase b kinase which in turn converts phosphorylase b to the more active phosphorylase a [33]. However, this phosphorylase activation is reversed after 5–15 minutes of contractions [33]. Phosphorylase can be reactivated during continued contractions by an increase in contraction frequency [150]. Phosphorylase activation, reversal, and reactivation fits the pattern of lactate release found in earlier studies as well as the lactate uptake pattern shown in Figure 4.5.

Another complementary explanation is the notion of a slower activation of oxidative metabolism relative to glycolysis as suggested by Stainsby [172]. A slower oxidative activation at the onset of contractions or an increase in contraction rate would allow a transient period of increased lactate release, or inhibited utilization. The suggestion is that if a muscle or a group of muscles can sustain a metabolic rate with only small declines in performance over time, lactate utilization at elevated blood lactate concentrations is greater at higher metabolic rates.

In conclusion, evidence from several different types of studies (exercising recovery, isotopic tracers, and in situ muscle) indicates that lactate utilization by skeletal muscle increases with increasing metabolic rate. The studies of lactate decline during exercising recovery in humans further suggest that lactate utilization increases to a maximal rate and then declines beyond a certain exercise intensity or metabolic rate. (Lactate utilization may also decline beyond some critical metabolic rate for in situ muscle. However, there are no data to verify this possibility.) That metabolic rate beyond which lactate utilization declines apparently coincides with an increase in endogenous lactate production by the muscle.

In intact animals, lactate utilization may be at least partly limited by factors external to the muscle itself. These factors include (a) increases in blood epinephrine with increasing metabolic rate [175] and/or (b) limited splanchnic blood flow and a subsequent decrease in lactate uptake by the splanchnic area [42, 51, 85, 156, 178, 179]. In in situ muscle preparations where cardiac output and whole body blood flow distribution are not challenged, local muscle blood flow could conceivably limit lactate uptake and utilization as discussed later. Significant elevations in blood catecholamines also occur as an artifact of surgical isolation of muscles during in situ muscle experiments [174].

MEMBRANE CHARACTERISTICS

Clear evidence of a carrier-mediated transport system for lactate has been presented for mammalian red cells [48, 49, 53, 82, 101], placenta [137], blood–brain barrier [142], enterocytes [184], Ehrlich ascites tumor cells [101, 167], sheep cardiac Purkinje strands [45], and rabbit and rat cardiac muscle [46, 126]. The notion of a lactate transporter has also been extended to skeletal muscle [105, 114, 123, 125, 129, 130, 192]. In fact, a recent case study [63] suggested a lactate transporter defect as a new disease of muscle.

In the past, investigators assumed that lactate moves rapidly across muscle membranes by simple diffusion [128]. However, there have been numerous reports of large gradients between muscle and blood or extracellular medium during exercise in humans [3, 66, 86, 104, 107, 113, 185], as well as during contractions of isolated [105, 121, 124, 125, 129, 163] and in situ muscle [35, 76, 77, 87, 88, 91, 109, 168–170]. Gradients between extracellular fluid and muscle during periods of elevated extramuscular lactate concentration have also been observed [71, 114, 134, 153, 192]. For example, Gladden and Yates [71] infused lactate into anesthetized dogs to raise the arterial blood lactate concentration to about 10 mM. During the infusion, the estimated ratio of intracellular muscle lactate to venous blood lactate averaged 0.65, indicative of a substantial gradient between blood and muscle. Also, McLane and Holloszy [134] perfused isolated rat hindlimbs with a perfusate containing 12 mM lactate. However, the plantaris muscle lactate concentration was only 3.2 millimoles per liter ($mmol \cdot l^{-1}$) of muscle water during the perfusion.

These large blood-to-muscle lactate gradients suggest, but do not prove, that there is a membrane hindrance to lactate translocation. Differences between intracellular and extracellular lactate concentration may simply reflect a steady-state distribution of lactate which might be determined by the transmembrane hydrogen ion gradient, as will be discussed in the following section. If this is the case, gradients of lactate concentration do not necessarily imply the presence of a membrane transport system.

If a lactate carrier plays a significant role in lactate transport, one would expect a saturation limit for lactate flux with continued increases in the transmembrane lactate concentration gradient. Indeed, saturation kinetics have been widely cited as evidence of a transport system for lactate [35, 103, 104, 109, 114]. Jorfeldt et al. [104] calculated lactate output by human leg muscle during light to heavy cycle exercise. Their results indicated that lactate output increased linearly as muscle lactate concentration increased from approximately 1 to 4 $mmol \cdot kg^{-1}$. However, above a muscle lactate concentration of 4 $mmol \cdot kg^{-1}$, there was a plateau in lactate output. Similarly, Karlsson et al. [109] indicated that lactate output from the contracting in situ dog gracilis reached a saturation point as muscle lactate concentration increased. Recently, saturation kinetics were reported again for the in situ dog gracilis during contractions by Connett et al. [35]; saturation occurred at a muscle lactate concentration of about 12 mmol·kg^{-1}.

In contrast, Hirche et al. [87, 88] found no plateau in lactate output by the contracting in situ dog gastrocnemius muscle. Lactate output increased linearly as muscle lactate concentration increased from approximately 1 to 30 mmol·l^{-1} of muscle water. McLane and Holloszy [134] also reported that lactate uptake by the resting rat hindlimb increased linearly with increasing perfusate lactate concentration between 6 and 26 mM; there was no evidence of a plateau in lactate uptake. Overall, studies of in situ blood perfused skeletal muscle have produced mixed results with regard to saturation kinetics.

Even if saturation of lactate translocation occurs, it does not necessarily confirm the existence of a lactate transport system. Saturation of lactate uptake with increasing external lactate concentration, depending on the type of measurements and their time frame, might reflect saturation of lactate utilization rather than saturation of a membrane transport system. The maximal rate of lactate transport across the muscle membrane may be faster than the maximal rate of lactate utilization by the muscle. Therefore, if the measurements are made in a steady state, maximal lactate uptake might be limited by the rate of lactate utilization rather than the rate of lactate transport. Similarly, in the case of lactate output, saturation could occur as a result of effects on the hydrogen ion gradient, number of perfused capillaries, or an uneven metabolism/perfusion ratio within the muscle tissue [35, 104].

For these reasons, membrane transport of lactate is best studied over short time intervals since it is most likely to be limiting at the onset of sudden changes in the transmembrane lactate gradient (see Fig. 4.2). Three studies [114, 130, 192] have made measurements that appear to describe membrane transport characteristics for lactate uptake by skeletal muscle. Koch et al. [114] studied the uptake of lactate over a short time span in quartered, incubated mouse diaphragms. Lactate uptake was determined at 15, 30, and 45 seconds after exposure to different external lactate concentrations, in the presence and absence of 20 mM α-cyano-4-hydroxycinnamate (cinnamate), a competitive inhibitor of lactate transport in other cell types. Their results suggested two modes of lactate entry into muscle: (*a*) a carrier system which has a K_m of 4 mM, saturates at about 10 mM, and accounts for about three-fourths of the transport at normal concentrations of lactate, and (*b*) free diffusion which accounts for about one-fourth of the membrane transfer when external lactate is low, and about half of the transfer when lactate concentration is 30 mM. From the data of Koch et al. [114], it can be estimated that at an extracellular lactate concentration of about 12 mM, the utilization rate was about 95 $\mu mol \cdot kg^{-1} \cdot min^{-1}$ as compared to an inward flux during the transient period of 200 $\mu mol \cdot kg^{-1} \cdot min^{-1}$ (about 140 due to the carrier and 60 by passive diffusion).

Mason and Thomas [130] studied frog sartorius muscles which were superfused with Ringer solutions containing lactate concentrations ranging from 5 to 60 mM. Using a microelectrode to measure intracellular pH in surface muscle fibers, they always observed intracellular acidification in response to the addition of lactate to the superfusate. Both the steady-state acidification and the maximal rate of acidification were measured at each external lactate concentration. Steady-state acidification was measured about 10 minutes or more after superfusion with a particular lactate solution was begun. The maximal rate of acidification was observed during the first 2 to 3 minutes of each superfusion period. At any constant external hydrogen ion concentration ($[H^+]$), the size and rate of intracellular acidification increased with increasing superfusate lactate concentration. In addition, an intracellular anion electrode gave compatible results in an accompanying series of experiments. As the superfusate lactate concentration was increased, the intracellular anion electrode qualitatively indicated a greater intracellular anion concentration. These results were interpreted to indicate that a significant component of lactate uptake in the frog sartorii was due to undissociated lactic acid diffusion, carrier cotransport of lactate and H^+ ions, or a combination of the two. Mason and Thomas [130] therefore assumed that their measurements of steady-state acidification reflected total lactate uptake while the maximal rate of acidification represented the peak rate of lactate uptake.

If the measurement technique of Mason and Thomas [130] for lactate uptake is accepted, their results show a nonlinear relationship between the peak rate of lactate uptake and extracellular lactate concentration. However, saturation was not observed with lactate concentrations from 5 to 60 mM. The nonlinear relationship between peak rate of lactate uptake and extracellular lactate was described well by a curve that calculated uptake as the sum of a carrier mechanism and a passive diffusion component. The carrier appeared to have a K_m of 10 mM at an extracellular pH of 7.35 and was quantitatively the more important lactate transport process in the physiological range of lactate concentrations and pH. At an extracellular pH of 7.35 and 20 mM lactate concentration, 64% of the lactate uptake was accounted for by the carrier system. SITS (4-acetamido-4'-isothiocyano-2,2'-stilbenedisulfonate, a blocker of inorganic anion exchange) did not affect the peak rate of lactate uptake with SITS concentrations from 20 to 100 μM. However, cinnamate (2–5 mM) caused a 39% decrease in the peak rate of lactate uptake. The cinnamate inhibition provides additional support for the presence of a lactate carrier system. However, cinnamate may not be entirely specific as an inhibitor of lactate transport [48].

In the most detailed characterization of skeletal muscle membrane transport of lactate to date, Watt et al. [192] used a dual tracer technique to study lactate transport in the perfused rat hindlimb. This tracer technique is designed to follow unidirectional uptake of lactate into tissue and does not attempt to determine the metabolic fate of lactate. Although possible effects of transfer of the lactate label to metabolites of lactate have not been reported, this technique is quite different from the radioactive tracer techniques referred to earlier. This method has been reviewed by Yudilevich and Mann [204] and previously applied to the study of lactate transport in perfused rabbit heart [126] and glucose and glutamine transport in the perfused rat hindlimb [97, 151]. In brief, a mixture of two tracers, one an extracellular marker ([^{3}H]mannitol) and the other the transportable substance being studied ([^{14}C]lactate in this case), is injected into the arterial inflow close to the tissue. The venous effluent is then collected in aliquots over a period of about 2 minutes; the unidirectional tracer uptake is the difference between the percentages of the doses of extracellular tracer and transportable tracer present in the venous effluent at any specific time. In the case of lactate, the unidirectional influx can be calculated from the average maximal tracer uptake, the perfusate flow, and the unlabeled arterial lactate concentration. Maximal lactate uptake usually occurred at about 20 seconds [192].

Primarily on the basis of dual tracer experiments in the presence of the known lactate transport blocker, cinnamate, Watt et al. [192] concluded that the transport of lactate across the sarcolemma of the rat hindlimb occurs by two major pathways. One pathway was nonsaturable and accounted for 70% of lactate movement at normal lactate concentrations and 90% of transport at 50 mM. The other pathway appeared to be saturable and was inhibited to varying degrees by 25 mM pyruvate, 5 mM cinnamate, 500 μM SITS, 1.0 mM amiloride (a blocker of Na^+/H^+ exchange), and 200 μM pCMBS (p-chloromercuriphenylsulfonic acid, a thiol group reagent). The latter is a known blocker of lactate transport in red blood cells [48, 49]. Watt et al. [192] emphasized the significance of their cinnamate experiments although, as noted earlier, the absolute specificity of cinnamate's inhibition of lactate transport has been questioned [48].

Although a major component of lactate transfer appeared to be non-carrier-mediated in nature, tracer lactate influx was less than that predicted from estimations of lactate permeability and sarcolemmal surface area. Simple diffusion did not appear to be a major route for lactate tracer influx. At a perfusate lactate concentration of 12 mM, the interpolated lactate influx for the rat hindlimb was 1332 μmol·kg^{-1}·min^{-1} [192] as compared to a utilization rate of 450 μmol·kg^{-1}·min^{-1} at the same perfusate lactate concentration [134]. The results of Watt et al. [192] differ from those of Koch et al. [114] and Mason and Thomas [130] in terms of the magnitude of utilization and influx of lactate as well as the relative importance of carrier versus noncarrier transport.

In another pertinent study, Juel [105] observed lactate efflux from mouse soleus muscles in vitro during 30 minutes of recovery from electrically stimulated contractions. Intramuscular lactate concentrations were increased approximately 10-fold above resting levels by stimulation prior to the recovery. Lactate efflux from the muscles was inhibited to varying degrees by cinnamate (4 mM), pCMBS (0.5 mM) and phloretin (0.6 mM), all known blockers of lactate carriers in other tissues. However, the anion-exchange inhibitors, SITS (0.5 mM, DIDS (4,4′-diisothiocyano-2,2′-stilbenedisulfonic acid, 0.05 mM) and tetrathionate (5 mM), did not appear to inhibit lactate efflux. These results indicated the existence of a lactate transporter in skeletal muscle that accounted for more than half of the lactate output during recovery from contractions.

In summary, there is solid evidence of a carrier-mediated transport system for lactate in skeletal muscle. This evidence is strongest in studies of isolated muscles in vitro [105, 114, 130]. The contribution of carrier-mediated lactate transport is estimated to be 50–75% of the total lactate uptake over the physiological range of lactate concentration. It has been suggested that an unstirred layer next to the membrane in these in vitro experiments might cause a curvilinear relationship between external lactate concentration and lactate uptake [130]. This could exaggerate the apparent contribution of a carrier to the lactate uptake process. However, the fact that known lactate transport blockers significantly reduce lactate uptake and output lends support to the concept of lactate carriers in skeletal muscle [105, 114, 130]. Since lactate transport blockers have similar effects on both lactate uptake [114, 130] and lactate output [105], the lactate carrier appears to be bidirectional and might be symmetrical as well.

In situ muscle studies of lactate uptake and output confound the observations of in vitro muscle studies with regard to a lactate carrier. Saturation kinetics for lactate transfer have been reported in some in situ studies [35, 103, 104, 109] but not in others [87, 88, 134]. There has been only one study [192] of perfused in situ muscle in which lactate transport blockers were used. In agreement with the in vitro muscle studies, this in situ muscle study reported evidence of a lactate carrier system. However, the contribution of this carrier to lactate uptake in the physiological range of lactate concentrations was estimated to be only 30% of the total lactate uptake. It should be noted that the perfusate used by Watt et al. [192] was a Krebs-Henseleit bicarbonate buffer containing 6% bovine serum albumin and no red blood cells.

More data are needed to evaluate the role of a skeletal muscle lactate carrier under varying physiological conditions. In the following sections, factors which might affect both lactate utilization and membrane transport of lactate are discussed.

HYDROGEN ION CONCENTRATION

There have been numerous reports of acid–base effects on lactate transfer (mostly lactate efflux) in isolated muscles [23, 121, 123–125, 129, 163], in situ muscles [67, 76, 87, 168, 170, 192], and intact men [41, 55, 56, 58, 78, 79, 102, 115, 132, 140, 185] at rest, during exercise, and during recovery. The isolated and in situ muscle studies have shown that extracellular alkalosis can increase the efflux of lactate by as much as 3-fold. Hydrogen ion concentration ($[H^+]$) could affect membrane transport, utilization, or both. Membrane transport effects are most likely linked to the transmembrane $[H^+]$ difference, whereas effects on lactate utilization are most likely related to the intramuscular $[H^+]$. The effects on lactate production can occur by way of influences on key enzymes in glycolysis. Alternatively, during muscle contractions, acid–base effects could change lactate production (or utilization) by decreasing the muscle's tension development and thereby its energy requirements [76].

Membrane Effects
One of the earliest observations of hydrogen ion effects was that of Mainwood et al. [125] in which lactate output from fatigued frog sartorius muscles varied with external $[H^+]$ in a bicarbonate buffered solution at constant P_{CO_2}. Mainwood et al. [123, 125] proposed four models that might explain their observations: (*a*) lactate anion diffusion mainly through membrane pores which might be affected by the hydrogen ion, (*b*) exchange of lactate for bicarbonate across the membrane possibly by way of a carrier, (*c*) hydrogen ion linked carrier transport of lactate, and (*d*) free diffusion of undissociated lactic acid. These models are illustrated in Figure 4.6.

Model A could contribute to lactate output because of a favorable electrochemical gradient for the lactate anion. However, lactate anion diffusion or transport seems unlikely in the case of lactate uptake since lactate would have to be actively transported against its electrochemical gradient [96, 123]. For example, at a normal membrane potential of -88 mV [39] and an intracellular lactate concentration of 1.5 mM, the Nernst equation predicts that an extracellular lactate concentration greater than 44 mM would be required to allow a passive inward leak of lactate anions. If the membrane potential were -60 mV (perhaps due to muscle fatigue), the extracellular lactate concentration would still have to be 10

FIGURE 4.6

Four models which might explain the effects of [H⁺] on lactate transfer across muscle membrane. See text for details. (Used with permission from Mainwood GW, Renaud JM, Mason MJ: The pH dependence of the contractile response of fatigued skeletal muscle. Can J Physiol Pharmacol 65:648–658, 1987.)

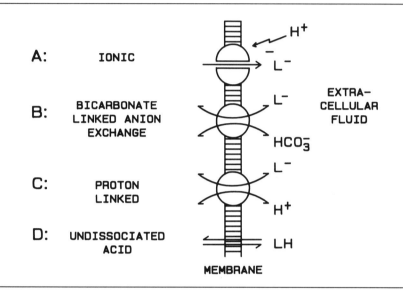

times greater than the intracellular lactate concentration to allow passive anionic diffusion inward.

Model B can be excluded because lactate efflux from the frog sartorius was shown to increase with a decrease in external [H⁺] independent of the buffer system used [124]. Models C and D remain as the most likely possible explanations for the effects of [H⁺] on lactate flux. Model C is presently indistinguishable from lactate anion:OH^{-1} exchange or transport of undissociated lactic acid.

As already described, Mason and Thomas [130] have provided evidence that both carrier-mediated transport and free diffusion (Models C and D) play a role in transmembrane movement of lactate. In the same study, they [130] also reported a significantly faster lactate uptake at any given external lactate concentration when the external pH was decreased from 7.35 to 6.8.

In an earlier study, Mason et al. [129] studied the effect of external propionate on lactate efflux from lactate-loaded (due to stimulation) frog muscle. The addition of propionate to the incubation medium caused a large increase in lactate efflux probably for two reasons: (*a*) an influx of propionic acid into the muscle increased intracellular hydrogen ion concentration ($[H^+]_i$), and (b) the simultaneous loss of propionic acid from the medium decreased the extracellular hydrogen ion concentration ($[H^+]_o$). The net effect would be an increased $[H^+]$ gradient across the muscle membrane.

All of these studies [123–125, 129, 130] of transmembrane $[H^+]$ and lactate transfer suggest that an increase in $[H^+]$ on either side of the membrane increases the concentration of undissociated lactic acid molecules (HL) on that side of the membrane. If all other conditions remain constant, this results in either an increased efflux of lactate *from* that side or a decreased influx of lactate *to* that side. On the other hand, a decrease in $[H^+]$ on either side of the membrane would decrease the HL concentration on that side by promoting dissociation of the molecule. This results in either a decreased efflux of lactate *from* that side or an increased influx *to* that side. In either case, the end result is a greater concentration gradient for HL across the membrane which enhances the net diffusion of HL down its concentration gradient. Even though HL is more than 99.5% dissociated in the physiological pH range, as shown in Figure 4.1, a decrease in pH from 7.4 to 6.8 more than doubles the HL concentration for any given lactate concentration.

These studies [123–125, 129, 130] are also compatible with Model C in Figure 4.6 which is sometimes referred to as an H^+-symport carrier system because lactate and an H^+ ion are carried together in the same direction. Changes in the transmembrane $[H^+]$ gradient would affect lactate transport by a symport carrier since the carrier can more readily obtain H^+ ions on the side with the greater $[H^+]$. An H^+-symport carrier system for lactate is indistinguishable from an OH^--antiport lactate carrier because cotransport of H^+ and lactate in the same direction cannot be distinguished from countertransport of lactate and OH^- in opposite directions.

That effects of $[H^+]$ gradients on lactate flux are due to membrane effects is verified by the data of Watt et al. [192]. As described above, they [192] used a dual tracer technique to follow unidirectional lactate influx in the perfused rat hindlimb. When perfusate pH was decreased from 7.4 to 6.8, lactate tracer influx was increased by 30% at 1 mM lactate and by 12% at 50 mM lactate. When perfusate pH was increased from 7.4 to 7.7, lactate tracer influx was decreased by about 20% at both 1 mM and 50 mM lactate.

Another interesting result of transmembrane $[H^+]$ differences does not require any direct effects on the *rate* of lactate flux across the muscle membrane. Roos [153] observed that the steady-state distribution of D-lactate between intracellular water and extracellular water for isolated rat hemidiaphragms varied with the transmembrane $[H^+]$ gradient. Variations in external pH over the range of about 6–8 hardly affected the

D-lactate distribution ratio as long as the extracellular to intracellular [H$^+$] ratio remained unchanged. Under normal conditions of external pH and P_{CO_2}, the intracellular D-lactate concentration averaged about 35% (40% for L-lactate) of the extracellular concentration. By changing the [H$^+$] gradient across the muscle membrane, the D-lactate distribution could be changed so that the intracellular concentration ranged from about 20–100% of the extracelllular concentration. Since Roos [152] observed similar distribution ratios for both D-lactate and L-lactate at normal pH and normal [H$^+$] gradient, it is assumed that the variation in distribution ratio observed for D-lactate with changes in transmembrane [H$^+$] would apply to L-lactate. (However, this cannot be accepted without reservation since there is evidence of stereospecificity of the lactate carrier [192].)

Roos's [152] explanation for the dependence of lactate distribution on the distribution of [H$^+$] is paraphrased below:

The dissociation of lactic acid (HL) into the lactate anion (L$^-$) and the hydrogen ion (H$^+$) occurs as follows:

$$HL \rightleftharpoons H^+ + L^-. \qquad\qquad 1$$

If the undissociated molecules (HL) are equilibrated across the cell membrane either by a carrier or by free diffusion, then

$$[HL]_i = [HL]_o, \qquad\qquad 2$$

where the subscripts i and o refer to inside and outside the cell, respectively. If the dissociation constant, K$'$, in intracellular water equals that in the extracellular water, then

$$K' = [H^+]_i[L^-]_i/[HL]_i = [H^+]_o[L^-]_o/[HL]_o. \qquad\qquad 3$$

Combining Equations 2 and 3,

$$[L^-]_i/[L^-]_o = [H^+]_o/[H^+]_i. \qquad\qquad 4$$

Over the physiological range of pH, [L$^-$] is much, much greater than [HL]; therefore,

$$[L^-]_i/[L^-]_o \approx [TL]_i/[TL]_o, \qquad\qquad 5$$

where [TL] indicates total lactate ([L$^-$] + [HL]). Combining Equations 4 and 5,

$$[TL]_i/[TL]_o = [H^+]_o/[H^+]_i. \qquad\qquad 6$$

At least one implication of the observations of Roos [152] is that even in a steady state in which the net flux of lactate is zero, the intracellular and extracellular concentrations of lactate are unlikely to be equal. Therefore, concentration differences between muscle and blood do not automatically imply a direct limitation in transport rate, but instead may reflect a usual distribution of lactate across the muscle membrane. Furthermore, it is conceivable that in a quasi-steady state, transport processes may be rapid enough to achieve a lactate distribution which is appropriate to the existing transmembrane conditions, and that net lactate output or uptake is limited by the transmembrane $[H^+]$ gradient. This gradient is obviously influenced by the interstitial fluid $[H^+]$, which could in turn be affected by blood $[H^+]$ and perfusion of the muscle, that is, the rate and distribution of flow to deliver or remove lactate and hydrogen ions to or from the interstitial space.

An important role for interstitial fluid $[H^+]$ can be derived from the study of Steinhagen et al. [183] which reports interstitial $[H^+]$ of in situ dog muscle at rest, during contractions, and during recovery. Interstitial fluid $[H^+]$ was higher than muscle venous $[H^+]$ at all times under all conditions. With normal acid–base balance, the difference between interstitial and venous $[H^+]$ widened from 8.9 nanomoles (nmol) per liter at rest ($\Delta pH = 0.07$) to 36 nmol ($\Delta pH = 0.2$) during contractions. This was apparently due to lactate efflux (accompanied by H^+ ions) into the interstitial space. In addition, this $[H^+]$ difference was increased further to 92 nmol ($\Delta pH = 0.30$) by metabolic acidosis due to L-arginine-hydrochloride infusion during muscle contractions. On the basis of studies already cited, increases in interstitial $[H^+]$ would obviously decrease lactate efflux from the muscle.

Utilization Effects
A different effect of $[H^+]$ is its role in regulating lactate production and possibly thereby lactate utilization. There are a number of studies that suggest possible effects on lactate utilization by way of changes in lactate production. In vitro enzyme studies have shown that changes in $[H^+]$ affect the activity of phosphofructokinase [50, 187, 188] and the conversion of phosphorylase b to phosphorylase a [25, 40, 116], with acidosis inhibiting and alkalosis promoting activation [96]. These enzyme studies have been borne out by studies of muscle metabolites in contracting in situ muscle [67, 76, 168, 170] and biopsies from exercising, intact man [185] in which lactate formation and glycogen usage is generally lower in acidosis. The effects of alkalosis on glycogen usage and lactate formation are not so definite, and it has been suggested that the regulatory enzymes of glycolysis may be more easily inhibited by acidosis in comparison to their activation by alkalosis [168]. None of these studies deal directly with the effects of $[H^+]$ on lactate utilization. However, the

assumption is that factors which inhibit lactate production in the presence of an adequate concentration of exogenous lactate will promote lactate utilization. In this context, Graham et al. [76] reported that acidosis resulted in net lactate uptake by in situ dog gastrocnemii after 20 minutes of contractions at 3 Hz. Under normal acid–base conditions, the muscles were still releasing lactate after 20 minutes of contractions.

Three other points concerning hydrogen ion effects on lactate translocation should be made; these points are especially pertinent to studies of whole animals. First, changes in blood [H+] can have confounding effects [140]. For example, blood alkalosis may promote lactate output from those muscles which have a high lactate concentration, but at the same time inhibit lactate uptake by those muscles which have a low lactate concentration. Second, acidosis is associated with an increase in blood catecholamine concentrations [56, 76, 138, 139, 154]. As noted previously, the catecholamines may stimulate glycolysis, which could inhibit lactate utilization. Third, while the effects of respiratory and nonrespiratory acid–base changes appear to be generally similar [132, 168, 170], there may be some subtle, but potentially confounding differences. It has been suggested that changes in extracellular [H+] due to variations in P_{CO_2} are more effective than nonrespiratory extracellular [H+] changes in altering intracellular [H+] [189]. This could occur because of a greater cell membrane permeability to CO_2 than to nonrespiratory acids. If this is the case, nonrespiratory [H+] changes should generate a greater transmembrane [H+] difference and therefore have a greater effect on membrane transfer of lactate. On the other hand, respiratory [H+] changes should cause a greater change in intracellular [H+] but a smaller change in transmembrane [H+] difference. This might translate into a greater effect on lactate production and thereby utilization, and a lesser effect on lactate translocation across the membrane.

PERFUSION

Studies of blood lactate decline during exercising recovery in humans [9, 12, 42, 51, 141, 178, 179] have frequently suggested that blood flow is a critical factor in increasing the rate of blood lactate decline. It has been proposed that moderate exercise during recovery increases the muscle blood flow which increases lactate output from the previously exercised muscles and transports this lactate more rapidly to lactate uptake sites which include resting muscles as well as the liver. In the case of lactate output, if all other factors remain constant, an increased blood flow should increase the transit rate through the capillary bed and thus maintain a lower capillary lactate concentration. This will in turn establish a greater intracellular to extracellular lactate concentration gradient and should promote lactate output. Conversely, for lactate uptake, an increased blood flow should maintain a higher extracellular to intracellular lactate gradient to increase lactate uptake. While this is a reasonable proposition, there have been few studies directly related to the role of blood flow in either lactate output or uptake.

Jorfeldt [103] found that the rate of lactate uptake by human forearm muscle during lactate infusion correlated more closely with the product of arterial lactate concentration and the muscle blood flow than with the arterial lactate concentration alone. This suggested that blood flow might play an important role in the uptake of lactate. During contractions of in situ dog gastrocnemius muscles, Graham et al. [77] found a low but significant correlation ($r = 0.50$) between lactate output and blood flow, as well as between muscle lactate concentration and blood flow. In contrast, Hirche et al. [87, 88] dismissed blood flow as an important determinant of lactate release in their studies of contracting, spontaneously perfused dog gastrocnemii. During 60 minutes of lactate infusion to an arterial concentration of 10 mM, Gladden and Yates [71] found no significant change in lactate uptake by resting dog gastrocnemius muscle even though blood flow varied by a factor of two, from 90 to 180 ml·kg^{-1}·min^{-1}. On the other hand, arteriovenous lactate difference during elevated blood lactate concentration typically remains small during increased metabolic rate (and increased lactate uptake) due to muscle contractions in the in situ dog gastrocnemius (Gladden, unpublished data). As a result, an increased blood flow is the major component of an increased lactate uptake with increasing $\dot{V}O_2$ during contractions.

Along with blood flow, capillary surface area or even the endothelial cells themselves could play a role in determining either lactate uptake or output by skeletal muscle, or other tissues [166]. There is growing evidence that endothelial cells are not simply passive barriers. Endothelial cells may be involved in active regulation of capillary transport of a variety of small solutes [166]. Hirche et al. [87] speculated that lactic acid with a relatively low molecular weight of 90 is not impeded by the capillary; however, there are apparently no data with which to confirm or refute this notion. Whether or not endothelial cells regulate the movement of the lactate anion or lactic acid molecules, the total capillary surface area within a particular muscle could play an important role in lactate uptake or output. Connett et al. [35] pointed out that the limiting surface area for lactate output from muscle is at the capillary; obviously the same holds for lactate uptake. If all other factors remain constant, lactate uptake or output for a given blood to intramuscular lactate concentration gradient will increase with a greater capillary surface area.

Jorfeldt [103] suggested that a correlation between lactate uptake and blood flow might occur because a larger blood flow implies a larger open capillary surface. More recently, Tesch and Wright [186] found a correlation between the pattern of postexercise blood lactate concentration and muscle capillary density in humans. Following 50 maximal voluntary knee extensions, the immediate postexercise blood lactate concentration was much higher and therefore much closer to the peak recovery value in subjects having a greater muscle capillary density as determined from biopsies of the vastus lateralis. This suggested that lactate was released more rapidly from muscles having a greater capillary density and therefore presumably a greater open capillary surface area at the onset of recovery. An increased capillary density might also allow a greater lactate uptake.

Mainwood et al. [122, 123] have emphasized that movements of lactate involve two processes in series. In the case of lactate uptake, the two processes are the influx of lactate from the blood into the interstitial space and the influx of lactate from the interstitial space into the muscle cell. Since a large, perhaps major, component of the lactate uptake involves either undissociated lactic acid or else coupled lactate and proton movement, maintenance of a high $[H^+]$ in the interstitial fluid will be important. In other words, an adequate blood flow with appropriate distribution will (a) ensure that a lactate gradient from the intersitital space into the cell is maintained as lactate moves from the interstitial space into the cell, and (b) ensure that an adequate supply of buffer (hydrogen ion source in this case) is delivered to the interstitial space as it becomes alkalotic because of the coupled movement of protons into the cell. For maximal lactate uptake, the blood flow must be matched to the lactate uptake in any particular area of the muscle. If capillaries are either not present or not adequately perfused, those muscle fibers which have a high lactate uptake may be limited by a decreased lactate gradient into the cell and a local alkalosis. These questions have not been sufficiently studied for either lactate output or uptake by muscle.

MUSCLE FIBER TYPE

It is well known that there are three basic mammalian muscle fiber types in terms of oxidative and glycolytic potential [73, 146, 168]. These fiber types are (a) fast glycolytic fibers (FG), which are better suited for glycolytic activity than oxidative activity (they have low concentrations of oxidative enzymes); (b) slow oxidative fibers (SO), which have high concentrations of oxidative enzymes and are therefore ideal for formation of ATP by oxidative phosphorylation; and (c) fast oxidative–glycolytic fibers (FOG), which are intermediate between FG and SO fiber types in terms of oxidative capability. Numerous studies [19, 20, 59, 98, 103, 108, 131, 180–182] have suggested that during exercise, glycolytic muscle fibers (FG) produce lactate which can diffuse into oxidative fibers (SO) directly or else diffuse into the blood, recirculate, and then diffuse into SO fibers where the lactate is oxidized. The metabolism of FOG fibers would be somewhere between the behavior of the FG and SO fibers; some FOG fibers might be producing lactate while some FOG fibers might be taking up and oxidizing lactate. This scheme is based on the known enzyme profiles of the fiber types and radioactive lactate tracer studies which indicate that muscle releases, takes up, and oxidizes lactate all at the same time. While the notion of lactate production by FG fibers along with concomitant uptake and oxidation of lactate by SO fibers appears reasonable, it is without direct proof, especially given the criticisms of lactate tracer studies which have been discussed earlier.

Strong indirect evidence to support this idea is the LDH profile of the respective fiber types [165]. LDH is composed of two subunits in a tetramere system in skeletal muscle; the two subunits are a muscle-specific type (M) and a heart-specific type (H). The M and H subunits can be combined in five different combinations resulting in five different LDH isozymes with different properties [44]. LDH isozymes with mostly H subunits favor oxidation of lactate, whereas LDH isozymes with mostly M subunits favor lactate formation. Total LDH activity is lower in muscles which are predominantly made up of slow-twitch fibers (analogous to SO), and the relative activity of H type LDH increases with increasing slow-twitch (SO) composition [165]. Schantz [160] has also suggested that lactate oxidation should be favored in SO fibers because of their higher malate−aspartate shuttle enzyme levels, especially their higher cytosolic malate dehydrogenase (cMDH) activities. Higher cMDH levels could keep the cytosolic NADH concentration low, thus facilitating the conversion of lactate to pyruvate [160].

In vitro studies of muscles of different fiber types support the idea of a greater tendency for predominantly SO muscles to oxidize lactate [4, 5]. For example, Baldwin et al. [4] studied the capacity of muscle homogenates containing different fiber types to oxidize lactate at concentrations ranging from 2 to 10 mM. Lactate oxidation was greater in oxidative muscles than in glycolytic muscles and was highly correlated with the total LDH H-isozyme activity. Greater lactate oxidation corresponded to higher H-isozyme activity. Baldwin et al. [4] speculated that highly oxidative muscle fibers would be stimulated to take up and oxidize lactate by (*a*) increased cellular lactate concentration due to influx from the blood and (*b*) increased oxidative activity by mitchondria due to contractions. Additional evidence for greater lactate uptake by oxidative muscles is given by the investigations of Bonen et al. (13, 14). They [14] reported low but significant correlations ($r = 0.54$) between the rate of blood lactate decline in humans during exercising recovery and the percentage of slow-twitch muscle fibers in the vastus lateralis as determined on muscle biopsies.

The evidence presented here (mostly indirect) indicates that lactate utilization should be greater in oxidative muscles than in glycolytic muscles. I am unaware of any direct evidence concerning possible differences in membrane transport capacity among the different fiber types. However, it is well established that highly oxidative muscle fibers have a greater capillary supply than do glycolytic fibers [81, 93, 95]. This greater capillary supply to oxidative muscle fibers might facilitate lactate uptake as noted above in the Perfusion section. However, it is interesting to note that even though oxidative fibers have a much greater total capillary supply than do glycolytic fibers, the glycolytic fibers have an oversupply of capillaries with reference to their oxidative capacity [93]. It has been suggested that the capillary supply of glycolytic muscle fibers may be more important for lactate transport than for oxygen transport [93, 95].

ENDURANCE TRAINING

It is well known that blood lactate concentration at a given absolute work rate as well as at a given percentage of $\dot{V}O_2max$ is lower following endurance training [92]. This has typically been attributed to a lower lactate production by skeletal muscle [92]. This decreased lactate production is in turn a product of an increased mitochondrial density, a concomitant increase in oxidative capacity, a decrease in muscle LDH activity, and a decrease in the percentage of the M-type isozyme of LDH [92].

Freminet et al. [64], in a study utilizing [^{14}C]lactate, found both a significantly increased lactate production and a greater lactate utilization in resting rats following training. Donovan and Brooks [52], also using radioactive lactate, refuted the role of decreased lactate production in the lower blood lactate concentration following training in exercising rats. Their study indicated that lactate production during exercise was unchanged by training while lactate clearance occurred at a faster rate in trained rats. Recently, Holloszy's group [62] used an in situ rat hindquarter preparation to study the effects of endurance exercise training on lactate production by skeletal muscle during concentrations induced by electrical stimulation. Their results provided direct evidence that lactate production was slower in trained muscles during contractile activity; the slower lactate production was accompanied by a slower rate of glycogen breakdown. These results are obviously at variance with the claim by Donovan and Brooks [52] that lactate production is unchanged by training. In addition, the radioactive tracer techniques used by Donovan and Brooks [52] and Freminet et al. [64] have been heavily criticized [29–31, 36, 158, 201]. Given these criticisms, the question of an increased clearance of lactate following training remains open.

There have been no direct assessments of the effect of training on lactate uptake by skeletal muscle. Aside from the Donovan and Brooks [52] study, it has been suggested that the rate of blood lactate decline during active recovery in humans following strenuous exercise may be faster in more well-trained subjects [12, 42, 68, 157]. Evans and Cureton [60] followed this suggestion by studying the effects of training on blood lactate decline during resting and exercising recovery. They found a greater rate of blood lactate disappearance at a given percentage of $\dot{V}o_2max$ (25%), but not at rest or at the same absolute work rate during recovery following training. The cause of the increased rate of blood lactate decline following training could be the ability to exercise at a greater work rate during recovery without increasing muscle lactate production and/or without reducing blood flow to lactate removal sites such as the liver.

The capacity of trained muscle to take up and utilize lactate in comparison to untrained muscle is unknown. However, it seems likely that endurance training would increase lactate utilization capacity. Sjodin [165] has shown that endurance training results in a decrease in the total LDH activity while at the same time the proportion of H-type isozyme is increased. In addition, the malate–aspartate shuttle enzymes are increased by endurance training [160]. As discussed previously for fiber type differences, an increase in the H-type isozyme component of LDH and an increase in the malate–aspartate shuttle enzymes should facilitate the conversion of lactate to pyruvate, and the subsequent oxidation of NADH, resulting in faster lactate utilization.

There is no direct evidence concerning the possible effects of endurance training on membrane transport processes for lactate. It is possible that membrane transport could be facilitated by the increased capillary density which has been reported to accompany endurance training [95, 159].

CONCLUSIONS

1. Lactate uptake is important because of the role of lactic acidosis and lactate in muscle fatigue and metabolism, as well as the clinical occurrence of lactic acidosis.
2. The rate of muscle lactate uptake is most likely limited by lactate utilization in the steady state. However, the rate of uptake may be limited by membrane transport processes during rapid changes in the transmembrane lactate concentration gradient.
3. There is little direct evidence relating to the role of metabolic and hormonal factors in the control of lactate utilization, but the following hypotheses have some merit: (*a*) Metabolic and hormonal factors which inhibit endogenous lactate production probably facilitate lactate utilization. (*b*) Activation of pyruvate dehydrogenase should enhance lactate utilization. (*c*) Ready availability of alternative substrates, for example, free fatty acids, may inhibit lactate utilization.
4. Several different types of experiments clearly show that increases in metabolic rate result in increases in lactate utilization, especially under conditions which do not promote endogenous lactate production. In

humans, there is indirect evidence that muscle lactate uptake is maximal at an exercise intensity which is just below the lactate threshold. Lactate uptake decreases at higher exercise intensities. A steady-state metabolic rate beyond which lactate uptake decreases has not yet been identified in studies of contracting in situ muscle.

5. There is a membrane carrier for lactate (lactic acid or lactate-H^+ symport, or lactate-OH^- antiport) in skeletal muscle. However, the exact contribution of this carrier to total lactate transport remains a topic of debate. In addition, there is no information concerning the physiological importance of this carrier during contractions, in different muscle fiber types, or following exercise training.

6. The transmembrane $[H^+]$ difference has a significant effect on the membrane transfer of lactate. As an example, under conditions of elevated extracellular lactate concentration, an increase in extracellular $[H^+]$ increases the extracellular concentration of undissociated lactic acid ($[HL]$). If the intracellular $[H^+]$ (and therefore intracellular $[HL]$) remains constant, lactate uptake will increase. This may be due to increased HL diffusion or to an increase in coupled lactate-H^+ symport (or lactate-OH^- antiport). On the other hand, an increased intracellular $[H^+]$ should influence membrane transport to reduce lactate uptake. However, an increase in intracellular $[H^+]$ will also inhibit glycolysis, and could perhaps increase lactate utilization. There is little evidence relating to this proposition.

7. There have been no direct tests of the role of muscle perfusion in lactate uptake. However, both an increased blood flow and an increased effective capillary density should promote lactate uptake. Increased blood flow should maintain a greater blood-to-muscle lactate concentration gradient and provide a source of hydrogen ions to reduce interstitial fluid alkalosis which may occur due to coupled lactate and proton uptake. Increased functional capillary density should increase the surface area for lactate transport and therefore increase lactate uptake for any given extracellular-to-intracellular lactate concentration gradient.

8. It seems likely that slow, oxidative muscle fibers have a greater capacity to take up and utilize lactate, but there is only indirect evidence to support this possibility.

9. Endurance-trained muscle should have a greater capacity for lactate uptake, but again there is little direct evidence to verify this idea.

ACKNOWLEDGMENTS

I appreciate the helpful discussions and advice of Drs. Graham Mainwood and Wendell Stainsby. I am also grateful to Drs. J. W. Yates and Ann Swank for their criticism of the original manuscript.

This work was supported by National Science Foundation Grant #RII-8610671 through the Kentucky EPSCoR Program.

REFERENCE

1. Ahlborg G, Hagenfeldt L, Wahren J: Substrate utilization by the inactive leg during one-leg or arm exercise. *J Appl Physiol* 39:718–723, 1975.
2. Ahlborg G, Hagenfeldt L, Wahren J: Influence of lactate infusion on glucose and FFA metabolism in man. *Scand J Clin Lab Invest* 36:193–201, 1976.
3. Åstrand P-O, Hultman E, Juhlin-Dannfelt A, Reynolds G: Disposal of lactate during and after strenuous exercise in humans. *J Appl Physiol* 61:338–343, 1986.
4. Baldwin KM, Hooker AM, Herrick RE: Lactate oxidative capacity in different types of muscle. *Biochem Biophys Res Commun* 83:151–157, 1978.
5. Bar U, Blanchaer MC: Glycogen and CO_2 production from glucose and lactate by red and white skeletal muscle. *Am J Physiol* 209:905–909, 1965.
6. Barbee RW, Stainsby WN, Chirtel SJ: Dynamics of O_2, CO_2, lactate and acid exchange during contractions and recovery. *J Appl Physiol* 54:1687–1692, 1983.
7. Barman, JM, Moreira MF, Consolazio F: Metabolic effects of local ischemia during muscular exercise. *Am J Physiol* 138:20–26, 1942.
8. Barr DP, Himwich HE: Studies in the physiology of muscular exercise. II. Comparison of arterial and venous blood following vigorous exercise. *J Biol Chem* 55:525–537, 1923.
9. Belcastro AN, Bonen A: Lactic acid removal rates during controlled and uncontrolled recovery exercise. *J Appl Physiol* 39:932–936, 1975.
10. Bersin RM, Arieff AI: Improved hemodynamic function during hypoxia with carbicarb, a new agent for the management of acidosis. *Circulation* 77:227–233, 1988.
11. Bihari D, Gimson AES, Lindridge J, Williams R: Lactic acidosis in fulminant hepatic failure. Some aspects of pathogenesis and prognosis. *J Hepatol* 1:405–416, 1985.
12. Bonen A, Belcastro AN: Comparison of self-selected recovery methods on lactic acid removal rates. *Med Sci Sports Exerc* 8:176–178, 1976.
13. Bonen A, Campbell CJ, Kirby RL, Belcastro AN: Relationship between slow-twitch muscle fibers and lactic acid removal. *Can J Appl Sport Sci* 3:160–162, 1978.
14. Bonen A, Campbell CJ, Kirby RL, Belcastro AN: A multiple regression model for blood lactate removal in man. *Pflügers Arch* 380:205–210, 1979.
15. Bonen A, Ness GW, Belcastro AN, Kirby RL: Mild exercise impedes glycogen repletion in muscle. *J Appl Physiol* 58:1622–1629, 1985.
16. Brevetti G, Chiariello M, Ferulano G, Policicchio A, Nevola E, Rossini A, Attisano T, Ambrosio G, Siliprandi N, Angelini C: Increases in walking distance in patients with peripheral vascular disease treated with L-carnitine: a double-blind, cross-over study. *Circulation* 77:767–773, 1988.
17. Brooks GA: Anaerobic threshold: review of the concept and directions for future research. *Med Sci Sports Exerc* 17:22–31, 1985.
18. Brooks GA: Lactate production under fully aerobic conditions: the lactate shuttle during rest and exercise. *Fed Proc* 45:2924–2929, 1986.
19. Brooks GA: The lactate shuttle during exercise and recovery. *Med Sci Sports Exerc* 18:360–368, 1986.
20. Brooks GA, Donovan CM, White TP: Estimation of anaerobic energy production and efficiency in rats during exercise. *J Appl Physiol* 56:520–525, 1984.
21. Cain SM: Appearance of excess lactate in anesthetized dogs during anemic and hypoxic hypoxia. *Am J Physiol* 209:604–610, 1965.
22. Carraro F, Klein S, Rosenblatt J, Wolfe RR: The effect of dichloroacetate on lactate concentration in exercising humans. *Physiologist* 30:227, 1987.

23. Cechetto D, Mainwood GW: Carbon dioxide and acid base balance in the isolated rat diaphragm. *Pflügers Arch* 376: 251–258, 1978.
24. Chapler CK, Stainsby WN: Carbohydrate metabolism in contracting dog skeletal muscle in situ. *Am J Physiol* 215:995–1004, 1968.
25. Chasiotis D, Hultman E, Sahlin K: Acidotic depression of cyclic AMP accumulation and phosphorylase b to a transformation in skeletal muscle of man. *J Physiol* 335:197–204, 1983.
26. Chasiotis D, Sahlin K, Hultman E: Regulation of glycogenolysis in human muscle in response to epinephrine infusion. *J Appl Physiol* 54:45–50, 1983.
27. Chirtel SJ, Barbee RW, Stainsby WN: Net O_2, CO_2, lactate, and acid exchange by muscle during progressive working contractions. *J Appl Physiol* 56:161–165, 1984.
28. Clark AS, Mitch WE, Goodman MN, Fagan JM, Goheer MA, Curnow RT: Dichloroacetate inhibits glycolysis and augments insulin-stimulated glycogen synthesis in rat muscle. *J Clin Invest* 79:588–594, 1987.
29. Cohen RD: The production and removal of lactate. In Bossart H, Perret C (eds): *Lactate in Acute Conditions.* New York, S. Karger, 1979, pp 10–19.
30. Cohen RD, Iles RA: Lactic acidosis: some physiological and clinical considerations. *Clin Sci Mol Med* 53:405–410, 1977.
31. Cohen RD, Woods HF: *Clinical and Biochemical Aspects of Lactic Acidosis.* London, Blackwell Scientific Publications, 1976.
32. Cohen RD, Woods HF: Lactic acidosis revisited. *Diabetes* 32:181–191, 1983.
33. Conlee RK, McLane JA, Rennie MJ, Winder WW, Holloszy JO: Reversal of phosphorylase activation in muscle despite continued contractile activity. *Am J Physiol* 237:R291–R296, 1979.
34. Connett RJ, Gayeski TEJ, Honig CR: Lactate accumulation in fully aerobic, working, dog gracilis muscle. *Am J Physiol* 246:H120–H128, 1984.
35. Connett RJ, Gayeski TEJ, Honig CR: Lactate efflux is unrelated to intracellular PO_2 in a working red muscle in situ. *J Appl Physiol* 61:402–408, 1986.
36. Connor H, Woods HF: Quantitative aspects of L($+$)-lactate metabolism in human beings. In *Metabolic Acidosis* (Ciba Foundation Symposium No. 87). London, Pitman Books, 1982, pp 214–227.
37. Corsi A, Zatti M, Midrio M, Granata AL: In situ oxidation of lactate by skeletal muscle during intermittent exercise. *FEBS Lett* 11:65–68, 1970.
38. Crabb DW, Yount EA, Harris RA: The metabolic effects of dichloroacetate. *Metabolism* 30:1024–1039, 1981.
39. Cunningham JN Jr, Carter NW, Rector FC Jr, Seldin DW: Resting transmembrane potential difference of skeletal muscle in normal subjects and severely ill patients. *J Clin Invest* 50:49–59, 1971.
40. Danforth WH: Activation of glycolytic pathway in muscle. In Chance B, Estabrook RW, Williamson JR (eds): *Control of Energy Metabolism.* London, Academic Press, 1965, pp 287–297.
41. Davies SF, Iber C, Keene SA, McArthur CD, Path MJ: Effect of respiratory alkalosis during exercise on blood lactate. *J Appl Physiol* 61:948–952, 1986.
42. Davies CTM, Knibbs AV, Musgrove J: The rate of lactic acid removal in relation to different baselines of recovery exercise. *Int Z Angew Physiol* 28:155–161, 1970.
43. Davis JA: Anaerobic threshold: review of the concept and directions for future research. *Med Sci Sports Exerc* 17:6–18, 1985.
44. Dawson DM, Goodfriend TL, Kaplan NO: Lactic dehydrogenases: functions of the two types. *Science* 143:929–933, 1964.
45. De Hemptinne A, Marrannes R, Vanheel B: Influence of organic acids on intracellular pH. *Am J Physiol* 245:C178–C183, 1983.

46. Dennis SC, Kohn MC, Anderson GJ, Garfinkel D: Kinetic analysis of monocarboxylate uptake into perfused rat hearts. *J Mol Cell Cardiol* 17:987–995, 1985.
47. Depocas F, Minaire Y, Chatonnet J: Rates of formation and oxidation of lactic acid in dogs at rest and during moderate exercise. *Can J Physiol Pharmacol* 47:603–610, 1969.
48. Deuticke B: Monocarboxylate transport in erythrocytes. *J Membr Biol* 70:89–103, 1982.
49. Deuticke B, Beyer E, Forst B: Discrimination of three parallel pathways of lactate transport in the human erythrocyte membrane by inhibitors and kinetic properties. *Biochim Biophys Acta* 684:96–110, 1982.
50. Dobson GP, Yamamoto E, Hochachka PW: Phosphofructokinase control in muscle: nature and reversal of pH-dependent ATP inhibition. *Am J Physiol* 250:R71–R76, 1986.
51. Dodd S, Powers SK, Callender T, Brooks E: Blood lactate disappearance at various intensities of recovery exercise. *J Appl Physiol* 57:1462–1465, 1984.
52. Donovan CM, Brooks GA: Endurance training affects lactate clearance, not lactate production. *Am J Physiol* 244:E83–E92, 1983.
53. Dubinsky WP, Racker E: The mechanisms of lactate transport in human erythrocytes. *J Membr Biol* 44:25–36, 1978.
54. Dunn RB, Critz JB: Uptake of lactate by dog skeletal muscle in vivo and the effect of free fatty acids. *Am J Physiol* 229:255–259, 1975.
55. Edwards RHT, Clode M: The effect of hyperventilation on the lactacidaemia of muscular exercise. *Clin Sci* 38:269–276, 1970.
56. Ehrsam RE, Heigenhauser GJF, Jones NL: Effect of respiratory acidosis on metabolism in exercise. *J Appl Physiol* 53:63–69, 1982.
57. Eldridge FL: Relationship between turnover rate and blood concentration of lactate in exercising dogs. *J Appl Physiol* 39:231–234, 1975.
58. Eldridge F, Salzer J: Effect of respiratory alkalosis on blood lactate and pyruvate in humans. *J Appl Physiol* 22:461–468, 1967.
59. Essen B, Pernow B, Gollnick PD, Saltin B: Muscle glycogen content and lactate uptake in exercising muscles. In Howald H, Poortmans JR (eds): *Metabolic Adaptations to Prolonged Physical Exercise.* Basel, Birkhauser, 1975, pp 130–134.
60. Evans BW, Cureton KJ: Effect of physical conditioning on blood lactate disappearance after supramaximal exercise. *Br J Sports Med* 17:40–45, 1983.
61. Evans OB: Dichloroacetate tissue concentrations and its relationship to hypolactatemia and pyruvate dehydrogenase activation. *Biochem Pharmacol* 31:3124–3126, 1982.
62. Favier RJ, Constable SH, Chen M, Holloszy JO: Endurance exercise training reduces lactate production. *J Appl Physiol* 61:885–889, 1986.
63. Fishbein WN: Lactate transporter defect: a new disease of muscle. *Science* 234:1254–1256, 1986.
64. Freminet A, Poyart C, Bursaux E, Tablon T: Effect of physical training on the rates of lactate turnover and oxidation in rats. In Howald H, Poortmans JR (eds): *Metabolic Adaptations to Prolonged Physical Exercise.* Basel, Birkhauser, 1975, pp 113–118.
65. Freyschuss U, Strandell T: Limb circulation during arm and leg exercise in supine position. *J Appl Physiol* 23:163–170, 1967.
66. Futre EMP, Noakes TD, Raine RI, Terblanche SE: Muscle glycogen repletion during active postexercise recovery. *Am J Physiol* 253:E305–E311, 1987.
67. Gimenez M, Florentz M: Effects of hypercapnia on the glycolytic metabolism, enzyme activity and myoglobin of stimulated skeletal muscle in the rat. *Bull Eur Physiopathol Respir* 15:269–284, 1979.
68. Gisolfi C, Robinson S, Turrell ES: Effects of aerobic work performed during recovery from exhausting work. *J Appl Physiol* 21:1767–1772, 1966.

69. Gladden LB: Current "anaerobic threshold" controversies. *Physiologist* 27:312–318, 1984.
70. Gladden LB, Stamford BA, Weltman A, Stainsby WN: Effect of lactic acid on isometric developed tension in canine skeletal muscle. *Fed Proc* 39:280, 1980.
71. Gladden LB, Yates JW: Lactic acid infusion in dogs: effects of varying infusate pH. *J Appl Physiol* 54:1254–1260, 1983.
72. Gollnick PD, Bayly WM, Hodgson DR: Exercise intensity, training, diet, and lactate concentration in muscle and blood. *Med Sci Sports Exerc* 18:334–340, 1986.
73. Gollnick PD, Hodgson DR: The identification of fiber types in skeletal muscle: a continual dilemma. In Pandolf KB, (ed): *Exercise and Sport Sciences Reviews*. New York, MacMillan, 1986, vol 14, pp 81–104.
74. Goodman MN, Ruderman NB, Aoki TT: Glucose and amino acid metabolism in perfused skeletal muscle. Effect of dichloroacetate. *Diabetes* 27:1065–1074, 1978.
75. Graf H, Leach W, Arieff AI: Effects of dichloroacetate in the treatment of hypoxic lactic acidosis in dogs. *J Clin Invest* 76:919–923, 1985.
76. Graham TE, Barclay JK, Wilson BA; Skeletal muscle lactate release and glycolytic intermediates during hypercapnia. *J Appl Physiol* 60:568–575, 1986.
77. Graham TE, Sinclair DG, Chapler CK: Metabolic intermediates and lactate diffusion in active dog skeletal muscle, *Am J Physiol* 231:766–771, 1976.
78. Graham T, Wilson BA, Sample M, Van Dijk J, Bonen A: The effects of hypercapnia on metabolic responses to progressive exhaustive work. *Med Sci Sports Exerc* 12:278–284, 1980.
79. Graham TE, Wilson BA, Sample M, Van Dijk J, Goslin B: The effects of hypercapnia on the metabolic response to steady-state exercise. *Med Sci Sports Exerc* 14:286–291, 1982.
80. Granata AL, Midrio M, Corsi A: Lactate oxidation by skeletal muscle during sustained contraction in vivo. *Pflügers Arch* 366:247–250, 1976.
81. Gray SD, Renkin EM: Microvascular supply in relation to fiber metabolic type in mixed skeletal muscles of rabbits. *Microvasc Res* 16:406–425, 1978.
82. Halestrap AP, Denton RM: Specific inhibition of pyruvate transport in rat liver mitochondria and human erythrocytes by α-cyano-4-hydroxycinnamate. *Biochem J* 138:313–316, 1974.
83. Harris P, Bateman M, Gloster J: The regional metabolism of lactate and pyruvate during exercise in patients with rheumatic heart disease. *Clin Sci* 23:545–560, 1962.
84. Hermansen L: Effect of metabolic changes on force generation in skeletal muscle during maximal exercise. In *Human Muscle Fatigue: Physiological Mechanisms* (Ciba Foundation Symposium No. 82). London, Pitman Medical, 1981, pp 75–88.
85. Hermansen L, Stensvold I: Production and removal of lactate during exercise in man. *Acta Physiol Scand* 86:191–201, 1972.
86. Hermansen L, Vaage O: Lactate disappearance and glycogen synthesis in human muscle after maximal exercise. *Am J Physiol* 233:E422–E429, 1977.
87. Hirche H, Hombach V, Langohr HD, Wacker U, Busse J: Lactic acid permeation rate in working gastrocnemii of dogs during metabolic alkalosis and acidosis. *Pflügers Arch* 356:209–222, 1975.
88. Hirche H, Wacker U, Langohr HD: Lactic acid formation in the working gastrocnemius of the dog. *Int Z Angew Physiol* 30:52–64, 1971.
89. Hogan MC, Cox RH, Welch HG: Lactate accumulation during incremental exercise with varied inspired oxygen fractions. *J Appl Physiol* 55:1134–1140, 1983.
90. Hogan MC, Welch HG: Effect of varied lactate levels on biocycle ergometer performance. *J Appl Physiol* 57:507–513, 1984.
91. Hogan MC, Welch HG: Effect of altered arterial O_2 tensions on muscle metabolism in dog skeletal muscle during fatiguing work. *Am J Physiol* 251:C216–C222, 1986.

92. Holloszy JO, Coyle EF: Adaptations of skeletal muscle to endurance exercise and their metabolic consequences. *J Appl Physiol* 56:831–838, 1984.

93. Hoppeler H, Kayar SR: Capillarity and oxidative capacity of muscles. *News Physiol Sci* 3:113–116, 1988.

94. Hubbard JL: The effect of exercise on lactate metabolism. *J Physiol* 231:1–18, 1973.

95. Hudlicka O, Hoppeler H, Uhlmann E: Relationship between the size of the capillary bed and oxidative capacity in various cat skeletal muscles. *Pflügers Arch* 410:369–375, 1987.

96. Hultman E, Sahlin K: Acid-base balance during exercise. In Hutton RS, Miller DI (eds): *Exercise and Sport Sciences Reviews.* Philadelphia, The Franklin Institute Press, 1980, vol 8, pp 41–128.

97. Hundal HS, Rennie MJ, Watt PW: Characteristics of L-glutamine transport in perfused rat skeletal muscle. *J Physiol* 393:283–305, 1987.

98. Issekutz B Jr, Shaw WAS, Issekutz AC: Lactate metabolism in resting and exercising dogs. *J Appl Physiol* 40:312–319, 1976.

99. Jacobs I: Lactate, muscle glycogen and exercise performance in man. *Acta Physiol Scand (Suppl)* 495:1–35, 1981.

100. Jervell O: Investigation of the concentration of lactic acid in blood and urine under physiologic and pathologic conditions. *Acta Med Scand (Suppl)* 24:1–135, 1928.

101. Johnson JH, Belt JA, Dubinsky WP, Zimniak A, Racker E: Inhibition of lactate transport in Ehrlich Ascites tumor cells and human erythrocytes by a synthetic anhydride of lactic acid. *Biochemistry* 19:3836–3840, 1980.

102. Jones NL, Sutton JR, Taylor R, Toews CJ: Effect of pH on cardiorespiratory and metabolic responses to exercise. *J Appl Physiol* 43:959–964, 1977.

103. Jorfeldt L: Metabolism of L(+)-lactate in human skeletal muscle during exercise. *Acta Physiol Scand (Suppl)* 338: 1–167, 1970.

104. Jorfeldt L, Juhlin-Dannfelt A, Karlsson J: Lactate release in relation to tissue lactate in human skeletal muscle during exercise. *J Appl Physiol* 44:350–352, 1978.

105. Juel C: Intracellular pH recovery and lactate efflux in mouse soleus muscles stimulated in vitro: the involvement of sodium/proton exchange and a lactate carrier. *Acta Physiol Scand* 132:363–371, 1988.

106. Juhlin-Dannfelt A: Metabolic effects of β-adrenoceptor blockade on skeletal muscle at rest and during exercise. *Acta Med Scand (Suppl)* 665:113–115, 1982.

107. Karlsson J, Bonde-Petersen F, Henriksson J, Knuttgen HG: Effects of previous exercise with arms or legs on metabolism and performance in exhaustive exercise. *J Appl Physiol* 38:763–767, 1975.

108. Karlsson J, Jacobs I: Onset of blood lactate accumulation during muscular exercise as a threshold concept. I. Theoretical considerations. *Int J Sports Med* 3:190–201, 1982.

109. Karlsson J, Rosell S, Saltin B: Carbohydrate and fat metabolism in contracting canine skeletal muscle. *Pflügers Arch* 331:57–69, 1972.

110. Katz A, Sahlin K: Regulation of lactic acid production during exercise. *J Appl Physiol* 65:509–518, 1988.

111. Katz A, Sahlin K: Effect of decreased oxygen availability on NADH and lactate contents in human skeletal muscle during exercise. *Acta Physiol Scand* 131:119–127, 1987.

112. Katz A, Sahlin K, Juhlin-Dannfelt A: Effect of β-adrenoceptor blockade on H^+ and K^+ flux in exercising humans. *J Appl Physiol* 59:336–341, 1985.

113. Knuttgen HG, Saltin B: Oxygen uptake, muscle high-energy phosphates, and lactate in exercise under acute hypoxic conditions in man. *Acta Physiol Scand* 87:368–376, 1973.

114. Koch A, Webster B, Lowell S: Cellular uptake of L-lactate in mouse diaphragm. *Biophys J* 36:775–796, 1981.
115. Kowalchuk JM, Heigenhauser GJF, Jones NL: Effect of pH on metabolic and cardiorespiratory responses during progressive exercise. *J Appl Physiol* 57:1558–1563, 1984.
116. Krebs EG, Love DS, Bratvold GE, Trayser KA, Meyer WL, Fischer EH: Purification and properties of rabbit skeletal muscle phosphorylase b kinase. *Biochemistry* 3:1022–1033, 1964.
117. Krebs HA, Hems R, Weidemann MJ, Speake RN: The fate of isotopic carbon in kidney cortex synthesizing glucose from lactate. *Biochem J* 101:242–249, 1966.
118. Kreisberg RA: Lactate homeostasis and lactic acidosis. *Ann Intern Med* 92:227–237, 1980.
119. Loubatieres AL, Ribes G, Valette G: Pharmacological agents and acute experimental hyperlactataemia in the dog. *Br J Pharmacol* 58:429P, 1976.
120. Loubatieres A, Ribes G, Valette G, Rondot A-M: Correction de l'hyperlactatémie et de l'acidose lactique expérimentales par le dichloroacétate de sodium. *C R Acad Sci Ser D (Paris)* 283:1803–1805, 1976.
121. Mainwood GW, Cechetto D: The effect of bicarbonate concentration on fatigue and recovery in isolated rat diaphragm muscle. *Can J Physiol Pharmacol* 58:624–632, 1980.
122. Mainwood GW, Renaud JM: The effect of acid-base balance on fatigue of skeletal muscle. *Can J Physiol Pharmacol* 63:403–416, 1985.
123. Mainwood GW, Renaud JM, Mason MJ: The pH dependence of the contractile response of fatigued skeletal muscle. *Can J Physiol Pharmacol* 65:648–658, 1987.
124. Mainwood GW, Worsley-Brown P: The effects of extracellular pH and buffer concentration on the efflux of lactate from frog sartorius muscle. *J Physiol* 250:1–22, 1975.
125. Mainwood GW, Worsley-Brown P, Paterson RA: The metabolic changes in frog sartorius muscles during recovery from fatigue at different external bicarbonate concentrations. *Can J Physiol Pharmacol* 50:143–155, 1972.
126. Mann GE, Zlokovic BV, Yudilevich DL: Evidence for a lactate transport system in the sarcolemmal membrane of the perfused rabbit heart: kinetics of unidirectional influx, carrier specificity and effects of glucagon. *Biochim Biophys Acta* 819:241–248, 1985.
127. Mansour TE: Phosphofructokinase activity in skeletal muscle extracts following administration of epinephrine. *J Biol Chem* 247:6057–6066, 1972.
128. Margaria R, Cerretelli P, Di Prampero PE, Massari C, Torelli G: Kinetics and mechanism of oxygen debt contraction in man. *J Appl Physiol* 18:371–377, 1963.
129. Mason MJ, Mainwood GW, Thoden JS: The influence of extracellular buffer concentration and propionate on lactate efflux from frog muscle. *Pflügers Arch* 406:472–479, 1986.
130. Mason MJ, Thomas RC: A microelectrode study of the mechanisms of L-lactate entry into and release from frog sartorius muscle. *J Physiol* 400:459–479, 1988.
131. Mazzeo RS, Brooks GA, Schoeller DA, Budinger TF: Disposal of blood [1-^{13}C]lactate in humans during rest and exercise. *J Appl Physiol* 60:232–241, 1986.
132. McCartney N, Heigenhauser GJF, Jones NL: Effects of pH on maximal power output and fatigue during short-term dynamic exercise. *J Appl Physiol* 55:225–229, 1983.
133. McGrail JC, Bonen A, Belcastro AN: Dependence of lactate removal on muscle metabolism in man. *Eur J Appl Physiol* 39:89–97, 1978.
134. McLane JA, Holloszy JO: Glycogen synthesis from lactate in the three types of skeletal muscle. *J Biol Chem* 254:6548–6553, 1979.
135. Merrill GF, Zambraski EJ, Grassl SM: Effect of dichloroacetate on plasma lactic acid in exercising dogs. *J Appl Physiol* 48:427–431, 1980.

136. Metzger JM, Fitts RH: Role of intracellular pH in muscle fatigue. *J Appl Physiol* 62:1392–1397, 1987.

137. Moll W, Girard H, Gros G: Facilitated diffusion of lactic acid in the guinea pig placenta. *Pflügers Arch* 385:229–238, 1980.

138. Morris ME, Millar RA: Blood pH/plasma catecholamine relationships: respiratory acidosis. *Br J Anaesth* 34:672–681, 1962.

139. Morris ME, Millar RA: Blood pH/plasma catecholamine relationships: non-respiratory acidosis. *Br J Anaesth* 34:682–689, 1962.

140. Morrow JA, Fell RD, Gladden LB: Respiratory alkalosis: no effect on blood lactate decline or exercise performance. *Eur J Appl Physiol* 58:175–181, 1988.

141. Newman EV, Dill DB, Edwards HT, Webster FA: The rate of lactic acid removal in exercise. *Am J Physiol* 118:457–462, 1937.

142. Oldendorf WH: Blood brain barrier permeability to lactate. *Eur Neurol* 6:49–55, 1972.

143. Omachi A, Lifson N: Metabolism of isotopic lactate by the isolated perfused dog gastrocnemius. *Am J Physiol* 185:35–40, 1956.

144. Park R, Arieff AI: Lactic acidosis: current concepts. *Clin Endocrinol Metab* 12:339–358, 1983.

145. Pearce FJ, Connett RJ: Effect of lactate and palmitate on substrate utilization of isolated rat soleus. *Am J Physiol* 238:C149–C159, 1980.

146. Peter JB, Barnard RJ, Edgerton VR, Gillespie CA, Stempel KA: Metabolic profiles of three types of skeletal muscle in guinea pigs and rabbits. *Biochemistry* 11:2627–2633, 1972.

147. Piiper J: Production of lactic acid in heavy exercise and acid-base balance. In Moret PR, Weber J, Haissly J-CL, Denolin H (eds): *Lactate: Physiologic, Methodologic and Pathologic Approach.* New York, Springer-Verlag, 1980, pp 35–45.

148. Poortmans JR, Bossche JD-V, Leclercq R: Lactate uptake by inactive forearm during progressive leg exercise. *J Appl Physiol* 45:835–839, 1978.

149. Rammal K, Strom G: The rate of lactate utilization in man during work and at rest. *Acta Physiol Scand* 17:452–456, 1949.

150. Rennie MJ, Fell RD, Ivy JL, Holloszy JO: Adrenaline reactivation of muscle phosphorylase after deactivation during phasic contractile activity. *Biosci Rep* 2:323–331, 1982.

151. Rennie MJ, Idstrom J-P, Mann GE, Schersten T, Bylund-Fellenius A-C: A paired-tracer dilution method for characterizing membrane transport in the perfused rat hindlimb. *Biochem J* 214:737–743, 1983.

152. Richter EA, Ruderman NB, Gavras H, Belur ER, Galbo H; Muscle glycogenolysis during exercise: dual control by epinephrine and contractions. *Am J Physiol* 242:E25–E32, 1982.

153. Roos A: Intracellular pH and distribution of weak acids across cell membranes. A study of D- and L-lactate and of DMO in rat diaphragm. *J Physiol* 249:1–25, 1975.

154. Rose CE Jr, Althaus JA, Kaiser DL, Miller ED, Carey RM: Acute hypoxemia and hypercapnia: increase in plasma catecholamines in conscious dogs. *Am J Physiol* 245:H924–H929, 1983.

155. Rovetto MJ, Whitmer JT, Neely JR: Comparison of the effects of anoxia and whole heart ischemia on carbohydrate utilization in isolated working rat hearts. *Circ Res* 32:699–711, 1973.

156. Rowell LB, Kraning KK II, Evans TO, Kennedy JW, Blackmon JR, Kusumi F: Splanchnic removal of lactate and pyruvate during prolonged exercise in man. *J Appl Physiol* 21:1773–1783, 1966.

157. Ryan WJ, Sutton JR, Toews CJ, Jones NL: Metabolism of infused L(+)-lactate during exercise. *Clin Sci* 56:139–146, 1979.

158. Sahlin K: Lactate production cannot be measured with tracer techniques (letter to the editor). *Am J Physiol* 252:E439–E440, 1987.
159. Saltin B, Gollnick PD: Skeletal muscle adaptability: significance for metabolism and performance. In Peachey LD (ed): *Handbook of Physiology: Skeletal Muscle.* Bethesda, MD, American Physiological Society, 1983, pp 555–631.
160. Schantz PG: Plasticity of human skeletal muscle with special reference to effects of physical training on enzyme levels of the NADH shuttles and phenotypic expression of slow and fast isoforms of myofibrillar proteins. *Acta Physiol Scand (Suppl)* 558:1–62, 1986.
161. Schneider SH, Komanicky PM, Goodman MN, Ruderman NB: Dichloroacetate: effects on exercise endurance in untrained rats. *Metabolism* 30:590–595, 1981.
162. Schwartz WB, Waters WC III. Lactate versus bicarbonate. A reconsideration of the therapy of metabolic acidosis (Editorial). *Am J Med* 32:831–834, 1962.
163. Seo Y: Effects of extracellular pH on lactate efflux from frog sartorius muscle. *Am J Physiol* 247:C175–C181, 1984.
164. Shiota M, Golden S, Katz J: Lactate metabolism in the perfused rat hindlimb. *Biochem J* 222:281–292, 1984.
165. Sjodin B: Lactate dehydrogenase in human skeletal muscle. *Acta Physiol Scand (Suppl)* 436:1–32, 1976.
166. Sparks HV Jr. Capillary endothelium: a metabolic barrier for solute transport. *Fed Proc* 44:2602, 1985.
167. Spencer TL, Lehninger AL: L-lactate transport in Ehrlich Ascites tumor cells. *Biochem J* 154:405–414, 1976.
168. Spriet LL, Lindinger MI, Heigenhauser GJF, Jones NL: Effects of alkalosis on skeletal muscle metabolism and performance during exercise. *Am J Physiol* 251:R833–R839, 1986.
169. Spriet LL, Matsos CG, Peters SJ, Heigenhauser GJF, Jones NL: Muscle metabolism and performance in perfused rat hindquarter during heavy exercise. *Am J Physiol* 248:C109–C118, 1985.
170. Spriet LL, Matsos CG, Peters SJ, Heigenhauser GJF, Jones NL: Effects of acidosis on rat muscle metabolism and performance during heavy exercise. *Am J Physiol* 248:C337–C347, 1985.
171. Spriet LL, Ren JM, Hultman E: Epinephrine infusion enhances muscle glycogenolysis during prolonged electrical stimulation. *J Appl Physiol* 64:1439–1444, 1988.
172. Stainsby WN: Biochemical and physiological bases for lactate production. *Med Sci Sports Exerc* 18:341–343, 1986.
173. Stainsby WN, Eitzman PD: Lactic acid output of cat gastrocnemius-plantaris during repetitive twitch contractions. *Med Sci Sports Exerc* 18:668–673, 1986.
174. Stainsby WN, Sumners C, Andrew GM: Plasma catecholamines and their effect on blood lactate and muscle lactate output. *J Appl Physiol* 57:321–325, 1984.
175. Stainsby WN, Sumners C, Eitzman PD: Effects of catecholamines on lactic acid output during progressive working contractions. *J Appl Physiol* 59:1809–1814, 1985.
176. Stainsby WN, Sumners C, Eitzman PD: Effects of adrenergic agonists and antagonists on muscle O_2 uptake and lactate metabolism. *J Appl Physiol* 62:1845–1851, 1987.
177. Stainsby WN, Welch HG: Lactate metabolism of contracting dog skeletal muscle in situ. *Am J Physiol* 211:177–183, 1966.
178. Stamford BA, Moffatt RJ, Weltman A, Maldonado C, Curtis M: Blood lactate disappearance after supramaximal one-legged exercise. *J Appl Physiol* 45:244–248, 1978.
179. Stamford BA, Weltman A, Moffatt R, Sady S: Exercise recovery above and below anaerobic threshold following maximal work. *J Appl Physiol* 51:840–844, 1981.
180. Stanley WC, Brooks GA: Measuring lactate production (letter to the editor) *Am J Physiol* 253:E472–E473, 1987.

181. Stanley WC, Gertz EW, Wisneski JA, Morris DL, Neese RA, Brooks GA: Systemic lactate kinetics during graded exercise in man. *Am J Physiol* 249:E595–E602, 1985.

182. Stanley WC, Gertz EW, Wisneski JA, Neese RA, Morris DL, Brooks GA: Lactate extraction during net lactate release in legs of humans during exercise. *J Appl Physiol* 60:1116–1120, 1986.

183. Steinhagen C, Hirche H, Nestle HW, Bovenkamp U, Hosselmann I: The interstitial pH of the working gastrocnemius muscle of the dog. *Pflügers Arch* 367:151–156, 1976.

184. Storelli C, Corcelli A, Cassano G, Hildmann B, Murer H, Lippe C: Polar distribution of sodium-dependent and sodium-independent transport system for L-lactate in the plasma membrane of rat enterocytes. *Pflügers Arch* 338:11–16, 1980.

185. Sutton JR, Jones NL, Toews CJ: Effect of pH on muscle glycolysis during exercise. *Clin Sci* 61:331–338, 1981.

186. Tesch PA, Wright JE: Recovery from short term intense exercise: its relation to capillary supply and blood lactate concentration. *Eur J Appl Physiol* 52:98–103, 1983.

187. Trivedi B, Danforth WH: Effect of pH on the kinetics of frog muscle phosphofructokinase. *J Biol Chem* 241:4110–4114, 1966.

188. Ui M: A role of phosphofructokinase in pH-dependent regulation of glycolysis. *Biochim Biophys Acta* 124:310–322, 1966.

189. Waddell WJ, Bates RG: Intracellular pH. *Physiol Rev* 49:285–329, 1969.

190. Wasserman K: The anaerobic threshold measurement to evaluate exercise performance. *Am Rev Respir Dis* 129:S35–S40, 1984.

191. Wasserman K: Anaerobiosis, lactate, and gas exchange during exercise: the issues. *Fed Proc* 45:2904–2909, 1986.

192. Watt PW, MacLennan PA, Hundal HS, Kuret CM, Rennie MJ: L(+) lactate transport in perfused rat skeletal muscle: kinetic characteristics and sensitivity to pH and transport inhibitors. *Biochim Biophys Acta* 944:213–222, 1988.

193. Welch HG: Effects of hypoxia and hyperoxia on human performance. In Pandolf KB (ed): *Exercise and Sport Sciences Reviews.* New York, MacMillan, 1987, vol 15, 191–221.

194. Welch HG, Bonde-Petersen F, Graham T, Klausen K, Secher N: Effects of hyperoxia on leg blood flow and metabolism during exercise. *J Appl Physiol* 42:385–390, 1977.

195. Welch HG, Stainsby WN: Oxygen debt in contracting dog skeletal muscle in situ. *Respir Physiol* 3:229–242, 1967.

196. Weltman A, Stamford BA, Fulco C: Recovery from maximal effort exercise: lactate disappearance and subsequent performance. *J Appl Physiol* 47:677–682, 1979.

197. Weltman A, Stamford BA, Moffatt RJ, Katch VL: Exercise recovery, lactate removal, and subsequent high intensity exercise performance. *Res Q* 48:786–796, 1977.

198. Whitehouse S, Randle PJ: Activation of pyruvate dehydrogenase in perfused rat heart by dichloroacetate. *Biochem J* 134:651–653, 1973.

199. Wildenthal K, Mierzwiak DS, Myers RW, Mitchell JF: Effects of acute lactic acidosis on left ventricular performance. *Am J Physiol* 214:1352–1359, 1968.

200. Wolfe BR, Graham TE, Barclay JK: Hyperoxia, mitochondrial redox state, and lactate metabolism of in situ canine muscle. *Am J Physiol* 253:C263–C268, 1987.

201. Wolfe RR, Jahoor F, Miyoshi H: Evaluation of the isotopic equilibration between lactate and pyruvate. *Am J Physiol* E532–E535, 1988.

202. Woll PJ, Record CO: Lactate elimination in man: effects of lactate concentration and hepatic dysfunction. *Eur J Clin Invest* 9:397–404, 1979.

203. Yates JW, Gladden LB, Cresanta MK: Effects of prior dynamic leg exercise on static effort of the elbow flexors. *J Appl Physiol* 55:891–896, 1983.

204. Yudilevich DL, Mann GE: Unidirectional uptake of substrates at the blood side of secretory epithelia: stomach, salivary gland, pancreas. *Fed Proc* 41:3045–3053, 1982.

5
Eccentric Action of Muscles: Physiology, Injury, and Adaptation

WILLIAM T. STAUBER, Ph.D.

Skeletal muscle performs multiple functions in humans, including bio-mechanical, thermogenic, and even cosmetic functions. In addition, muscle is composed of protein and serves as a protein reservoir for times of extreme need. The function most frequently discussed in physiology is generally the mechanical one, since all interactions of humans with their environment, including breathing, require coordinated muscle actions.

In performing movements, skeletal muscles are required to function as motors, springs, shock absorbers, and stabilizers. Classical muscle physiology has focused its attention, for the most part, on the motor (muscle shortening) and stabilizer (tension development) functions, referred to as concentric and isometric muscle actions, respectively. Most frequently, electrophysiology, muscle mechanics, and energetics were investigated using muscles studied under in vitro conditions where the muscle was active and allowed to shorten (concentric muscle action) or kept at a constant external length (isometric muscle action). That is not to say that the importance of spring and shock absorption functions (eccentric muscle action) was ignored even in the early studies of muscle physiology [1, 2, 68]. Within the last 10 years, there has been increased interest in how muscles resist externally applied forces and how eccentric muscle action leads to delayed-onset muscle soreness. However, it has been difficult to develop a clear picture of the importance of eccentric muscle actions and any resultant muscle adaptation because, in part, the subject has been discussed under quite diverse topics that include classification some of which do not even exist in standard medical reference systems (these include stretch–shortening cycles [78], eccentric exercise [28], downhill walking [5] and running [109], negative work production [8], lengthening contractions [90], and decelerator muscle function [59]).

To add to the difficulty described above, some confusion exists in terminology used to define this subject. What is the best designation for an active muscle which is stretched by an imposed load? The simplest method is to describe the work performed. So, for a muscle that was stretched by an external load, work would be absorbed or be negative. In contrast, the work performed by a muscle that was shortening would be positive. Using this convention, special terms would be needed for

157

muscle actions at fixed lengths (isometric) where no external work is performed but internal work varies with the tension developed by the muscle. The terms *concentric* and *eccentric* are widely used to describe the shortening and lengthening actions of muscles, but they are not without difficulty. Use of *eccentric* can result in strange phrases such as "eccentric exercise" or "eccentric contractions." (The words *concentric* and *eccentric* seem to have originated in 1953 in a paper by Asmussen [8]. The spelling used at that time was "excentric," which might have eliminated some confusion if it were still used today.) Other terms have been suggested, such as "resisted muscle shortening" and "resisted muscle lengthening" [119], which are accurate but cumbersome. Still others used are *isometric*, *miometric*, and *pliometric* [75]. To simplify matters, Cavanagh suggested the modification of terminology currently in vogue but with slight variation [23]. Active muscles can be simply referred to as performing isometric action, concentric action (shortening), and eccentric action (lengthening). This review will follow Cavanagh's terminology except where specific examples require the terminology used by the original investigators.

The focus of this discussion will be on the physiology of eccentric muscle action, the possible dysfunction produced by eccentric muscle action and the adaptive nature of activities which include eccentric muscle action both of a chronic and acute nature. The emphasis will be on human responses, although results of animal research will be presented in areas where insufficient evidence exists for humans. Lastly, some consideration will be given to the possibility of decelerator deficits and abnormal adaptation from exercises involving repetitive eccentric muscle action and the potential use of these exercises in rehabilitation.

PHYSIOLOGY

Much is known about the physiology of active human skeletal muscle under conditions of resisted shortening (concentric action) [130]. The variation of tension as a function of shortening velocity is a fundamental property of muscle mechanics (as described by the Hill equation [55]; it appears in abbreviated form in almost every textbook on physiology). Simply stated, the tension developed by an active muscle decreases as the shortening velocity increases (concentric muscle action). If the external force overcomes the ability of the muscle to actively resist, the muscle lengthens (eccentric muscle action) but only after producing additional tension [68]. (The origin of this additional tension has been debated often and was recently reviewed in detail [23].) One theory explaining the force–velocity relationship is the cross-bridge theory of muscle action [60]. This theory will be used to account for the active tension which exceeds that tension recorded for the concentric muscle action when a muscle is tetanized and stretched.

Force–Velocity

According to the cross-bridge theory [60] the active force generated by a single cross-bridge within a sarcomere results from the binding of actin and myosin by high-affinity electrostatic bonds, cross-bridge movement (tension and shortening), and the dissociation of actin and myosin in the presence of adenosine triphosphate (ATP) (relaxation) with the subsequent recharging of the myosin for the next cycle. The rate of shortening of a sarcomere is dependent on the ability of many myosins to move to their next respective actin along the thin filaments. The shortening process is opposed by the force of the load which tends to lengthen the sarcomere. For each cross-bridge cycle, energy is consumed, even if, as with isometric muscle actions, the external length of the muscle remains constant (tension-time heat or internal work).

At rest myosin exists in a preenergized or a high-energy form and tropomyosin rests on the binding sites of actin, preventing cross-bridge formation. When the muscle is activated by processes of excitation–contraction coupling, binding of myosin to actin automatically takes place because the inhibition imposed by the tropomyosin on the actin binding site is removed by the interaction of calcium with troponin. Normally cross-bridges form and sarcomere shortening or tension results as the potential energy stored in the preenergized myosin becomes transformed into the mechanical events of cross-bridge action (tension or shortening). If, however, immediately after the binding reaction occurs the cross-bridge is forcibly pulled backward, the actin–myosin bond would break before transduction of energy could occur. This separation of the cross-bridge would require more force than recorded from normal cross-bridge cycling. The energized myosin, which has not lost its potential energy, could reattach only to be pulled apart again if the external force is maintained. Each of these attachment–separation reactions produces a recorded tension (resistance to stretch) by the muscle but with no apparent energy consumption because the cross-bridge has not cycled but continues to remain in the high-energy form. The tension recorded at a given sarcomere length would be greater than that during isometric action and independent of velocity until the velocity of stretch exceeded the binding rate of the cross-bridges (this situation is what Loeb [85] referred to as "the pulling apart of two parallel strings of permanent magnets"). On the other hand, if the stretch were performed at very slow velocities, a few of the cross-bridges would have time to cycle (shorten) and reduce the net tension recorded in response to the stretch. Such a force–velocity relationship was proposed early in the history of muscle mechanics [3] and seems to be valid for intact human muscle [77].

Muscle Injury

The model of the cross-bridge detachment is helpful in understanding how injury can occur from forced muscle lengthening of an active muscle (eccentric action) as well as in explaining some observations of muscle action in humans. However, it has definite limitations. For instance, it does not explain muscle responses to very brief stretches which may involve actual physical lengthening of the myofilaments [49]. Even so, the model provides a conceptual framework to model how myofibers generate more tension when undergoing eccentric muscle action, an event which occurs in everyday human performance.

The first report that human muscles could develop more dynamic tension during eccentric muscle action came from the laboratory of one of the pioneers in exercise science. Singh and Karpovich [112] demonstrated that human muscles under voluntary control could develop more dynamic tension during eccentric muscle action than during concentric or isometric muscle actions. Using a constant velocity motor coupled to a force transducer, they were able to measure the effective force of the elbow flexors and extensors as a function of elbow position during maximal voluntary efforts. At all positions throughout the range of motion, the effective force recorded during the eccentric muscle action of the elbow flexors was greater than during the isometric or concentric muscle action. The motor allowed movement to occur around the elbow joint at approximately 18°/second for a total of 90°, and the force of the muscles resisting the device was maintained for about 5 seconds. This period of sustained force, while the muscle was changing length through a functional range, was more than 10 times greater than that described for the series elastic component [24] and certainly much greater than cross-bridge time [27].

Similar results of elevated force throughout the range of motion were obtained during slow speed testing of the human knee extensors [11], but they are not as impressive. This is due in part to the muscle group selected and most likely to its neural control. Slightly different relationships seem to exist for different muscle groups. For example, the elbow extensors [112] produced elevated force during the first part of the range of motion (i.e., closer to full elbow extension) during eccentric muscle action and later fell to isometric levels instead of remaining elevated as if fatigue had occurred. In general, the overall force–velocity relation for human muscle groups more or less followed the predictions based on experiments with isolated muscles except that less force is produced during the eccentric action than expected [66, 77].

This deviation from in vitro muscle actions is not unique to eccentric muscle actions. Even concentric muscle actions deviate from the expected force–velocity relationship at very slow velocities [43, 98]. It may be that the central nervous system monitors the tension-time integral and limits access to the physiological potential under certain conditions. There is some indirect evidence that the central nervous system does override the innate ability of muscles to produce approximately 100% more force during their eccentric action than during isometric action [32].

If one studies the force output of the knee extensors in patients with spasticity, the force produced, even at low speeds, is always dramatically higher during the eccentric action than concentric action [72, 73] more similar to the muscle actions recorded in vitro. Likewise, if innervated human muscles are driven by external stimulators, as for example in spinal-cord-injured patients without spasticity, the force recorded during the eccentric muscle action, even at slow velocities, approaches twice the force during the concentric muscle action under the same stimulation parameters and electrode placement [126]. Thus, the stimulator, by directly stimulating the motor nerves in the muscle, circumvents the proposed inhibitory mechanism limiting physiological potential.

In summary, the force–velocity relationship for a group of human muscles is similar in shape but not magnitude to that recorded for isolated muscles. Yet muscles under voluntary control (as in the case of amputees possessing cineplastic tunnels allowing direct access to the muscle tendon [103]) almost duplicated the force–velocity relationship described by the Hill equation for concentric muscle action. Thus, the mechanism of inhibition of physiological potential which is proposed to account for differences during eccentric muscle action needs further discussion and research.

ENERGETICS

Since muscle is a biological machine that converts chemical energy into tension and work, consideration of the energy requirements for eccentric muscle actions needs some discussion in order to differentiate the various muscle actions further. Here the reference to muscle energetics deals solely with differences in utilization between similar muscles performing different functions rather than with the processes of energy utilization or their variation within the different fiber types. All aspects of muscle energetics have been reviewed in detail elsewhere [102].

During early investigations on the energetics of muscle, it was found that the physiological cost of performing negative work (eccentric muscle action) was substantially less than that of performing positive work, at least during cycling activities involving the lower extremities [3]. This difference in metabolic cost between concentric and eccentric muscle action became greater as the speed of the cycling increased, ranging from 10 to 30% less energy for the production of a comparable amount of negative work [74]. One explanation for this difference was that fewer muscle fibers were actually used during the production of negative work on the cycle ergometer [3]. It has been demonstrated that under comparable work loads the electromyographic (EMG) activity of muscles involved in eccentric action is less compared to concentric action (the EMG records reflect the number of action potentials in a muscle which indicates the recruitment and activation of the muscle fibers that compose the muscle). At the same time, the amount of EMG activity can be directly related to force output for concentric muscle action [13]. Thus, there is support for the concept of reduced muscle activation during negative work by a given muscle.

Another aspect of muscle energetics needs some comment. Less energy is consumed during the performance of negative work in an isolated muscle which is tetanized by an external stimulation device [102] than is required for its positive counterpart. Here the number of muscle fibers is not a variable since the entire muscle is activated maximally. During eccentric muscle action, energy consumption as measured by either energy liberation or high-energy phosphate hydrolysis can be as low as one-fourth that of concentric during action [102]. Thus, two aspects of reduced energy cost are operational during eccentric actions of human muscles: (a) altered recruitment of motor units (reduced EMG) and (b) decreased energy utilization of the active muscles which develop tension while being stretched.

The observation that fewer fibers are recruited for eccentric muscle action indicates that the central nervous system can, and does, utilize the ability of muscles to generate greater tensions when it becomes more efficient to do so. In other words, "the brain is able to exploit the biomechanical properties of the body" [50].

MOTOR CONTROL

It should be clear from the preceding discussion that the central nervous system has different control programs for using muscles for different purposes (e.g., shock absorption or stabilization). With regard to force output, it has been demonstrated that muscle tension is directly related to the integrated electrical activity (EMG) in a muscle during concentric, eccentric, or isometric action [13]. However, it was noted that the EMG activity was less in an active muscle which was being forcibly stretched (eccentric action) than one shortening at the same constant load [13]. Thus raising and lowering the same weight require different motor strategies as would cycling activities performing positive and negative work [8] at the same submaximal work output. It is important to emphasize again that greater EMG activity accompanies concentric muscle action against the same (submaximal) load used for the eccentric action.

In contrast to the submaximal effort, during maximal efforts, the EMG activity remains constant while the force varies according to the force–velocity relationship [77]. It is of interest to note that the maximal force developed during eccentric muscle action never exceeded about 140% of the maximum value recorded for any concentric action. This deviation in human muscle performance from that of isolated muscles must be a function of central nervous system action, since stimulation of a muscle by an external muscle stimulator results in the same high forces as seen in isolated muscles. In patients with spastic paresis, results similar to those seen for an electrical stimulator have been reported [72, 73]. Thus, some physiological mechanism apparently prevents the development of the full force potential during normal actions involving muscle lengthening in untrained individuals. This central nervous system response may protect the muscle from complete rupture during shock absorption activities.

A reference to neurology might be useful to account for this observation. In patients with spasticity characterized by an increased muscle activation in response to passive stretch, muscle tension increases in response to stretch up to a point where a sudden release occurs as tension falls off dramatically. This "clasped knife reflex," described in most standard textbooks of neurology [96], is linked to the function of the muscle force transducer, the Golgi tendon organ. However, recent research has questioned the role of the Golgi tendon organ in such a reflex because extremely small forces such as generated by a single muscle fiber [51] can elicit a response in the receptor. It should be noted that the "clasped knife reflex" results after a rather substantial length change has occurred. Perhaps the classic description of a role for the Golgi tendon organ in preventing excessive muscle forces by overriding the voluntary nerve may be operational for maximal sustained efforts only after a certain length change has occurred; thus although the central nervous system has a mechanism for utilization of eccentric action to minimize energy costs, it also has a protective circuit to prevent excessive forces which might tear the muscles apart.

In contrast to the eccentric muscle action just described, the regulation of muscle stiffness (springlike function) or muscle stretch prior to shortening appears to be quite different [78]. This is probably quite obvious to the sport's practitioner, who recognizes that the strategies and preparation are different for lowering a weight or rebounding the same weight at the end of the range of motion. Two different features seem to characterize the stretch–shortening cycle: (*a*) EMG activity appears to increase as the muscle lengthens, reaching a maximum just prior to the concentric muscle action; and (*b*) the tension drops if time is allowed to pass between the stretch and shortening phases. Here one sees a drop in force if the stretch is held for about 1 second [78]. The observations of the physiology of the stretch–shortening cycle indicate that the control of muscle elasticity may be quite different from that of muscle shock absorption, even though both have eccentric muscle actions.

In considering the muscle as an elastic tissue, repetitive stretching under high loads might be expected to lead to its rupture. Muscle fibers are no exception and ruptures can occur at different sites along the fibers, including the region where the muscle fiber connects to the tendon (myotendinous junction) [44]. It would be interesting to know whether the force required to rupture a muscle must exceed the limits imposed by the protective reflexes, if they are indeed operative, or must exceed some tension–time integral which could occur at different force levels over different time periods. One mechanism of rupture could result if fatigue of the reflexes were to occur while the other would require fatigue of the tissue. Perhaps the site of injury could be different and explain the myotendinous tears in one experimental model [44] and midfiber ruptures in others [120]. There is little information on the mechanism of such injuries.

INJURY

Damage to active muscles is a common occurrence in sports and ranges from completely torn muscles to damaged fibers [101]. Mechanical trauma seems to be the most common cause of injury following exercise or sports, especially after eccentric muscle action [122]. Following mechanical muscle trauma, there is a period of perceived pain which varies in both quality and duration with the type of injury. In this review, exercise-induced muscle damage will be discussed together with muscle soreness, since they are difficult to separate from each other and are so interrelated in the scientific literature.

For some time it has been recognized that certain types of exercise produce delayed-onset muscle soreness which appears 1–2 days after the cessation of the actual exercise bout [122]. In fact, delayed-onset muscle soreness is so common that it is rare to find an individual who has not experienced it some time in his or her life. Delayed-onset muscle soreness, which follows bouts of exercise which involve deceleration or eccentric muscle actions [4, 109], is not to be confused with exertional pain (pain during exercise) or that seen following fatigue which has a metabolic origin [35]. In fact, it was the persistence of muscle soreness reported after exercise that led early investigators to postulate that muscle injury had occurred [55]. However, it must be emphasized that pain can have a variety of origins not related to tissue damage [35].

What evidence exists to support muscle injury results to a greater degree from eccentric as opposed to concentric or isometric muscle action? Asmussen [7] first indicated that pain and soreness are particularly associated with muscles which performed eccentric actions. Similarly, Talag [122] surmised that pain, which occurred 1–2 days after eccentric but not concentric or isometric muscle actions, was related to tissue changes, although no data were presented to support the tissue response mediating the pain sensation. Remmers and Kaljot [104] provided the link between exercise and muscle damage by demonstrating that serum levels of the muscle enzyme glutamic oxalacetic transaminase (GOT) were markedly elevated following strenuous exercise in human subjects involving running and forced marches. In other words, cellular damage of such magnitude that intracellular proteins (GOT) could leak out was apparently due to certain exercises.

In exercises using combined concentric and eccentric actions, Tidus and Ianuzzo [125] observed that serum enzyme activity and delayed muscle soreness were both related to the intensity and duration of the exercise with the intensity producing the more pronounced effect. In a series of studies, Armstrong et al. [6, 109] demonstrated the relationship among soreness, serum enzyme changes, and myofiber damage by studying downhill running in both humans and animals. By using downhill running, which, like downhill walking [5], requires more eccentric muscle action than level running [86], they were able to establish that pain was linked to muscle damage in humans and at the same time observe the inflammatory response in rats [6] subjected to similar running activities. Thus, as with other instances of tissue damage, soreness may reflect the presence of inflammation.

Once muscle damage has been confirmed in animals, the observations of unstable oxygen uptake [71] and of increased muscle activation (IEMG) [93] during moderate periods of negative work performance could be given new meaning. Klausen and Knuttgen [71] first observed that subjects cycling against a special cycle ergometer using only eccentric muscle action at a steady power output never achieved a steady oxygen uptake, but rather oxygen uptake increased throughout the exercise bout. Yet at the time when the activity reached exhaustion (exhaustion being defined as the inability to produce forces necessary to resist the pedals) none of the other signs of exhaustion such as elevations in blood lactate and heart rate were present. In a different study in which subjects performed stepping exercises, the leg which resisted the step down or was engaged in the eccentric actions required increased electrical activation of the quadriceps muscles for the generation of a given muscular force. In a more recent study, Dick and Cavanagh [30] reported both an increase in oxygen uptake and an increase in electrical activation during the performance of constant-velocity downhill running. They referred to this phenomenon as an upward drifting oxygen uptake during prolonged submaximal downhill running. It was hypothesized [30] that during downhill running, increased motor unit recruitment occurred within the active muscles in order to maintain a constant force output in the muscles which were undergoing intracellular damage. As damage occurred, the muscles were still active, generating action potentials (IEMG) and using metabolic energy (oxygen consumption), but with diminishing force output, which required additional muscle fibers to participate [30]. With the possible visualization of ongoing muscle damage as hypothesized in this study, pain appeared to reach a maximum after 48 hours.

Why do the markers of muscle injury, the muscle enzymes, appear in the circulation at a much later time than the occurrence of the actual exercise insult and differ still further in time from the pain experience? One possibility is that they are not related to each other at all but occur by different mechanisms. If the pain receptors, which are primarily located in muscle connective tissue between fibers [112], are stimulated in response to connective tissue damage, independent of myofiber damage, pain could result when both components are injured or only when the connective tissue part is. In the case of myopathic conditions, there does exist a dissociation between muscle pain and damage with the exception of the inflammatory diseases which can be painful [34]. In marked contrast, many connective tissue disorders are accompanied by pain [106], including myofascial syndromes, fasciitis, fibrositis syndrome, and the common overuse problems of connective tissue frequently seen in athletes such as tendonitis, bursitis, ligament strains, and others. Thus, pain in damaged muscle following exercise may result from overuse of the connective tissue component around the active muscle rather than from injury to the myofiber itself. These important differences between connective tissue and myofibers may be useful to explain the response of the muscles to multiple episodes of trauma where pain occurs in the absence of indicators of myofiber damage.

For the present; three aspects of muscle tissue damage need to be differentiated from each other: (*a*) direct myofiber damage, (*b*) delayed myofiber damage, and (*c*) connective tissue or fascial damage. Direct myofiber damage occurs during the activity or can be observed immediately after the activity is completed. Delayed myofiber damage, on the other hand, occurs after the exercise insult has been completed and may even commence a day or more following the initial event. Connective tissue damage is less well defined but certainly involves collagen and other extracellular matrix components as well as the interconnections between adjacent muscle cells. Each will be considered separately below.

Direct Myofiber Damage
Direct myofiber damage can be defined as an alteration in muscle fiber structure or function which can be observed immediately after the exercise bout has been completed. The structural abnormalities might in-

clude sarcomere derangement, swollen mitochondria, fragmented or swollen sarcoplasmic reticular elements, dilated T-tubules, and lesions in the plasma membrane. The physiological alterations would manifest themselves by faulty excitation–contraction (E–C) coupling, impaired calcium transport, abnormal energetics, and the inability to produce tension. Unfortunately, most of these structural and functional alterations commonly occur in response to fatigue such as dilated T-tubules, swollen mitochondria [74], impaired E–C coupling [33], and decreased force output [14]. Nevertheless, in nonfatigued muscle following eccentric muscle action, these same alterations may indicate myofiber damage resulted directly from the muscle action.

Unfortunately, few investigators evaluate their subjects immediately after the exercise bout for signs of myofiber damage or pathology—they usually wait at least 24 hours. Friden et al. [39] observed that following intense cycling involving eccentric muscle action, the morphology of the vastus lateralis demonstrated focal disturbances of the striated pattern with Z band streaming and broadening, most often in the type II (fast-twitch) muscle fibers, and affecting up to 50% of the fibers examined [39]. At the same time, muscle strength (force output) was diminished during maximal knee extension exercises as would be expected if the high-threshold motor units (type II) had been damaged. This relationship between force and sarcomere derangement may indicate that a failure of the contractile mechanism had occurred at the level of the sarcomere as a result of eccentric muscle actions. In contrast, after a downhill run of 30 minutes serum myoglobin levels were elevated significantly by 6 hours [21], indicating that myofiber plasma membranes may be disrupted or some myofibers were actually broken. More severe damage was noted after a marathon [129], although one must also consider the possibility of the coexistence of metabolic alterations due to shifts in pH and energy store depletion for the origin of this damage. Still, some myofiber rupture was evident with organelles such as mitochondria actually free in the extracellular space [54]. In contrast, in untrained individuals performing arm exercises, damage was not reported immediately afterward but was seen to increase for days after the exercise ceased [64]. Thus, unless there is a difference in the response to exercise by muscles of the upper extremity versus the lower extremity, no clear picture of direct myofiber damage emerges and further studies are needed.

Delayed Myofiber Damage

Delayed myofiber damage is probably the best established injury resulting from eccentric muscle action [64]. In this case, the signs of muscle damage begin at the end of the exercise period and continue for a period of days following the cessation of all activity. The two most clearly described signs of muscle damage of a delayed nature are the following: (a) Muscle-specific enzymes, such as creatine kinase and lactate dehydrogenase, are released after the exercise is over—this release can often continue for days after the cessation of exercise [64]; and (b) the uptake of the radioisotope technetium (^{99m}Tc) pyrophosphate by muscle, seen after whole-body scintigraphy, is indicative of cellular membrane damage expressed as increased permeability [52]. The observation of increased entrance of ^{99m}Tc pyrophosphate helps rule out the possibility of muscle enzyme release by some cell-mediated process. Thus, the release of intracellular enzymes indicates that damage to the cell membrane of the myofiber is present. Sometimes, the release of muscle-specific intracellular enzymes can continually rise for 5–7 days after the exercise bout, especially in untrained individuals, [36] as if a progressive deterioration of the sarcolemma continues unchecked. The magnitude of enzyme release can approach that seen in myopathic conditions [97]. Even in well-trained marathon runners, the creatine kinase levels remained high for 4 days [105].

Morphologically myofibrillar damage can be seen up to 3 days post-exercise, indicating that the contractile unit is degraded for an extended time [38, 39]. One possible explanation is that the initial exercise caused some minor damage, direct myofiber damage, which activated a secondary response by the immune system to perform its surveillance activity. The resultant attack and destruction of muscle fibers then followed the arrival and action of lymphoid cells. There is some evidence from research conducted on animals to support this concept [120], and lymphoid involvement in muscle regeneration has been suggested [37] as well. In human muscle, however, lymphoid attack is less clear. In a recent study [64], release of creatine kinase and uptake of technetium pyrophosphate was followed for up to 20 days after an exercise bout. The increase in plasma creatine kinase paralleled the increase uptake of technetium pyrophosphate into the exercised muscles. Type II muscle fibers were preferentially involved in at least one individual, and it was noted that only after 7 days, infiltration by mononuclear cells corresponded with regeneration arriving by day 20. It was concluded by Jones et al. [64] that the infiltration by mononuclear cells is considered a response to damage rather than a cause. However, the number of cytotoxic cells seen in the animal studies is quite small [120] and could have been overlooked in the biopsy samples since specific markers were not used. Besides it is possible that if only one natural killer cell is sufficient to destroy a myofiber, it could be easily missed.

Alternatively, direct mechanical damage to the sarcoplasmic reticulum could lead to calcium leakage and protein degradation due to the action of the intracellular calcium-activated proteases. The role of these destructive enzymes in muscle biochemistry has not been defined. But limited proteolysis of the myofiber could in turn lead to cellular death as the unit proceeds to be damaged. Such a calcium-mediated theory of cell death has been proposed to account for myocardial necrosis following ischemia. The term "calcium paradox" [131] is used specifically to characterize this process of myofiber degeneration because of the prominent role that calcium plays.

Following severe exercise, degenerative fibers are seen to persist until perhaps a week or two in severely stressed muscles [54]. During this postexercise time, necrosis, degeneration, and other aspects of actual muscle pathology and indications of inflammation are evident. The worst case of muscle damage can exist in a condition referred to as exertional rhabdomyolitis which can be severe enough to require hospitalization [104, 108]. Fortunately, this severe condition is rare and does not seem to continue after a period of rest has occurred [104].

Connective Tissue Damage

The connective tissues of skeletal muscle form sheaths around various bundles of muscles and include the endomysium, perimysium, and epimysium. The endomysium is perhaps the most important for the present discussion, since it forms a sheath around each myofiber and may interconnect adjacent myofibers [17]. The surface of a myofiber is composed of an endomysial fibrous network, a basal lamina, and the sarcolemma (plasma membrane) [62]. The endomysium and basal lamina are so intimately related physically that they probably should be considered, from a mechanical viewpoint, as a single elastic structure. In human muscle, the components that make up this complex consist of type IV and V collagen, fibronectin, laminin, and various specific proteoglycans [12]. The physiology of these extracellular structures is not well understood, but they seem to be intimately involved in growth, adaptation, and certain disease processes.

There are distinct differences in content and composition of the endomysium in different fiber types of animals [79]. The type I (slow-twitch) muscle fibers have a more robust connective tissue than the type II (fast-twitch) fibers [80]. This should come as no surprise since the texture of red and white meat from animals is known to differ accordingly. If the same relationships exists for human muscle, then type II fibers might be more susceptible to stretch-induced injury due to a less developed endomysium than type I fibers.

Following exercise involving eccentric muscle action, evidence for connective tissue degradation accompanied reports of muscle soreness [4]. The elevated urinary excretion of hydroxyproline in humans following this exercise was interpreted to indicate an increased catabolism of collagen. The amino acid hydroxyproline is a unique component of mature collagens, and its presence in urine can only occur from degradation of existing collagens. Since the collagen component of the connective tissue is the primary passive elastic element, it would be expected to demonstrate overuse or strain damage as connective tissue elsewhere might. However, only limited research in this area exists for any clear interpretation. Yet, it may be the most important component of the postexercise injury reaction. Connective tissue disorders can produce pain, inflammatory responses, and stiffness or decreased range of motion—all common postexercise responses [57]. In fact many aspects of the postexercise inflammatory state in muscle, including the cellular infiltration, are almost indistinguishable from the myopathic condition polymyositis.

Certainly the concept of connective tissue damage has been mentioned before [7, 76], but evidence for degradation as opposed to mechanical disruption is limited to studies on collagen degradation and proteoglycan disappearance. Collagen breakdown products, in particular hydroxyproline, increase after exercise involving eccentric actions and were accompanied by delayed soreness [4]. In fact, the soreness followed the appearance of hydroxyproline in the urine. In contrast, the proteoglycan component of the extracellular matrix surrounding rat muscles subjected to forced lengthening as a means of injuring muscle showed noticeable histological variation by 24 hours [42]. It is reasonable to assume then that collagen and other components of the endomysium are disrupted when active muscles are forcibly stretched.

Since peptide fragments of collagen [99] can mediate monocyte migration, the inflammatory cell invasion seen in exercise-injured muscles may be mediated by some degradation product released from the endomysium. This association of increased collagen degradation and inflammatory cell arrival would suggest that extracellular proteolysis preceded and proteases were free to act in the extracellular space. One additional substrate for extracellular protease action might be the kininogens. The production of kinins could be responsible in part for the pain. In addition to histamine, the local liberation of kinins produces pain [107]. Kinins are released by the action of proteases on kininogens, and it is conceivable that the same proteases (chymase, plasminogen activator, lysosomal proteases, etc.) involved in endomysium destruction also produce kinins. Further research is needed to provide more substance to the model presented of connective tissue damage ("torn tissue" hypothesis).

MECHANISM OF INJURY

Injury of muscle from repeated eccentric actions somehow involves the mechanical forces of stretch in tearing the tissue. The most severe case would be an entire fiber rupture; it serves as a useful starting point of discussion. Studies have been performed on muscle to determine at what point rupture occurs. By stretching a muscle which was activated by electrical stimulation, it was evident that the magnitude of the applied force and not the velocity of the stretch was important in producing a lesion; the injury was most often observed at the interface between myofiber and the connective tissue—the myotendinous junction [44]. However, the stretch necessary for breakage often occurred at muscle lengths greater than those within the physiological range. In other studies, McCully and Faulkner [90] observed that tension was a causative agent of injury and as few as 15 eccentric muscle actions produced muscular damage. In these studies, fatigue was not a contributing factor. Thus, some direct influence of stretch on the muscle unit was considered. It is obvious that some degree of confusion exists as to the amount and type of stimulus needed to produce muscle damage. Presently it is best to accept that there may be damage that occurs at the onset of activity due to weakness from past usage and later as the activity continues to tax the system.

When a muscle is active and stretched the following components could break under tension: (*a*) The connective tissue linking adjacent myofibers (the struts) could break; (*b*) the basal lamina could be peeled off the fiber, exposing a patch of plasma membrane; (*c*) the plasma membrane could rupture; (*d*) a sarcomere could be pulled apart and perhaps disrupt the adjacent sarcoplasmic reticulum or plasma membrane; and (*e*) a myofiber could break in two without disrupting the basal lamina. Of course there are combinations of the above. The premise of this presentation is that the damage can occur in two places: in the region of the endomysium between two fibers and in the myofiber at the level of the sarcomeres. The endomysial damage could result from the inability of the connective tissue to withstand the repetitive microtrauma of stretch.

In contrast, all injury could result from selective errors in calcium handling. Inability of the sarcoplasmic reticulum to relax a muscle at the appropriate speed could result in a rigor-type state and the muscle would behave as a purely elastic element. If only one fiber (myofiber rigor) or one myofibril (induction of segmental hypercontraction) were involved in the rigor, then a shear force would develop between adjacent units and rupture or myofilament damage could easily result. Some tearing between myofilaments has been proposed to result from shearing forces [124]. Thus as the force resisted by a unit of muscle increased, microtrauma could result. If, on the other hand, the damage were small, perhaps a break in the T-tubule for example, and not repaired immediately, then calcium would enter the cell and cause a delayed-onset myofiber necrosis [131].

Exposure of muscle to a calcium ionophore induces histologic evidence of damage [31] not much different from that seen following eccentric muscle action. Administration of drugs such as verapamil to reduce calcium accumulation actually prevented experimental rhabdomyolysis [63, 100, 118] or necrosis of muscle. Thus, it is not surprising that in patients with exertional muscle pain syndrome, verapamil provided a striking improvement in the ability of these patients to perform exercises without pain [82]. It is quite possible that the drug acted at multiple sites both extracellular and intramuscular. However, little information is available to suggest such a role of calcium antagonists in prevention of exercise-induced muscle damage. In addition, such calcium-antagonist drugs produce a variety of responses, including local anesthesia [82]. It remains to be seen if cellular damage can be prevented or reduced by calcium-antagonist application following exercise as it is in other experimental models of muscle damage.

ADAPTATION–MALADAPTATION FROM ECCENTRIC MUSCLE ACTION

It should now be clear that some sort of damage can occur in a muscle in response to even a single bout of exercise which involves eccentric muscle action. Since human muscle function is preserved throughout life and athletes are not more dysfunctional as a result of long-term training, the muscle damage from mechanical forces is either insignificant or serves as a stimulus for repair and adaptation. If one considers the response of normal skin or even bone [20] to submaximal mechanical strains, it is clear that both structures adapt to resist further insult. It seems likely that muscle would repair and adapt to mechanical microdamage in much the same way. In order to understand the processes involved in muscle adaptation, it is useful to compare the response of muscle to a single exercise bout with the chronic adaptation seen in individuals who are well trained or have experienced multiple insults to their muscles.

In untrained individuals exercising for the first time or in trained individuals performing novel tasks, some limited muscle dysfunction can be seen immediately after the exercise is completed. Soreness and swelling are the first to be noted along with other indicators of muscle damage, if the appropriate measurements are taken. Initially, a measurable loss of range of motion [25] can be evident especially after exhausting eccentric muscle action. This loss in muscle extensibility cannot be accounted for by a muscle spasm since there is no increase in the electrical activity of the exercised muscle at rest [57]; the muscle, however, does appear to be swollen. Howell et al. [57] have suggested that an analogy to a water balloon within a nylon stocking might be useful to describe the lost motion. The presence of additional water in the balloon would stretch the stocking to its full length and limit the range of motion by pulling on the fascial components. Since pain receptors are located in the fascia (connective tissue) surrounding muscle [116] and group IV sensory fibers terminate as free nerve endings in this region [91], it is reasonable to postulate that increased fluid pressures in the tissue produce pain [41]. This is a useful model because similar conditions of swollen muscles of greater magnitude constitute compartment syndromes in which marked muscle damage can be evident. Compartment syndromes are characterized by increased pressure in an area bound by bone or fascia. Therefore, following exercise, a miniature compartment syndrome could result.

In patients with chronic compartment syndromes, the interstitial fluid pressures often exceed 15 mm Hg [92]. If the pressures are large enough, obvious microcirculatory imbalances result and lymphatic drainage is impaired. The concept of a localized swollen compartment resulting from exercise is appealing because it does not identify the cellular constituents responsible for the swelling but instead focuses attention on the possibility of impaired extracellular fluid movement and decreased nutrient supply at a local level as another alternative mechanism for continued muscle damage.

It is a common experience with untrained individuals who begin to lift weights that limitations in range of motion can be observed immediately after their first exercise session even before soreness is experienced [25]. Perhaps water is squeezed out of the vascular system and is temporarily bound in the extracellular space by some component or metabolite. The amount of water-binding material, acting like a sponge, initially determines the amount of swelling. The subsequent breakdown of connective tissue, the accumulation of metabolites, and the release of muscle-specific proteins and intracellular ions over the following hours or days add an additional osmotic force and lead to further fluid accumulation. Although tissue swelling was of interest in some of the earliest studies of muscle soreness [56, 122], only recently have measurements of fluid pressure been made in muscles after exercise [128].

The goal of these studies was to investigate the possibility that osmotic pressure differences would cause localized edema and might be a source of pain following exercise. The exercises consisted of either concentric or eccentric muscle actions of the ankle dorsiflexors of human volunteers. The load was identical for the two exercises but an assistant lowered or raised the exercise device so that only the desired muscle action was exercised. Intramuscular fluid pressures were measured before, during, and after the exercises [41]. The tissue fluid pressure was found to be elevated in the muscles exercised using eccentric muscle actions but not in those using concentric actions. The fluid pressure accompanied by pain continued to be elevated for 2 days following the exercise. In contrast, only stiffness was experienced in the muscles that were exercised using concentric muscle actions. Furthermore, as noted earlier, soreness could not be produced in trained weight lifters [57]. Yet body-builders have pronounced swelling of the muscles (the so-called pump) after an exercise session; this swollen state can often last for days without pain. So one unexplored area for potential adaptation is the nature of the extracellular compartment, its compliance to exercise training, and its relationship to pain.

Since pain is perceived by the central nervous system and usually serves as a stimulus for a variety of protective reflexes, it is possible that some reorganization of the motor control system might result to prevent the reoccurrence of pain. It is well known that pain or injury without pain can directly alter the muscles' ability to produce maximal strength, leading eventually to muscle weakness [121]. In the case of muscle swelling or delayed-onset muscle soreness, it is quite possible that the central nervous system, after experiencing pain, responds by evoking an alternative motor program. The resulting muscle action distributes the forces over a greater number of muscle fibers which are activated at submaximal levels. Such rapid alterations are commonly seen in altered gait patterns after banging one's shin but rarely do they continue long after the pain subsides.

If the central nervous system were to use a different motor program which employed a greater number of muscle fibers, then the metabolic cost of the identical workload would increase because of the activation and shortening heats required for the additional fibers to participate. In studies specifically looking at the training effect of downhill running on the development of delayed-onset muscle soreness, oxygen uptake either remained the same or decreased slightly [110]. Further proof that no central adaptation resulted from the pain experienced after eccentric muscle action came from a study designed to compare the effect of a single bout of exercise on the appearance of common indicators of muscle damage (soreness and serum creatine kinase). In this study, one leg was exercised and 7 days later either the same leg or opposite leg was exercised using the same procedure. No additional protection was imparted to the contralateral leg and thus only the ipsilateral leg revealed any adaptive responses. At first this study seems at odds with that of Singh and Karpovich [113], who reported some cross-over training when elbow flexors were exercised using a velocity-controlled dynamometer. However, no special care was taken to ensure inactivity of the contralateral musculature during the exercise. Thus some bilateral exercise training probably resulted. So while the central nervous system seems to respond to ongoing damage with increasing recruitment of motor units [30], no apparent training response remains after a single exercise session.

MYOFIBER REPAIR

Another response which might result in tissue swelling is the release of muscle-specific proteins indicative of cellular damage. Much attention has been given to the myofiber damage leading to the rise in muscle-specific enzymes in the serum. Although only about 5% of the myofibers show overt signs of injury or rupture following exercise in rats [6], almost 50% of the fibers examined for ultrastructural injury in humans demonstrated some intracellular damage [40]. As seen in the rat, the broken fibers can be increased in number up to 30% by increasing the tension applied to the active muscle [89, 120]. Without a continuous structure to exert force against, the myofiber, even if activated, would not generate any useful force; an observed decline in force capability of the entire muscle would result [89, 29]. Restoration would require regenerative responses if the muscle were to return to normal function without residual loss in force capacity.

Muscle regeneration does occur in exercise-damaged muscles [89, 24] and has been reviewed in detail elsewhere [24, 58]. For optimal regeneration, the process requires an intact basal lamina, an uninterrupted vascular supply, and a functional nerve. If any of these components are themselves damaged, then regeneration proceeds at a slower rate and may not be complete. The incomplete repair may actually contain scar tissue as sometimes occurs after contusions and intramuscular bleeding [84]. Normally, myofiber rupture following eccentric muscle action is not accompanied by bleeding or nerve injury and in most cases the muscle has a relatively intact basal lamina [42]. The reattachment of the broken muscle can proceed along this basal lamina and is characterized by a budding or outgrowth of the sarcoplasm of the remaining fiber. Numerous similarities to those seen in myotubes during muscle development can be observed in the regenerating myofiber [15] including many nuclei in the region of the budding. Although the origin of the nuclei in the muscle buds still remains controversial, it is thought that they represent satellite cell nuclei. Satellite cells were demonstrated in rats to be the precursors of myoblasts during regeneration in vivo [114, 115]. Since satellite cells are located under the basal lamina of an adult muscle fiber and appear as dormant cells, their role in regeneration and repair has been postulated for quite some time. In addition, recent interest has developed concerning a specific growth factor which is released as a result of injury [16] and may activate various cells including satellite cells to aid in the repair of the broken myofiber.

In contrast, little is known as to the mechanism of intracellular repair of a damaged sarcomere or myofibril which appears to be the most common injury seen [40]. Is the myofibril degraded and replaced or is there a repair system to restore individual components? In muscles which are increasing their length because the muscle is under a constant stretch, sarcomeres seem to be added at the ends of the myofibril [46]. But this is a special case of constant tension and although injury may be more prevalent at the myotendinous junction [44], other adaptive mechanisms must be operative for sarcomere repair along the entire length of a myofiber. Friden has noted that changes in fine structure of sarcomeres in human muscles do occur in response to eccentric muscle action and training [40].

Myofibers have the ability to be repaired and remain functional after damage from the forces encountered from eccentric muscle actions. Under normal situations of intact innervation, the newly repaired muscle is not different physiologically from its uninjured precursor. Thus, there is no reason to believe that a special injury-resistant muscle fiber is manufactured in response to myofiber damage or that a hypertrophic muscle would develop from a single exercise session. Yet a single bout of exercise somehow serves to prevent muscle damage from a subsequent exercise session for as long as 6 weeks [21].

CONNECTIVE TISSUE

The regions that actually swell following muscle damage are the endomysium and perimysium where the pain receptors are located. The endomysium and perimysium are composed of connective tissue and represent the passive elastic component of skeletal muscle. Unlike cardiac muscle [67], no major mechanical function has been attributed to the connective tissue of skeletal muscles over most of its useful length. However, elaboration or reorganization of the connective tissue could increase the shock absorption capability and spare the myofibers from excessive loads. The adverse effects of scarring illustrate the limitations that connective tissue proliferation could provide. After a single exercise insult scarring does not take place. Instead fibroblasts or myofibers are stimulated to produce different connective tissue constituents, particularly proteoglycans which bind water [69]. In rats injured by forced muscle lengthening, dramatic changes in proteoglycans of the extracellular matrix occurred as early as 12 hours following injury [42]. As the content and quality of proteoglycans changed, so too would their ability to function together as a shock absorber. Thus, the dynamics of the extracellular space may be the single most important element in the injury repair process providing protection from further damage and may range from mild adaptive thickening to actual fibrosis.

TRAINING

Athletes by virtue of specific sports or training design subject themselves to repetitive eccentric muscle actions followed by specific adaptations. For example, Howell et al. [57] were unable to induce soreness in trained weight lifters. Yet, trained runners had resting levels of serum enzymes indicative of muscle damage that were elevated above those of an untrained group [36]. But, unlike the untrained group, the trained runners showed little additional rise in the serum content of those enzymes after an exhausting downhill run, and no soreness was reported. Thus, training induces some adaptive change in the muscle which somehow lessens myofiber damage and pain.

The first possibility is that the additional tension per myofiber during eccentric muscle action serves as a stimulus for muscle hypertrophy. The resulting muscle fibers by virtue of their larger size can resist injury. This is an attractive hypothesis which would support the common belief that performance of negative work produces larger muscles. Since muscles grow in response to tension [45], even passive tension [10], this hypothesis is reasonable. The relationship between tension and muscle growth was demonstrated in a variety of studies on animals [46] and even in myoblasts grown in cell culture [127]. It was also noted that the fibroblast activity was increased at the same time [83], indicating a synergistic role of the connective tissue with muscle growth. From the standpoint of muscle growth promotion, the increased tension per myofiber seen during eccentric muscle action would seem optimal. However, there is little evidence that increased hypertrophy results from training which includes a large amount of negative work. Body-builders, who often advocate eccentric muscle actions, have no larger muscle fibers than weight lifters [123] who often avoid lowering weights.

Perhaps the adaptation to eccentric muscle action does not involve the myofiber to any greater degree than isometric or concentric actions but influences the connective tissue in the fascial elements. The development of connective tissue has a distinct advantage in that it does not consume energy during eccentric muscle action yet can resist large forces as experienced in tendons and ligaments. The disadvantage of connective tissue production is that excessive amounts may actually inhibit motion or increase the oxygen cost of work performed by antagonist muscles.

Small changes in the endomysium around each muscle fiber shortly after a single exercise bout could protect the muscle from myofiber rupture but not necessarily from sarcomere or fascial damage. No direct evidence is available to support this hypothesis. Still, enzyme leakage was prevented from muscles which had 1 week before experienced a bout of damaging exercise [95]. Pain and decreased force output were still present at the end of the second exercise session in the exercised muscles. If exercise training was more regular over a 5-week period, endomysial connective tissue stimulation was evident in previously untrained individuals [19].

In chronically trained animals and human individuals, there is evidence to support the idea that a modification of connective tissue occurs around muscles which experience eccentric muscle actions [79, 88]. MacDougall et al. [88] reported that connective tissue content was greater in body-builders, paralleling their increased myofiber size. In biopsied muscles from ultra-marathon runners, increased connective tissue was observed at the ultrastructural level and was suggestive of microfibrosis [112]. Further analysis of muscles from body-builders [87] and marathon runners [54] demonstrate evidence of ongoing degeneration and regeneration of muscle. Thus, continued damage and repair are part of the long-training effect of repeated eccentric muscle actions. It may well be that the observed changes in the body-builders' physique with long-term training are due to the gradual deposition of connective tissue between the muscles and not to a continued increase in myofiber size—an area where more study is needed.

CLINICAL APPLICATIONS

The important role of eccentric muscle action in deceleration of the body during walking and running is now well recognized. Since anterior knee pain is a common problem with runners, possible errors in deceleration or maladaptation to repetitive eccentric muscle action have been suggested as a contributing factor [59]. With the advent of machines such as the Kin/Com that could test eccentric muscle actions, force deficits during eccentric muscle action are being reported. For example, in patients with anterior knee pain syndrome, a specific force deficit during the performance of eccentric muscle action but not concentric could be demonstrated [11]. Often the deficit in eccentric muscle action was eliminated after only 2–4 weeks of exercise training which emphasized control of the decelerator function. This inability of a muscle group to adequately decelerate a limb or the body could lead to more serious problems than painful articulations. Such decelerator defects may subject ligaments, cartilage, and bones to additional forces if they are required to absorb the forces normally absorbed by muscles. The result could be a decelerator injury seen in many sports.

Chronic training involving eccentric muscle action can lead to a variety of overuse syndromes such as tendonitis. It should not be surprising that graded exercises involving eccentric muscle actions might be useful in restoration of function in people with "tennis elbow." It has become common to use this type of exercise in rehabilitation programs in sports medicine [117]. The exact balance between just enough eccentric muscle action for positive adaptation and too much leading to exacerbation needs further study.

Finally, a unique clinical application of eccentric muscle action has appeared for the classification and treatment of patients with spasticity [72]. In patients with spastic paresis, performance of concentric muscle action is inhibited by the stretch activation of the antagonistic muscles. Antagonistic muscle activation during voluntary movement inhibits muscle function by serving as a mechanical resistance to the agonist action and by inhibiting agonist activation through interneurons in the spinal cord. Training using only eccentric muscle actions eliminates the inhibitory actions and allows for a marked improvement in muscle strength and function. Thus, evaluation and training using eccentric muscle actions may have special applications in neurology.

SUMMARY

Eccentric muscle action deserves special consideration from the standpoint of physiology, adaptation, and training. The function of muscles as shock absorbers or springs seems to be quite different from other actions described in classical descriptions of muscle biology. This uniqueness certainly requires a more careful understanding of muscle as a unit consisting of myofibers and fascia which may work together or in opposition in response to chronic or acute stimuli. In addition, the stretch–shortening cycle is a special case of its own. However, from the standpoint of maximum human performance, there remain tremendous gaps in our understanding of the role of eccentric muscle action and its use in athletic training. How much is good? Does microfibrosis represent a problem of overtraining and eventually limit performance, or is it advantageous for success? Is the body-builder really developing muscle or connective tissue separating muscles? How does eccentric muscle action sometimes produce pain but not always? It would appear that much work is needed before a complete understanding of eccentric muscle action is obtained. This brief review has been designed to encourage research, argument, and discussion.

ACKNOWLEDGMENTS

Special thanks goes to Francoise D. Stauber for critically reviewing the manuscript, Valerie K. Fritz for her excellent assistance, and John A. Firth for his continued encouragement. This project was supported in part by funds from Comptex, Inc.

REFERENCES

1. Abbott BC, Aubert XM, Hill AV: The absorption of work by a muscle stretched during a single twitch of a short tetanus. *Proc R Soc Lond (Biol)* 139:86–104, 1951.
2. Abbott BC, Aubert XM: Changes of energy in a muscle during very slow stretches. *Proc R Soc Lond (Biol)* 139:104–117, 1951.
3. Abbott BC, Bigland B, Ritchie JM: The physiological cost of negative work. *J Physiol* 117:380–390, 1952.
4. Abraham WM: Factors in delayed muscle soreness. *Med Sci Sports* 9:11–20, 1977.
5. Armstrong BW, Hurt HH, Workman JM: Downhill walking as a possible form of negative work. *Am J Physiol* 211:1264–1268, 1966.

6. Armstrong RB, Ogilvie RW, Schwane JA: Eccentric exercise-induced injury to rat skeletal muscle. *J Appl Physiol* 54:80–93, 1983.

7. Asmusen E: Observations on experimental muscular soreness. *Acta Rheum Scand* 2:109–116, 1952.

8. Asmussen E: Positive and negative muscular work. *Acta Physiol Scand* 28:365–382, 1953.

9. Aura O, Komi PV: Effects of prestretch on mechanical efficiency of positive work and on elastic behavior of skeletal muscle in stretch-shortening cycle exercise. *Int J Sports Med* 7:137–143, 1986.

10. Barnett JG, Holly RG, Ashmore CR: Stretch-induced growth in chicken wing muscles: biochemical and morphological characterization. *Am J Physiol* 239:C39-C46, 1980.

11. Bennett JG, Stauber WT: Evaluation and treatment of anterior knee pain using eccentric exercise. *Med Sci Sports Exerc* 18:526–530, 1986.

12. Bertolotto A, Palmucci L, Doriguzzi C, Mongini E, Gagnor M, del Rosso M, Tarone G: Laminin and fibronection distribution in normal and pathological human muscle. *J Neurol Sci* 60:377–382, 1983.

13. Bigland B, Lippold OCJ: The relation between force, velocity and integrated electrical activity in human muscles. *J Physiol* 123:214–224, 1954.

14. Bigland-Ritchie B: EMG/Force relations and fatigue of human voluntary contractions. In Miller DI (ed): *Exercise and Sport Sciences Reviews*. Philadelphia, The Franklin Institute, 1981, vol 9, pp 75–117.

15. Bischoff R: Proliferation of muscle satellite cells on intact myofibers in culture. *Dev Biol* 115:129–139, 1986.

16. Bischoff R: A satellite cell mitogen from crushed adult muscle. *Dev Biol* 115:140–147, 1986.

17. Borg TK, Caufield JB: Morphology of connective tissue in skeletal muscle. *Tissue Cell* 12:197–207, 1980.

18. Borg TK, Klevay LM, Gay RE, Siegel R, Bergin ME: Alteration of connectie tissue network of striated muscle in copper deficient rats. *J Mol Cell Cardiol* 17:1173–1183, 1985.

19. Brzank VKD, Pieper KS: Die Wirkung intensiver, kraftbetonter Trainingsbleastungen auf die Feinstruktur der menschlichen Skelettmuskelkapillare. *Anat Anz* 161:243–248, 1986.

20. Burr DB, Martin RB, Schaffler MB, Radin EL: Bone remodeling in response to in vivo fatigue microdamage. *J Biomech* 18:189–200, 1985.

21. Byrnes WC, Clarkson PM, White JS, Hsieh SS, Frykman PN, Maughan RJ: Delayed onset muscle soreness following repeated bouts of downhill running. *J Appl Physiol* 59:710–715, 1985.

22. Carlson BM, Faulkner JA: The regeneration of skeletal muscle fibers following injury: a review. *Med Sci Sports Exerc* 15:187–198, 1983.

23. Cavanagh PR: On "muscle action" vs "muscle contraction." *J Biomech* 21:69, 1988.

24. Chapman AE: The mechanical properties of human muscle. In Terjung RL (ed): *Exercise and Sport Sciences Reviews*. New York, Macmillan, 1985, vol 13, pp 443–501.

25. Clarkson PM, Tremblay I: Rapid adaptation to exercise induced muscle damage. *Med Sci Sports Exerc* 19:S36, 1987.

26. Clarkson PM, Byrnes WC, Gillisson E, Harper E: Adaptation to exercise-induced muscle damage. *Clin Sci* 73:383–386, 1987.

27. Curtin N, Gilbert C, Kretzschmar KM, Wilkie DR: The effect of the performance of work on total energy output and metabolism during muscular contraction. *J Physiol* 238:455–472, 1974.

28. Curwin S, Stanish WD: *Tendinitis: Its Etiology and Treatment.* Lexington, Collamore Press, 1984, pp 1–189.
29. Davies CT, White MJ: Muscle weakness following eccentric work in man. *Pflügers Arch* 392:168–171, 1981.
30. Dick RW, Cavanagh PR: An explanation of the upward drift in oxygen uptake during prolonged sub-maximal downhill running. *Med Sci Sports Exerc* 19:310–317, 1987.
31. Duncan CJ: Role of calcium in triggering rapid ultrastructural damage in muscle: a study with chemically skinned fibers. *J Cell Sci* 87:581–594, 1987.
32. Edman KAP, Elizinga G, Noble MIM: The effect of stretch on contracting skeletal muscle fibers. In Sugi H, Pollack GH (eds): *Cross-Bridge Mechanism in Muscle Contraction.* Baltimore, University Park Press, 1979, pp 297–309.
33. Edwards RHT, Hill DK, Jones DA, Merton PA: Fatigue of long duration in human skeletal muscle after exercise. *J Physiol* 272:769–778, 1977.
34. Edwards RHT, Jones DA: Diseases of skeletal muscle. In *Handbook of Physiology: Vol. 10. Skeletal Muscle.* Baltimore, Williams & Wilkins, 1983, pp 633–672.
35. Edwards RHT: Muscle fatigue and pain. *Acta Med Scand(Suppl)* 711:179–188, 1987.
36. Evans WJ, Meredith CN, Cannon JG, Dinarello CA, Frontera WR, Hughes VA, Jones BH, Knuttgen HG: Metabolic changes following eccentric exercise in trained and untrained men. *J Appl Physiol* 61:1864–1868, 1986.
37. Field EJ: The development of the conducting system in the heart of sheep. *Br Heart J* 13:129–147, 1951.
38. Friden J, Sjostrom M, Ekblom B: A morphological study of delayed muscle soreness. *Experientia* 37:506–507, 1981.
39. Friden J, Sjostrom M, Ekblom B: Myofibrillar damage following intense eccentric exercise in man. *Int J Sports Med* 4:170–176, 1983.
40. Friden J: Changes in human skeletal muscle induced by long-term eccentric exercise. *Cell Tissue Res* 236:365–372, 1984.
41. Friden J, Sfakianos PN, Hargens AR: Muscle soreness and intramuscular fluid pressure: comparison between eccentric and concentric load. *J Appl Physiol* 61:2175–2179, 1986.
42. Fritz VK, Stauber WT: Characterization of muscles injured by forced lengthening: II. Proteoglycans. *Med Sci Sports Exerc* 20:354–361, 1988.
43. Froese EA, Houston ME: Torque-velocity characteristics and muscle fiber type in human vastas lateralis. *J Appl Physiol* 59:309–314, 1985.
44. Garrett WE, Nikolaou PK, Ribbeck BM, Glisson RR, Seaber AV: The effect of muscle architecture on the biomechanical failure properties of skeletal muscle under passive extension. *Am J Sports Med* 16:7–12, 1988.
45. Goldberg AL, Etlinger JD, Goldspink DF, Jablecki C: Mechanism of work-induced hypertrophy of skeletal muscle. *Med Sci Sports* 7:185–198, 1975.
46. Goldspink G: Growth of muscle. In Goldspink DF (ed): *Development and Specialization of Skeletal Muscle.* London, Cambridge University Press, 1981, pp 19–35.
47. Gollnick PD, King DW: Effect of exercise and training on mitochondria of rat skeletal muscle. *Am J Physiol* 216:1502–1509, 1969.
48. Hansen KN, Bjerre-Knudsen J, Brodthagen U, Jordal R, Paulev PE: Muscle cell leakage due to long distance training. *Eur J Appl Physiol* 48:177–178, 1982.
49. Harrington WF: On the origin of the contractile force in skeletal muscle. *Proc Natl Acad Sci USA* 76:5066–5070, 1979.
50. Hasan Z, Enoka RM, Stuart DG: The interface between biomechanics and neurophysiology in the study of movement: some recent approaches. In Terjung RL (ed): *Exercise Sports Sciences Reviews.* New York, Macmillan, 1985, vol 13, pp 169–234.

51. Hasan Z, Stuart DG: Mammalian muscle receptors. In Davidoff RA (ed): *Handbook of the Spinal Cord*: Vols. 2 and 3. Anatomy and Physiology. New York, Marcel Dekker, 1984, pp 559–607.

52. Haseman MK, Kriss JP: Selective, symmetric, skeletal muscle uptake of Tc–99m pyrophosphate in rhabdomyolysis. *Clin Nucl Med* 10:180–183, 1985.

53. Heppenstall RB, Sapega AA, Scott R, Shenton D, Park YS, Maris J, Chance B: The compartment syndrome. An experimental and clinical study of muscular energy metabolism using phosphorus nuclear magnetic resonance spectroscopy. *Clin Orthop* 226:138–155, 1988.

54. Hikada RS, Staron RS, Hagerman FC, Sherman WM, Costill DL: Muscle fiber necrosis associated with human marathon runners. *J Neurol Sci* 59:185–203, 1983.

55. Hill AV: The heat of shortening and the dynamic constants of muscle. *Proc R Soc Lond (Biol)* 126:136–195, 1938.

56. Hough T: Ergographic studies in muscular soreness. *Am J Physiol* 7:76–92, 1902.

57. Howell JN, Chila AG, Ford G, David D, Gates T: An electromyographic study of elbow motion during postexercise muscle soreness. *J Appl Physiol* 58:1713–1718, 1985.

58. Hudgson P, Field EJ: Regeneration of muscle. In Bourne GH (ed): *The Structure and Function of Muscle*, ed 2. New York, Academic Press, 1973, vol 2, pp 312–363.

59. Hughston JC, Walsh WM, Puddu G: *Patellar Subluxation and Dislocation*. Philadelphia, W. B. Saunders, 1984, vol 5, pp 1–191.

60. Huxley HE: The mechanism of muscular contraction. *Science* 164:1356–1366, 1969.

61. Huxley HE: General discussion. In Sugi H, Pollack GH, (eds): *Cross-Bridge Mechanism in Muscle Contracting*. Baltimore, University Park Press, 1979, p 638.

62. Ishikawa H, Sawada H, Yamada E: Surface and internal morphology of skeletal muscle. In *Handbook of Physiology*: Section 10. Skeletal Muscle. Bethesda, MD, American Physiological Society, 1983, pp 1–22.

63. Jones DA, Jackson MJ, McPhail G, Edards RHT: Experimental mouse muscle damage: the importance of external calcium. *Clin Sci* 66:317–322, 1984.

64. Jones DA, Newham DJ, Round JM, Tolfree SEJ. Experimental human muscle damage: morphological changes in relation to other indices of damage. *J Physiol* 375:435–448, 1986.

65. Jones DA, Newham DJ, Clarkson PM: Skeletal muscle stiffness and pain following eccentric exercise of the elbow flexors. *Pain* 30:233–242, 1987.

66. Jorgensen K: Force–velocity relationship in human elbow flexors and extensors. In Komi PV (ed): *International Series on Biomechanics*: Vol. 1A. Biomechanics V-A. Baltimore, University Park Press, 1976, pp 145–151.

67. Katz AM: *Physiology of the Heart*. New York, Raven Press, 1977, pp 132–136.

68. Katz B: The relation between force and speed in muscular contraction. *J Physiol* 96:45–64, 1939.

69. Katz EP, Wachtel EJ, Maroudas A: Extrafibrillar proteoglycans osmotically regulate the molecular packing of collagen in cartilage. *Biochim Biophys Acta* 882:136–139, 1986.

70. King SW, Statland BE, Savory J: The effect of a short burst of exercise on activity values of enzymes in sera of healthy young men. *Clin Chim Acta* 72:211–218, 1976.

71. Klausen K, Knuttgen H: Effect of training on oxygen consumption in negative muscular work. *Acta Physiol Scand* 83:319–323, 1971.

72. Knutsson E: Analysis of spastic paresis. In *Proceedings of the Tenth International Congress of the World Confederation for Physical Therapy*. Sydney 1987, pp 629–633.

73. Knutsson E, Gransberg L, Martensson A: Facilitation and inhibition of maximal voluntary contractions by the activation of muscle stretch reflexes in patients with spastic paresis. *EEG Clin Neurophysiol*, in press.

74. Knuttgen HG: Human performance in high-intensity exercise with concentric and eccentric muscle contractions. *Int J Sports Med (Suppl)* 7:6–9, 1986.

75. Knuttgen HG, Kraemer WJ: Terminology and measurement in exercise performance. *J Appl Sport Res* 1:1–10, 1987.

76. Komi PV, Buskirk ER: Measurement of eccentric and concentric conditioning on tension and electrical activity in human muscle. *Ergonomics* 15:417–434, 1972.

77. Komi PV: Relationship between muscle tension, EMG, and velocity of contraction under concentric and eccentric work. In Desmedt JE (ed): *New Developments in Electromyography and Clinical Neurophysiology.* Karger, Basel, 1973, vol 1, pp 596–606.

78. Komi PV: Physiological and biomechanical correlates of muscle function: effects of muscle structure and stretch-shortening cycle on force and speed. In Terjung RL (ed): *Exercise and Sport Sciences Reviews.* Lexington, MA, Collamore Press, 1984, vol 12, pp 81–121.

79. Kovanen V, Suominen H, Heikkinen E: Connective tissue of "fast" and "slow" skeletal muscle in rats—effects of endurance training. *Acta Physiol Scand* 108:173–180, 1980.

80. Kovanen V, Suominen H, Heikkinen E: Mechanical properties of fast and slow skeletal muscle with special reference to collagen and endurance training. *J Biomech* 17:725–735, 1984.

81. Kumazawa T, Mizumura K: Thin-fibre receptors responding to mechanical, chemical and thermal stimulation in skeletal muscle of the dog. *J Physiol* 273:179–194, 1977.

82. Lane RJM, Turnbull DM, Welch JL, Walton SJ: A double-blind, placebo-controlled, crossover study of verapamil in exertional muscle pain. *Muscle Nerve* 9:635–641 1986.

83. Laurent GJ, Millward DJ: Protein turnover during skeletal muscle hypertrophy. *Fed Proc* 39:42–47, 1980.

84. Lehto M, Jaarvinen M, Nelimarkka O: Scar formation after skeletal muscle injury. A histological and autoradiographical study in rats. *Arch Orthop Trauma Surg* 104:366–370, 1986.

85. Loeb GE: The control and responses of mammalian muscle spindles during normally executed motor tasks. In Terjung RL (ed): *Exercise and Sport Sciences Reviews.* Lexington, MA, Collamore Press, 1984, vol 12, pp 157–204.

86. MacDougall JD, Sale DG, Elder GCB, Sutton JR: Muscle ultra-structural characteristics of elite powerlifters and bodybuilders. *Eur J Appl Physiol* 48:117–126, 1982.

87. MacDougall JD, Sale DG, Alway SE, Sutton JR: Muscle fiber number in biceps brachii in bodybuilders and control subjects. *J Appl Physiol* 57:1399–1403, 1984.

88. Margaria R: Positive and negative work performances and their efficiencies in human locomotion. In Cumming GR, Snidal D, Taylor AW (eds): *Environmental Effects on Work Performance.* Edmonton, Canadian Association of Sports Sciences, 1972, pp 215–228.

89. McCully KK, Faulkner JA: Injury to skeletal muscle fibers of mice following lengthening contractions. *J Appl Physiol* 59:119–126, 1985.

90. McCully KK, Faulkner JA: Characteristics of lengthening contractions associated with injury to skeletal muscle fibers. *J Appl Physiol* 61:293–299, 1986.

91. Mense S, Schmidt RF: Activation of group IV afferent units from muscle by algesic agents. *Brain Res* 72:305–310, 1974.

92. Mubarak SJ: Exertional compartment syndromes. In Mubarak SJ, Hargens AR (eds): *Compartment Syndromes and Volkman's Contracture.* Philadelphia, W. B. Saunders, 1981, pp 209–226.

93. Newham DJ, Mills KR, Quigley BM, Edwards RHT: Pain and fatigue after concentric and eccentric muscle contractions. *Clin Sci* 64:55–62, 1983.

94. Newham DJ, McPhail G, Mills KR, Edwards RHT: Ultrastructural changes after concentric and eccentric contractions of human muscle. *J Neurol Sci* 61:109–122, 1983.

95. Newham DJ, Clarkson PM: Repeated high-force eccentric exercise: effects on muscle pain and damage. *J Appl Physiol* 63:1381–1386, 1987.

96. Patton HD, Sundstein JW, Crill WE, Swanson PD: *Introduction to Basic Neurology.* Philadelphia, W. B. Saunders, 1976, pp 131–132.

97. Pennington RJT: Biochemical aspects of muscle disease. In Walton JN (ed): *Disorders of Voluntary Muscle.* Edinburgh, Churchill Livingstone, 1981, pp 417–444.

98. Perrine JJ, Edgerton VR: Muscle force–velocity and power–velocity relationships under isokinetic loading. *Med Sci Sports Exerc* 10:159–166, 1978.

99. Postlethwaite AE, Kang AH: Colalgen- and collagen peptide-induced chemotaxis of human blood monocytes. *J Exp Med* 143:1299–1307, 1976.

100. Publicover SF, Duncan CJ, Smith JL: The use of A23187 to demonstrate the role of intracellular calcium in causing ultrastructural damage in mammalian cells. *J Neuropathol Exp Neurol* 37:S544–557, 1978.

101. Radin EL: Role of muscles in protecting athletes from injury. *Acta Med Scand (Suppl)* 711:143–147, 1986.

102. Rall JA: Energetic aspects of skeletal muscle contraction: implications of fiber types. In Terjung RL (ed): *Exercise and Sport Sciences Reviews.* New York, Macmillan, 1985, vol 13, pp 33–74.

103. Ralston HJ, Pollissar MJ, Inman VT, Close JR, Feinstein B: Dynamic features of human isolated voluntary muscle in isometric and free contractions. *J Appl Physiol* 1:526–533, 1949.

104. Remmers AR, Kaljot V: Serum transaminase levels. Effect of strenuous and prolonged physical exercise on healthy young subjects. *JAMA* 185:968–970, 1963.

105. Rodnan GP, Schumacher HR: *Primer on the Rheumatic Diseases,* ed. 8. Atlanta, GA, Arthritis Foundation, 1983, pp 217.

106. Rogers MA, Stull GA, Apple RS: Creatine kinase isoenzyme activities in men and women following a marathon race. *Med Sci Sports Exerc* 17:679–682, 1985.

107. Schmidt RF, Thews G: *Human Physiology.* Berlin, Springer-Verlag, 1983, p 425.

108. Schmitt HP, Bersch W, Feutstel HP: Acute abdominal rhabdomyolysis after body building exercise: is there a "rectus abdominus syndrome"? *Muscle Nerve* 6:228–232, 1983.

109. Schwane JA, Johnson SR, Vandenakker CB, Armstrong RB: Delayed-onset muscular soreness and plasma CPK and LDH activities after downhill running. *Med Sci Sports Exerc* 15:51–56, 1983.

110. Schwane JA, Williams JS, Sloan JH: Effects of training on delayed muscle soreness creatine kinase activity after running. *Med Sci Sports Exerc* 19:584–590, 1987.

111. Siegel AJ, Warhol MJ, Lang G: Muscle injury and repair in ultra-long distance runners. In Sutton JR, Brock RM (eds): *Sports Medicine for the Mature Athlete.* Indianapolis, Benchmark Press, 1986, pp 35–43.

112. Singh M, Karpovich PV: Isotonic and isometric forces of forearm flexors and extensors. *J Appl Physiol* 21:1435–1437, 1966.

113. Singh M, Karpovich PV: Effect of eccentric training of agonists on antagonistic muscles. *J Appl Physiol* 23:742–745, 1967.

114. Snow MH: Myogenic cell formation in regeneration rat skeletal muscle injured by mincing. I. A fine structural study. *Anat Rec* 188:181–200, 1977.

115. Snow MH: Myogenic cell formation in regeneration rat skeletal muscle injured by mincing. II. An autoradiographic study. *Anat Rec* 188:200–218, 1977.

116. Stacy MJ: Free nerve endings in skeletal muscle of the cat. *J Anat* 105:231–254, 1969.
117. Stanish WD, Rubinovich RM, Curwin S: Eccentric exercise in chronic tendinitis. *Clin Orthop* 208:65–68, 1986.
118. Statham HE, Duncan CJ, Smith JL: The effect of the ionophore A23187 on the ultrastructure and electrophysiological properties of frog skeletal muscle. *Cell Tissue Res* 173:193–209, 1976.
119. Stauber WT: Editor's note. *Recent Advances in Robotic Dynamometry* 3:6, 1987.
120. Stauber WT, Fritz VK, Vogelbach DW, Dahlmann B: Characterization of muscles injured by forced lengthening. I. Cellular infiltrates. *Med Sci Sports Exerc* 20:345–353, 1988.
121. Stokes M, Young A: The contribution of reflex inhibition to arthrogenous muscle weakness. *Clin Sci* 67:7–14, 1984.
122. Talag TS: Residual muscular soreness as influenced by concentric, eccentric and static contractions. *Res Q* 44:458–469, 1973.
123. Tesch PA, Larson L: Muscle hypertrophy in bodybuilders. *Eur J Appl Physiol* 49:301–306, 1982.
124. Tidball JG, Daniel TL: Elastic energy storage in rigored skeletal muscle cells under physiological loading conditions. *Am J Physiol* 250:R56-R64, 1986.
125. Tidus PM, Ianuzzo CD: Effects of intensity and duration of muscular exercise on delayed soreness and serum enzyme activities. *Med Sci Sports Exerc* 15:461–465, 1983.
126. Triolo R, Robinson D, Gardner E, Betz R: The eccentric strength of electrically stimulated paralyzed muscle. *IEEE Trans Biomed Eng* 651–652, 1987.
127. Vandenburgh HH, Kaufman S: In vitro skeletal muscle hypertrophy and Na pump activity. In Pette D (ed): *Plasticity of Muscle*. Berlin, Walter de Gruyter, 1980, pp 493–506.
128. Wallensten R, Eklund B: Intramuscular pressures and muscle metabolism after short-term and long-term exercise. *Int J Sports Med* 4:231–235, 1983.
129. Warholl MJ, Siegel AJ, Evans WJ, Silverman LM: Skeletal muscle injury and repair in marathon runners after competition. *Am J Pathol* 118:331–339, 1985.
130. Wilkie DR: The relation between force and velocity in human muscle. *J Physiol* 110:249–280, 1950.
131. Wrogemann K, Pena SDJ: Mitochondrial calcium overload: a general mechanism for cell-necrosis in muscle diseases. *Lancet* 1:672–674, 1976.
132. Yoshimura T, Tsujihata M, Satoh A, Mori M, Hazama R, Kinoshita N, Takashima H, Nagataki S: Ultrastructural study of the effect of calcium ionophore, A23187, on rat muscle. *Acta Neuropathol (Berl)* 69:184–192, 1986.

6
Determining Muscle's Force and Action in Multi-Articular Movement

FELIX E. ZAJAC, Ph.D.
MICHAEL E. GORDON, M.S.

INTRODUCTION

Knowledge of muscle forces and their action on the body is fundamental for improving the diagnosis and treatment of persons with movement disabilities and analyzing the techniques used by Olympic-caliber athletes to achieve exceptional performance. Muscle forces can sometimes be recorded directly or can be computed from electromyographic (EMG) signals. Alternatively, muscle forces can be estimated using models of multijoint dynamics, either alone or together with kinematic and reaction force data. Once muscle force is determined, the next step is to determine the body motion caused by the muscle force.

The direction of the torque exerted by a muscle, determined by the muscle's anatomical location, is often used to infer the muscle's action on movement of the body. For example, a muscle that develops a flexor torque is assumed to flex the spanned joint. For tasks in which only one joint of the body is free to rotate in a single direction, any muscle spanning the joint and exerting a flexor torque will indeed act to flex the joint.

For multijoint movement, however, extreme caution should be exercised when anatomy alone is used to infer the action of a muscle, since a muscle acts to accelerate all joints, whether spanned or not. For example, soleus exerts only an ankle extensor torque, yet it can accelerate the knee into extension with more vigor than it accelerates the ankle into extension. Biarticular muscles can have a multitude of actions. For example, gastrocnemius, which exerts both ankle-extensor and knee-flexor torques, can act to (*a*) extend the ankle and flex the knee, (*b*) flex the ankle (*sic*) and flex the knee, or (*c*) extend the ankle and extend the knee (*sic*). Since a muscle's action depends on the position of the body and on the muscle's interaction with external objects (such as the ground), it can vary among motor tasks, and even during a single motor task.

Classified either by its action on joint rotation or by the direction of its torque(s), a muscle can be said to assist (or hinder) the motor task and can also be said to work in concert with (or in opposition to) other muscles. At times, a muscle is called an *agonist* if its torque is in the same

187

FIGURE 6.1

System dynamics. The excitation of muscles received from the nervous system is manifested in their electromyograms (EMGs), the "inputs" to the dynamic system. The forces developed by muscles and transmitted to their tendons (forces) depend on the integrated dynamical properties of the muscles and tendons (musculotendon dynamics) and on the joint angles (ϕ) and velocities ($\dot{\phi}$). Forces are linear in torques by the relations among the muscles and the joint centers of rotation (joint geometry), which depend on joint angles. Torques cause rotary motion of the joints, which are the joint angular accelerations ($\ddot{\phi}$) and velocities ($\dot{\phi}$), and joint angles (ϕ).

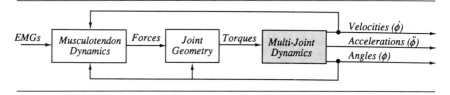

direction as the net torque that muscles must develop to produce the motion. Two muscles can also be called an *agonist–antagonist pair* if their torques are in opposite directions. Alternatively, the actions caused by a muscle can be used to determine agonist–antagonist relationships. Because muscles that work together need not function identically, it may be best to study how muscles work as *synergists* rather than as *agonists*.

MUSCLE FORCE DURING MOVEMENT

Muscle forces can sometimes be measured directly. Often this is not possible, and instead muscle forces are estimated by processing the recorded EMG signals. Another indirect approach is to apply static optimization to estimate what each muscle force must be to produce the required torques, which are computed from measurements of body motion and external reaction forces. Muscle forces can also be estimated without measurement of EMG signals, body motion, or reaction forces by applying dynamic optimization techniques to a model of the system dynamics (Fig. 6.1) and the task being performed.

Recording Tendon Force

Tendon force has been recorded in animals during a variety of motor tasks [117, 118]. One method is to measure the strain, which is proportional to force, in a metal transducer shaped as a buckle and through which the tendon passes [11, 117, 118]. Another method is to use a liquid metal strain gauge placed in parallel with the tendon [18, 106]. With either technique, the net force delivered to the tendon from all of the muscle's motor units is recorded. This net force is usually assumed to be the sum of the forces generated by the motor units, though it may not be if some units absorb mechanical energy from others. Obviously, only those muscles with well-defined external tendons are candidates, and the technique has limited potential in humans.

Estimating Force from the Electromyogram

The estimation of force from an EMG signal [58] is most often based on a Hill-type model of muscle dynamics [55, 125]. In such models, muscle force depends on the neural excitation (EMG signal) and the length and velocity (rate of shortening or lengthening) of the muscle fibers. As Hill noted long ago, tendon stretch affects the length and velocity of muscle fibers. Therefore, muscle force must be computed from a model that includes both muscle and tendon (Figs. 6.1 and 6.2**A**). The model must be a dynamic one because force depends on its past trajectory [125]. With a model of the attachment of muscle and tendon to the body, muscle-fiber length and velocity can be calculated from the joint angles and velocities. Therefore, the model has EMG activity, joint angles, and joint velocities as inputs, and force as the output (Figs. 6.1 and 6.2**A**).

A consequence of this type of model for muscle dynamics is the well-known, steady-state proportional relation between the force and the smoothed EMG signal observed in isometric contractions [77]. The estimation of muscle forces from EMG signals has been used to gain insight into muscle's "active state" [43], neural control of human locomotion [104, 105], and energy storage in series musculotendon elastic structures during human walking [56] and jumping [13]. Forces in muscles during walking, estimated from EMG signals, have been shown to compare favorably with estimates computed from measurements of body motion and external reaction forces, as described below [57, 93, 105].

Systems Dynamics and Net Muscle Torques

Before we review other methods used to estimate muscle forces, let us review the *natural* flow of kinetic and kinematic events occurring in the body (i.e., the system dynamics; Fig. 6.1). The nervous system excites the muscular system, and this excitation is manifested in the EMG signals. Excitation of the muscular system leads to the development of forces, which are related to torques at the joints by the juxtaposition of the muscles to the joints. Torques cause angular accelerations of the joints which, after time, cause the joint angular velocities and angles to change. Thus, the natural flow of events is efferent: from the nervous system, to the muscular system to the skeletal system.

To scrutinize the natural flow of events further, let us assume that m muscles are producing movement of n joints, where $m > n$ (Fig. 6.2**A**).

FIGURE 6.2

*Comparison of direct (**A**) and inverse (**B**) system dynamics. **A**, Muscle excitations are the inputs, body motions are the outputs, and thus the flow of events is natural. If all the elements are modeled (i.e., musculotendon dynamics, moment arms R(ϕs), and multijoint dynamics), and if the criterion by which performance is judged is specified mathematically, dynamic optimization can be applied to find all the "inputs" (EMG[1] . . . EMG[m]), and thus all the "outputs" (i.e., F^1 . . . F^m; T_1^{mus} . . . T_n^{mus}; $\ddot{\phi}_1$ . . . $\ddot{\phi}_n$; $\dot{\phi}_1$ . . . $\dot{\phi}_n$; ϕ_1 . . . ϕ_n). **B**, Body positions are the inputs, and thus the flow of events is inverted. Some variation of the inverse dynamics approach is used to find the net muscle torques (T_1^{mus} . . . T_n^{mus}) derived from f^{-1} ($\ddot{\phi}$ s, $\dot{\phi}$ s, ϕ s), measurements of ϕ_1 . . . ϕ_n, and computations of $\dot{\phi}_1$ . . . $\dot{\phi}_n$ and $\ddot{\phi}_1$ . . . $\ddot{\phi}_n$ (see text). Individual muscle forces are not uniquely determined from net muscle torques and static optimization is used to find a "best" set of muscle forces (see text).*

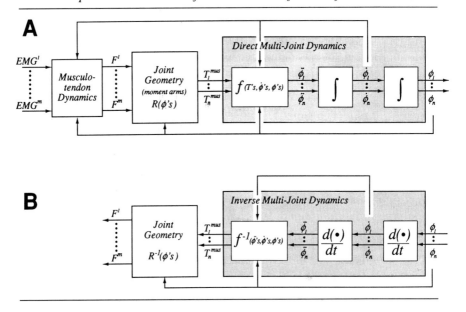

Thus, *m* EMG signals (EMG[1] . . . EMG[m]) generate *m* muscle forces (F^1 . . . F^m), which are trajectory dependent (i.e., dynamic, given by musculotendon dynamics). Each muscle force generates a torque about all the joints it spans. Each torque is the product of muscle force and its *moment arm* (the muscle's shortest distance from the joint). The sum of the torques developed by all muscles spanning a joint is the *net muscle torque*; so for *n* joints there are *n* net muscle torques (T_1^{mus} . . . T_n^{mus}) (see Appendix A for discussion of muscle force, moment of muscle force, moment arm, and torque).

These net muscle torques produce motion of the joints, which is given by the direct multijoint dynamics of the system (Fig. 6.2**A**). The reason the dynamics is referred to as "direct dynamics" is that it specifies the *natural* sequence in which motion occurs. Thus, the net muscle torques, in combination with torques due to gravity and current motion of the joints (not shown in Fig. 6.2**A**; see figure legend), accelerate the joints of the body instantly ($\ddot{\phi}_1 \ldots \ddot{\phi}_n$). However, joint angular velocities ($\dot{\phi}_1 \ldots \dot{\phi}_n$) and joint angles ($\phi_1 \ldots \phi_n$) do not change instantly, but develop over time (Fig. 6.2**A**, integral symbols). Thus, motion of the joints is dynamical.

In summary, the actual sequence of events in nature is that the muscle excitations are the inputs, and all the other variables can be considered the outputs (Fig. 6.2**A**). By definition, all the outputs can be calculated if the inputs are known. So given an initial value for all independent outputs (e.g., muscle forces and the joint angles and velocities), the trajectory of muscle forces and body motion is known if the EMG trajectory is given.

Estimating Net Muscle Torques from Inverse Dynamics
Inverse dynamics can be employed to estimate the net torque that muscles must have produced to have generated the movement [17, 22]. Thus, the natural, direct multijoint dynamics are inverted and used to compute the n net muscle torques ($T_1^{mus} \ldots T_n^{mus}$), given that the kinematics ($\ddot{\phi}_1 \ldots \ddot{\phi}_n; \dot{\phi}_1 \ldots \dot{\phi}_n; \phi_1 \ldots \phi_n$) are known (Fig. 6.2, compare the direct multijoint dynamics with the inverse multijoint dynamics). Thus recorded data of joint angles versus time can be differentiated once to yield velocities versus time, or a second time to yield joint accelerations versus time. Once joint angular positions, velocities, and accelerations are calculated, then net joint torques can be computed.

However, reaction force data are often used to compute the net muscle torques [17, 20, 34, 81, 101, 120, 121, 128]. External reaction forces serve as a measure of the inertia forces of the body segments, which obviates modeling of the whole body [17, 34, 81]. In gait, for example, net ankle muscle torques can be computed from ground reaction forces, from a model of the foot, and from estimates of the acceleration of the foot [17, 101, 120]. Thus, neither the mass distribution of all segments proximal to the ankle, nor their accelerations, would have to be measured or computed. And acceleration data are especially noisy because position data are differentiated twice [20, 120]. Thus, the inertia force of all the segments proximal to the ankle, including the large inertia force of the trunk [68], does not have to be estimated from kinematic data.

This variation of the inverse dynamics approach to compute net muscle torques continues to be widely used in studies of many tasks, for example, in studies of human and animal gait [2, 20, 29, 101, 104, 105,

120, 121], jumping [1, 13, 76], sitting [113], and pedaling [46, 66, 91]. The reason for calculating net muscle torques, rather than examining recordings of body motion alone, is that finding net muscle torques makes it easier to infer which muscles need to generate force, and how much force. Knowledge of net muscle torques needed at the hip, knee, and ankle during walking, for example, can be helpful in the quantitative assessment of amputee and pathological gait, and in the design of subsequent rehabilitation strategies [22, 29, 85, 119–121].

Estimating Force Using Static Optimization
Once net muscle torques are computed, determining individual muscle forces is often not straightforward because the number of muscles m may exceed the number of joints n. In this case, there is not enough information to uniquely determine the individual muscle forces, and many solutions are possible (e.g., $R^{-1}(\phi\ s)$ does not exist even though $R(\phi\ s)$ does; see Fig. 6.2A, **B**). It's much like being asked to solve for x and y given only that $x + y = 6$. A solution can be found, however, if enough muscles are observed or assumed to be inactive so that the number of active muscles does not exceed the number of joints.

Static optimization can also be employed to find the muscles forces from the net muscle torques [27, 100, 103, 110]. With this approach, a mathematical description of what the body is trying to optimize at a specific instant, the cost function, is defined. Using relatively simple algorithms, a solution which minimizes the cost function is found, and the individual muscle forces are determined. Then the algorithm is repeated to find a solution corresponding to another instant of the motor task. A commonly used cost function is the sum of muscle stresses, where each stress is weighted by an exponent that is the same for each muscle [27, 28]. (Muscle stress is the force in muscle divided by its physiological cross-sectional area.)

The choice of a suitable cost function is critical to this approach, and the cost function determines what kinds of results are possible. For example, a minimal stress cost function cannot result in the coactivation of antagonist muscles, a strategy that might be useful for improving measures of performance unrelated to simple energetic efficiency.

Nevertheless, because static optimization is based on well-developed theories [79], computational algorithms are commercially available to readily solve such problems. Static optimization has been used to find the distribution of forces of limb muscles during walking, jumping, and cartwheeling [28, 29, 32, 47, 98, 102, 110, 116], of elbow and knee muscles during isometric and isokinetic tasks [4, 27, 33, 54, 103], of trunk muscles during posture [12], of facial muscles during biting [95], and of finger muscles during flexion [19]. Limitations of the approach include the somewhat arbitrary choice of a cost function [28, 33, 54,

100]; its sensitivity to parameters, such as muscle cross-sectional area [16]; and the resolution of the kinematic recordings or torque computations [98].

Estimating Force from Direct Dynamics

If recordings of EMG signals are available, a model of the system dynamics can be used to generate muscle forces and body motion (Fig. 6.2**A**). A simulation of human walking, partially based on the "central pattern generator" theory of locomotion [105], has employed this approach, though the effort to date seems, understandably, to have been in constructing and validating the simulation rather than in analyzing the simulation to gain fundamental understanding of human gait.

We have empathy because our past experience in using eight muscles to drive a four-segment model of the body to jump has indicated how critical muscle timing is [62]. We found it virtually impossible to find EMG inputs by trial and error that produce physiological trajectories, even when we based the simulation EMG inputs on measured EMG signals. The reason is, of course, that control of a four-segment, inverted pendulum is difficult (e.g., balancing a one-segment broom on one's hand is hard enough). In fact, we have recently found that a change by 5 milliseconds in the excitation of vastis lateralis from its optimal pattern, as determined by dynamic optimization, causes the propulsion phase of the jump to be very uncoordinated [97]. Nevertheless, having used the trial-and-error approach, we had gained insight into muscle, tendon, and body-segmental energetics [62]. Still, we feel that the application of dynamic optimization provides much greater insight and should therefore be used when possible.

Estimating Force Using Dynamic Optimization

The application of dynamic optimization to models of the system dynamics (Fig. 6.2**A**) is potentially the most powerful method for studying muscle forces during human movement. The power of the method derives from the scope of the modeling: Not only is there a model of the system dynamics, but also a model of what the motor task is attempting to achieve (the performance criterion) [9, 52, 127]. As with the cost function associated with static optimization, the performance criterion is often ambiguous, though reasonable conjectures are at times possible (e.g., maximum-height vertical jumping) [76, 127, 129].

A dynamic optimization algorithm uses a model of the system dynamics to find the inputs (e.g., EMGs), and all the outputs (e.g., forces), that maximize the performance of the whole task as defined by some single criterion. For some movements, alternative performance criteria may lead to similar neural control strategies (inputs) [90, 114]. One difference between static and dynamic optimization is that static optimization calculates the inputs at only a single instant of time, independent of the past or the future. And the algorithm is run repeatedly to find the inputs at other instants. In contrast, a dynamic optimization algorithm is run once and computes the inputs (and outputs) for all times during the motor task.

Once a solution to a dynamic optimization problem is found, a wealth of information is available to compare with experimental data. Because there is a model of the system dynamics, the complete history of muscle excitations, muscle forces, external reaction forces, joint angles, joint velocities, and joint accelerations can be calculated. Thus the model can be used to understand all aspects of muscle and multijoint coordination. Not only would all muscle forces and their contributions to movement be known, but the neural control strategy for the coordination of the motor task would be known as well.

Dynamic optimization can thus provide a deep understanding of the sensitivity of the solution to assumptions made in formulating the model [76, 97, 123, 127], including assumptions of neural connectivity. For instance, the structure of the central nervous system (CNS) through which control must pass could be assumed to be a one-to-one mapping between the higher CNS structures and the muscles (motoneuronal pools). In this case, the model is permitting the independent excitation of muscles [127]. Or the CNS could be assumed to be constrained by some CNS network, which has fewer inputs than there are motoneuronal pools. In this case, the muscle excitation pattern found by the optimization would be different than the one found in the absence of the network. Also, performance of the motor task would be less when the network exists because performance is always greater in the absence of constraints [9].

Should the optimization results provide a good match with experimentally observed trajectories, then both the motion itself and the control strategy being used would appear to have been well modeled. In this case, one might as well "pack one's bags and go home," because the intellectual part of the job would seem to be done. Of course computer simulation of movement is never perfect. So, the challenge is to identify, perhaps through additional experiments, the significant inaccuracies of the current modeling data. Development of a next-generation, more complex model would then be justified to better comprehend the motor task, and to eliminate known inadequacies of the current-generation model.

Though dynamic optimization has been used to study jumping [53, 76, 97, 123], walking [23, 30], kicking [50], posture [24], and arm movements [38, 92], its full potential has not yet been realized. This is because solving dynamic optimization problems can be extremely difficult, especially if many body segments and muscles are modeled. In fact, the techniques needed to implement suitable dynamic optimization algorithms are at the forefront of control system theory [76, 97].

A MOTOR TASK'S DYNAMIC EQUATIONS OF MOTION

Though muscle force can be found using any of the approaches reviewed in the previous section, an important question still remains: What is the contribution of a muscle's force to the body motion, particularly the angular accelerations of the joints? The answer can be found by applying mechanics to derive the direct multijoint dynamics (Fig. 6.2**A**). However, except for studies that apply dynamic optimization, the governing dynamical equations are usually not formulated to answer this question. And even when formulated, the dynamical equations are rarely analyzed in depth to ascertain the action of muscle on body motion.

The analysis of muscle action using the dynamical equations is worthwhile because the equations may differ among motor tasks, even though the mechanical properties of the body segments and joints are usually assumed to remain the same. Muscle action is therefore task dependent. The equations may differ because the body segments and the environment interact, just as the body segments interact among themselves, and all these interactions determine the dynamical equations [67, 72].

Though the subject of dynamics is beyond the scope of this view, this section reviews the dynamics of several motor tasks to convey the essence of the principles involved. Also discussed are the assumptions about body-segmental interactions made in studying multiarticular movement and muscle coordination. Using these same assumptions in subsequent sections, we present the dynamical equations for the simplest example of a multiarticular motor task, the two-joint system. These equations are then discussed to illustrate how multijoint movement differs from single-joint movement and to show how muscle action, as described in textbooks, can lead to misinterpretations of muscle action during multiarticular movement.

Modeling Body Segments and Joints

Coordination studies almost always assume that the body segments are rigid. Although rarely stated explicitly, the reason is that intersegmental motion is believed to be dominated by the relative movement among the body segments rather than by movement of parts within a body segment. We believe the "rigid-body" assumption is currently appropriate, except perhaps when the body impacts rigid objects, as evident by the subsequent shock-wave propagation in the body [31].

The least restrictive representation of the motion of one body segment relative to an adjacent segment allows both rotation and translation (Fig.

FIGURE 6.3

Number of degrees of freedom (df) *of a joint.* **A,** *The maximum number of* df *of a joint is 6.* θ_1, θ_2, *and* θ_3 *specify the orientation of the upper body segment relative to the lower segment.* x, y, *and* z *specify the translation of the upper segment with respect to the lower segment (i.e., the position of* P *relative to* O. **B,** *A ball-and-socket joint has only 3* df *(i.e.,* θ_1, θ_2, *and* θ_3) *since* P *and* O *coincide.* **C,** *A pin joint has 1* df *(i.e.,* θ) *since the upper segment rotates in a plane, and about a fixed axis.*

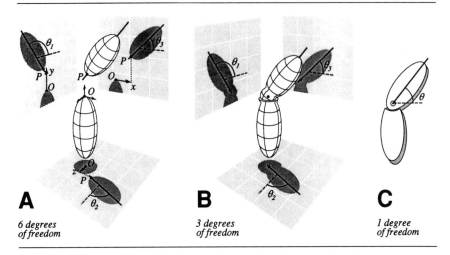

A

6 degrees of freedom

B

3 degrees of freedom

C

1 degree of freedom

6.3**A**). Thus, the number of degrees of freedom *(df)* of each joint is at most 6: 3 associated with the orientation of one segment relative to the other (θ_1, θ_2, θ_3 in Fig. 6.3**A**), and 3 with the position of a point in one segment relative to the other segment (*x, y, z* in Fig. 6.3**A**). In studies of joint mechanics, where the emphasis is on stresses and strains in joint structures, it may be necessary to assume 6 *df* for each joint [3, 22, 74, 112]. Some studies that use static optimization to find muscle forces also assume 6 *df* joints [29, 100].

For sound practical reasons, models of joints are kept as simple as possible, and coordination studies almost always assume frictionless ball-and-socket joints or pin joints (Fig. 6.3**B,C**) [6, 51]. Translational motion within a joint, assumed to be small, is generally ignored. In studies of walking, the hip is often assumed to be a ball-and-socket joint (Fig. 6.3**B**), in which case the pelvis is assumed to rotate relative to the femur [80]. Thus, the relative location of the two segments can be described by three angles (Fig. 6.3**B**). In vertical jumping, for example, the hip may even be assumed to be a pin joint, which has only 1 *df* (θ in Fig. 6.3**C**), because sagittal plane motion is assumed to dominate performance of the motor task [13, 123, 127]. A pin-joint hip has also been used to study coordination of walking, where the focus is on sagittal-plane motion [23, 30, 101, 120, 121]. When a joint is assumed to have less than 6 *df*, the implications are that joint structures such as bone, ligaments, and menisci, for example, constrain the joint to have less than 6 *df* and, except for these effects, affect intersegmental dynamics in no other way.[a]

Because frictional losses in joints are assumed negligible, the joint reaction forces do not have to appear in the dynamical equations [72] (e.g., see equations in references 19, 30, 60, 97). Expressions for joint forces are often found, however, in the derivation of the dynamical equations [26, 75, 83, 94, 96]. If frictional losses in joints are high, such as in pathology, then joint reaction forces would have to appear explicitly in these equations. As a consequence, the net effect of muscle force on joint rotation would depend not only on the torque developed by the muscle, but also on its contribution to the magnitude and direction of the compressive forces produced between the articular surfaces of the joint (Appendix A) [51, 72].

Determining the Degrees of Freedom of a Motor Task and Choosing a Set of Generalized Coordinates
The minimum number of coordinates needed to specify both the position and orientation of the segments of the body and the external objects with which it contacts during performance of a motor task is the number of *df* of the task [72]. Any minimal set of coordinates is called a set of generalized coordinates; generalized refers to the fact that they need not be only positional or only angular coordinates.

The *df* for the body during a motor task is at most $N + 6$, where N is the total *df* for the joints in the mechanical system, including the body joints. Constraints on the configuration of the mechanical system due to its interaction with the environment reduce the *df* during motor tasks. For example, in Fig. 6.4**A**, there are three pin joints, so $N = 3$ and there are at most 9 *df* for the body. However, the task is a planar free fall, and remaining in the plane imposes three constraints. Thus there are 6 *df* during planar free fall; one possible set of generalized coordinates is shown, consisting of two Cartesian coordinates to specify the point P (i.e., x_p, y_p) and four angular coordinates to specify the orientation of the segments (i.e., θ_1, θ_2, θ_3, θ_4). Other variables could be used for the generalized coordinates, such as the position of a point other than P, or intersegmental angles.

---

[a]Sometimes these structures are assumed to generate passive torques that act, additionally, to hinder joint rotation (e.g., to prevent joint hyperextension) (51, 52, 122).

FIGURE 6.4

Number of degrees of freedom (df) *of a planar motor task (e.g., landing, jumping) whose parts form an open kinematic linkage. In* **A**, **B**, *and* **C**, *the body parts involved in the task are assumed to consist of three pin joints and four segments. The number of* df *of these body parts is four (i.e., θ_1, θ_2, θ_3, θ_4).* **A**, *The number of* df *of the task is 6; 4 to specify the orientation of the segments (θ_1, θ_2, θ_3, θ_4) and 2 (x_p, y_p) to specify the rectilinear position of the body with respect to the ground reference frame* (x, y). **B**, *The number of* df *of the task is 4 (θ_1, θ_2, θ_3, θ_4) since (x_p, y_p) are stationary.* **C**, *the number of* df *of the task is only 3 (θ_2, θ_3, θ_4), since the foot is stationary. Notice that the number of* df *of the task can be greater than, equal to, or less than the number of* df *of the body parts (**A**, **B**, and **C**, respectively).*

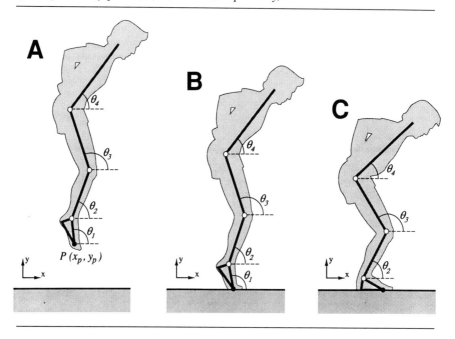

The *df* of a motor task may vary from start to finish, such as during falling and landing (Fig. 6.4**A**–**C**). The *df* decrease by 2 when the toes first make contact with the ground (Fig. 6.4**B**), and the number decreases by 1 more when the sole of the feet make contact (Fig. 6.4**C**). In vertical jumping, this sequence is reversed, and the *df* increase during the task.

The above are considered examples of an "open linkage" because one end of the "chain" of the rigid bodies is free to move. During some motor tasks, the body interacts with the environment to form a "closed linkage." For example, while seated on a bicycle, the position of the hip may remain stationary, as does the axis of rotation of the crankshaft (Fig. 6.5). The

FIGURE 6.5
Number of degrees of freedom (df) *of a planar motor task (pedaling,* insert) *whose parts form a closed kinematic linkage. In* **A** *and* **B** *the body parts involved in the task are assumed to consist of three pin joints (hip, knee, and ankle) and three segments (thigh, shank, and foot) of each leg. The number of* df *of the body parts participating in the task is thus 6, 3 for each leg.* **A,** *The two legs are assumed to pedal symmetrically and deliver power only during the downstroke. The task is thus specified by motion of either one of the two legs. The number of* df *of the task is 2. One of many sets of generalized coordinates is* (θ_{1R}, θ_0), *where* θ_{1R} *is the orientation of the right foot and* θ_0 *is the orientation of the crank.* **B,** *The two legs are assumed to mechanically interact through the crank. The number of* df *of the task is one greater than in* **A,** *and the one additional generalized coordinate could be* θ_{1L}, *the orientation of the left foot. Notice that in both* **A** *and* **B,** *the number of* df *of the task is less than the number of* df *of the body parts because constraints are imposed on the configuration of the participatory body parts.*

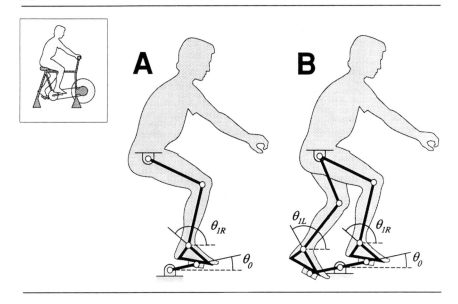

effect of a closed linkage is that there are additional constraints on the configuration, and thus the *df* are further reduced. One possible model of interlimb coordination of pedaling a stationary ergometer might assume that the hips are stationary, that the limbs are symmetrically controlled except for being 180° out of phase, and that each limb delivers power to the crank only during the power stroke (Fig. 6.5**A**). Thus the *df* of this model of pedaling is 2, and a set of generalized coordinates could be the crank and right pedal (foot) angles (i.e., θ_0 and θ_{1R}, Fig. 6.5**A**). If mechanical coupling of the limbs is to be analyzed (Fig. 6.5**B**), then the *df* of the task increases by 1, and the left pedal angle (θ_{1L}) could be added as a generalized coordinate. An alternative set of generalized coordinates could be the knee and hip angles of the right side, and the knee (or hip) angle of the left leg, since orientation of all other joint angles and the crank would then be specified.

For some multiarticular, single *df* tasks, the generalized coordinate need not be a joint angle. The bilaterally symmetrical leg press, where the hips are assumed stationary, and the feet flat and fixed to a foot plate, has 1 *df*, and thus only one generalized coordinate (Fig. 6.6). The orientation of the foot plate (θ) is an appropriate generalized coordinate since all other parts that can move (the foot, the shank, and the thigh) are uniquely located by this coordinate. The orientation of the link at the other end (i.e., the thigh) is also an appropriate choice, as are either the knee or ankle angle.

Finding the Dynamic Equations of Motion
Once the linkage system among the body segments and external objects is defined and a set of generalized coordinates specified for the motor task, the governing dynamic equations of motion for the motor task can be written [72]. Once written, muscular control and motion of the motor task can be analyzed quantitatively. Since a set of generalized coordinates is nonunique, there are other ways of expressing the dynamic equations. However, the motion described by any set of equations is independent of the choice of generalized coordinates (i.e., the body and objects move the same way no matter how the motion is described).

For each generalized coordinate, there is a corresponding equation of motion [72]. Therefore, if the *df* change during a motor task, the dynamic equations also change. Since deriving just one set of equations is time consuming, especially if three-dimension motion is to be studied, often the coordination of only one part of a motor task is studied, for example the propulsion [76, 97] or the airborne [53] phase of jumping.

Different methods are available to derive the dynamic equations of motion for a motor task. In the commonly used Newton-Euler method [26, 75, 83, 94, 96], the multijoint system is "broken apart," and free-body diagrams are constructed to show the external forces and torques acting on the each rigid-body segment. Equations for the linear accelerations of the segments are written using Newton's second law, and expressions for the angular accelerations are written using Euler's equations. One disadvantage of this method is that many extra equations must be written and then, often with considerable effort, combined to form the governing dynamic equations. An advantage, however, is that

FIGURE 6.6

1-df, *multiarticular motor task (leg press,* insert*). Though the hip, knee, and ankle can move, the configuration constraint imposed on the task reduces the task to 1* df. *One possible generalized coordinate is* θ, *which although not a coordinate of the body, when known specifies all joint angles of the participatory body parts as well as the height of the weight.*

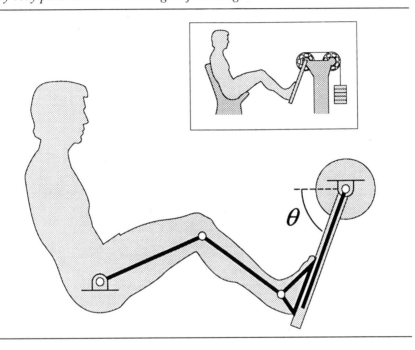

sometimes these extraneous equations provide useful information (e.g., joint reaction forces). Although equations are not derived in this chapter, our discussions make use of D'Alembert's principle. Rather than thinking of a force causing an acceleration ($F = ma$), the use of D'Alembert's principle converts dynamics problems into statics problems by defining an inertia force ($F^* = -ma$) that places a rigid body into "equilibrium" ($F + F^* = 0$).

The Lagrangian method and Kane's method [72], also referred to as Lagrange's form of D'Alembert's principle [67, 70], are both based on the generalized coordinate concept. Kane's method is particularly advantageous when deriving equations for a task with many *df*, or if forces which are noncontributory to the motion, such as the equal and opposite forces acting at the joints and at the ground, are of no interest.

HOW THE DYNAMICS OF SINGLE- AND MULTIJOINT TASKS DIFFER

Our knowledge of how forces control the motion of one segment (e.g., an inverted pendulum) is often used to infer mechanisms of control of multiarticular motor tasks. However, there are basic differences between the dynamics of multi- and single-*df* movement that must be recognized. The fundamental difference is forces on each segment caused by motion of the other segment. To illustrate this difference, we compare two simple models of standing. In the first model, the knee and hip joints are locked by external braces, and the body is represented as a single segment (Fig. 6.7). In the second model, the knee is allowed to bend, and the body is represented by two segments (Fig. 6.9). In this section we use the orientation angles of each segment with respect to horizontal, to focus on the effects of forces due to the motion of the other segment. In subsequent sections we use joint angles, to facilitate understanding of muscle control of joint motion.

Dynamics of a One-Joint, 1-df Task

For a one-segment 1-*df* representation of the standing body, assume that soleus and tibialis anterior can develop forces to control the sway of the body (Fig. 6.7**A**). The net effect of these forces on the one-segment body is to exert a torque on the segment (T^{mus} in Fig 6.7**B**; Appendixes A and C). Similarly, the net effect of gravity (body weight) is that it also exerts a torque on the segment (T^{grav} in Fig 6.7**B**; Appendix B). If the body is in static equilibrium, these torques (T^{mus} and T^{grav}) are equal and opposite. If not, the body is accelerating, creating an inertia torque on the segment $\bar{I}\ddot{\theta}$ (not shown in Fig. 6.7**B**; Appendix B), which is the net difference of T^{mus} and T^{grav} (i.e., $T^{net} = T^{mus} - T^{grav}$). The one dynamic equation of motion can be expressed as a "torque balance equation" (Appendix C):

$$(\bar{I})\ddot{\theta} = T^{mus} - T^{grav} = T^{net}, \tag{1}$$

where θ is the one generalized coordinate.

Notice from Equation 1 that the net torque on the shank (T^{net}) is proportional to the angular acceleration of the shank ($\ddot{\theta}$) and the constant of proportionality is $\bar{I}$. The angular acceleration of the body is therefore

$$\ddot{\theta} = \left(\frac{1}{\bar{I}}\right) T^{mus} - \left(\frac{1}{\bar{I}}\right) T^{grav} = \left(\frac{1}{\bar{I}}\right) T^{net}. \tag{2}$$

Just as the net torque equals the difference of the muscle and gravity torques, the (net) acceleration is the difference of the acceleration due to the muscle torque, and the acceleration due to the gravity torque.

FIGURE 6.7

One-joint, 1-df *sagittal-plane model of standing.* **A,** *Feet are assumed to always be flat on the ground, and knees and hips "locked." The distributed mass of the body is* m, *whose mass center is assumed to be located a distance of* l *from the pin-joint ankle and to have a moment of inertia about the mass center of* I *(not shown). Only muscles crossing the ankle (e.g., soleus [SOL] and tibialis anterior [TA]) contribute to body motion.* **B,** *The net effect of each ankle muscle is to generate a torque on the segment (Appendix A). The summed torques from all ankle muscles is* T^mus *(e.g.,* T^mus = T^SOL − T^TA*). Gravity also develops a torque (*T^grav*), which opposes* T^mus *when the body lean forwards.* θ *is chosen as the generalized coordinate.*

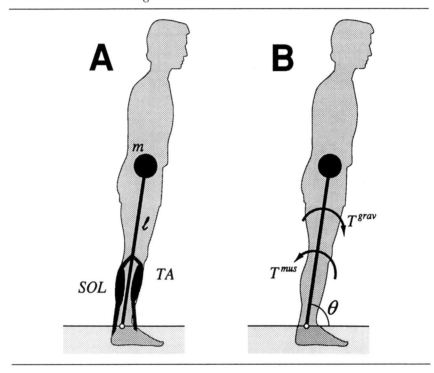

Therefore, there is a linear relationship between the net acceleration and the muscle and gravity torques (Fig. 6.8). Notice that soleus (SOL) and tibialis anterior (TA) act in opposition. The torque produced from soleus (T^{SOL}) acts instantaneously to accelerate the one body segment posteriorly (i.e., $+T^{SOL} > 0$, and thus causes $\ddot{\theta}$ to increase), and tibialis anterior torque (T^{TA}) acts instantaneously to accelerate the segment anteriorly (i.e., $-T^{TA} < 0$, and thus acts to decrease $\ddot{\theta}$, or to accelerate the segment anteriorly, or equivalently, to decelerate the segment). Thus,

FIGURE 6.8

Block diagram of the 1-df model of standing. Torques developed from each ankle muscle sum to produce the net muscle torque ($T^{mus} = T^{SOL} - T^{TA}$). The net muscle torque sums with the gravity torque (T^{grav}) to produce the net torque (T^{net}) acting on the segment. T^{net}, including each component of T^{net}, produces an instantaneous angular acceleration of the body ($\ddot{\theta}$). The body's angular velocity ($\dot{\theta}$) and orientation (θ) depends on the trajectory of $\ddot{\theta}$ and $\dot{\theta}$, respectively (i.e., refer to integrals). The mechanical system is nonlinear because gravity affects torque generation nonlinearly ($T^{grav} = T^g \cos\theta$).

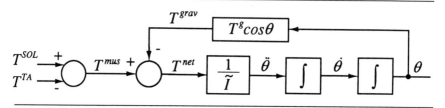

torques from muscles sum to produce the net muscle torque (T^{mus}) acting on the segment. Torque from gravity acts instantaneously to hinder posterior acceleration when the body leans forward (i.e., $\cos\theta > 0$) and acts to assist posterior acceleration when the body leans backward (i.e., $\cos\theta < 0$).

Although there is a linear relationship between the angular acceleration and the torques, this is *not* a linear system [71]. The nonlinearity is due to the gravity torque, which depends on the cosine of the segment angle. Therefore, no simple relationship between the torques and the velocity or position of the segment exists. In a linear system, the motion resulting from each input acting alone can be summed to find the motion when all the inputs act together. This is known as superposition.

Suppose this one segment model was being used to understand the action of soleus during standing posture, and the body motion and muscle torques for an experimental trial were determined. It would be natural to wonder how the motion would differ if, for example, soleus had developed 20% more torque throughout the trial. If the dynamical equation were linear, it would be straightforward to answer this question using superposition.

Although the dynamics are not linear, one might assume the system to be linear if the range of motion during the trial was sufficiently small. However, unless the assumption of linearity can be justified, it is necessary to simulate the trial, using the dynamical equation, to determine the change in body motion resulting from a 20% increase in soleus torque.

When gravity does not affect the mechanics of a one-segment, 1-*df* motor task (e.g., during spaceflight, or during horizontal movement of the forearm), the mechanical system is linear, and segment positions, velocities, and accelerations are all affected proportionally by changes in muscle torque. However, in multiarticular tasks, the mechanical system is nonlinear, even when the task is conducted in a gravity-free environment (see below). Thus, in more complex tasks, only the accelerations, and not the positions or velocities, remain proportional to the muscle torques.

Dynamics of a Two-Joint, 2-df Task
For the two-segment, 2-*df* model of the standing body (Fig. 6.9**A**), muscles crossing the ankle add to the net torque acting on the shank, and muscles crossing the knee add to the net torques acting on both segments (Appendix A). In Fig. 6.9**B**, T_1^{mus} is therefore the net muscle torque acting on the shank, and T_2^{mus} is the net muscle torque acting on the thigh. When in static equilibrium, these net muscle torques balance the torques from gravity (Fig. 6.9**B**; $T_1^{grav} = T_1^{mus}$, and $T_2^{grav} = T_2^{mus}$). Otherwise the body is accelerating, and inertia torques and torques induced from motion of the other segment are generated (not shown in Fig. 6.9**B**). The dynamic equations of motion can be expressed as a "torque balance equation" for segment 1 (Equation 3a) and a "torque balance equation" for segment 2 (Equation 3b) with (θ_1, θ_2) as the two generalized coordinates (Appendix D):

$$[\tilde{I}_1] \ \ddot{\theta}_1 + [\tilde{I}_{cs} \ cos(\theta_1 - \theta_2)] \ \ddot{\theta}_2 \ = \ T_1^{net} \qquad (3a)$$

$$[\tilde{I}_2] \ \ddot{\theta}_2 + [\tilde{I}_{cs} \ cos(\theta_1 - \theta_2)] \ \ddot{\theta}_1 \ = \ T_2^{net} \qquad (3b)$$

where

$$T_1^{net} = T_1^{mus} - T_1^{grav} - [\tilde{I}_{cs} \ sin(\theta_1 - \theta_2)] \ \dot{\theta}_2^2$$

$$T_2^{net} = T_2^{mus} - T_2^{grav} + [\tilde{I}_{cs} \ sin(\theta_1 - \theta_2)] \ \dot{\theta}_1^2,$$

and T_1^{net} and T_2^{net} are the net torques accelerating the segments. Notice that the accelerations are proportional to the net torques (T_1^{net}, T_2^{net}).

A fundamental difference of the 2-*df* and 1-*df* systems is the presence of torques from the motion of the other segment (Appendix E). For the one-segment, 1-*df* system, the net torque is the difference of the gravity and muscle torques acting on the segment (see Equation 1). For the 2-*df* system, the net torque (T_1^{net}), for example, contains an additional term due to the angular velocity of segment 2 $(\dot{\theta}_2)$; similarly, the net torque (T_2^{net}) contains a term due to the angular velocity of segment 1 $(\dot{\theta}_1)$. For the 1-*df* task, the inertia torque of the segment equals the net torque acting on the segment. For the 2-*df* task, however, this is not the

FIGURE 6.9

Two-joint, 2-df model of standing. **A,** *The body is modeled by a shank segment (mass* m_1*, length* ρ_1*, and mass center location from ankle* l_1*) and an upper segment (mass* m_2 *and c.m. location from knee* l_2*).* **B,** *Ankle and knee muscles develop torque on the shank. Their summed torque is* T_1^{mus}*. For the sign convention assumed, extensor muscles of the ankle and knee develop a positive torque on the shank. Knee muscles also develop torque on the upper segment; extensor muscles contributing negatively to* T_2^{mus}*. Similarly, gravity produces a torque on both segments,* T_1^{grav} *and* T_2^{grav}*. The orientations of the two segments* (θ_1, θ_2) *are chosen to be the generalized coordinates.*

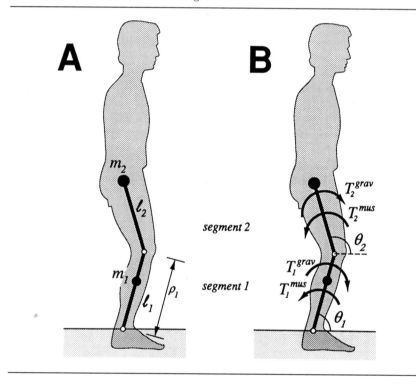

case. Notice that the left-hand side of Equations 3a and 3b contains both the angular acceleration of segment 1 ($\ddot{\theta}_1$), and the angular acceleration of segment 2 ($\ddot{\theta}_2$).

The torques exerted on one segment due to the motion of the other segment depend not only on the angular acceleration and velocity of the other segment, but also on the relative orientation of the two segments ($\theta_1 - \theta_2$). Notice from Equations 3a and 3b that the torque from angular acceleration of the other segment is maximum when the segments are colinear (i.e., $cos(\theta_1 - \theta_2) = 1$), and zero when perpendicular (i.e., $cos(\theta_1 - \theta_2) = 0$). The opposite is true for the torque from the angular velocity of the other segment (i.e., it is maximum when the segments are perpendicular, when $sin(\theta_1 - \theta_2) = 1$, and zero when colinear, when $sin(\theta_1 - \theta_2) = 0$).

Using Equations 3a and 3b the angular acceleration of each segment caused by the net torques can be found:

$$\ddot{\theta}_1 = \frac{1}{\beta} \left\{ \left[\frac{1}{\tilde{I}_1} \right] T_1^{\text{net}} - \left[\frac{\tilde{I}_{cs} \, cos(\theta_1 - \theta_2)}{\tilde{I}_1 \tilde{I}_2} \right] T_2^{\text{net}} \right\} \tag{4a}$$

$$\ddot{\theta}_2 = \frac{1}{\beta} \left\{ \left[\frac{1}{\tilde{I}_2} \right] T_2^{\text{net}} - \left[\frac{\tilde{I}_{cs} \, cos(\theta_1 - \theta_2)}{\tilde{I}_1 \tilde{I}_2} \right] T_1^{\text{net}} \right\} \tag{4b}$$

where

$$\beta = [\tilde{I}_1 \tilde{I}_2 - \tilde{I}_{cs}^2 \, cos^2(\theta_1 - \theta_2)] / (\tilde{I}_1 \tilde{I}_2) > 0 \text{ for all } (\theta_1 - \theta_2).$$

Notice that the angular accelerations of both segments depend on T_1^{net} and T_2^{net}. Consequently, muscles such as soleus, which contribute only to T_1^{net}, act to accelerate both segments 2 and 1. In fact, the effect on the other segment can be large. For example, in upright posture, T^{SOL} (or for that matter any term contributing to T_1^{net}) can act to accelerate the thigh (segment 2) about the same as it acts to accelerate the shank (segment 1) [42].

Even with just one extra segment, there is a large increase in the complexity of the dynamics (Fig. 6.10). The ways that one segment affects the motion of the other are indicated by heavy lines. Notice that in the absence of the dynamic coupling, the flow of events in the two segments would be independent. Therefore, segment 1 could be controlled by exciting muscles crossing the ankle (to control T_1^{net}), and segment 2 could be controlled by exciting muscles crossing the hip (to control T_2^{net}). However, dynamical coupling must always exist since $cos(\theta_1 - \theta_2)$ and $sin(\theta_1 - \theta_2)$ cannot both be zero.[b]

For a two-joint, as for a one-joint, system, there is a linear relationship between torque and acceleration. Should the torque from any one muscle change, the angular accelerations of all the segments would change proportionally.

However, there is no linear relationship between the segment's angular velocities and the torques, or between the segment's orientations and

[b]Actually, β also depends on $cos(\theta_1 - \theta_2)$ (see Fig. 6.10 and Equations 4a and 4b).

FIGURE 6.10

Block diagram of the 2-df model of standing. Notice how much more complex the dynamics are when the body is assumed to be articulated (compare with Fig. 6.8). If the segments were to move independently of one another, the heavily outlined boxes would be absent (i.e., no dynamic coupling would exist). The block diagram of the two-segment dynamics would then be the sum of two, one-segment block diagrams (thin lines; compare with Fig. 6.8). Dynamic coupling always exists, however, and is significant (see text). Notice that the torques acting on one segment affect the angular acceleration of both segments viz the feed-forward $\cos(\theta_1 - \theta_2)$ terms, that the angular velocities of the segments generate torques on the segments viz the feedback $\sin(\theta_1 - \theta_2)$ terms, and that the segmental orientations affect the feed-forward gain because β depends on θ_1 and θ_2 (see Equations 4a and 4b). Observe that the dynamics are nonlinear even in the absence of gravity (i.e., when $T_1{}^g = T_2{}^g = 0$).

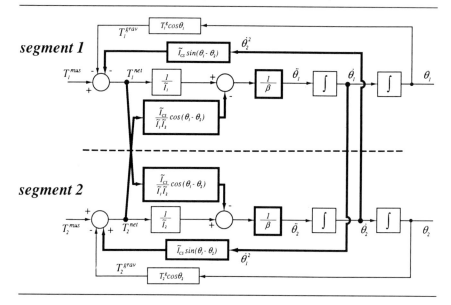

the torques. The system dynamics contain several nonlinearities (Fig. 6.10, sines and cosines). Therefore, superposition does not apply. So, a computer simulation of the task is required to determine how force (or torque) developed by a muscle affects the angular velocities and orientations of the segments. Similarly, forces and joint angular velocities and angles are nonlinearly related.

In other multijoint systems, it can be shown that dynamic coupling exists across all segments [26, 42, 67, 72, 96, 97, 124]. For example, in a planar analysis of standing or walking, the trunk exhibits coupling to both the thigh and the shank, and the shank and thigh to the trunk. Again, torques arising from angular acceleration of another segment are maximum when the two segments are colinear, and angular-velocity induced-torques are maximum when the two segments are perpendicular. For example, during standing, soleus will act to accelerate the pelvis the most when the pelvis's center of mass is colinear with the shank's. The old saying, the "shank bone is connected to the thigh bone, the thigh bone is connected to the hip bone, the hip bone etc." shows perhaps that intersegmental coupling is generally recognized, though we believe its effect on how muscles act to accelerate the segments is less appreciated (see section entitled "Muscle Action on Joint Motion").

Are the Dynamical Interactions Among Segments Significant?
The answer is yes. First, we mentioned briefly above that soleus can act to angularly accelerate the thigh by the same amount that it acts to accelerate the shank near upright posture when humans stand flat-footed. The consequence of this is that soleus acts two times more powerfully to accelerate the knee into extension than it does the ankle (see next section). This analysis is based on a two-segment model of a person. Fortunately, this result appears robust, being insensitive to both typical anthropometrical variations found among children and adults, and to the number of segments used to model the head−arms−trunk segment [42, 73]. Other results to be presented in the next section are likewise robust, unless otherwise stated.

Analyzing a variety of movements in animals and humans has indicated that intersegmental coupling is indeed significant. For example, analysis of arm movements, based on a two-segment model, has shown that angular velocity of one joint induces a significant torque at the other joint, even when the reaching task is conducted slowly [60]. Similarly, the torque induced from angular acceleration of the other joint was found to be significant during these forearm and upper arm movements. Intersegmental (or joint) motion has also been found to affect the torques that need to be developed by ankle and knee muscles in the cat's swing leg during gait [63]. Dynamic analysis of cat paw shaking has revealed that proximal muscles have to counter the torques induced by motion of the distal segments [64]; these findings have led to hypotheses about neural control of knee and ankle muscles during the paw shake [65]. Finally, in human gait studies, intersegmental dynamic interactions are deemed, *prima facie*, significant [17, 20, 22, 101, 120, 121].

MUSCLE ACTION ON JOINT MOTION

In this section, we review the relation between muscle torques and the joint angular accelerations they cause. It is important to recognize that muscle acts to accelerate all the joints of the body, and the acceleration of an unspanned joint can greatly exceed that of a spanned joint. Further, multiarticular muscles may accelerate a spanned joint in the direction opposite to that of the torque it applies to the joint. Because muscle action is task dependent, it is necessary to use the task-specific dynamic equations to find muscle's action on the body. Therefore, as an example, the two-segment model of standing posture is used again, although the equations are expressed in joint rather than segmental coordinates. With this model, soleus acts to accelerate the knee (the unspanned joint) into extension twice as much as it acts to accelerate the ankle (the spanned joint) into extension. Although gastrocnemius exerts a knee flexor torque, it can act to accelerate the knee into extension.

Two-Joint Dynamic Equations

Consider again the two-segment model of standing posture, with the equations expressed using the joint angles (ϕ_a and ϕ_k, Fig. 6.11A). The dynamic equations in joint space (see Equations 8a and 8b in Appendix F) become on rearrangement:

$$\ddot{\phi}_a = \frac{1}{\gamma}\left\{ \left[\frac{1}{\tilde{I}_a}\right] T_a{}^{net} - \left[\frac{\tilde{I}_{cj}}{\tilde{I}_a\tilde{I}_k}\right] T_k{}^{net} \right\} \tag{5a}$$

$$\ddot{\phi}_k = \frac{1}{\gamma}\left\{ \left[\frac{1}{\tilde{I}_k}\right] T_k{}^{net} - \left[\frac{\tilde{I}_{cj}}{\tilde{I}_a\tilde{I}_k}\right] T_a{}^{net} \right\} \tag{5b}$$

where

$$T_a{}^{net} = T_a{}^{mus} - T_a{}^{grav} + T_a\,(\dot{\phi}_a,\,\phi_k,\,\dot{\phi}_k)$$
$$T_k{}^{net} = T_k{}^{mus} - T_k{}^{grav} + T_k\,(\dot{\phi}_a^2,\,\phi_k)$$

and

$$\gamma = [\tilde{I}_a\tilde{I}_k - I_{cj}^2]\,/\,[\tilde{I}_a\tilde{I}_k] > 0 \text{ for all } \phi_k.$$

The structure of these equations, expressed in joint coordinates, is similar to the structure of Equations 4a and 4b, which are the equations expressed in segmental coordinates. Again, torques from muscle, gravity, and velocity sum to produce the net torques ($T_a{}^{net}$, $T_k{}^{net}$). Torques from muscles crossing the ankle sum to produce $T_a{}^{mus}$, the total muscle torque at the ankle. Similarly, torques from muscles crossing the knee sum to produce $T_k{}^{mus}$, the total muscle torque at the knee. The sign convention is that torques in the direction of joint extension are positive; thus soleus torque (T^{SOL}, Fig. 6.11A) is positive, and biceps femoris (BFsh) torque (T^{BFsh}, Fig. 6.11B) is negative.

FIGURE 6.11

*Relationships among torques generated by uni- and biarticular muscles. **A**, ϕ_k and ϕ_a define the knee and ankle joint angles. Soleus (SOL) produces an ankle-extensor torque ($T^{SOL} > 0$). **B**, Biceps-femoris, short-head (BFsh) generates a knee-flexor torque ($T^{BFsh} < 0$). **C**, Gastrocnemius (GAS) develops both an ankle-extensor torque ($T_a^{GAS} > 0$) and a knee-flexor torque ($T_k^{GAS} < 0$). Gastrocnemius can be considered to be the sum of two uniarticular muscles, an ankle-extensor muscle like soleus and a knee-flexor muscle like biceps femoris. The ratio of the magnitude of gastrocnemius's torque at the knee to the ankle is equal to the ratio of gastrocnemius's moment arm at the knee to the ankle (i.e., $r_k^{GAS} : r_a^{GAS}$). F^{GAS} is the force developed by gastrocnemius.*

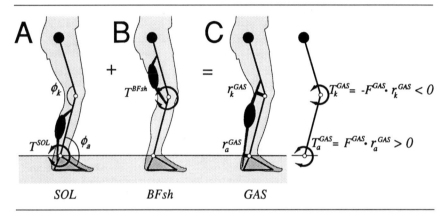

Notice that the angular accelerations of both the ankle and the knee depend on T_a^{net} and T_k^{net}. A consequence of this is that muscles such as the soleus, which contribute to only T_a^{net}, act to accelerate both the knee and the ankle joints. Again, it should be emphasized that only the relation between joint angular acceleration and torque is linear.

Uniarticular Muscle Crossing a Pin Joint

A uniarticular muscle crossing a pin joint will always act to accelerate the joint in the direction of the muscle's torque. Thus a muscle like the soleus, which develops an extensor torque at the ankle, will accelerate the ankle into extension. The certainty of the conclusion follows from energetic arguments [7, 8, 73]. That is, the soleus, acting alone to generate force on a body initially at rest, must *initially* shorten to perform work to initiate movement of the body. In order to shorten, the ankle must move *initially* into extension. However, all the energy developed by the soleus, even initially, does not have to be spent on initiating movement of the ankle; some energy, and perhaps a lot, can be expended on initiating movement of other joints.

Analysis of the dynamical equations leads to the same conclusion [42, 124]. For example, since the soleus contributes only to T_a^{net}, the ankle angular acceleration caused by the soleus can be found from the coefficient of T_a^{net} in Equation 5a. Since $\bar{I}_a > 0$ and $\gamma > 0$, and $T^{SOL} > 0$, the soleus accelerates the ankle into extension. Similarly, the uniarticular biceps femoris, which produces a negative (flexor) torque at the knee and thus contributes to T_k^{net}, accelerates the knee into flexion (since $\bar{I}_k > 0$ and $T^{BFsh} < 0$). More generally, it can be shown from analysis of the structure of the dynamic equations that a uniarticular muscle crossing a pin joint will always accelerate the joint in the direction of the muscle torque, regardless of the task [42, 124].

The dynamic equations can also be analyzed to study the action of uniarticular muscles on unspanned joints [41, 42, 73, 124, 126]. For example, the sign of the knee angular acceleration caused by the soleus for the two-joint model of standing depends on the sign of $\bar{I}_{cj}$ in Equation 5b, which can be positive, negative, or zero, depending on ϕ_k and the inertial parameters of the two segments.

The action on unspanned joints can be powerful [42, 124]. For example, for positions near upright posture, the soleus accelerates the knee into extension twice as much as the ankle (Fig. 6.12). Notice that with the knee more flexed, the soleus's action on the knee lessens, and when flexed beyond 90° ($\phi_k < 90°$), the soleus's action at the ankle dominates. Similarly, using Equation 5a, the biceps femoris accelerates the ankle into flexion (dorsiflexion), though its action at the ankle is less than its action at the knee, and the ratio of knee and ankle accelerations varies little with knee angle. The qualitative nature of these actions is insensitive to the inertial parameters of the body and the number of segments used to represent flat-footed standing posture [42].

Biarticular Muscle Crossing Two Pin Joints

A biarticular muscle crossing two pin joints accelerates at most one spanned joint at a time in a direction opposite to its torque at that joint [7, 8, 41, 42, 124, 126]. Energetic arguments can be invoked to show that muscle can shorten in three possible ways when acting alone on the body [7, 8]. For example, gastrocnemius can accelerate either (*a*) the knee into flexion and the ankle into extension (plantarflexion), (*b*) the knee into extension and the ankle into extension, or (*c*) the knee into flexion and the ankle into flexion (dorsiflexion). These three possibilities are also consistent with analysis of the dynamical equations [41, 42, 124, 126]. For example, gastrocnemius behaves as soleus and biceps femoris acting together since gastrocnemius develops a flexor knee torque (T_k^{GAS}) and an extensor ankle torque (T_a^{GAS}) (Fig. 6.11). Since soleus accelerates both joints into extension, and biceps femoris accelerates both joints into flexion, the net action of gastrocnemius on either one (but

FIGURE 6.12

The effect of soleus (SOL) on angular acceleration of the knee relative to the ankle. Soleus's effect on knee and ankle angular acceleration depends on the knee angle (ϕ_k), and thus so does the ratio of the two accelerations (see text). Notice that when the knee is flexed less than 90° (i.e., $\phi_k > 90°$), SOL accelerates the knee (into extension) more than it accelerates the ankle (into extension) (bold line is above the dotted line).

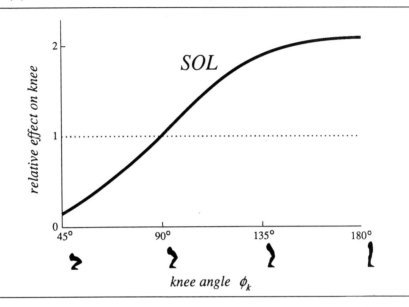

not both) of the joints can be opposite to the direction of its torque at that joint.

The dynamic equations of motion can be analyzed in detail to ascertain which of the three possible ways a biarticular muscle will act if, in addition, the muscle's moment arms at the spanned joints are given [42, 124]. For example, the action of gastrocnemius on the ankle is given by the sum of the accelerations caused by gastrocnemius's ankle torque (T_a^{GAS}) and its knee torque (T_k^{GAS}), and can be computed from Equation 5a by setting $T_a^{net} = T_a^{GAS}$ and $T_k^{net} = T_k^{GAS}$. Thus, the ratio of knee to ankle torque developed by gastrocnemius ($T_k^{GAS} : T_a^{GAS}$), or, equivalently, the ratio of its moment arm at the knee to ankle ($r_k^{GAS} : r_a^{GAS}$) (Fig. 6.11C), influences the net action of gastrocnemius on the ankle, as well as on the knee (see Equation 5b). Therefore, for a specific body configuration (knee angle ϕ_k in this example), the action of gastrocnemius to accelerate the knee and ankle can be found if its moment–arm ratio ($r_k^{GAS} : r_a^{GAS}$) is also specified.

Results from this model of standing and others (42) suggest that gastrocnemius may indeed act, at times, either to accelerate the ankle into flexion (dorsiflexion) or to accelerate the knee into extension (Fig. 6.13). Notice that all three possible combinations of ankle and knee action can occur. Assuming the knee-to-ankle moment–arm ratio is about 0.5 in the human (M. G. Hoy, personal communication, 1988), gastrocnemius's action will be sensitive to model structure (e.g., a two- versus three-segment model of standing) and parameters (e.g., moment arms). Thus, gastrocnemius's action may vary among people, and even for the same person, gastrocnemius may act differently when the body is in different flat-footed postures (Fig. 6.13). Using fundamentally the same approach outlined here, Andrews [8] found that hamstrings and rectus femoris also act in three ways during pedaling. Perhaps this is why limb biarticular muscles are considered enigmatic, and their function during motor tasks sometimes appears paradoxical [8, 15, 21, 46, 61, 69, 82, 86, 115].

In fact, it may be that biarticular muscles are well suited to transferring power among joints [14, 34, 35, 45, 56, 58, 87, 107, 128] rather than to accelerating joints. For example, gastrocnemius's action on the knee and ankle will be small, since it operates near the regional boundaries shown in Figure 6.13 [7, 8].

Uniarticular Muscle Crossing a Ball-and-Socket Joint
Even though for pin joints the acceleration of the spanned joint caused by a uniarticular muscle is in the same direction as the applied torque, this result does not necessarily hold for more complex joints, such as a ball-and-socket joint (B. J. Fregly and F. E. Zajac, unpublished analysis, 1988). For example, gluteus maximus, which crosses the ball-and-socket hip joint and generates both an extensor and an abductor torque [80], will not necessarily accelerate the hip simultaneously into extension and abduction. Energetic arguments require only that the muscle shorten, and there are many possible joint accelerations consistent with such a shortening. For instance, its extensor torque might accelerate the hip into adduction which, when added to the hypothetically small abductor acceleration caused by the muscle's abductor torque, may produce a net acceleration of adduction. The reason torque can cause angular accelerations around axes different from the axis around which torque is generated is the same as the reason why a biarticular muscle can accelerate a spanned joint in the direction opposite to its applied torque: It is a result of dynamic coupling. To ascertain even a qualitative action for gluteus maximus, or for other uniarticular muscles crossing complex joints, demands deriving the dynamic equations for the specific motor task under study.

FIGURE 6.13

Directionality of gastrocnemius's (GAS's) action on the angular acceleration of the ankle and the knee as a function of GAS's moment–arm ratio ($r_k^{GAS}:r_a^{GAS}$) and knee angle (ϕ_k). **A,** *GAS's action on ankle angular acceleration.* The bold line *separates the regions where GAS accelerates the ankle into extension (i.e.,* ankle extends*) and into flexion (i.e.,* ankle flexes*). Between $135° < \phi_k < 180°$, and for ratios less than 0.5, GAS accelerates the ankle into extension because its ankle-extensor torque dominates the action at the ankle. For ratios greater than 0.5, GAS accelerates the ankle into flexion because the ankle extensor action produced from its ankle-extensor torque is less than the ankle flexor action produced from GAS's knee-flexor torque (see text).* **B,** *GAS's action on knee angular acceleration. For moment–arm ratios greater than about 0.5, GAS accelerates the knee into flexion (i.e.,* knee flexes*), regardless of how much the knee is flexed, because its knee-flexor torque dominates. For moment–arm ratios less than 0.5, GAS accelerates the knee into extension (i.e.,* knee extends*) because the knee flexor effect caused by its knee-flexor torque is less than the knee extensor action generated by its ankle-extensor torque.* **C,** *Regions showing the three possible actions of GAS. Notice that between $135° < \phi_k < 180°$, slight variations of GAS's moment–arm ratio around the nominal 0.5 may cause GAS to have a different action on either ankle or knee rotation, or on both.*

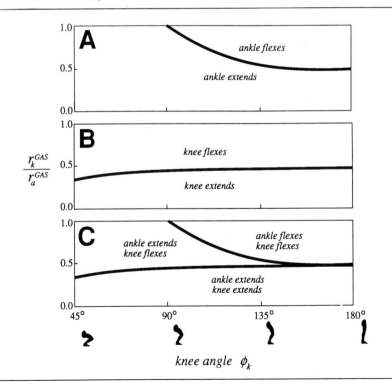

Anatomical Classification and Its Connotation for Movement: Reasons to Be Cautious

Though textbooks [5, 25, 108] use anatomy to correctly infer the directionality of torque developed by a muscle, their stated inference of muscle action may be erroneous. Using an anatomical classification, a muscle is called either a flexor or an extensor muscle, depending only on its torque. The interpretation is that muscle y defined anatomically as a *flexor muscle* of joint z, will act *to flex* joint z. Thus, "to flex" needs to be defined. A common interpretation is that if a muscle were acting alone from all other muscles, then it would, on development of force, move the joint into flexion. And if the muscle should develop more force, the joint would move faster and further into flexion and, as long as no other forces act on the body, the joint would in no way move into extension. When do we know with certainty that this interpretation is correct?

This classical interpretation is correct when the body is constrained so that only one joint, the joint under consideration, can move, and in only one direction. Only muscles crossing that joint will act to "move" the joint. If there are no other forces acting on the body, the mechanical system is linear. Thus the force developed by an anatomically defined flexor muscle will indeed accelerate the joint from rest into flexion and, at a later time, the joint will be flexing (i.e., moving with a certain velocity into flexion) and will have moved into flexion. If the muscle develops more force, the joint will accelerate into flexion faster, flex faster, and move to a flexed position faster. Even for biarticular muscles, no ambiguity arises since the other spanned joint will have been constrained from moving. And no ambiguity occurs for uniarticular muscles crossing a ball-and-socket joint either, because the joint is constrained from moving in the other directions and is only allowed to move in one direction (e.g., flex/extend).

In multiarticular motor tasks, however, the classical interpretation should be subjected to analysis. As we have repeatedly emphasized, there is no simple relationship among joint angle, joint velocity, and an individual torque acting alone because the mechanical system is nonlinear and superposition does not apply. However, the joint acceleration and the individual torque are linearly related. Thus, statements like "muscle y flexes joint z" or "the action of muscle y is to flex joint z" should be interpreted as "muscle y acts *to accelerate* joint z into flexion." Previously, we avoided using "*to flex*" for fear of causing ambiguity.

We have also emphasized that the way in which a muscle acts to accelerate a joint cannot necessarily be inferred from anatomy. For example, gastrocnemius can at times extend the knee, and at other times dorsiflex the ankle, even though it develops always a knee flexor torque and an ankle extensor torque. And a uniarticular muscle, like gluteus maximus, may flex the ball-and-socket hip at times, or adduct the hip at other times, even though it develops extension torque and abduction torque.

Finally, muscle action, as inferred by anatomical classification, conveys the notion that muscles do not instantaneously affect unspanned joints. Muscles do indeed act to accelerate all joints; at times, such as in standing, muscles crossing the ankle can extend or flex the knee much more than they flex or extend the ankle. Clearly, muscle action on body motion is a topic worthy of more careful scrutiny than appears in textbooks.

MUSCLE AGONIST–ANTAGONIST GROUPS AND SYNERGIES

Muscle function on the body during a motor task can be analyzed to determine if a muscle assists or hinders the desired task, and to determine if a muscle functions identically or oppositely to other muscles. When torque is used to define muscle function, a muscle is called an *agonist* if its torque is in the same direction as the net muscle torque, or two muscles are called an *agonist–antagonist pair* if their torques are in opposition signs [6–8, 80]. Alternatively, the joint accelerations caused by muscle may be used to determine agonist/antagonist relationships [7, 8, 124, 126]. We believe that using acceleration to classify agonist/antagonist function rather than torque will lead to a better understanding of muscle coordination [42, 124]. However, because muscles that work together need not function identically, it may be best to study how muscles work *synergistically* [41, 48, 84, 88] rather than *agonistically*, in accomplishing the motor task.

For single-joint motor tasks, the use of torque to define muscle function is consistent with the use of acceleration, and thus "agonist–antagonist" is unambiguous. In the control of elbow flexion/extension with the arm horizontal, for example, only the elbow is free to move. Thus whether the muscles are uni- or biarticular is immaterial, since each muscle develops either a flexor or an extensor elbow torque and thus acts to accelerate the elbow either into flexion or extension, respectively. Thus the relation between agonists, antagonists and task performance is easily related to whether the muscle is a flexor or extensor muscle, as defined by anatomy. In such highly constrained tasks, therefore, classifying muscles into agonist–antagonist groups is a convenient and meaningful way to view muscles and has lead to the elucidation of neural control mechanisms [39, 40, 44, 111], though such mechanisms may not necessarily operate during multiarticular tasks [49, 78].

Uniarticular muscles crossing a pin joint can also be consistently classified as agonists or antagonists. For example, if the ankle is assumed to be a pin joint, then soleus and tibialis anterior are opposites in the anatomical sense because the former exerts an ankle extensor torque, and the latter exerts an ankle flexor torque. It is simple to show that when they exert torques of equal magnitudes, all the joint accelerations caused by tibialis anterior are exactly opposite to all the joint accelerations caused by soleus. Thus soleus and tibialis anterior function oppositely when function is defined either anatomically (by torque), or dynamically (by acceleration). Thus, when EMG activity is recorded in such muscles, it may well be because the task requires joint stiffening [59].

With the exception of uniarticular muscles crossing a pin joint, the use of torque to define muscle function in tasks with many degrees of freedom can lead to different agonist/antagonist relationships than the use of acceleration [7, 8, 41, 42, 124, 126]. For example, consider hamstrings and rectus femoris. Anatomically they are antagonists because their torques at both the hip and the knee are opposite. However, they would not necessarily act to accelerate the joints oppositely should the ratio of their hip-to-knee torques be unequal. Thus although their torques have opposite signs, hamstrings and rectus femoris may both act, for example, in flat-footed postures, to extend the knee [42]. Similarly, the action of a uniarticular muscle crossing a ball-and-socket joint depends on the ratio of its three torque components. Thus uniarticular muscles which are anatomical opposites may not act to accelerate the body oppositely.

While we feel that muscle coordination is best understood when dynamic equations are used to analyze accelerations caused by muscle, it can be useful to compare a muscle's torque with the net muscle torque required to perform the task. For example, if a net ankle extensor torque is required, tibialis anterior would be an antagonist to the task, since it exerts an ankle flexor torque. If both an ankle-extensor and a knee-flexor torque is required, gastrocnemius would be an agonist at both joints because it contributes positively to both muscle torques. Indeed, such analyses have fostered insight into why some muscles are excited and others not during task performance [8, 34, 35, 69, 70, 73, 80, 120, 121].

The limitation of comparing the directions of torques developed by muscles to the directions required of muscles in the task is that coordination of muscles is discussed in the context of their ability to develop the required torques. However, such discussions do not provide insight into the action that these torques have on accelerating the joints. For example, soleus may be an agonist to fulfill the requirement of the task that ankle extensor torque be generated, but that does not necessarily mean that soleus (or any other muscle generating ankle extensor torque) is acting primarily to extend the ankle, even if the ankle should be accelerating into extension. Soleus may instead be acting mostly to accelerate the knee into extension (Fig. 6.12). And furthermore, though the net torque at the ankle is an extensor torque, the net acceleration of the ankle, resulting from torques at all the joints, need not be in extension.

If agonist–antagonist comparisons based on directionality of the torques needed and produced among muscles at joints can lead to misconceptions of coordination of joint movement, do agonist–antagonist comparisons based on the directionality of muscle action to accelerate joints have utility? For highly constrained tasks, it may be useful to use the dynamical equations of motion to find groups of muscles that accelerate the joints identically or oppositely. Obviously, single-joint, 1-*df* tasks fulfill this requirement. But some multiarticular tasks do also. For example, in the leg press (Fig. 6.6), there is only 1 *df*, so all lower limb muscles either accelerate the weight up ($\ddot{\theta} > 0$) or down ($\ddot{\theta} < 0$), and knowledge of a muscle's action on the weight specifies exactly how it will accelerate each of the three joints.

For tasks with many degrees of freedom, it may not be useful to identify agonist/antagonist groups because muscles may work together, yet not act identically. For example, in standing posture, muscles must actually work together even though their action on joints oppose one another [41, 42, 84, 89]. That is, a muscle must be excited even though its action at some of the joints is in opposition to task requirements. To counter the muscle's undesired action, a *synergistic* muscle must be excited. Since muscles need not act identically to work together, it may be best to study how muscles work as *synergists* rather than as *agonists*.

CONCLUSIONS

1. Dynamic optimization is the most powerful method for determining muscle forces and how they coordinate movement, because both the dynamics and what the task is attempting to achieve must be modeled.
2. A muscle acts to accelerate not only the joints it spans, but the unspanned joints as well. The angular acceleration of unspanned joints can exceed that of spanned joints.
3. Muscle's action is *task dependent* because the dynamic equations describing the relation among forces and motion depend on the interactions among the body segments and the environment.
4. Anatomy determines muscle-torque directionality, which is *task independent*. Therefore, extreme caution must be exercised when anatomy is used to infer muscle action during movement.
5. Since muscles need not function identically as agonists/antagonists to work together, it may be best to study how muscles work as *synergists* rather than as *agonists*.

ACKNOWLEDGMENTS

We thank J. Peter Loan for his assistance in analyzing two-joint dynamics, including the generation of Figures 6.12 and 6.13; David Delp for many discussions on the visual presentation and on the preparation of the figures; Kristin Bennett for assistance in manuscript preparation; and Scott Delp, Melissa Hoy, Gerald Loeb, Marcus Pandy, and Eric Topp for their careful review of an earlier draft. We especially appreciate discussions with Marcus Pandy on optimization and direct and inverse dynamics, and with Eric Topp on degrees of freedom and dynamics. The work was supported by the National Institutes of Health Grant NS17662, the Alfred P. Sloan Foundation, and the Veterans Administration.

APPENDIX A: MUSCLE FORCE, MOMENT, COUPLE AND TORQUE

Although muscle develops force (see Muscle Force During Movement section), often other terms are used in the biomechanics and motor control literature, for example, "moment of muscle force" about a joint, a muscle's "force couple," a muscle's "joint reaction force," the "torque of the force couple" of a muscle, the "joint torque" developed by a muscle, and the muscle's "torque at the joint." The relation among these terms [6, 34–37, 72, 81, 99] is reviewed here for uniarticular muscles, though similar relations apply to bi- and multiarticular muscles.

Assuming uniform tension along a straight line path from muscle's "effective" origin to its "effective" insertion (Fig. 6.14A), the muscle exerts a force F_i^{mus} acting on segment i at the effective origin, and an opposite force $-F_i^{mus}$ on segment $i - 1$ at the effective insertion (Fig. 6.14B).

The set of forces shown in Figure 6.14B is equivalent to the same forces acting at the joint, together with a force couple of torque T_i^{mus} acting on segment i, and a force couple of torque $-T_i^{mus}$ acting on segment $i - 1$ (Fig. 6.14C). A force couple is a pair of equal and opposite forces. A special property of a force couple is that its moment about any point is the same, and is called the *torque* of the force couple. Because the moment of a force about its point of application is zero, T_i^{mus} is equal in magnitude and direction to the moment of muscle force F_i^{mus} about the joint center. And $-T_i^{mus}$ is equal to the moment of muscle force $-F_i^{mus}$ about the joint center.

If the joint allows for translation of the two adjacent segments, or if frictional forces are significant, both the muscle's force and the torque acting on each segment must be included in a dynamic analysis. Otherwise, the muscle forces sum to zero at the joint, and only the two segment torques contribute to the motion. Because the torque on segment $i-1$ is exactly opposite to the torque on segment i, the muscle acts as a mechanical torque actuator would, such as those used in robotics [26, 60]. Therefore, the combination of these two segment torques is called

FIGURE 6.14

Relations among a uniarticular muscle (A), the force it exerts on each of the two adjacent segments (B), the equivalent joint reaction forces and torques of the force couples acting on the two segments (C), and the equivalent joint-torque (D).

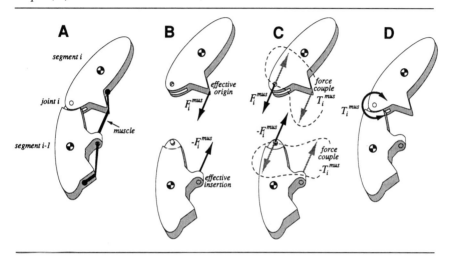

the muscle's *joint-torque* (Fig. 6.14**D**), or the *torque of the muscle at the joint*; these terms are often used in coordination studies [10, 30, 47, 60, 98, 109]. For brevity, we refer simply to the muscle's *torque* in this chapter.

Similarly, one can shown that a biarticular muscle acts as two uniarticular muscles. So, for frictionless pin- and ball-and-socket joints, a biarticular muscle acts as two "torque actuators," one at each of the spanned joints.

APPENDIX B: GRAVITY AND INERTIA FORCES, COUPLES AND TORQUES

With at least one point of one of the body segments stationary, every force acting on a segment is accompanied by an equal and opposite reaction force that also acts on the segment. For example, consider a segment connected to another segment by a joint (the upper joint in Fig. 6.15), and to the ground by another joint (the lower joint). Suppose only two external forces act on this segment: the reaction force F_{jr} at the upper joint, and the force from gravity $m_1 g$ (Fig. 6.15). In addition, the internal inertia force $-m_1 a_1$ of the segment acts on itself, as does its inertia torque $-I_1 \ddot{\theta}_1$ (Fig. 6.15). Notice that three equal and opposite

FIGURE 6.15

For each force acting on a segment, there is an equal and opposite reaction force that also acts on the segment. The force and its reaction force are a force couple. The moment of the force couple about any point is the same, and is called the torque of the couple.

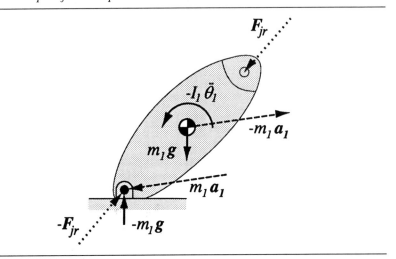

reaction forces appear at the lower joint: two in reaction to the external forces (*i.e.*, $-F_{jr}$ and m_1g), and one in reaction to the inertia force (*i.e.*, m_1a_1).

Thus, because of the reaction forces, both external and inertia forces occur in pairs. Each pair constitutes a force couple which has a torque associated with it (see Appendix A). For example, the torque of the gravity force couple acting on this segment equals the moment of the gravity force about the lower joint. So, for frictionless pin- and ball-and-socket joints, and with at least one point of the body stationary, the net effect of gravity and inertia on the motion of the segments is given by their torques.

APPENDIX C: DYNAMIC EQUATION OF A ROTATING PLANAR SEGMENT

The dynamic equation of the rotating planar segment shown in Figure 6.7 is as follows:

$$(\tilde{I})\ddot{\theta} = T^{\text{mus}} - T^{\text{grav}} = T^{\text{net}}. \tag{1}$$

The segment has a mass m, and its mass center is located a distance l from the joint, and the segment is oriented at an angle θ with respect to horizontal. Muscle torques T^{SOL} and T^{TA} act in opposition; therefore,

$$T^{\text{mus}} = T^{\text{SOL}} - T^{\text{TA}}.$$

The net and gravity torques are, respectively,

$$T^{\text{net}} = (\tilde{I})\ddot{\theta} = (I + ml^2)\ddot{\theta} \quad \text{and} \quad T^{\text{grav}} = mgl\cos\theta = T^g\cos\theta.$$

APPENDIX D: DYNAMIC EQUATIONS FOR TWO ROTATING PLANAR SEGMENTS

The dynamic equation for the two-segment system shown in Figure 6.9 can be derived from the recursive equations in reference 75. The equations are as follows:

$$(\tilde{I}_1)\ddot{\theta}_1 + [\tilde{I}_{cs}\cos(\theta_1 - \theta_2)]\ddot{\theta}_2 = T_1^{\text{mus}} - T_1^{\text{grav}} - [\tilde{I}_{cs}\sin(\theta_1 - \theta_2)]\dot{\theta}_2^2. \quad (3a)$$
$$(\tilde{I}_2)\ddot{\theta}_2 + [\tilde{I}_{cs}\cos(\theta_1 - \theta_2)]\ddot{\theta}_1 = T_2^{\text{mus}} - T_2^{\text{grav}} + [\tilde{I}_{cs}\sin(\theta_1 - \theta_2)]\dot{\theta}_1^2. \quad (3b)$$

Our notation is m_i for the mass of segment i, ρ_1 for the length of segment 1, l_i for the distance from the joint nearest to the ground to the mass center, I_i for the moment of inertia about the mass center, and θ_i for the angle of the segment with respect to horizontal. Thus,

$$\tilde{I}_1 = I_1 + m_1 l_1^2, + m_2 \rho_1^2, \quad \tilde{I}_2 = I_2 + m_2 l_2^2, \quad \tilde{I}_{cs} = m_2 l_2 \rho_1,$$
$$T_1^{\text{grav}} = T_1^g\cos\theta_1 = g(m_1 l_1 + m_2\rho_1)\cos(\theta_1),$$
$$T_2^{\text{grav}} = T_2^g\cos\theta_2 = g(m_2 l_2)\cos(\theta_2).$$

APPENDIX E: ANALYSIS OF DYNAMIC COUPLING

The forces acting on segment 2 are the gravity force $m_2 g$, and the joint reaction force F_{jr}, as well as the inertia force $-m_2 a_2$ (Fig. 6.16). The coupling arises on segment 2 because its own acceleration, a_2, is a function of θ_1, $\dot{\theta}_1$, and $\ddot{\theta}_1$. Therefore, the coupling on segment 2 occurs for purely kinematic reasons; that is, the inertia force of segment 2 depends on the kinematics of segment 1.

In contrast, coupling from segment 2 on segment 1 occurs because of joint reaction forces. The forces acting on segment 1 are the gravity force $m_1 g$ and the reaction force at each of the two joints $(-F_{\text{jr}}, F_{\text{gr}})$. Therefore, since the acceleration of segment 1 does not depend on θ_2 or its time derivatives, the coupling on segment 1 occurs because both the inertia force of segment 2 $(-m_2 a_2)$ and its gravity force $(m_2 g)$ have reactionary forces at the joints.

FIGURE 6.16
Dynamic coupling arises because inertia and gravity forces may be transmitted via the joints to the other segments, and because the inertia force of one segment may depend on the kinematics of other segments.

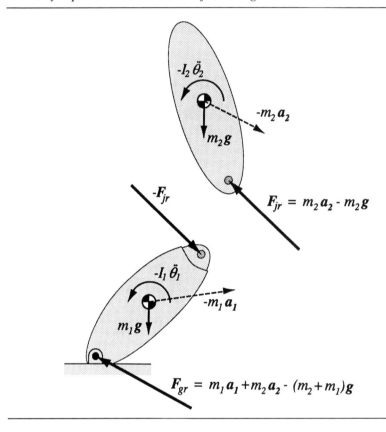

$$-I_2 \ddot{\theta}_2$$
$$-m_2 a_2$$
$$m_2 g$$
$$-F_{jr}$$
$$F_{jr} = m_2 a_2 - m_2 g$$
$$-I_1 \ddot{\theta}_1$$
$$-m_1 a_1$$
$$m_1 g$$
$$F_{gr} = m_1 a_1 + m_2 a_2 - (m_2 + m_1)g$$

APPENDIX F: DYNAMIC EQUATIONS OF TWO SEGMENTS IN JOINT SPACE

Although the equations of motion can be derived directly in joint space [26], the equations are easily converted from segment to joint coordinates. The segment and joint coordinates, and torques are related by:

$$\theta_1 = \phi_a,$$
$$\theta_2 = \phi_a - \phi_k + \pi. \qquad \qquad T_1^{net} = T_a^{net} + T_k^{net},$$
$$T_2^{net} = -T_k^{net}. \qquad (6)$$

Therefore,

$$\ddot{\theta}_1 = \ddot{\phi}_a, \qquad \dot{\theta}_1 = \dot{\phi}_a, \qquad \ddot{\theta}_2 = \ddot{\phi}_a - \ddot{\phi}_k, \qquad \dot{\theta}_2 = \dot{\phi}_a - \dot{\phi}_k, \qquad (7)$$
$$cos(\theta_1 - \theta_2) = -cos(\phi_k), \qquad sin(\theta_1 - \theta_2) = -sin(\phi_k).$$

Substituting Equations 6 and 7 into Equations 3a and 3b, the dynamic equations in joint coordinates are as follows:

$$(\tilde{I}_a)\, \ddot{\phi}_a + (\tilde{I}_{cj})\, \ddot{\phi}_k = T_a^{net} \qquad (8a)$$
$$(\tilde{I}_k)\, \ddot{\phi}_k + (\tilde{I}_{cj})\, \ddot{\phi}_a = T_k^{net} \qquad (8b)$$

where

$$\tilde{I}_a = \tilde{I}_1 + \tilde{I}_2 - 2\tilde{I}_{cs}\, cos\phi_k, \qquad \tilde{I}_k = \tilde{I}_2, \qquad \tilde{I}_{cj} = \tilde{I}_{cs}cos\phi_k - \tilde{I}_2,$$

and

$$T_a^{net} = T_a^{mus} - T_a^{grav} + T_a(\dot{\phi}_a, \phi_k, \dot{\phi}_k),$$
$$T_k^{net} = T_k^{mus} - T_k^{grav} + T_k(\dot{\phi}_a^2, \phi_k),$$
$$T_a^{mus} = T_1^{mus} + T_2^{mus},$$
$$T_k^{mus} = -T_2^{mus},$$
$$T_a^{grav} = T_1^{grav} + T_2^{grav},$$
$$T_k^{grav} = -T_2^{grav},$$
$$T_a(\dot{\phi}_a, \phi_k, \dot{\phi}_k) = \tilde{I}_{cs}sin(\phi_k)\,(\dot{\phi}_k^2 - 2\dot{\phi}_a\dot{\phi}_k),$$
$$T_k(\dot{\phi}_a^2, \phi_k) = \tilde{I}_{cs}sin(\phi_k)\,\dot{\phi}_a^2.$$

REFERENCES

1. Alexander RMcN: The mechanics of jumping by a dog (*Canis familiaris*). *J Zool (Lond)* 173:549–573, 1974.
2. Alexander RMcN, Vernon A: The mechanics of hopping by kangaroos (*Macropodidae*). *J Zool (Lond)* 177:265–303, 1975.
3. An KN, Chao EY: Kinematic analysis of human movement. *Ann Biomed Eng* 12:585–597, 1984.
4. An KN, Kwak BM, Chao EY, Morrey BF: Determination of muscle and joint forces: a new technique to solve the indeterminate problem. *J Biomech Eng* 106:364–367, 1984.
5. Anderson JE: *Grant's Atlas of Anatomy*, ed 8. Baltimore, Williams & Wilkins, 1983.
6. Andrews JG: On the relationship between resultant joint torques and muscular activity. *Med Sci Sports Exerc* 14:361–367, 1982.
7. Andrews JG: A general method for determining the functional role of a muscle. *J Biomech Eng* 107:348–353, 1985.
8. Andrews JG: The functional role of the hamstrings and quadriceps during cycling: Lombard's paradox revisited. *J Biomech* 20:565–575, 1987.
9. Athans M, Falb PL: *Optimal Control: An Introduction to the Theory and Its Application*. New York, McGraw-Hill, 1966, p 879.
10. Atkeson CG, Hollerbach JM: Kinematic features of unrestrained vertical arm movements. *J Neurosci* 5:2318–2330, 1985.

11. Barry D, Ahmed AM: Design and performance of a modified buckle transducer for the measurement of ligament tension. *J Biomech Eng* 108:149–152, 1986.
12. Bean JC, Chaffin DB, Schultz AB: Biomechanical model calculation of muscle contraction forces: a double linear programming method. *J Biomech* 21: 59–66, 1988.
13. Bobbert MF, Huijing PA, van Ingen Schenau, GJ: A model of the human triceps surae muscle-tendon complex applied to jumping. *J Biomech* 19: 887–898, 1986.
14. Bobbert MF, Huijing PA, van Ingen Schenau GJ: An estimation of power output and work done by the human triceps surae muscle-tendon complex in jumping. *J Biomech* 19:899–906, 1986.
15. Bock WJ: Mechanics of one- and two-joint muscles. *Am Mus Novit* 2319:1–45, 1968.
16. Brand RA, Pedersen DR, Friederich JA: The sensitivity of muscle force predictions to changes in physiologic cross-sectional area. *J Biomech* 19:589–596, 1986.
17. Bresler B, Frankel JP: The forces and the moments in the leg during level walking. *Trans ASME (Am Soc Mech Eng) J Biomech Eng* 72:27–35, 1950.
18. Brown TD, Sigal L, Njus GO, Njus NM, Singerman RJ, Brand RA: Dynamic performance characteristics of the liquid metal strain gauge. *J Biomech* 19:165–173, 1986.
19. Buchner HJ, Hines MJ, Hemami HA: Dynamic model for finger interphalangeal coordination. *J Biomech* 21:459–468, 1988.
20. Cappozzo A, Leo T, Pedotti A: A general computing method for the analysis of human locomotion. *J Biomech* 8:307–320, 1975.
21. Carlsoo S, Molbech S: The functions of certain two-joint muscles in a closed muscular chain. *Acta Morphol Neerl Scand* 6:377–386, 1966.
22. Chao EYS: Biomechanics of the human gait. In Schmid-Schonbein GW, Woo SLY, Zweifach BW (eds): *Frontiers in Biomechanics*. New York, Springer-Verlag, 1986, pp 225–244.
23. Chow CK, Jacobson DH: Studies of human locomotion via optimal programming. *Math Biosci* 10:239–306, 1971.
24. Chow CK, Jacobson DH: Further studies of human locomotion: postural stability and control. *Math Biosci* 15:93–108, 1972.
25. Cooper JM, Adrian M, Glassow RB: *Kinesiology*, ed 5. St. Louis, Mosby, 1982, p 452.
26. Craig JJ: *Introduction to Robotics: Mechanics and Controls*. Reading, MA, Addison-Wesley, 1986, p 303.
27. Crowninshield D: Use of optimization techniques to predict muscle forces. *J Biomech Eng* 100:88–92, 1978.
28. Crowninshield RD, Brand RA: A physiologically based criterion of muscle force prediction in locomotion. *J Biomech* 14:793–801, 1981.
29. Crowninshield RD, Johnston RC, Andrews JG, Brand RA: A biomechanical investigation of the human hip. *J Biomech* 11:75–85, 1978.
30. Davy DT, Audu ML: A dynamic optimization technique for predicting muscle forces in the swing phase of gait. *J Biomech* 20:187–201, 1987.
31. Dickinson, JA, Cook SD, Leinhardt TM: The measurement of shock waves following heel strike when running. *J Biomech* 18:415–422, 1985.
32. Dul J, Johnson GE, Shiavi R, Townsend MA: Muscular synergism-II. A minimum-fatigue criterion for load sharing between synergistic muscles. *J Biomech* 17:675–684, 1984.
33. Dul J, Townsend MA, Shiavi R, Johnson GE: Muscular synergism—I. On criteria for load sharing between synergistic muscles. *J Biomech* 17:663–673, 1984.
34. Elftman H: Forces and energy changes in the leg during walking. *Am J Physiol* 125:339–356, 1939.
35. Elftman H: The function of muscles in locomotion. *Am J Physiol* 125:357–366, 1939.
36. Elftman H: The action of muscles in the body. *Biol Symp* 3:191–209, 1941.
37. Elftman H: Biomechanics of muscle. *J Bone Joint Surg* 48A:363–377, 1966.
38. Flash T, Hogan N: The coordination of arm movements: An experimentally confirmed mathematical model. *J Neurosci* 5:1688–1703, 1985.

39. Ghez C, Gordon J: Trajectory control in targeted force impulses: I. Role of opposing muscles. *Exp Brain Res* 67:225–240, 1987.
40. Ghez C, Martin JH: The control of rapid limb movement in the cat: III. Agonist–antagonist coupling. *Exp Brain Res* 45:115–125, 1982.
41. Gordon ME, Zajac FE, Hoy MG: Postural synergies dictated by segmental accelerations from muscles and physical constraints. *Soc Neurosci Abstr* 12:1425, 1986.
42. Gordon ME, Zajac FE, Khang G, Loan JP: Intersegmental and mass center accelerations induced by lower extremity muscles: theory and methodology with emphasis on quasivertical standing postures. In Spilker RL, Simon BR (eds): *Proc Symposium Computational Methods Bioengineering: 1988 ASME Winter Annual Meeting/Chicago.* New York, American Society of Mechanical Engineers, 1988, BED-Vol 9, pp. 481–492.
43. Gottlieb GL, Agarwal GC: Dynamic relationship between isometric muscle tension and the electromyogram in man. *J Appl Physiol* 30:345–351, 1971.
44. Gottlieb GL, Corcos DM, Agarwal GC: Strategies for the control of voluntary movements. *Behav Brain Sci* (in press).
45. Gregoire L, Veeger HE, Huijing PA, van Ingen Schenau GJ: Role of mono- and biarticular muscles in explosive movements. *Int J Sports Med* 5:301–305, 1984.
46. Gregor RJ, Cavanagh PR, LaFortune M: Knee flexor moments during propulsion in cycling—a creative solution to Lombard's Paradox. *J Biomech* 18:307–316, 1985.
47. Hardt DE: Determining muscle forces in the leg during normal walking—an application and evaluation of optimization methods. *J Biomech Eng* 100:72–78, 1978.
48. Hasan Z, Enoka RM, Stuart DG: The interface between biomechanics and neurophysiology in the study of movement: some recent approaches. In Terjung RL (ed): *Exercise and Sport Sciences Reviews.* New York: Macmillan, 1985, pp. 169–234.
49. Hasan Z, Stuart DG: Animal solutions to problems of movement control: The role of proprioceptors. *Annu Rev Neurosci* 11:199–223, 1988.
50. Hatze H: The complete optimization of a human motion. *Math Biosci* 28:99–135, 1976.
51. Hatze H: A complete set of control equations for the human musculo-skeletal system. *J Biomech* 10:799–805, 1977.
52. Hatze H: Neuromusculoskeletal control systems modeling—a critical survey of recent developments. *IEEE Trans Auto Control* AC-25:375–385, 1980.
53. Hatze H: A comprehensive model for human motion simulation and its application to the take-off phase of the long jump. *J Biomech* 14:135–142, 1981.
54. Herzog H: Individual muscle force prediction in athletic movements. Ph.D. dissertation, University of Iowa, Ames, 1985.
55. Hill AV: The heat of shortening and the dynamic constants of muscle. *Proc R Soc Lond (Biol)* 126:136–195, 1938.
56. Hof AL, Geelen BA, Van Den Berg JW: Calf muscle moment, work and efficiency in level walking: role of series elasticity. *J Biomech* 16:523–537, 1983.
57. Hof AL, Pronk CNA, van Best JA: Comparison between EMG to force processing and kinetic analysis for the calf muscle moment in walking and stepping. *J Biomech* 20:167–178, 1987.
58. Hof AL, Van Den Berg JW: EMG to force processing I: an electrical analogue of the Hill muscle model. *J Biomech* 14:747–758, 1981.
59. Hogan N: The mechanics of multi-joint posture and movement control. *Biol Cybern* 52:315–331, 1985.
60. Hollerbach JM, Flash T: Dynamic interactions between limb segments during planar arm movement. *Biol Cybern* 44:67–77, 1982.
61. Houtz SJ, Fischer FJ: An analysis of muscle action and joint excursion during exercise on a stationary bicycle. *J Bone Joint Surg* 41-A:123–131, 1959.
62. Hoy MG, Zajac FE, Topp EL, Cady CT, Levine WS: Synergistic control of uniarticular and biarticular muscles in human jumping: a computer simulation study. *Soc Neurosci Abstr* 12:1425, 1986.

63. Hoy MG, Zernicke RF: Modulation of limb dynamics in the swing phase of locomotion. *J Biomech* 18:49–60, 1985.
64. Hoy MG, Zernicke RF: The role of intersegmental dynamics during rapid limb oscillations. *J Biomech* 19:867–877, 1986.
65. Hoy MG, Zernicke RF, Smith JL: Contrasting roles of inertial and muscle moments at knee and ankle during paw-shake response. *J Neurophysiol* 54:1282–1294, 1985.
66. Hull M, Davis RR: Measurement of pedal loading in bicycling: 1. Instrumentation. *J Biomech* 14:843–856, 1981.
67. Huston RL, Passerello CE, Harlow MW: Dynamics of multirigid-body systems. *J Appl Mech* 45:889–894, 1978.
68. Inman VT, Ralston HJ, Todd F: *Human Walking*. Baltimore, Williams & Wilkins, 1981, p 154.
69. Jorge M, Hull L: Analysis of EMG measurements during bicycle pedaling. *J Biomech* 19:683–694, 1986.
70. Ju MS, Mansour, JM: Simulation of the double limb support phase of human gait. *J Biomech Eng* 110:223–229, 1988.
71. Kailath T: *Linear Systems*. Englewood Cliffs, Prentice-Hall, 1980, p 682.
72. Kane TR, Levinson DA: *Dynamics: Theory and Applications*. New York, McGraw-Hill, 1985, p 379.
73. Khang G: Paraplegic standing controlled by functional neuromuscular stimulation: computer model, control-system design, and simulation studies. Ph.D dissertation, Stanford University, Stanford, CA, 1988, p 115.
74. Kinzel GL, Gutkowski LJ: Joint models, degrees of freedom, and anatomical motion measurement. *J Biomech Eng* 105:55–62, 1983.
75. Koozekanani SH, Barin K, McGhee RB, Chang HT: A recursive free-body approach to computer simulation of human postural dynamics. *IEEE Trans Biomed Eng* 30:787–792, 1983.
76. Levine WS, Zajac FE, Belzer MR, Zomlefer MR: Ankle controls that produce a maximal vertical jump when other joints are locked. *IEEE Trans Auto Control* AC-28:1008–1016, 1983.
77. Lippold OCJ: The relation between integrated action potentials in a human muscle and its isometric tension. *J Physiol* 117:492–499, 1952.
78. Loeb GE: Hard lessons in motor control from the mammalian spinal cord. *Trends Neurosci* 10:108–113, 1987.
79. Luenberger DG: *Linear and Nonlinear Programming*. Reading, Addison-Wesley, 1984, p 491.
80. Mansour JM, Pereira JM: Quantitative functional anatomy of the lower limb with application to human gait. *J Biomech* 20:51–58, 1987.
81. Manter JT: The dynamics of quadrupedal walking. *J Exp Biol* 15:522–540, 1938.
82. Markee JE, Logue JT, Williams M, Stanton WB, Wrenn RN, Walker LB: Two-joint muscles of the thigh. *J Bone Joint Surg* 37-A:125–142, 1955.
83. Marshall RN, Jensen RK, Wood GA: A general Newtonian simulation of an *n*-segment open chain model. *J Biomech* 18:359–367, 1985.
84. McCollum G, Nashner M: Mechanics of stance and locomotion in physiological coordinates: a biomechanical model taking into account the physiology of muscle contraction and the activation patterns of muscle synergies. *Soc Neurosci Abstr* 8:284, 1982.
85. Miller D: Resultant lower extremity joint moments in below-knee amputees during running stance. *J Biomech* 20:529–541, 1987.
86. Morrison JB: The mechanics of the knee joint in relation to normal walking. *J Biomech* 3:51–61, 1970.
87. Morrison JB: The mechanics of muscle function in locomotion. *J Biomech* 3:431–451, 1970.
88. Nashner LM: Fixed patterns of rapid postural responses among leg muscles during stance. *Exp Brain Res* 30:13–24, 1977.

89. Nashner LM, McCollum G: The organization of human postural movements: a formal basis and experimental synthesis. *Behav Brain Sci* 8:135–172, 1985.

90. Nelson WL: Physical principles for economies of skilled movements. *Biol Cybern* 46:135–147, 1983.

91. Newmiller J, Hull ML, Zajac FE: A mechanically decoupled two force component bicycle pedal dynamometer. *J Biomech* 21:375–386, 1988.

92. Oǧuztöreli MN, Stein RB: Optimal control of antagonistic muscles. *Biol Cybern* 48:91–99, 1983.

93. Olney SJ, Winter DA: Prediction of knee and ankle moments of force in walking from EMG and kinematic data. *J Biomech* 18:9–20, 1985.

94. Orin DF, McGhee RB, Vukobratovic M, Hartoch G: Kinematic and kinetic analysis of open-chain linkages utilizing Newton-Euler methods. *Math Biosci* 43:107–130, 1979.

95. Osborn JW, Baragar FA: Predicted pattern of human muscle activity during clenching derived from a computer assisted model: symmetric vertical bite forces. *J Biomech* 18:599–612, 1985.

96. Pandy MG, Berme N: A numerical method for simulating the dynamics of human walking. *J Biomech* (in press).

97. Pandy MG, Zajac FE, Hoy MG, Topp ER, Tashman S, Stevenson PJ, Cady C, Sim E, Levine WS: Sub-optimal control of a maximum-height, countermovement jump. In Stein JL (ed): *Proceedings Symposium Modeling and Control Issues in Biomechanical Systems: 1988 ASME Winter Annual Meeting/Chicago*. New York, American Society of Mechanical Engineers, 1988, DSC-Vol 12, pp 27–44.

98. Patriarco AG, Mann RW, Simon SR, Mansour JM: An evaluation of the approaches of optimization models in the prediction of muscle forces during human gait. *J Biomech* 14:513–525, 1981.

99. Paul JP: Letter to the editor: torques produce tension. *J Biomech* 11:87, 1978.

100. Pedersen DR, Brand RA, Cheng C, Arora JS: Direct comparison of muscle force predictions using linear and nonlinear programming. *J Biomech Eng* 109:192–199, 1987.

101. Pedotti A: A study of motor coordination and neuromuscular activities in human locomotion. *Biol Cybern* 26:53–62, 1977.

102. Pedotti A, Krishnan VV, Stark L: Optimization of muscle-force sequencing in human locomotion. *Math Biosci* 38:57–76, 1978.

103. Penrod DD, Davy DT, Singh DP: An optimization approach to tendon force analysis. *J Biomech* 7:123–129, 1974.

104. Pierrynowski MR, Morrison JB: Estimating the muscle forces generated in the human lower extremity when walking: a physiological solution. *Math Biosci* 75:43–68, 1985.

105. Pierrynowski MR, Morrison JB: A physiological model for the evaluation of muscular forces in human locomotion: theoretical aspects. *Math Biosci* 75:69–102, 1985.

106. Riemersma DJ, Lammertink Jos LMA: Calibration of the mercury-in-silastic strain gauge in tendon load experiments. *J Biomech* 21:469–476, 1988.

107. Robertson DGE, Winter DA: Mechanical energy generation, absorption and transfer amongst segments during walking. *J Biomech* 13:845–854, 1980.

108. Romanes GJ (ed): *Cunningham's Textbook of Anatomy*, ed 12. Oxford, Oxford University Press, 1981, p 1078.

109. Romick-Allen R, Schultz AB: Biomechanics of reactions to impending falls. *J Biomech* 21:591–600, 1988.

110. Seireg A, Arvikar RJ: The prediction of muscular load sharing and joint forces in the lower extremities during walking. *J Biomech* 8:89–102, 1975.

111. Sherrington CS: Flexion-reflex of the limb, crossed extension-reflexes, and reflex stepping and standing. *J Physiol* 40:28–121, 1910.

112. Shiavi R, Limbird T, Frazer M, Stivers K, Strauss A, Abramovitz J: Helical motion

analysis of the knee—II. Kinematics of uninjured and injured knees during walking and pivoting. *J Biomech* 20:653–665, 1987.

113. Son K, Miller JAA, Schultz AB: The mechanical role of the trunk and lower extremities in a seated weight-moving task in the sagittal plane. *J Biomech Eng* 110:97–103, 1988.

114. Stein RB, Oğuztöreli MN, Capaday C: What is optimized in muscular movements? In Jones NL, McCartney N, McComas AJ (eds): *Human Muscle Power*. Champaign, IL, Human Kinetics, 1986, pp 131–150.

115. Suzuki S, Watanabe S, Homma S: EMG activity and kinematics of human cycling movements at different constant velocities. *Brain Res* 240:245–258, 1982.

116. Vaughan CL, Hay JG, Andrews JG: Closed loop problems in biomechanics. Part II—An optimization approach. *J Biomech* 15:201–210, 1982.

117. Walmsley B, Hodgson JA, Burke RE: Forces produced by medial gastrocnemius and soleus muscles during locomotion in freely moving cats. *J Neurophysiol* 41:1203–1216, 1978.

118. Whiting WC, Gregor RJ, Roy RR, Edgerton VR: A technique for estimating mechanical work of individual muscles in the cat during treadmill locomotion. *J Biomech* 17:685–694, 1984.

119. Winter DA: The locomotion laboratory as a clinical assessment system. *Med Prog Technol* 4:95–106, 1976.

120. Winter DA: *Biomechanics of Human Movement*. New York, Wiley, 1979, p 202.

121. Winter DA: *The Biomechanics and Motor Control of Human Gait*. Waterloo, University of Waterloo Press, 1987, p 72.

122. Yoon YS, Mansour JM: The passive elastic moment at the hip. *J Biomech* 15:905–910, 1982.

123. Zajac FE: Thigh muscle activity in cats during maximal height jumps. *J Neurophysiol* 53:979–993, 1985.

124. Zajac FE: Dynamics of limb movement: interpretation of EMG signals and the effects of musculotendon forces on body acceleration. In Butler DL, Torzilli PA (eds): *ASME 1987 Biomechanics Symposium in Cincinnati*. New York: The American Society of Mechanical Engineers, 1987, vol. AMD-84:391–394.

125. Zajac FE: Muscle and tendon properties: models, scaling, and application to biomechanics and motor control. *CRC Crit Rev Biomed Eng*, in press.

126. Zajac FE, Gordon ME, Hoy MG: Physiological classification of muscles into agonist–antagonist muscle action groups: theory and methodology based on mechanics. *Soc Neurosci Abstr* 12:1424, 1986.

127. Zajac FE, Levine WS: Novel experimental and theoretical approaches to study the neural control of locomotion and jumping. In Talbott R, Humphrey D (eds): *Posture and Movement: Perspective for Integrating Sensory and Motor Research on the Mammalian Nervous System*. New York, Raven Press, 1979, pp 259–279.

128. Zarrugh MY: Kinematic prediction of intersegment loads and power at the joints of the leg in walking. *J Biomech* 14:713–725, 1981.

129. Zomlefer MR, Ho R, Levine WS, Zajac FE: The use of optimal control in the study of a normal physiological movement. *Proceedings of the 1975 IEEE Conference on Decision and Control in Houston*. New York: The Institute of Electrical and Electronic Engineers, 1975, pp 402–407.

7
Impedance Cardiography: Noninvasive Assessment of Human Central Hemodynamics at Rest and During Exercise

DANIEL S. MILES, Ph.D.
ROBERT W. GOTSHALL, Ph.D.

Few of us are partial to any invasive procedure to assess our cardiac status, and fewer still have the fortitude to catheterize their own heart as Forssman did in 1929 [55]. Yet, there is no question that assessment of the mechanical pumping activity of the heart provides information of critical importance for evaluation of the circulatory system. The use of electrical impedance to assess the cardiac status has developed into a relatively simple, repeatable, atraumatic, cost-effective, and, most important, noninvasive procedure to assess the cardiac pump on a beat-by-beat basis. This review summarizes selected literature, primarily of the 1980s, to provide a perspective on the use of electrical impedance to assess human cardiac performance in basic and applied physiology, as well as clinical practice.

Historical Perspective

Electrical impedance has been used to evaluate heart function and a host of other divergent physiological events since the early 1900s [55]. Reviews on the detection of physiological events by evaluation of impedance changes have been presented by Geddes and Baker [25], Miller and Horvath [72], Baker [3], Mohapatra [78], Lamberts et al. [55], Penney [88], and Schuster and Schuster [97]. This review differs from previously published material in that it summarizes the 1980s work with special consideration given to our current understanding of the impedance waveform genesis, advances in waveform conditioning, and applications at rest and during exercise which provide relevant information concerning myocardial function.

The earlier measurements of the changes in electrical impedance resulting from the activity of the heart have been labeled dielectrography, radiocardiography, rheocardiography, and cardiographie à haute fréquence. Nyboer [82] was a pioneer in suggesting the use of a thoracic tetrapolar electrode arrangement and should be credited with proposing the term electrical impedance plethysmography. In the simplest terms,

Nyboer considered the impedance tracing to be a plethysmogram and related the changes observed in thoracic impedance to a change in thoracic blood volume (stroke volume). The work of Kubicek et al. [49–52] in the early 1960s, while developing a noninvasive method to assess cardiac function suitable for astronauts, led to a refinement of the stroke volume equation and the first commercially available impedance cardiograph. Since 1960, considerable progress has been made in validating, refining, and interpreting the impedance cardiogram [55, 78].

Acquisition of the Impedance Waveform
Ohm's law is the basis for the electrical impedance technique. It describes the relationship between current (I), voltage (V), and resistance (R), or impedance (Z).

$$R = V/I \qquad Z = V/I$$

This relationship is true for direct current (dc) as well as alternating current (ac) circuits. The term R applies to dc, whereas Z applies to ac and may change with the frequency. Impedance is a complex term consisting of resistance and reactance (capacitive resistance). The impedance of mammalian tissue is primarily resistive at the frequencies used in impedance cardiographs.

Because of safety considerations [3, 78], currents from dc to 5 kHz are not used to measure impedance changes. Furthermore, the operational frequency applied to the thorax must be greater than the highest frequency component found in any bioelectric signal [3, 78]. The electrocardiogram (ECG) and electroencephalogram maximum frequencies do not exceed 100 Hz. The input impedance of the voltage measuring circuit must be very high (ideally infinite) compared to the tissue impedance between the voltage electrodes to ensure that polarization impedances at the electrodes are negligible. Given the constraints of safety and bioelectric signals, most impedance instruments have employed frequencies within the range of 20–100 kHz at constant current levels from 20 μA to 10 mA root mean square, respectively.

For effective impedance measurements, electrodes must be attached in such a way to encompass the physiological event under consideration [40, 43]. For measuring stroke volume, four electrodes are attached to the chest and neck, as shown in Figure 7.1. The electrodes have traditionally been numbered consecutively with electrode #1 cephalad and electrode #4 caudal. The outer two electrodes should be spaced at least 3 cm from the inner electrodes to avoid nonlinearities in the electrical field [3, 55, 78]. In those cases where neck length is small, as with infants or individuals with a large body build such as football players, a strip of electrode tape can be placed on the forehead for the #1 electrode. The

FIGURE 7.1

Placement of four circumferential impedance leads. A constant sinusoidal alternating current is introduced through electrodes #1 and #4. Electrodes #2 and #3 detect changes in voltage.

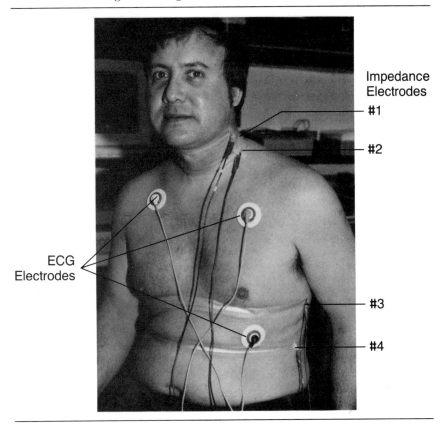

most commonly used electrode material is manufactured by 3M Company, St. Paul, Minnesota, and is constructed from 1 mil aluminum deposited on a polyester film and bonded to an adhesive backing.

Most commercially available impedance cardiography units introduce a constant, sinusoidal ac current through electrodes #1 and #4. This establishes an electrical field between the outer two electrodes while the inner electrodes detect changes in the voltage ($V = IZ$) with which to determine changes in Z. The impedance signal is composed of three components relevant to the determination of stroke volume (Fig. 7.2). The largest component is the basal thoracic impedance (Z_o) and reflects the conductance of the total thoracic mass (tissues, fluid, air). Resistivity

FIGURE 7.2
Magnitude of the component parts of the impedance signal.

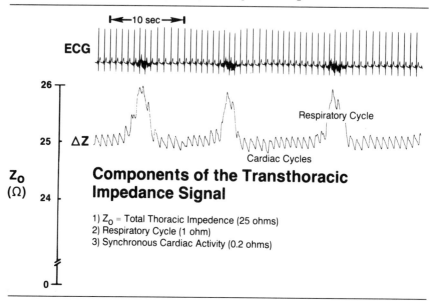

Components of the Transthoracic Impedance Signal

1) Z_0 = Total Thoracic Impedence (25 ohms)
2) Respiratory Cycle (1 ohm)
3) Synchronous Cardiac Activity (0.2 ohms)

values ($\Omega \cdot cm$) vary for blood (150), cardiac muscle (750), lung (1275), and fat (2500) tissue [25]. An average value for Z_0 in a healthy man is about 25 ohms, while values for women are slightly greater, averaging 30 ohms [15, 66, 67]. Respiratory activity induces approximately a 3% change in the thoracic impedance signal; impedance increases with inspiration and decreases with expiration. The third component, which is synchronous with the cardiac activity, comprises $< 1\%$ of the basal impedance level. This value decreases by 0.1–0.15 ohms (ΔZ) during the systolic portion of the cardiac cycle in an adult human at rest.

Typical signal outputs from an impedance cardiograph are Z_0, ΔZ, and dZ/dt (the first derivative of ΔZ with respect to time). A normal impedance cardiogram is presented in Figure 7.3 together with an ECG and phonocardiogram (PCG). The ΔZ and dZ/dt waveforms are traditionally recorded with negative values upward, and this convention will be followed throughout this review. The ΔZ waveform appears similar to a normal aortic pressure tracing, and dZ/dt is similar to an aortic flow waveform.

Cardiac Events That Affect the dZ/dt Waveform
The thoracic impedance waveform is the complex result of a number of physiological events [8, 27, 35, 48, 55, 78, 85]. Consequently, there is no definitive statement which accounts for its genesis, but at least two

FIGURE 7.3

Typical recording of changes in impedance (ΔZ) and the first derivative of ΔZ (dZ/dt) together with the electrocardiogram (ECG) and phonocardiogram (PCG).

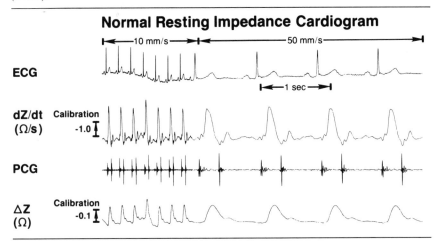

Normal Resting Impedance Cardiogram

major contributors are recognized. The major components are changes in blood volume within tissues between the measuring electrodes and changes in erythrocyte orientation as aortic blood flow velocity changes [55, 78].

The differentiated impedance cardiogram (*dZ/dt* waveform) is most frequently used to calculate stroke volume because of sharp demarcation of the points of interest and stability of the *dZ/dt* tracing during respiration. A normal impedance cardiogram is presented in Figure 7.4 with the most commonly used designations for the points and waves. Not all investigators use the same terminology, which contributes to confusion in labeling the impedance signal and makes comparative evaluations between studies difficult. The physiological events in the cardiac cycle which correlate with changes in the *dZ/dt* waveform can be identified by comparison with the ECG and PCG.

The A wave of the *dZ/dt* recording follows the P wave of the ECG and corresponds to atrial systole. The C wave appears after the QRS complex and reflects the rate of blood flow ejection from the left ventricle. A linear relationship has been demonstrated in dogs, using an electromagnetic flow probe, between *dZ/dt* and peak flow in the ascending aorta [52]. The O wave occurs after the T wave of the ECG and corresponds with rapid ventricular filling during diastole.

The B point occurs immediately after the aortic valve opens, and the X and Y points coincide with closing of the aortic and pulmonic valves,

FIGURE 7.4

Terminology used to designate the points and waves of the impedance cardiogram.

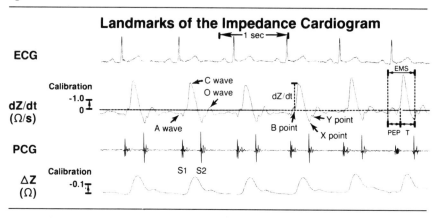

respectively. The correlation between movement of the heart valves and the associated *dZ/dt* peaks have been confirmed by M-mode echocardiography [78]. The B, X, and Y points occur synchronously with the corresponding heart sounds monitored by phonocardiography and are valuable for timing intervals within the cardiac cycle [53, 67, 94].

Components of the Impedance Equation for Calculating Stroke Volume

The decrease in thoracic impedance generated by the ejection of blood from the heart has been quantitatively related to the volume of blood ejected [3, 55, 78, 88]. The most widely used equation to calculate stroke volume from the impedance signal is that derived by Kubicek et al. [51, 52]. This equation is:

$$SV = \text{rho} \cdot \left(\frac{L}{Z_o}\right)^2 \cdot dZ/dt \cdot T,$$

where

SV = stroke volume (ml),
rho = resistivity of blood (ohm·cm),
L = distance between the detection electrodes #2 and #3 (cm),
Z_o = baseline thoracic impedance (ohm),
dZ/dt = first derivative of the change in thoracic impedance (ΔZ, ohm/second),
T = left ventricular ejection time (seconds),
SV = $(\Omega \cdot \text{cm})(\text{cm}^2/\Omega^2)(\Omega/\text{second})(\text{second})$ = $\text{cm}^3(\text{ml})$.

As an example, stroke volume calculated from the impedance tracing in Figure 7.4 is as follows:

$$SV = (135\ \Omega\text{·cm}) \left(\frac{25\ \text{cm}}{27\ \Omega}\right)^2 (3.0\ \Omega/\text{second})(0.25\ \text{second}) = 87\ \text{ml}$$

Stroke volume calculated manually by this formula on a beat-by-beat basis can be reported as individual stroke outputs, or several stroke volumes (4–10 beats) can be averaged to yield an average stroke volume over a time period. Cardiac output, expressed as a beat-by-beat output or averaged over several beats, is calculated from the stroke volume and heart rate.

BLOOD RESISTIVITY. The preferred value for blood resistivity (rho) is controversial. Because blood resistivity varies with the hematocrit, several investigators have proposed the calculation of a hematocrit-based rho, and several different formulas for this calculation have been presented [26, 42, 79]. The most widely used formula for calculating rho from the hematocrit is that derived by Geddes and Sadler [26] and is

$$rho = 53.2e^{0.22\ \text{Hct}}$$

with the hematocrit (Hct) expressed in percent.

However, Quail et al. [92] evaluated in vivo changes of rho as hematocrit was varied over a wide range and found that rho changed little as hematocrit was varied. They concluded that a constant rho of 135 ohm·cm could be used for the canine [92, 104], rabbit [104], and human [104]. We have utilized 135 ohm·cm in rats [34] and canine pups [31] in studies involving hemorrhage and found close agreement between cardiac outputs determined by impedance and thermodilution.

ELECTRODE DISTANCE. The distance (*L*) between leads #2 and #3 is measured in centimeters. In earlier studies, *L* was measured as the average of the anterior and posterior distances between leads #2 and #3. Mohapatra [78] and Lamberts et al. [55] recommend measuring on the anterior thorax along the sternum between leads #2 and #3 as first indicated by Denniston et al. [12]. The use of calipers has been suggested [55, 78] to avoid the influence of the topography of the chest on *L*. We have routinely used the topographical distance on the anterior thorax for determining *L* [67, 69, 34]. A comparative study of the two methods of determining *L* has not been published; therefore, it is recommended that each laboratory standardize its measurement of *L*.

BASELINE THORACIC IMPEDANCE. The baseline thoracic impedance (Z_o) is the electrical impedance about which changes in impedance due to respiration and cardiac function occur. The Z_o is determined by the relative amounts of air and tissue in the thorax and, therefore, will be changed by lung volume or thoracic fluid [19]. The value of Z_o influences the height of the *dZ/dt* signal [14] such that subjects with lower Z_o values have smaller *dZ/dt* deflections during cardiac ejection, and conversely. Thus, the inclusion of Z_o in the denominator of the stroke volume equation normalizes its effect on *dZ/dt*.

Values for Z_o vary since each individual will have a different baseline thoracic impedance. The Z_o depends upon the length between the electrodes and the cross-sectional area (*L/A*). However, some generalizations can be made. The Z_o value for a healthy young man with an *L* of approximately 25 cm would be around 24–25 ohms [66]. A value of Z_o for a healthy young woman would be higher and approximately 30–33 ohms [66]. Z_o can also be affected by posture, being lower when the subject is supine than when upright, due to blood and organ movement into the thoracic compartment [19]. In addition, the smaller the thoracic circumference, the higher the Z_o. For example, neonates can have Z_o values above 45 ohms [108], adult rats above 100 ohms and neonatal rats above 200 ohms (unpublished observations).

RATE OF CHANGE IN IMPEDANCE. The maximum rate of change of impedance (*dZ/dt*) during systole is represented by the height of *dZ/dt*. This is shown in Figure 7.4. Traditionally, this has been measured as the distance above the zero impedance baseline during a brief period of voluntary apnea. However, as discussed by Doerr et al. [15], during spontaneous breathing the *dZ/dt* recording may rise and fall around the zero baseline as shown in Figure 7.5. Therefore, if the height of *dZ/dt* is always referenced to the zero baseline, *dZ/dt* will be over- or underestimated depending on the location of the oscillating *dZ/dt* signal within the respiratory cycle (Fig. 7.5). To correctly measure *dZ/dt*, the onset of ejection should be taken as the beginning of the rapid upstroke of *dZ/dt* corresponding to the B point, without regard to the zero baseline.

FIGURE 7.5
Oscillation of the dZ/dt *waveform around the zero baseline.*

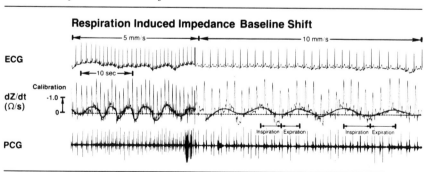

VENTRICULAR EJECTION TIME. Left ventricular ejection time (T) is measured from the rapid upstroke of dZ/dt (B point) to the nadir of the downward deflection (X point) shown in Figure 7.4. This corresponds to the time of ejection within the cardiac cycle as shown by the PCG. Several studies have verified this measurement of T from the impedance dZ/dt recording in comparison with both direct [94] and indirect [41] measurements. Often, however, the characteristics of the dZ/dt waveform are altered and the traditional indicators of the end of ejection are not evident on the dZ/dt recording (Figure 7.9**B**). Therefore, we suggest recording a PCG simultaneously to verify the end of ejection.

Because impedance cardiography permits the accurate measurement of left ventricular ejection time, other time intervals within the cardiac cycle can be measured or calculated from just the impedance tracing and ECG. These are also shown in Figure 7.4. The total electrical–mechanical systole (*EMS*) is measured from the beginning of ventricular electrical activity (Q wave of the ECG) to the closing of the aortic valve (X point on dZ/dt). By subtracting T from *EMS*, the preejection period (PEP) can be determined. These systolic time intervals (*STI*) can be used to further evaluate cardiac function at rest or during exercise [67, 104].

EVALUATION OF THE ASSUMPTIONS OF THE STROKE VOLUME EQUATION. There are three main assumptions which underly the derivation of the impedance stroke volume equation. First, the decrease in impedance during systole is due to a change in aortic blood volume (plethysmographic); second, the thorax is a cylindrical conductor composed of two parallel conducting paths, one path through the tissues and the other through the blood; third, there is no significant arterial run-off from the thorax during systole. Since a detailed discussion of assumption validity is beyond the scope of this presentation, the interested reader is referred to the following reviews [55, 78, 88].

Most investigators agree that dZ/dt is primarily the result of the ejection of blood from the left ventricle. It is still not clear, however, if this impedance change is solely due to a change in aortic blood volume. Lamberts et al. [55] and Visser et al. [110, 111] have demonstrated, fairly convincingly, that as much as 60% of dZ/dt is generated by the velocity of the ejected blood. This velocity-dependent change in blood resistivity as reflected in dZ/dt is related to the reorientation of erythrocytes [55, 110, 111] as blood begins to flow. Since the stroke volume equation as proposed by Kubicek et al. [51, 52] was derived on the basis of a change in blood volume and not velocity, it is not yet understood how this finding affects the stroke volume equation. We do know, however, that the Kubicek equation, although largely empirical in nature, yields values for stroke volume that correlate well with other techniques for determining stroke volume (Tables 7.1–7.4).

The two-compartment, parallel-conductor model of the thorax (i.e., tissue resistivity and blood resistivity) used in the derivation of the stroke volume equation represents the thorax as a parallel connection of tissue and blood impedance with the blood impedance varying coincident with the ejection of blood from the heart. Vissar et al. [109] tested this two-compartment, parallel-conductor model in a series of eloquent experiments involving exchange transfusion with stroma-free hemoglobin. They concluded that the thoracic impedance changes were adequately described by the two-compartment model. Therefore, this aspect of the stroke volume equation derivation was valid. Multicompartment models have been investigated [85] without improvement in the results of the technique.

Implicit within the assumption that dZ/dt is the result of a change in blood volume in the thorax is the concept that the volume of blood ejected from the ventricle must remain within the thorax during systole to be measured. Since blood continues to flow into and out of the thorax throughout the cardiac cycle, some accounting of this volume loss (or gain) must be made. The equation derived by Kubicek et al. [51, 52] estimates stroke volume from the change in thoracic impedance as though there were no arterial run-off during systole. Simply described, the peak ejection dZ/dt is projected over the entire systolic period (T), and this accounts for the continued arterial run-off during systole. This particular aspect of the stroke volume equation has not been fully evaluated. However, the close correlation of the impedance technique with other techniques for estimating stroke volume suggests that this assumption does not normally present significant error. In circumstances when the ejection pattern is altered (e.g., valvular disease, heart failure), there could be a significant error due to this assumption.

The impedance technique assumes that the cardiogenic change in thoracic impedance is due to an alteration in blood volume within the thorax. As we have discussed, there is significant evidence that velocity-induced blood impedance changes dominate the dZ/dt value. This might explain why the cardiogenic impedance change is predominantly localized in the ascending aorta, location of the highest velocity of blood flow during left ventricular ejection, and why the impedance signal is relatively immune to the continued flow of blood into or out of the thorax throughout the cardiac cycle. This concept has not been investigated experimentally.

Alternative Stroke Volume Equation

While the Kubicek et al. equation [51, 52] is the most widely used stroke volume equation, other equations have been proposed [7, 62]. For the most part, these have not significantly altered the calculation of stroke volume. However, the equation derived by Sramek and modified by Bernstein [7] is becoming more widely used, mainly because it is incorporated within a commercially available impedance cardiographic instrument. This equation is based on modeling the thorax as a truncated cone as opposed to a uniform cylinder and is expressed as follows [7]:

$$SV = \Delta \cdot \frac{(0.17Ht)^3}{4.2} \cdot \left(\frac{dZ/dt}{Z_o}\right) \cdot T.$$

This equation was derived based on the thorax as a truncated cone rather than a cylinder. The delta term (Δ) was introduced by Bernstein [7] to account for the effect of the body habitus on cardiac output calculations. Delta is unitless and varies according to the percent deviation of the subject's weight from an assumed ideal body weight. L is replaced in this equation by 0.17 Ht, where Ht is the subject's height in cm.

Both the Kubicek and Sramek formulas have the same form:

$$SV = k \cdot (dZ/dt) \cdot T$$

The major difference between the two equations, therefore, is the value assigned to k. The underlying assumptions as to the generation of dZ/dt are the same. The major differences in the calculation of k are that, in the Sramek equation,

1. delta is used;
2. blood resistivity (rho) is not utilized;
3. L or its estimate, 0.17 Ht, is cubed;
4. Z_o is included to the first power.

The reputed benefits from the Sramek equation are that it accounts for the morphology of the subject, makes the use of L more reproducible, and reduces the effect of changes in Z_o on the calculation [7, 62].

Comparisons of stroke volumes calculated with this equation with invasive techniques in patients have shown good agreement [1, 6]. We have also observed similar results in patients; however, we have observed [32], as have others [11], that this formula overestimates stroke volume in young healthy individuals. The reason for these contradictory results is not evident from the existing data. A comprehensive evaluation of the various stroke volume formulas has not been published.

Technical Improvements in Methodology
The thoracic electrical impedance varies with both respiration and stroke output. To reduce the effect of respiration on the dZ/dt recording, a short period of apnea is frequently employed. In a number of situations (e.g., patients, exercise), an apneic period may not be feasible and the measurement of dZ/dt must occur during respiration. Apnea becomes increasingly difficult as respiratory effort is increased, such as during

strenuous exercise levels. In addition, the impedance recording can suffer from motion artifact as the subject moves. For example, walking or running on a treadmill creates movement of internal organs, as well as movement of the electrodes. This can make the impedance recording unreadable. As a consequence of these unwanted variations in thoracic impedance, the use of impedance cardiography is often limited.

A number of investigators have addressed this motion artifact problem and have applied signal conditioning techniques to the thoracic impedance signal [80, 98, 115]. The most promising technique is ensemble-averaging. Ensemble-averaging is a signal-processing technique used to suppress random portions of a signal while leaving the periodic portions intact. Waveforms are controlled and an average waveform calculated. In this manner, nonperiodic waveforms such as motion artifacts, electrical noise, and respiratory-induced baseline shifts are gradually averaged and cancelled out, leaving the periodic dZ/dt signal intact.

Muzi et al. [80] have described an ensemble-averaging technique applied to the impedance cardiogram. The cardiac values determined by ensemble-averaging compared well ($r = 0.97$) with the same parameters calculated manually, and were equally effective at rest and during supine or seated exercise. Zhang et al. [115] adapted an ensemble-averaging technique for eliminating motion artifacts during treadmill exercise. Impedance ensemble-averaged cardiac output values agreed well with CO_2-rebreathing values ($r > 0.90$) during three levels of treadmill exercise. Use of signal conditioning techniques would appear to extend the usefulness of the impedance cardiographic technique into areas where, previously, signal artifacts limited the reliability of the results. Unfortunately, these ensemble-averaging programs are not yet available commercially.

Other techniques to reduce signal artifacts in the impedance cardiogram might be the use of electrode configurations other than the traditional four-band electrode system [6, 89, 91]. Proposed changes in the electrode system include the use of spot electrodes instead of the traditional band electrodes. The impedance signal with each of these electrode configurations [6, 89, 91] is not significantly different from that derived using band electrodes. The calculated values are the same, and motion artifact may be reduced. Therefore, substitution of spot electrodes for band electrodes may be of some value. We routinely use a spot electrode on the forehead for lead #1 and a spot electrode on the lower abdomen for lead #4 at rest and during exercise (Fig. 7.6) without any apparent loss of signal fidelity (band electrodes were utilized for leads #2 and #3).

Accuracy of Impedance Cardiac Output in Resting Individuals
A number of investigations in the 1980s have evaluated the accuracy of

FIGURE 7.6
Substitution of a spot electrode on the forehead for lead #1 and lower abdomen for lead #4.

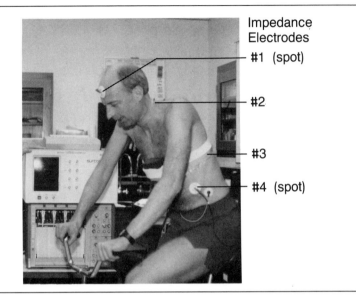

Impedance
Electrodes

#1 (spot)

#2

#3

#4 (spot)

cardiac output measured by impedance in resting individuals (Table 7.1). Impedance values have been compared to those obtained by thermodilution [1, 6, 16, 30, 34, 71, 80, 102, 105], M-mode echocardiography [2], Doppler ultrasound [5], left ventriculography [18], electromagnetic flow probe [21, 104], direct Fick [69], dye dilution [73], isotope dilution [113], and radionuclide angiocardiography [114]. Results have been compared in rats, pups, dogs, rabbits, children, healthy young and elderly adults, and patients. The correlation between impedance and the other procedures has generally been greater than 0.70. The vast majority of investigators agree that the impedance technique can accurately track the magnitude and direction of changes in cardiac output. Some controversy exists, however, on whether the absolute values are accurate. The conclusion reached by 14 of the 18 studies cited in Table 7.1 (78%) supports the accuracy of the impedance technique. This has also been the conclusion of a similar percentage of investigators in the previous two decades that the impedance technique has been used [55, 78]. Standardization in obtaining and analyzing the impedance waveform and identification of patients and situations in which impedance is reliable will further clarify its role.

Recent literature has encouraged investigators to pursue lines of re-

TABLE 7.1
Validation of Transthoracic Electrical Impedance at Rest: 1981–1988

Investigator	Population	N	Reference Standard	r	Comments	Investigator Conclusion
Appel 1986 [1]	Patients	16	Thermodilution	0.83	Difficulties arose with dysrhythmias, tachycardia, metal in the chest or chest wall, sepsis, hypertension, oily skin. Sramek-Bernstein equation used; NCCOM-3 monitor.	Absolute and trending of cardiac output supported.
Aust 1982 [2]	Healthy 21–26 yrs	6	M-mode Echocardiography	0.83	Amezinium metilsulfate and placebo administered 80° head-up tilt.	Valid information about changes in stroke volume.
Barbacki 1981 [5]	Children 8–14 yrs	15	Doppler ultrasound	0.50	Impedance cardiogram obtained during momentary interruption of respiration.	Absolute values are valid.
Bernstein 1986 [6]	Patients 34–91 yrs	17	Thermodilution	0.88	Critically ill medical and surgical patients. NCCOM-3 monitor.	Absolute values acceptable.
Donovan 1986 [16]	Patients 20–70 yrs	20	Thermodilution	0.63	Measurements made at end-expiration. Critically ill patients.	Cardiac output unsatisfactory.
Ebert 1984 [18]	Patients 48–72 yrs	14	Left ventriculography	0.79	Impedance analogue data recorded throughout the injection. Breathhold at end-inspiration.	Absolute values are reliable.
Ehlert 1982 [21]	Canine	14	Electromagnetic flow probe	0.80	Data obtained during end-expiratory apnea.	Absolute values cannot be obtained; suitable for measuring changes in cardiac output.
Goldstein 1986 [30]	Patients Healthy	21 34	Thermodilution	0.86	Intensive care unit and cardiology patients. Manipulation used: cardiac pacing, ergonovine, dipyridamole, isoproterenol, tilt, and valsalva.	Absolute measures, percent changes, and differential changes of cardiac output are vaild.

Gotshall 1987 [34]	Neonatal and adult rats	24	Thermodilution	0.73	Highest impedance voltage step-down transformer used. Hemorrhage and blood reinfusion.	Absolute and relative changes valid.
Miles 1986 [71]	Pups	7	Thermodilution	0.76	Exposure to 12% and 8% O_2.	Absolute values are valid.
Miles 1988 [69]	Children 2 mos–14 yrs	37	Direct Fick	0.84	Diagnostic heart catheterization, congenital heart defects, atrial septal defect, ventricular septal defect, patent ductus arteriosus, no shunts.	Accurate without shunts or valvular insufficiency and in the presence of intra- or extracardiac left–right shunting.
Milson 1983 [73]	Pregnant adults	10	Dye dilution	0.93	Elective cesarean section.	Accurate for measurement of changes in stroke volume.
Muzi 1985 [80]	Patients	14	Thermodilution	0.87	Analyzed by ensemble-averaging.	Absolute values accurate.
Spinelli 1983 [102]	Canine 7–21 kg	10	Thermodilution	0.84	Beats recorded during two respiratory cycles. Positive pressure respirator used. Bilateral vagotomy performed.	Directional and relative changes in stroke volume can be followed on a beat-by-beat basis.
Traugott 1981 [104]	Dog, man, rabbit	3	Electromagnetic flow probe	0.98	Suggested that the best estimate of rho in vivo within the normal hematocrit range is 135 ohm·cm.	Absolute values can be obtained.
Tremper 1986 [105]	Canine	5	Thermodilution	0.84	In vivo NCCOM calibration. Hypotension, hemorrhage, resuscitation.	Accurate values and trends obtained.
Williams 1980 [113]	Patients 69–95 yrs	40	Isotopic indicator dilution	0.77	Semisupine.	Absolute values accurate and highly repeatable.
Williams 1985 [114]	Patients 69–95 yrs	45	Radionuclide angiocardiography	0.90	Agreement excellent for patients in sinus rhythm, without valvular lesions, severe airways obstruction, or right bundle branch block. Systolic time intervals recorded.	Absolute values accurate.

search not foreseen by earlier pioneers in the field. The diversity and uniqueness of impedance cardiography to assess cardiovascular function under a variety of resting conditions is demonstrated in Table 7.2. The accurate trending of cardiac output by impedance has proved particularly useful in clinical medicine [44, 86, 90, 97]. In many instances, the clinician is more concerned with how the therapeutic intervention is affecting cardiac output rather than with the precise value. From our experience and this literature review, we believe cardiac output measured by impedance is usually within ± 15% of the more standard invasive techniques, which in themselves are accurate within ± 15% [3, 55, 78].

The impedance technique has also proved to be equally effective for applied physiologists and clinicians in measuring cardiac output and stroke volume during water immersion [99], sleep [9], and during high-frequency jet ventilation [33]. The unique ability to assess stroke volume on a beat-by-beat basis has presented an opportunity to examine autonomic reflex mechanisms during the performance of such procedures as the Valsalva maneuver [101], head-up tilt [19], carotid body stimulation [29], and lower body negative pressure [22].

Accuracy of Impedance Cardiac Output in Exercising Individuals
An impressive number of investigations have used impedance cardiography to assess myocardial pumping and contractility qualities during exercise. The literature presented in Table 7.3 reflects only studies pub-

TABLE 7.2
Application of Transthoracic Electrical Impedance to Evaluate Cardiopulmonary Functions in the 1980s

Clinical Assessment

Burn injury [90][a]
Anesthesiology [86]
Dental surgery [13]
Mitral valve diseases [84]
Cardiac failure [44]
Renal hemodialysis [61]
Magnesium and potassium deficiency [58]
Newborn infants [23, 54, 69]
Pregnancy [11]
Valsalva maneuver [101]
Psychological stress [98]

Applied Physiology

Sleep [9]
Thoracic blood volume [19]
Thoracic fluid compartments [56]
Lower body negative pressure [22]
Electrical neuromuscular stimulation [28]
High-frequency jet ventilation [33]
Pulmonary diffusing capacity [63]
Anti-G suit inflation [57]
Blood pooling [100]
Water immersion [99]
Carotid baroreceptor stimulation [29]

[a] Reference number.

TABLE 7.3
Validation of Transthoracic Electrical Impedance During Exercise: 1981–1987

Author	Population	N	Reference Method	r	Exercise Modality	Remarks	Investigator Conclusion
Du Quesnay 1987 [17]	Healthy, mean 21.4 yrs	5	CO_2 rebreathing	0.93	Cycle ergometer 50, 100, 150, 200 W	Impedance cardiogram (ZCG) obtained end-expiratory, end-inspiratory breathhold and normal breathing. Quality tracings obtained during exercise.	Respiratory cycle does not influence the calculation of stroke volume.
Edmunds 1982 [20]	Healthy, mean 29 yrs 11.8 yrs	9	CO_2 rebreathing	0.92 0.88	Treadmill walking; cycle ergometer	No difficulty with motion artifacts. Cardiac output measured at total lung capacity, functional residual capacity, and residual volume.	Cardiac output not affected by lung volume. Absolute values are accurate.
Hatcher 1986 [36]	Healthy, mean 20.4 yrs	60	CO_2 rebreathing	0.75	Cycle ergometer; exercise to exhaustion	ZCG collected during a brief voluntary end-expiratory apnea.	Impedance cardiac output independent of lung volume. Reliable over a large range of workloads.
Hetherington 1985 [38]	Patients with previous myocardial infarction	20 15	Direct Fick	0.93	Cycle ergometer (supine). Progressive test starting at 30 W	ZCG obtained at the end of each workload. Reproducibility evaluated.	Impedance technique was accurate and reproducible.
Miles 1981 [66]	Healthy, mean 29 yrs	10	CO_2 rebreathing	0.57	Arm-crank ergometer 10, 20, 30 W	ZCG recorded during arm-cranking and during exercise pause.	Valid estimation of cardiac output by impedance was supported.
Milsom 1982 [74]	Healthy, mean 25 yrs	11	Dye dilution	0.82	Leg-cycling movements with legs raised	Recorded during end-expiratory apnea; techniques compared 1 minute after exercise.	Relative changes in stroke volume were possible. Absolute values not recommended.
Miyamoto 1981 [76]	Healthy	6	CO_2 rebreathing	0.91	Cycle ergometer 90, 180 W	Rest and exercise measurement made by a computer-based system.	Ensemble averaging eliminates respiratory and motion artifacts.
Qu 1986 [91] Zhang 1986 [115]	Healthy 23–45 yrs	10	CO_2 rebreathing	0.95	Treadmill 3–4 mph, 0–10% grade	Ensemble averaging employed. Band and spot electrode signals compared.	Spot electrode can provide an accurate impedance signal.
Teo 1985 [103]	Patients	20	Direct Fick	0.93	Cycle ergometer (supine)	Movement stopped and breath held at end-expiration.	Results are accurate and reproducible.

lished between 1981 and 1988. In general, the types of exercise employed and conclusions reached by these investigators have been echoed in previous summaries of the earlier research [55, 78].

The majority of the recent exercise validation studies have been conducted with healthy adults in their 20s (Table 7.3). The reference methods have included dye dilution and direct Fick, with the CO_2 rebreathing technique as the most commonly used standard. Lower body exercise using the cycle ergometer has been employed the most extensively. Treadmill walking and arm-crank ergometry have also been used. The correlations between cardiac output measured by impedance and by the other standards, in general, have averaged 0.86. The exercise intensity has ranged from very light to maximal. Similar to the validation studies in resting individuals, roughly 75% of these investigators have concluded that the absolute values for cardiac output measured by impedance are accurate. There is almost total unanimity that the relative changes in cardiac output can be accurately measured. A further number of recent publications have also used impedance to measure exercise cardiac output without corroboration with another methodology (Table 7.4). Thus, while some investigators feel further validation of the impedance technique is necessary, others have already accepted it.

A number of these studies have used pauses in the exercise to obtain quality impedance cardiograms. A word of caution must be raised, however, about assessing central hemodynamics during an exercise pause (Fig. 7.7). Although the impedance motion artifacts may be reduced, significant changes in cardiac output, stroke volume, and heart rate can occur even within an exercise pause as brief as 5–10 seconds. At low power outputs (10–30 W) during upper body exercise, stroke volume is maintained during the pause, but heart rate falls significantly [66] (Fig. 7.8). Therefore, the exercise pause stroke volume must be multiplied by the exercise heart rate to avoid an underestimation of the exercise cardiac output. At intensities of exercise which exceed an oxygen uptake of 1.0 l/minute during either upper or lower body exercise, stroke volume, as well as heart rate, falls immediately during an exercise pause [67]. As stroke volume and heart rate fall, estimation of the exercise cardiac output using values collected during a pause is inappropriate. The fall in stroke volume most likely results from venous pooling due to vasodilation of skeletal muscle and loss of the skeletal muscle pump for venous return. Without the use of some type of waveform conditioning (i.e., ensemble-averaging) during moderate to strenuous exercise, the impedance cardiogram should be recorded for 30 seconds to obtain a minimum of 4–5 acceptable heart beats clear of artifacts with which to calculate stroke volume.

FIGURE 7.7
Reduction of motion artifact in the dZ/dt *waveform with an exercise pause.*

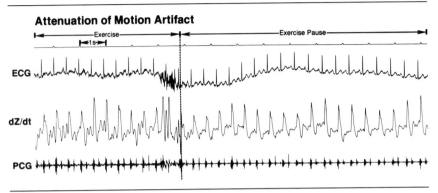

FIGURE 7.8
Changes in cardiac output ($\dot{Q}$), stroke volume (SV), and heart rate (HR) during an exercise pause with an arm-crank or cycle ergometer.

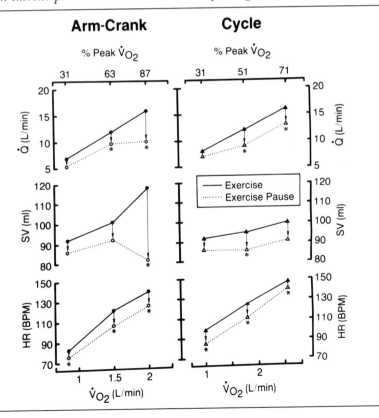

TABLE 7.4
Applications of Transthoracic Impedance During Exercise from 1981–1988.

Investigator	Population	N	Exercise Modality	Comments	Investigator Conclusion
Hetherington 1986 [39]	Patients, mean 52 yrs	27	Cycle ergometer, upright position, 20–218 W	Evaluate training regimen following myocardial infarction. Impedance cardiogram (ZCG) taken at rest and immediately after each workload. Subjects stopped pedaling and held their breath.	Conventional training HR may be too high for those individuals with an abnormal stroke volume response.
Hetherington 1987 [37]	Healthy, mean 49 yrs	9	Incremental loads to maximum		
Miles 1987 [65]	Healthy, mean 24 yrs	17	Leg extension	Twelve repetitions to exhaustion. ZCG throughout exercise. Systolic time intervals calculated.	Leg extension exercise has a substantial static component which affects peripheral resistance and venous return.
Miles 1984 [67]	Healthy, mean 28 yrs	9	Arm-crank and cycle ergometer	25, 74, 98 W arm-crank exercise; 49, 98, 147 W cycle exercise. ZCG obtained during and immediately after exercise.	A pause in exercise is useful to obtain a relatively artifact-free ZCG.
Miles 1988 [68]	Healthy, mean 26 yrs	10	Cardiopulmonary resuscitation, Resusci-Anne manikin	The role of ventilator, one-man, and compressor were performed continuously for 10 minutes.	The roles of compressor and one-man elicit the greatest cardiovascular, metabolic, and ventilatory demands.
Miles 1988 [64]	Healthy, mean 24 yrs	10	Cycle ergometer 120, 180 W	ZCG recorded during exercise and cardiac output measured during DL_{CO} 15-second breathhold maneuver.	Stroke volume was reduced at rest, during exercise and recovery by the breathhold maneuver.

Miyamoto 1983 [75]	Healthy, 23–28 yrs	4	Cycle ergometer; upright and supine, 50 and 100 W	Transient and steady-state hemodynamics assessed. Computer-based automated system used.	Ensemble averaging used to reduce motion artifact.
Miyamoto 1982 [77]	Healthy, 24–28 yrs	4	Cycle ergometer 60 and 120 W	Ensembly averaging used. Transient responses evaluated.	The concept of cardiodynamics hyperpnea was supported.
Muzi 1985 [80]	Healthy, 20–25 yrs	6	Cycle ergometer, supine and seated, 60 and 120 W	ZCG recorded at the end of exercise. Hand digitized and ensemble averaged, data compared.	Ensemble averaging recommended to facilitate data collection.
Nakazono 1985 [81]	Healthy, 22–25 yrs	4	Cycle ergometer 30–90 rpm	Passive limb movement exercise. Ensemble-averaging.	Hyperpnea during passive exercise mediated by reflexes from the moving limbs or the right heart.
Panigrahi 1983 [83]	Patients over 65 yrs	17	Cycle ergometer 50, 100, 150 W	Physical training after acute myocardial infarct. Stop exercise for 5–10 seconds to record ZCG.	Physical training resulted in peripheral adaptions and improved left ventricular hemodynamics.
Penney 1985 [89]	Healthy, 20–38 yrs	10	Cycle ergometer, supine 25, 50, 75, 100 W	ZCG recorded during and after exercise. Valsalva maneuver performed. Spot electrode, band electrode array compared.	Spot electrodes appear to provide similar information and are more convenient than band electrodes.
Veigl 1983 [107]	Healthy, 23–26 yrs	8	Cycle ergometer 49, 98, 147 W	Exercise stopped for 10 seconds to obtain ZCG. Protocol repeated three times on separate days.	Hemodynamics were very reproducible and correlated well with the workload.
Wilde 1981 [112]	Wheelchair dependent	9	Wheelchair ergometer 10, 20, 30 W	ZCG recorded immediately after exercise. Systolic time intervals calculated.	Myocardial pump and contractility indices can be obtained.

Clinical Applications of Impedance Cardiography

There are many clinical settings [24, 97] in which impedance cardiography could and does provide significant information (Table 7.2). For the purposes of this review, we will discuss impedance waveform analysis and exercise stress testing as examples of how impedance cardiography might permit physicians to more fully assess cardiac functional capabilities.

IMPEDANCE WAVEFORM ANALYSIS. As previously described, the impedance cardiogram is generated by events occurring throughout the cardiac cycle. For the quantification of stroke volume, only the events occurring within ventricular systole are needed. However, various investigators have noted that the characteristics of the impedance waveform have demonstrated marked departures from the norm in various patients during both ventricular systole (LBBB, asynchronous ventricles) [50, 60] and diastole (valvular disease) which correlated with the patient's specific cardiac disease [16, 53, 84, 96].

Characteristic changes in the diastolic "O" wave have been noted since early in the development of impedance cardiography. An example of an elevated "O" wave is shown in Figure 7.9**D**. Kubicek et al. [50] observed an increase in the "O" wave amplitude in patients with coronary artery disease during exercise. Lababidi et al. [53] suggested that since the "O" wave was associated with mitral valve opening and ventricular filling, an increase in amplitude might be associated with atrial enlargement. Correspondingly, Donovan et al. [16] measured an increase in pulmonary wedge pressure associated with the presence of an exaggerated "O" wave in patients. Ramos et al. [93] identified a large "O" wave as an indicator of poor prognosis in patients with heart failure. Thus, an elevated "O" wave may be associated with an impairment in ventricular function resulting in atrial congestion and enlargement.

Several investigators [47, 84, 95] have demonstrated characteristic changes in the "O" wave associated with mitral valve disease. For example, Parulkar et al. [84] have shown that mitral stenosis was associated with a wide, M-shaped "O" wave and mitral insufficienty by an "O" wave of large amplitude. They quantitated these changes and demonstrated high correlations with the severity of valvular disease. Thus, both systolic and diastolic cardiac function are represented in the impedance cardiogram and can be evaluated with the impedance technique. However, more investigations of the physiological and pathological significance of alterations of the "O" wave are needed to ascertain the full significance of these observations.

Alterations in aortic valve function can also affect the impedance waveform. For example, Schieken et al. [96] have evaluated the impedance cardiogram in patients with aortic valve insufficiency ($n = 44$). Aortic valve regurgitation produced a characteristic alteration of the systolic

FIGURE 7.9

Variations in the dZ/dt *waveform of known and unknown origin.*

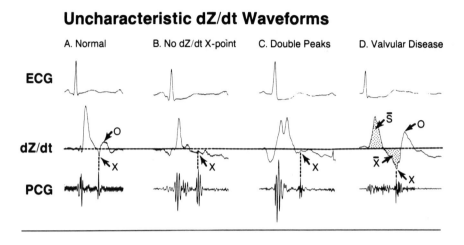

Uncharacteristic dZ/dt Waveforms

dZ/dt waveform which was interpreted as due to an aortic regurgitant fraction (Fig. 7.9**D**). A regurgitant fraction (*RF*) was calculated from the ratio of the area $\bar{S}$ to the area $\bar{X}$. The difference between cardiac output measured by direct Fick or angiography was used to calculate the aortic valvular regurgitant fraction, which was closely related to the derived impedance *RF* ($r = 0.90$). No other studies of aortic valvular stenosis have been reported, and more data are needed to evaluate the full implications of aortic valvular disease on the impedance cardiogram and the accurate quantification of cardiac function. The results of these studies reemphasize that care should be taken when interpreting impedance cardiac outputs in patients with valvular disease.

Occasionally, two distinct peaks occur in the *dZ/dt* waveform during systole (Fig. 7.9**C**). We, and others [50, 60], have observed these in both normal subjects and patients. Double peaks in the *dZ/dt* waveform could be the result of asynchrony between left and right ventricles [50] or the result of an abnormal left ventricular ejection pattern (dyssynergy) [60]. The waveform does not provide information to distinguish between these two possibilities. Unfortunately, the presence of these double peaks may alter the accuracy of the stroke volume calculation; however, the extent to which this may occur has not been evaluated.

CARDIAC PUMP FUNCTION DURING EXERCISE STRESS TESTING. Single determinations of cardiac function do not necessarily indicate the loss of cardiac pumping capability in cardiac patients, since cardiac output at rest may be normal. Measurement of the ability of the heart to respond to stress is more revealing of true cardiac status. Thus, exercise stress testing is a valuable clinical tool, for it enables the physician to assess cardiac reserve and better quantify cardiac impairment. However, the majority of the information regarding cardiac function during stress tests has come from the ECG analysis, heart rate, and patient symptoms. A more complete cardiac functional profile could be obtained if the routine measurement of stroke volume and cardiac output were added to exercise stress testing. This would enable the clinician to ascertain the pumping capability of the heart and better direct the patient's cardiac rehabilitation program. In addition, the measurement of cardiac output during exercise stress testing allows some evaluation of the vascular system and its control since changes in peripheral resistance can be calculated from cardiac output and blood pressure.

Several investigators [4, 37–39, 103] have demonstrated that the hemodynamic information derived from impedance cardiography during exercise stress testing can yield unique information about cardiac function in heart disease. The study by Hetherington et al. [37] is an example of this approach to exercise stress testing. Impedance cardiography was used to study the stroke volume and cardiac output in 39 patients, who were 8–10 weeks postmyocardial infarction. These authors had previously validated the use of impedance with the direct Fick method in subjects exercising to maximum [38]. Nine healthy age-matched men were controls. Subjects performed progressive workloads of upright cycle exercise to symptom-limited maximums. The patients could be classified into three groups on the basis of their stroke volume response to the exercise (Fig. 7.10). Group 1 ($n = 14$) had a normal stroke volume response; group 2 ($n = 13$) had a stroke volume increase and then a stroke volume decrease as heart rate exceeded 100 BPM; and group 3 ($n = 12$) failed to increase stroke volume with exercise. Calculations of peripheral resistance indicated that group 3 patients also failed to lower vascular resistance during exercise. This study demonstrated that characterization of patient groups by stroke volume response to exercise identified those individuals with reduced ventricular function and increased vascular resistance, which was not apparent by other clinical data. Such information may be important in planning patient management, including exercise prescription and drug therapy.

Balasubramanian and Hoon [4] used a novel approach with impedance cardiography to assess cardiac function of ischemic heart disease (IHD) patients during submaximal exercise. Thirty-two men with IHD were studied on the treadmill to 85% of predicted maximum heart rate or until symptoms developed. These investigators focused on the Z_o and not on stroke volume changes. Since decreases in Z_o indicate accumulation of fluid (or loss of air) in the thorax, and vice versa [19], they

FIGURE 7.10
Responses of stroke volume and heart rate to progressive cycle exercise in control and patient populations.

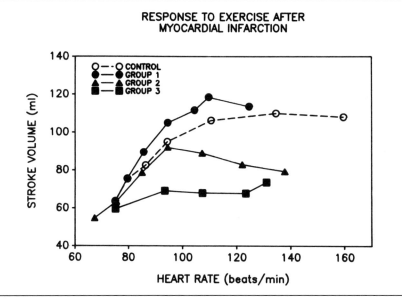

hypothesized that a dysfunctioning heart (in particular, the left ventricle) would not pump sufficiently during exercise to match cardiac output with venous return and fluid would accumulate in the thorax.

The patients were categorized into two groups and compared to normals. Group 1 had IHD with ECG ST-segment depression, and Group 2 were patients free of IHD but with preexcitation syndrome (PES) and ST-segment depression. As shown in Figure 7.11, Z_o did not change in normals or PES subjects, but decreased in IHD patients. Both PES and IHD patients demonstrated ST-segment depression. Thus, this type of analysis would be of value to differentiate false-positive exercise tests from true ST-segment changes reflective of IHD.

IMPEDANCE EJECTION FRACTION INDEX. Preliminary findings reported as abstracts by Judy et al. [45, 46] and papers by others [58, 87] have demonstrated that an index of left ventricular ejection fraction may be calculated from the impedance cardiogram. Judy et al. [45] have reported strong correlations between left ventricular ejection fraction measured by impedance (*ZEF*) and single-pass radionuclide angiocardiography in patients with IHD or heart failure ($r = 0.72-0.88$). Once *ZEF* and *SV* are determined, left ventricular end-diastolic volume

FIGURE 7.11

The use of submaximal exercise to identify ischemic heart disease (IHD). Normal subjects were compared to patients with preexcitation syndrome (PES) or IHD.

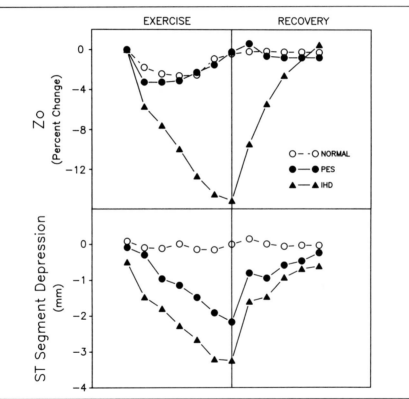

($EDV = SV/ZEF$) and end-systolic volume ($ESV = EDV - SV$) can be used to construct a Frank-Starling curve. This information would be most helpful for identifying cardiac dysfunction and for serial assessment of therapeutic progress. Unfortunately, our own evaluation of this index indicated it was not satisfactory [70]. We evaluated 46 men and 49 women patients with a variety of cardiac problems who were scheduled for the measurement of ejection fraction by multiple-gated equilibrium nuclear angiocardiography (MUGA). Correlations between ZEF and ejection fractions obtained by MUGA were unacceptably low ($r < 0.10$). We concluded that the currently proposed ZEF should not be used to make a clinical diagnosis. However, as this procedure evolves, it may prove to be of clinical value in assessing changes in left ventricular ejection fraction.

Conclusion

The impedance technique, as true of all methods used to measure cardiac output, has limitations as to the patient population or situation to which it can be accurately applied. New applications are continually emerging as investigators take advantage of its noninvasive nature to assess cardiac output and stroke volume on a beat-by-beat basis.

The impedance waveform is most easily obtained and evaluated under resting conditions. Quality tracings are difficult to obtain during moderate to strenuous exercise; however, the introduction of an exercise pause or signal-averaging procedures are valuable in reducing exercise-induced artifacts. The technique's greatest strength is assessment of directional changes in SV and cardiac output. In general, cardiac output obtained by impedance has a high intrasubject reproducibility and will agree within 15% to values obtained by the more traditional methods, which are themselves accurate to within 15% when compared with each other.

The studies presented show that cardiovascular information, which should aid the clinician in management of the cardiac patient, is obtainable from the impedance cardiogram during exercise. The combination of waveform analysis with SV and Z_o measurements represents a simple, noninvasive technique to profile cardiac function and evaluate cardiac reserve capabilities.

ACKNOWLEDGMENTS

We would like to thank Michael H. Cox, Ph.D, Thomas J. Ebert, M.D., Ph.D., and Mary Anne B. Frey, Ph.D., for their constructive criticism of the manuscript. Various aspects of this work were supported by grants from the Miami Valley Chapter of the American Heart Association, the American Lung Association, and the Dayton Area Heart Association.

REFERENCES

1. Appel PL, Kram HB, MacKabee J, Fleming AW, Shoemaker WC: Comparison of measurements of cardiac output by bioimpedance and thermodilution in severely ill surgical patients. *Crit Care Med* 14:933–935, 1986.
2. Aust PE, Belz GG, Belz G, Koch W: Comparison of impedance cardiography and echocardiography for measurement of stroke volume. *Eur J Clin Pharmacol* 23:475–477, 1982.
3. Baker LE: Electrical impedance pneumography. In Rolfe P (ed): *Noninvasive Physiological Measurements*. New York, Academic Press, 1979, pp 65–94.
4. Balasubramanian V, Hoon RS: Changes in transthoracic electrical impedance during submaximal treadmill exercise in patients with ischemic heart disease—a preliminary report. *Am Heart J* 91:43–49, 1976.
5. Barbacki M, Gluck A, Sandhage K: Estimation of the correlation between the transcutaneous aortic flow velocity curve and impedance cardiogram in normal children. *Cor Vasa* 23:291–298, 1981.
6. Bernstein DP: Continuous noninvasive real-time monitoring of stroke volume and cardiac output by thoracic electrical bioimpedance. *Crit Care Med* 14:898–901, 1986.
7. Bernstein DP: A new stroke volume equation for thoracic electrical bioimpedance: theory and rationale. *Crit Care Med* 14:904–909, 1986.
8. Bonjer FH, Van Den Berg JW, Dirken MNJ: The origin of the variations of body impedance occurring during the cardiac cycle. *Circulation* 6:415–420, 1952.
9. Bunnell DE, Bevier WC, Horvath SM. Effects of exhaustive submaximal exercise on cardiovascular function during sleep. *J Appl Physiol* 58:1909–1913, 1985.
10. Davies P, Francis RI, Docker MF, Watt JM, Crawford JS: Analysis of impedance cardiography longitudinally applied in pregnancy. *Br J Obstet Gynecol* 93:717–720, 1986.
11. DeMey C, Enterling D: Noninvasive assessment of cardiac performance by impedance cardiography: disagreement between two equations to estimate stroke volume. *Aviat Space Environ Med* 59:57–62, 1988.
12. Denniston JC, Maher JT, Reeves JT, Cruz JT, Cymerman A, Grover RF: Measurement of cardiac output by electrical impedance at rest and during exercise. *J Appl Physiol* 40:91–95, 1976.
13. Dionne RA, Driscoll EJ, Butler DP, Wirdzek PR, Sweet JP: Evaluation by thoracic impedance cardiography of diazepam, placebo, and two drug combinations for intravenous sedation of dental outpatients. *J Oral Maxillofac Surg* 41:782–788, 1983.
14. Djordjevich L, Sadove MS: Experimental study of the relationship between the base impedance and its time derivative in impedance plethysmography. *Med Phys* 8:76–78, 1981.
15. Doerr BM, Miles DS, Frey MAB: Influence of respiration on stroke volume determined by impedance cardiography. *Aviat Space Environ Med* 52:394–398, 1981.
16. Donovan KD, Dobb GJ, Woods WPD, Hockings BE: Comparison of transthoracic electrical impedance and thermodilution methods for measuring cardiac output. *Crit Care Med* 14:1038–1044, 1986.
17. DuQuesnay MC, Stoute GJ, Hughson RL: Cardiac output in exercise by impedance cardiography during breath holding and normal breathing. *J Appl Physiol* 62:101–107, 1987.
18. Ebert TJ, Eckberg DL, Vetrovec GM, Cowley MJ: Impedance cardiograms reliably estimate beat-by-beat changes of left ventricular stroke volume in humans. *Cardiovasc Res* 18:354–360, 1984.

19. Ebert TJ, Smith JJ, Barney JA, Merrill DC, Smith GK: The use of thoracic impedance for determining thoracic blood volume changes in man. *Aviat Space Environ Med* 57:49–53, 1986.

20. Edmunds AT, Godfrey S, Tooley M: Cardiac output measured by transthoracic impedance cardiography at rest, during exercise and at various lung volumes. *Clin Sci* 63:107–113, 1982.

21. Ehlert RE, Schmidt HD: An experimental evaluation of impedance cardiographic and electromagnetic measurements of stroke volumes. *J Med Eng Technol* 6:193–200, 1982.

22. Frey MAB, Mathes KL, Hoffler GW: Aerobic fitness in women and responses to lower body negative pressure. *Aviat Space Environ Med* 58:1149–1152, 1987.

23. Freyschuss U, Gentz J, Noack G, Persson B: Circulatory adaptation in newborn infants of strictly controlled diabetic mothers. *Acta Pediat Scand* 71:209–215, 1982.

24. Gastfriend RJ, Van De Water JM, Leonard ML, Macko P, Lynch PR: Impedance cardiography: current status and clinical applications. *Am Surg* 52:636–640, 1986.

25. Geddes LA, Baker LE: Detection of physiological events by impedance. In *Principles of Applied Biomedical Instrumentation*, ed 2. New York, John Wiley & Sons, 1975, pp 276–410.

26. Geddes LA, Sadler C: The specific resistance of blood at body temperature. *Med Bio Eng* 11:336–339, 1973.

27. Geddes LE, Baker LE: Thoracic impedance changes following saline injection into right and left ventricles. *J Appl Physiol* 33:278–281, 1972.

28. Glaser RM, Rattan SN, Davis GM, Servidio FJ, Figoni SF, Gupta SC, Suryaprasad AG: Central hemodynamic responses to lower-limb FNS. *Proc IEEE* 615–617, 1987.

29. Goldstein DS, Keiser HR: Pressor and depressor responses after cholinergic blockade in humans. *Am Heart J* 107:974–979, 1984.

30. Goldstein DS, Cannon III RO, Zimlichman R, Keiser HR: Clinical evaluation of impedance cardiography. *Clin Physiol* 6:235–251, 1986.

31. Gotshall RW, Miles DS: Noninvasive assessment of cardiac output by impedance cardiography in the newborn canine. *Crit Care Med* 17:63–65, 1989.

32. Gotshall RW, Wood VC, Miles DS: Comparison of two impedance cardiographic techniques for measuring cardiac output in critically ill patients. *Crit Care Med*, in press.

33. Gotshall RW, Miles DS, Sexson WR, Spohn WA, Courtney SE: Oscillatory cardiopulmonary effects of high-frequency jet ventilation. *Respiration* 49:283–291, 1986.

34. Gotshall RW, Breay-Pilcher JC, Boelcskevy BD: Cardiac output in adult and neonatal rats utilizing impedance cardiography. *Am J Physiol* 253:H1298–1304, 1987.

35. Harley A: Observations on the origin of the impedance cardiogram. *Br Heart J* 37:550, 1975.

36. Hatcher DD, Srb OD: Comparison of two noninvasive techniques for estimating cardiac output during exercise. *J Appl Physiol* 61:155–159, 1986.

37. Hetherington M, Teo KK, Haennel RG, Rossall RE, Kappagoda T: Response to upright exercise after myocardial infarction. *Cardiovasc Res* 21:399–406, 1987.

38. Hetherington M, Teo KK, Haennel R, Greenwood P, Rossall RE, Kappagoda T: Use of impedance cardiography in evaluating the exercise response of patients with left ventricular dysfunction. *Eur Heart J* 6:1016–1024, 1985.

39. Hetherington M, Haennel R, Teo KK, Kappagoda T: Importance of considering ventricular function when prescribing exercise after acute myocardial infarction. *Am J Cardiol* 58:891–895, 1986.

40. Hill DW, Mohapatra SN: The current status of electrical impedance techniques for the monitoring of cardiac output and limb blood flow. In *IEEE Medical Electronics Monographs*. England, Peregrinus, 1977, pp 23–58.

41. Hill DW, Merrifield AJ: Left ventricular ejection and the heather index measured by non-invasive methods during postural changes in man. *Acta Anaesthiol Scand* 20:313–320, 1976.

42. Hill DW, Thompson FD: The effect of haematocrit on the resistivity of human blood at 37°C and 100 kHz. *Med Biol Eng* 13:132–186, 1975.

43. Hill DW: The role of electrical impedance methods for the monitoring of central and peripheral blood flow changes. In Rolfe P (ed): *Noninvasive Physiological Measurements*. New York, Academic Press, 1979, pp 95–112.

44. Hubbard WN, Fish DR, McBrien DJ: The use of impedance cardiography in heart failure. *Int J Cardiol* 12:71–79, 1986.

45. Judy WV, Hall JH, Elliott WC: Influence of acute angina on exercise cardiodynamics (abstract). *Fed Proc* 41:1751, 1982.

46. Judy WV, Hall JH, Elliott WC: Left ventricular ejection fraction measured by the impedance cardiographic method (abstract). *Fed Proc* 42:1006, 1983.

47. Karnegis JN, Kubicek WG: Physiological correlates of the cardiac thoracic impedance waveform. *Am Heart J* 79:519–523, 1970.

48. Kosicki J, Chen L, Hobbie R, Patterson R, Ackerman E: Contributions to the impedance cardiogram waveform. *Ann Biomed Eng* 14:67–80, 1986.

49. Kubicek WG, From AHL, Patterson RP, Witsoe DA, Castaneda A, Lillehei RC, Ersek R: Impedance cardiography as a noninvasive means to monitor cardiac function. *J Assoc Adv Med Instrum* 4:79–84, 1970.

50. Kubicek WG, Kottke FJ, Ramos MU, Patterson RP, Witsoe DA, LaBrec JW, Remole W, Layman TE, Schoening H, Smith D: The Minnesota impedance cardiograph—theory and applications. *Biomed Eng* 9:410–416, 1974.

51. Kubicek WG, Karnegis JN, Patterson RP, Witsoe DA, Mattson RH: Development and evaluation of an impedance cardiac output system. *Aerospace Med* 37:1208–1212, 1966.

52. Kubicek WG, Patterson RP, Witsoe DA: Impedance cardiography as a noninvasive method of monitoring cardiac function and other parameters of the cardiovascular system. *Ann NY Acad Sci* 170:724–732, 1970.

53. Lababidi Z, Ehmke DA, Durnin RE, Leaverton PE, Lauer RM: The first derivative thoracic impedance cardiogram. *Circulation* 41:651–658, 1970.

54. Lababidi Z, Ehmke DA, Durnin RE, Leaverton PE, Lauer RM: Evaluation of impedance cardiac output in children. *Pediatrics* 47:870–879, 1971.

55. Lamberts R, Visser KR, Zijlstra WG. *Impedance Cardiography*. Assen, the Netherlands, Van Grocum, 1984.

56. Larsen FF, Mogensen L, Tedner B: Transthoracic electrical impedance at 1 and 100 kHz—a means for separating thoracic fluid compartments? *Clin Physiol* 7:105–113, 1987.

57. Logan JS, Veghte JH, Frey MAB, Robillard LMJ, Mann BL, Luciani RJ: Cardiac function monitored by impedance cardiography during changing seatback angles and anti-g suit inflation. *Aviat Space Environ Med* 54:328–333, 1983.

58. Lücker PW, Witzmann HK: Influence of magnesium and potassium deficiency on renal elimination and cardiovascular function demonstrated by impedance cardiography. *Magnesium* 3:265–273, 1984.

59. Lücker PW, Venitz J, Adolph S, Hey B: Measurement of the effect of cardiovascular drugs by impedance cardiography in healthy subjects. *Methods Find Exp Clin Pharmacol* 8:443–448, 1986.

60. Luisada AA, Perez GL, Kitapci H, Knighten V: Abnormal left ventricular contraction revealed by impedance cardiograms and arterial tracings in bundle branch blocks and old myocardial infarcts. *Angiology* 32:439–447, 1981.

61. Mansell MA, Crowther A, Laker MF, Wing AJ: The effect of hyperacetatemia on cardiac output during regular hemodialysis. *Clin Nephrol* 18:130–134, 1982.

62. Mapleson WW, Chiledat RT, Blewett MC, Lunn JN: Analysis of the thoracic impedance waveform for estimation of cardiac output. *Br J Anaesth* 49:185–189, 1977.

63. Miles DA, Enoch AD, Grevey SC: Interpretation of changes in DL_{CO} and pulmonary function after running five miles. *Respir Physiol* 66:135–145, 1986.

64. Miles DS, Gotshall RW, Motta MR, Duncan CA: Single-breath DL_{CO} maneuver causes cardiac output to fall during and after cycling. *J Appl Physiol* 65:41–45, 1988.

65. Miles DS, Owens JJ, Golden JC, Gotshall RW: Central and peripheral hemodynamics during maximal leg extension exercise. *Eur J Appl Physiol* 56:12–17, 1987.

66. Miles DS, Sawka MN, Wilde SW, Doerr BM, Frey MAB, Glaser RM: Estimation of cardiac output by electrical impedance during arm exercise in women. *J Appl Physiol* 51:1488–1492, 1981.

67. Miles DS, Sawka MN, Hanpeter DE, Foster Jr JE, Doerr BM, Frey MAB: Central hemodynamics during progressive upper- and lower-body exercise and recovery. *J Appl Physiol* 57:366–370, 1984.

68. Miles DS, Underwood Jr. PD, Nolan DJ, Frey MAB, Gotshall RW: Metabolic, hemodynamic, and respiratory responses to performing cardiopulmonary resuscitation. *Can J Appl Sport Sci* 9:141–147, 1984.

69. Miles DS, Gotshall RW, Golden JC, Tuuri DT, Beekman III RH, Dillon T: Accuracy of electrical impedance cardiography for measuring cardiac output in children with congenital heart defects. *Am J Cardiol* 61:612–616, 1988.

70. Miles DS, Gotshall RW, Quinones JD, Wulfeck DW, Kreitzer RD: Impedance cardiography fails to accurately measure left ventricular ejection fraction. *Crit Care Med*, in press.

71. Miles DS, Gotshall RW, Sexson WR: Evaluation of impedance cardiography in the canine pup. *J Appl Physiol* 60:260–265, 1986.

72. Miller JC, Horvath SM: Impedance cardiography. *Psychophysiology* 15:80–91, 1978.

73. Milsom I, Forssman L, Biber B, Dottori O, Silvertsson R: Measurement of cardiac stroke volume during cesarean section: a comparison between impedance cardiography and the dye dilution technique. *Acta Anaesthesiol Scand* 27:421–426, 1983.

74. Milsom I, Silvertsson R, Biber B, Olsson T: Measurement of stroke volume with impedance cardiography. *Clin Physiol* 2:409–417, 1982.

75. Miyamoto Y, Higuchi J, Abe Y, Hiura T, Nakazono Y, Mikami T: Dynamics of cardiac output and systolic time intervals in supine and upright exercise. *J Appl Physiol* 55:1674–1681, 1983.

76. Miyamoto Y, Higuchi J, Abe Y, Hiura T, Nakazono Y, Mikami T: Continuous determination of cardiac output during exercise by the use of impedance plethysmography. *Med Biol Eng Comput* 19:638–644, 1981.

77. Miyamoto Y, Hiura T, Tamura T, Nakamura T, Higuchi J, Mikami T: Dynamics of cardiac, respiratory, and metabolic function in men in response to step work load. *J Appl Physiol* 52:1198–1208, 1982.

78. Mohapatra SN: *Non-Invasive Cardiovascular Monitoring By Electrical Impedance Technique.* London, Pitman Medical, 1981.

79. Mohapatra SN, Costeloe KL, Hill DW: Blood resistivity and its implications for the calculation of cardiac output by the thoracic electrical impedance technique. *Intensive Care Med* 3:63–67, 1977.

80. Muzi M, Ebert TJ, Tristani FE, Jeutter DC, Barney JA, Smith JJ: Determination of cardiac output using ensemble-averaged impedance cardiograms. *J Appl Physiol* 58:200–205, 1985.
81. Nakazono Y, Miyamoto Y: Cardiorespiratory dynamics in men in response to passive work. *Jpn J Physiol* 35:33–43, 1985.
82. Nyboer J: *Electrical Impedance Plethysmography.* Springfield, IL, Charles C. Thomas, 1970.
83. Panigrahi G, Pedersen A, Boudoulas H: Effect of physical training on exercise hemodynamics in patients with stable coronary artery disease. The use of impedance cardiography. *J Med* 14:363–373, 1983.
84. Parulkar GB, Jindal GD, Bhardwaj R, Suraokar S, Dharani JB: Impedance cardiography in mitral valve diseases. *Indian Heart J* 37:37–42, 1985.
85. Patterson RP: Sources of the thoracic cardiogenic electrical impedance signal as determined by a model. *Med Biol Eng Comput* 232:411–417, 1985.
86. Pedersen T, Engbaek J, Ording H, Viby-Mogensen J: Effect of vecuronium and pancuronium on cardiac performance and transmural myocardial perfusion during ketamine anaesthesia. *Acta Anaesthiol Scand* 28:443–446, 1984.
87. Pederson T: Cardiac performance measured by impedance cardiography and radionuclide angiography. *Methods Find Exp Clin Pharmacol* 6:717–720, 1984.
88. Penney BC: Theory and cardiac applications of electrical impedance measurements. *CRC Crit Rev Biomed Eng* 13:227–281, 1985.
89. Penney BC, Patwardhan NA, Wheeler HB: Simplified electrode array for impedance cardiography. *Med Biol Eng Comput* 23:1–7, 1985.
90. Porter JM, PG Shakespeare: Cardiac output after burn injury. *R Coll Surg Engl* 66:33–35, 1984.
91. Qu M, Zhang Y, Webster JG, Tompkins WJ: Motion artifact from spot and band electrodes during impedance cardiography. *IEEE Trans Biomed Eng* 33:1029–1036, 1986.
92. Quail AW, Traugott FMK, Porges WL, White SW: Thoracic resistivity for stroke volume calculation in impedance cardiography. *J Appl Physiol* 50:191–195,1981.
93. Ramos MU: An abnormal early diastolic impedance waveform: a predictor of poor prognosis in the cardiac patient? *Am Heart J* 94:274–281, 1977.
94. Rasmussen JP, Sorensen B, Kann T: Evaluation of impedance cardiography as a non-invasive means of measuring systolic time intervals and cardiac output. *Acta Anaesthesiol Scand* 19:210–218, 1975.
95. Schieken RM, Patel MR, Falsetti HL, Lauer RM: Effect of mitral valvular regurgitation on transthoracic impedance cardiogram. *Br Heart J* 45:166–172, 1981.
96. Schieken RM, Patel MR, Falsetti HL, Barnes RW, Lauer RM: Effect of aortic valvular regurgitation upon the impedance cardiogram. *Br Heart J* 40:958–963, 1978.
97. Schuster CJ, Schuster HP: Application of impedance cardiography in critical care medicine. *Resuscitation* 11:255–274, 1984.
98. Sherwood A, Allen MT, Obrist PA: Evaluation of beta-adrenergic influences on cardiovascular and metabolic adjustments to physical and psychological stress. *Psychophysiology* 23:99–104, 1986.
99. Shiraki K, Konda N, Sagawa S, Lin YC, Hong SK: Cardiac output by impedance during head-out water immersion. *Undersea Biomed Res* 13:247–256, 1986.
100. Shuartz E, Gaume JG, White RT, Reibold RC: Hemodynamic responses during prolonged sitting. *J Appl Physiol: Respir Environ Exerc Physiol* 54:1673–1680, 1983.
101. Smith SA, Salih MM, Littler WA: Assessment of beat to beat changes in cardiac output during the Valsalva manoeuvre using electrical bioimpedance cardiography. *Clin Sci* 72:423–428, 1987.

102. Spinelli JC, Valentinuzzi ME: Stroke volume in the dog: measurements by the impedance technique and thermodilution. *Med Prog Technol* 10:45–53, 1983.
103. Teo KK, Hetherington MD, Haennel RG, Greenwood PV, Rossall RE, Kapppagoda T: Cardiac output measured by impedance cardiography during maximal exercise tests. *Cardiovasc Res* 19:737–743, 1985.
104. Traugott FM, Quail AW, White SW: Evaluation of blood resistivity in vivo for impedance cardiography in man, dog and rabbit. *Med Biol Eng Comput* 19:547–552, 1981.
105. Tremper KK, Hufstedler SM, Barker SJ, Zaccari J, Harris D, Anderson S, Roohk V: Continuous noninvasive estimation of cardiac output by electrical bioimpedance: an experimental study in dogs. *Crit Care Med* 14:231–233, 1986.
106. Vanfraechem JHP: Stroke volume and systolic time interval adjustments during bicycle exercise. *J Appl Physiol* 46:588–592, 1979.
107. Veigl VL, Judy WV: Reproducibility of haemodynamic measurements by impedance cardiography. *Cardiovasc Res* 17:728–734, 1983.
108. Victorin L, Olsson T: Transthoracic impedance; IV. Studies of the infant during the first two hours of life. *Acta Pediatr Scand* 207S:49–56, 1970.
109. Visser KR, Lamberts R, Zijlstra WG: Investigation of the parallel conductor model of impedance cardiography by means of exchange transfusion with stroma free haemoglobin solution in the dog. *Cardiovasc Res* 21:637–645, 1987.
110. Visser KR, Lamberts R, Poelmann AM, Zijlstra WG: Origin of the impedance cardiogram investigated in the dog by exchange transfusion with a stroma-free haemoglobin solution. *Pflügers Arch* 368:169–171, 1977.
111. Visser KR, Lamberts R, Korsten HH, Zijlstra WG: Observations on blood flow related electrical impedance changes in rigid tubes. *Pflügers Arch* 366:289–291, 1976.
112. Wilde SW, Miles DS, Durbin RJ, Sawka MN, Suryapresad AG, Glaser RM: Evaluation of myocardial performance during wheelchair ergometer exercise. *Am J Physical Med* 60:277–291, 1981.
113. Williams BO, Caird FI: Impedance cardiography and cardiac output in the elderly. *Age Ageing* 9:47–52, 1980.
114. Williams BO, Caird FI: Accuracy of the impedance cardiogram in the measurement of cardiac output in the elderly. *Age Ageing* 14:277–281, 1985.
115. Zhang Y, Qu M, Webster JG, Tompkins WJ, Ward BA, Bassett DR Jr: Cardiac output monitoring by impedance cardiography during treadmill exercise. *IEEE Trans Biomed Eng* 33:1037–1041, 1986.

8
Acute Polycythemia and Human Performance During Exercise and Exposure to Extreme Environments

MICHAEL N. SAWKA, Ph.D.
ANDREW J. YOUNG, Ph.D.

In this chapter, the influence of acute polycythemia on human performance during exercise and exposure to extreme environments is examined. In addition, we describe how an individual's aerobic fitness and acclimation state might modify his or her ergogenic response to erythrocyte infusion. Readers are encouraged to also read two earlier reviews by Gledhill [14, 15] concerning the effect of erythrocyte infusion on athletic performance. Several world-class endurance athletes have recently been accused of using erythrocyte infusions (homologous and autologous), or "blood doping," as an ergogenic aid. These athletes were participants in endurance events which require high aerobic power and which make considerable thermoregulatory demands for heat dissipation. Data are presented in this chapter substantiating that erythrocyte infusion improves exercise performance [3, 6, 11, 18, 67], increases maximal aerobic power [18, 27, 33, 37, 52, 57], and reduces thermoregulatory strain [19, 20, 43, 45] in normoxic environments. Likewise, data suggest that for some individuals erythrocyte infusion can improve exercise performance in hypoxic environments [35, 38, 39]. The potential adverse health effects of high hematocrits combined with exercise in extreme environments, however, have not been systematically evaluated.

Acute polycythemia can improve a person's ability to perform physical exercise and to tolerate some environmental extremes. It is not our intention to advocate the use of erythrocyte infusion as an ergogenic aid for athletic competition; in fact, we believe that practice to be unethical and do not condone its use for athletes. The American College of Sports Medicine [1] has recently taken the position that "blood doping as an ergogenic aid for athletic competition is unethical and unjustifiable, but that autologous red blood cell (RBC) infusion is an acceptable procedure to induce erythrocythemia in clinically controlled conditions for the purpose of legitimate scientific inquiry." Furthermore, there may be special situations in which hard physical labor must be performed in protective clothing or adverse environments (e.g., nuclear reactor clean-up, fire-fighting, and mountain search and rescue operations). In such situations, acute polycythemia could increase the probability of performing a task and thereby increase the safety of the civilian population. Finally, research on acute polycythemia is encouraged since it provides a tool to further the understanding of physiological control mechanisms in response to physical exercise and environmental extremes.

METHODOLOGY AND INFUSION EFFECTS

Acute polycythemia can be induced by the infusion of erythrocytes produced by oneself (autologous infusion) or another individual (homologous infusion). Autologous infusions are preferable because, even with the most careful laboratory testing, homologous transfusions have the risks of disease transmission (e.g., hepatitis or acquired immune deficiency syndrome) as well as blood type incompatibility. To induce acute polycythemia via autologous infusion, several blood units are removed from an individual by phlebotomy, stored, and then infused. Each phlebotomy is usually spaced by several weeks so that normal hematocrit can be reestablished prior to the next phlebotomy or the infusion. If autologous infusions are employed, cryopreservation procedures can be used to store the erythrocytes for several months or longer.

Erythrocyte infusion will acutely increase hemoglobin concentration and hematocrit. For a given infused erythrocyte volume, the magnitude of the hemoglobin increase can be quite variable between subjects [48]. For example, on the basis of the data from 21 subjects, the erythrocyte product of two blood units increased hemoglobin from 2 to 18% after infusion [48]. Spriet et al. [52] recently reported that infusing the erythrocyte product of two blood units increased hemoglobin by approximately 8% and infusing the product of three blood units increased hemoglobin by approximately 10%. Berglund et al. [4] reported that infusing the erythrocyte product of three blood units increased hemoglobin concentration by about 8%. On the other hand, Robertson et al. [39] found that infusing the product of four blood units increased hemoglobin concentration by about 28%. In those subjects, resting hematocrit was increased from 43 to 55 divisions (1% of the column of packed cells and plasma in the centrifuge tube), which approaches the high end of normal values for humans.

As hematocrit increases, so does the oxygen-carrying capacity of a given volume of blood. On the other hand, the higher the hematocrit the greater the blood viscosity, so that blood flow for a given driving pressure will be reduced [5]. This trade-off between oxygen-carrying capacity and blood flow has resulted in the development of the concept of an "optimal hematocrit." The optimal hematocrit is the level at which the greatest amount of oxygen can be delivered to the metabolically active tissues for a given driving pressure. For humans, the optimal hematocrit is often reported as approximating 40–45 divisions [5, 23, 54]. The recent data of Spriet et al. [52], however, suggest that the optimal hematocrit for athletic humans could be at least 51 divisions. In addition, when the hematocrit is about 63 divisions, deformation of the erythrocyte occurs and the ability to transfer oxygen is reduced [5]. These data suggest that the erythrocyte product of 2–3 blood units will provide the optimal hematocrit change to increase oxygen delivery to the active skeletal muscle during exercise.

After erythrocyte infusion, the acute increase in hematocrit gradually declines toward base line levels during the subsequent weeks. Pace et al. [35] found an initial 11% increase in hematocrit (infusion of 500 ml of fresh homologous erythrocytes) that was still increased by 6% at 40 days and did not return to base line levels until 60 days posttransfusion. Gledhill et al. [14] found an initial 8% increase in hematocrit (infusion of 450 ml of autologous erythrocytes) that did not return to control levels until 120 days postinfusion. These reported elevations in hematocrit for 60–120 days are not surprising since the erythrocyte has a life span of approximately 120 days. The magnitude of the polycythemia and its time course have been generally monitored by the indices of hemoglobin concentration and hematocrit.

Both of these indices of polycythemia (hemoglobin concentration and hematocrit) are influenced by the independent effects of erythrocyte volume and plasma volume. Surprisingly few studies concerning erythrocyte infusion and exercise performance have attempted to actually measure blood volume [27, 43, 45]. It is generally thought that the infusion of extra erythrocytes will result in a compensatory reduction in plasma volume to maintain the preinfusion blood volume [21, 32]; this is because the erythrocytes do not exert an in vitro oncotic pressure. Therefore, if erythrocytes are infused with saline, it might be expected that hematocrit changes would provide a reasonable index of erythrocyte volume changes.

Sawka et al. [43] measured blood volume in non-heat-acclimated subjects on several days prior to and 24 hours postinfusion. Their subjects were infused with the erythrocyte product of two blood units in a saline solution containing 50% hematocrit. They found that at rest the increased erythrocyte volume (222 ml) was associated ($r = -0.72$) with a reduced plasma volume (265 ml) to maintain the same blood volume as during the preinfusion measurements. Figure 8.1 presents the individual data showing this relationship. The reduction in plasma volume was accompanied by a 15–20 g reduction in total circulating protein mass. The loss of this amount of protein will reduce oncotic pressure sufficiently to account for the observed plasma volume reduction [49].

FIGURE 8.1

Relationship between percent change in erythrocyte volume and percent change in plasma volume after erythrocyte infusion in non-heat-acclimated subjects. (Data are from Sawka MN, Dennis RC, Gonzalez RR, Young AJ, Muza SR, Martin JW, Wenger CB, Francesconi RP, Pandolf KB, Valeri CR: Influence of polycythemia on blood volume and thermoregulation during exercise−heat stress. J Appl Physiol *62:1165−1169, 1987.)*

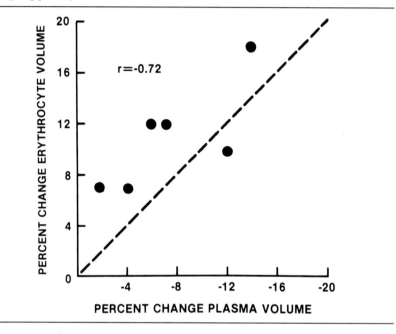

In a subsequent study, Sawka et al. [45] measured plasma volume in heat-acclimated subjects several days prior to and 24 hours postinfusion. Their subjects were infused with the erythrocyte product of two blood units in a saline solution containing 60% hematocrit. They found that the increased erythrocyte volume (187 ml) was associated with a slightly increased plasma volume (140 ml) during rest and exercise. The increased plasma volume was accompanied by a 20-g increase in total circulating protein mass. Therefore, the small plasma volume expansion was probably oncotically mediated. This increased plasma volume in heat-acclimated subjects after erythrocyte infusion is striking since those investigators previously reported a reduced plasma volume in non-heat-acclimated subjects after erythrocyte infusion. Therefore, heat acclimation may modify humans' total circulating protein mass and plasma volume response to erythrocyte reinfusion. Figure 8.2 presents the total circulating protein mass and plasma volume responses to erythrocyte infusion for both non-acclimated [43] and heat-acclimated [45] subjects during both rest and exercise–heat stress. Finally, Kanstrup and Ekblom [27] have reported that for five very fit (maximum oxygen uptake [$\dot{V}O_2max$] = 64 ml·kg^{-1}·min^{-1}) subjects the infusion of an unspecified volume of erythrocytes and saline resulted in an increased blood volume. Examination of their data, however, did not allow determination of whether the increase of blood volume was accompanied by an increase of plasma volume.

Heat acclimation has been associated with an increased amount of intravascular protein [50, 51]; perhaps extravascular protein was also increased and the infusion "washed" these additional extravascular proteins into the intravascular space where they were retained. Wasserman and Mayerson [64] have shown that infusion of isotonic saline to expand plasma volume can increase the total circulating protein mass by "washing" protein out of the interstitial space and into the lymph for return to the intravascular space. Those investigators reasoned that the mass of extravascular protein available to mix with the filtrate will influence the change in total circulating protein mass [64]. Consistent with the findings of Sawka et al. [45], Valeri and Altschule [59] report that erythrocyte transfusion increased plasma volume and intravascular albumin in trauma patients who had been transported from Southeast Asia during the preceding 2 weeks. These individuals were probably heat acclimated from living in a warm climate. Similar findings were reported from an animal study that was primarily conducted in the summer months in a warm–humid vivarium [60]. It seems possible that an individual's level of heat acclimation can alter one's protein mass and therefore plasma volume responses to erythrocyte infusion.

These results demonstrate that changes in hematocrit or hemoglobin do not always provide an accurate index of changes in erythrocyte volume for acute polycythemia studies. The subjects' state of heat acclimation and perhaps their level of aerobic fitness might modify their plasma volume response and therefore these indices after erythrocyte reinfusion. As a result, the importance of obtaining actual plasma volume and/or erythrocyte volume measurements during erythrocyte reinfusion studies needs to be stressed.

EXERCISE PERFORMANCE AND MAXIMAL AEROBIC POWER

A fundamental question is to what extent might erythrocyte infusion improve exercise performance. This question is difficult to answer from the reported literature because of differences between studies regarding exercise tasks, subject status, environmental conditions, as well as ex-

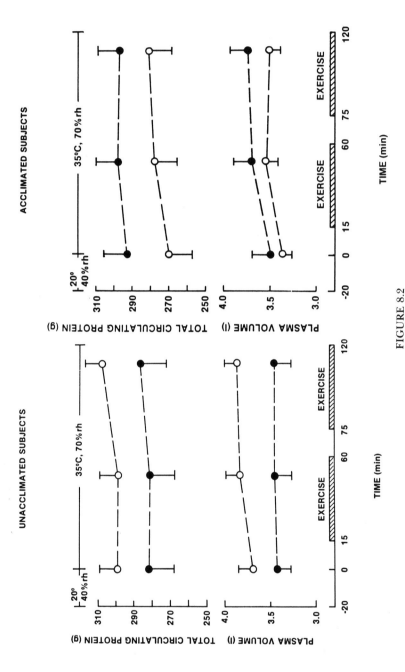

FIGURE 8.2

FIGURE 8.2
*Plasma volume and total circulating protein mass responses to erythrocyte infu-
sion for unacclimated and heat-acclimated subjects. (Data for unacclimated
subjects are from Sawka MN, Dennis RC, Gonzalez RR, Young AJ, Muza
SR, Martin JW, Wenger CB, Francesconi RP, Pandolf KB, Valeri CR: Influence of polycythemia on blood volume and thermoregulation during exercise—heat stress.* J Appl Physiol *62:1165–1169, 1987. Data for heat-
acclimated subjects are from Sawka MN, Gonzalez RR, Young AJ, Muza SR,
Pandolf KB, Latzka WA, Valeri CR, Dennis RC: Polycythemia and hydration: effects on thermoregulation and blood volume during exercise—heat stress.*
Am J Physiol (Reg Int Comp Physiol) *255:R456–R463, 1988.)*

perimental designs. A number of investigators have reported that race
times are faster after erythrocyte infusion [3, 6, 18, 67]. During running
races, improvements of approximately 5 [18], 6 [66], and 7 [6] seconds
per kilometer have been reported. Interestingly, the largest improvement in running performance was observed in experiments conducted
at a terrestrial altitude of 1550 m above sea level [6]. During a 15-k cross-
country ski race, acute polycythemia was found to improve performance
times by 5% compared to control values. The criterion of race time to
evaluate exercise performance, however, can be influenced by many
nonphysiological factors (e.g., motivation and pacing). As a result, many
erythrocyte infusion studies have employed the physiological criterion
of maximal aerobic power to evaluate exercise performance.

Maximal aerobic power (or maximal oxygen uptake) is defined as the
maximal rate at which oxygen can be taken up by the body tissues during
physical exercise [2, 31, 56]. For this determination, oxygen uptake is
measured as an individual performs progressively more intense exercise,
such as running at an increasing treadmill grade or pedaling against
increasing resistance on a cycle ergometer, until exhaustion. The individual's ability to sustain the exercise is dependent on the circulatory
system's ability to deliver oxygen and the capacity of the skeletal muscle
mitochondria to use oxygen and produce adenosine triphosphate.
Therefore, the oxygen uptake provides a measurement of aerobic caloric
expenditure which will increase linearly with the increase of exercise
intensity. Eventually the oxygen uptake will not increase with the increase
of exercise intensity, and the oxygen uptake begins to "level off" or
plateau. This leveling off of oxygen uptake despite increased exercise
intensity is used as the physiological criterion signifying individuals have
achieved their "true" maximal aerobic power [2, 31, 56].

Maximal aerobic power is used as the primary index of an individual's cardiorespiratory fitness, and is dependent on both central circulatory (oxygen delivery) and peripheral (oxygen extraction) factors. The Fick equation can be employed to describe these relationships for oxygen uptake:

$$\dot{V}O_2 = HR \times SV \times CaO_2 - C\bar{v}O_2, \tag{1}$$

where $\dot{V}O_2$ is oxygen uptake; HR is heart rate; SV is stroke volume; CaO_2 is oxygen content of arterial blood; and $C\bar{v}O_2$ is oxygen content in mixed venous blood. This equation can be simplified by substituting cardiac output ($\dot{Q}$) as the product of heart rate and stroke volume:

$$\dot{V}O_2 = \dot{Q} \times CaO_2 - C\bar{v}O_2 \tag{2}$$

Typical values for rest, moderate exercise, and maximal exercise are as follows:

> rest: $0.25\,l \cdot min^{-1} = 6\,l \cdot min^{-1} \times 0.042$
> $l\,O_2 \cdot$ liter of blood^{-1};
> moderate exercise: $2.24\,l \cdot min^{-1} = 16\,l \cdot min^{-1} \times 0.140$
> $l\,O_2 \cdot$ liter of blood^{-1};
> maximal exercise: $4.00\,l \cdot min^{-1} = 25\,l \cdot min^{-1} \times 0.160$
> $l\,O_2 \cdot$ liter of blood^{-1}.

It should be noted that from rest to maximal exercise the 16-fold increase in maximal oxygen uptake is accomplished by a 4-fold increase in cardiac output and an almost 4-fold increase in arteriovenous oxygen difference. Therefore, a high maximal oxygen uptake value requires considerable central and peripheral cardiovascular support.

Oxygen uptake represents the aerobic caloric expenditure per unit time, and is proportional to the individual's body mass during weight-bearing exercise. All other things being equal, the larger the body mass the larger the absolute ($l \cdot min^{-1}$) oxygen uptake during weight-bearing exercise. Therefore, the measured absolute maximal oxygen uptake is divided by the individual's body weight to facilitate comparisons between individuals and to provide normative data. For providing an index of aerobic fitness, $\dot{V}O_2max$ values are often expressed as milliliters of oxygen per kilogram of body weight per minute. An individual's maximal aerobic power ($\dot{V}O_2max$ in $ml \cdot kg^{-1} \cdot min^{-1}$) is closely related to his or her ability to perform endurance (aerobic) exercise [2, 17].

Buick et al. [7] were the first to demonstrate conclusively that acute polycythemia increased an individual's maximal aerobic power. Subsequent studies have confirmed these findings in normoxic [18, 27, 33,

37, 52, 57] as well as hypoxic [38, 39] environments. The physiological mechanism primarily responsible for the increased maximal aerobic power is an elevated arterial oxygen content [15]. However, other mechanisms such as blood volume expansion [15, 27, 45], increased maximal cardiac output [57], and improved blood buffering capacity [7, 52] have also been hypothesized to contribute to the overall ergogenic effect. Regardless of the physiological mechanism(s) responsible, surprisingly little detailed information is available to describe the magnitude of increase in maximal aerobic power elicited by acute polycythemia.

In a recent paper [48], data from four separate investigations [7, 33, 37, 57] were compiled and the influence of erythrocyte infusion on maximal aerobic power reanalyzed. The database was compiled from the results of studies in which: (*a*) the reinfused autologous erythrocytes were the product of two blood units; (*b*) the erythrocytes were preserved by freezing; (*c*) the infusion did not precede reestablishment of normocythemia; and (*d*) the maximal oxygen uptake was measured 24–72 hours after infusion. This time period enables sufficient equilibration of body fluids between compartments after the infusion and is well within the period of peak ergogenic effects [3, 15, 33].

Table 8.1 presents a description of the 30 subjects who participated in the four investigations and whose data were used in the analyses. For each study that employed control experiments, $\dot{V}O_2$max was not altered by saline infusion [7, 33, 37, 57]. Figure 8.3 presents the individual data for maximal aerobic power (ml $O_2 \cdot kg^{-1} \cdot min^{-1}$) measured before and shortly after (24–72 hours) erythrocyte infusion [48]. Maximal aerobic power was increased from a mean of 60.6 ($\pm$ 16.3) to a mean of 65.4 ($\pm$ 16.1) ml $O_2 \cdot kg^{-1} \cdot min^{-1}$ and there were greater increases from pre- to postinfusion in Studies 2 and 3 than in Studies 1 and 4. A correlation coefficient of 0.99 was found between the pre- and postinfusion values. Figure 8.4 presents the relationship between an individual's aerobic fitness (reflected by the initial maximal aerobic power normalized for body weight) and the absolute ($l \cdot min^{-1}$) increase in maximal oxygen uptake subsequent to erythrocyte infusion [48]. In Study 1 there was a smaller increase than in Study 3, and in Study 4 there was a smaller increase than in Studies 2 and 3. These data suggest that moderately fit, or perhaps moderately trained (aerobically) individuals (Studies 2 and 3) have an accentuated increase in maximal oxygen uptake after erythrocyte infusion.

Hemoglobin data were compiled and analyzed for Studies 1, 2, and 3. Erythrocyte infusion resulted in an increased hemoglobin concentration (a mean of 1.36 [$\pm$ 0.55g] Hb$\cdot$100 ml of blood^{-1}) which corresponds to a mean of 10% ($\pm$ 5) increase. No differences were found among the three studies for the increase in hemoglobin concentration after infusion. As shown in Figure 8.5 [48], the relationship between the absolute change

TABLE 8.1
Description of the Subject Population and Test Methods

Study	n	Sex	Age in Years	Height in cm	Weight in kg	Percent Body Fat	Exercise Mode	Initial Maximal Aerobic Power (ml $O_2 \cdot kg^{-1} \cdot min^{-1}$)
1. Buick et al. [7]	11	M					Treadmill	
Mean			21	175	64	7		80
SD			3	4	5	1		6
2. Thomson et al. [57]	4	M					Treadmill	
Mean			23	177	71	—		56
SD			1	7	6	—		7
3. Muza et al. [33]	6	M					Treadmill	
Mean			30	182	79	15		54
SD			7	4	9	5		5
4. Robertson et al. [37]	9	F					Cycle	
Mean			23	167	56	—		43
SD			2	7	3	—		4

FIGURE 8.3

Individual data for maximal aerobic power values measured before and after erythrocyte infusion. Broken line *represents line of equality.* Squares = *group 1;* triangles = *group 2;* circles = *group 3;* hexagons = *group 4. (From Sawka MN, Young AJ, Muza SR, Gonzalez RR, Pandolf KB: Erythrocyte reinfusion and maximal aerobic power: an examination of modifying factors.* JAMA 257:1496–1499, 1987.)

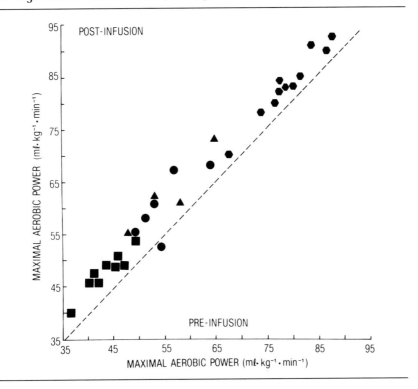

in an individual's hemoglobin concentration and the concomitant change in maximal aerobic power ($lO_2 \cdot min^{-1}$) was not statistically significant. This is not to say that the increased oxygen-carrying capacity does not mediate the increased maximal aerobic power, but rather that erythrocyte infusion also affects other physiological determinants of maximal aerobic power.

Erythrocyte infusion increased maximal oxygen uptake for 29 of the 30 subjects. The magnitude of the increase in maximal oxygen uptake was related to the subject's initial fitness level. Individuals with an initial maximal aerobic power between 50 and 65 ml $O_2 \cdot kg^{-1} \cdot min^{-1}$ appear to experience the greatest response to erythrocyte infusion (Fig. 8.3),

FIGURE 8.4

Individual data for the relationship between initial (preinfusion) maximal aerobic power and absolute change in maximal oxygen uptake after erythrocyte infusion. Broken line *represents no change in maximal oxygen uptake.* Squares = *group 1;* triangles = *group 2;* circles = *group 3;* hexagons = *group 4. (From Sawka MN, Young AJ, Muza SR, Gonzalez RR, Pandolf KB: Erythrocyte reinfusion and maximal aerobic power: an examination of modifying factors.* JAMA *257:1496–1499, 1987.)*

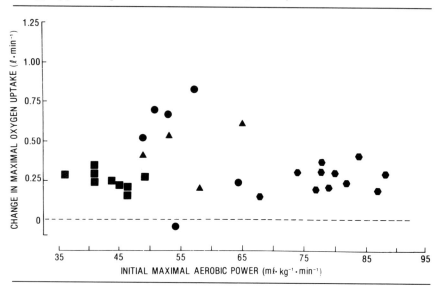

since their maximal oxygen uptake increased by a mean of 0.515 (± 0.204) $l \cdot min^{-1}$. These moderately to highly fit individuals were probably sufficiently trained to have a greater potential to increase both oxygen delivery and extraction to optimally increase their oxygen uptake after erythrocyte infusion [9, 25]. Individuals with an initial maximal aerobic power below 50 and above 65 ml $O_2 \cdot kg^{-1} \cdot min^{-1}$ displayed a very homogeneous but blunted (relative to the moderately fit subjects) increase in $\dot{V}O_2max$ of about 0.250 $l \cdot min^{-1}$ after erythrocyte infusion (Fig. 8.4).

The physiological mechanism(s) responsible for the blunted increase in $\dot{V}O_2max$ after erythrocyte infusion are probably different for the low-fit and highly fit groups. The low fit individuals may not have had the central reserves (ability to increase cardiac output and deliver oxygen) or peripheral reserves (ability to extract and use the oxygen delivered at the skeletal muscle) during maximal effort exercise to fully benefit from the increased arterial oxygen content available after erythrocyte infusion. In contrast, the very fit individuals might already be effectively

FIGURE 8.5

Individual data for the relationship between absolute change in hemoglobin concentration and absolute change in maximal oxygen uptake after erythrocyte infusion. Broken line *represents no change in maximal oxygen uptake.* Squares = *group 1;* triangles = *group 2;* circles = *group 3;* hexagons = *group 4. (From Sawka MN, Young AJ, Muza SR, Gonzalez RR, Pandolf KB: Erythrocyte reinfusion and maximal aerobic power: an examination of modifying factors.* JAMA *257:1496–1499, 1987.)*

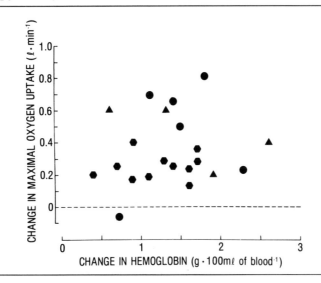

using (without erythrocyte infusion) a comparatively larger portion of their potential central and peripheral reserves during maximal exercise.

The blunted increase in $\dot{V}O_2$max by highly fit subjects (i.e. greater than 65 ml $O_2 \cdot kg^{-1} \cdot min^{-1}$) may be due to an exercise-induced arterial hypoxemia [10, 16]. Dempsey et al. [10] reported that in highly trained endurance runners there was a tendency for arterial blood to desaturate at maximal exercise and therefore limit their aerobic performance. The arterial hypoxemia they noted, with the increased alveolar-to-arterial (A–a) PO_2 difference (22–35 mm Hg), during high-intensity exercise was attributed to a diffusion limitation and an inadequate hyperventilatory response to heavy exercise. A diffusion limitation may occur either when the erythrocyte transit time in the pulmonary capillary decreases (increased pulmonary capillary blood flow) or the blood–gas barrier thickens, so that the O_2 diffusing across the blood–gas barrier does not have time to equilibrate with the capillary blood. Dempsey [10] suggests that during maximal exercise a highly fit subject may experience a decrease in the erythrocyte transit time in the pulmonary capillary to the point that diffusion limitation occurs. Other explanations for the increasing A–a PO_2 difference include a pulmonary venous admixture and a ventilation to perfusion inequality; however, their contributions to the A–a difference during exercise at sea level are minimal [61, 62]. Gledhill et al. [16] have reported that acute polycythemia does not reduce the magnitude of exercise-induced arterial hypoxemia in highly fit subjects.

Erythrocyte infusion increased hemoglobin concentration by approximately 1.36 g·100 ml of blood^{-1} [48], which corresponds to an increased arterial oxygen content (at 100% saturation) of approximately 1.82 ml O_2·100 ml of blood^{-1} (1.36 g Hb × 1.34 ml O_2·g Hb^{-1}). It is likely that a fit subject may have achieved an average cardiac output of approximately 30l·min^{-1} during maximal exercise [41]. If maximal exercise elicited a theoretical cardiac output of 30 l·min^{-1}, the increased arterial oxygen content would result in an additional 0.546 l O_2·min^{-1} available to the tissues after erythrocyte infusion. Also, if erythrocyte infusion increased maximal cardiac output [14], then an even greater increment in the volume of oxygen available to the tissues would be produced. However, an increased $\dot{V}O_2$max is also dependent on the peripheral tissue's ability to extract and use the additional oxygen which is made available [25]. Overall, erythrocyte infusion increased $\dot{V}O_2$max by an average of 0.357 (± 0.216) l·min^{-1}, which represents about 65% of the theoretical maximal potential for increase at a cardiac output of 30 l ·min^{-1}.

Surprisingly, no relationship was found between the increase in hemoglobin concentration and the increase in $\dot{V}O_2$max [48]. The lack of a statistically significant relationship may be due in part to the homogeneity in the volume of infused erythrocytes; each subject received the product of two blood units. However, the range of increases in hemoglobin concentration after erythrocyte infusion was fairly wide (0.6–2.6 g Hb·100 ml of blood^{-1}). Alternatively, there may be differences between individuals in the amount of additional oxygen that is made available to contracting skeletal musculature during maximal exercise. For example, erythrocyte infusion may cause varied effects on maximal cardiac output as well as vasomotor responses (at a given cardiac output) directing blood to the contracting musculature. Several studies, however, report that erythrocyte infusion does not increase the cardiac output during near-maximal or maximal exercise [12, 37, 38, 40, 52, 57]. The mechanisms by which erythrocyte infusion might increase maximal cardiac output would be an expanded blood volume causing an increased myocardial preload, increased myocardial oxygenation, or a reduced negative inotropic effect from reduced anaerobiosis. Furthermore, some subjects may not have sufficient peripheral tissue adaptations, such as available gas exchange surface area (capillary-to-muscle-fiber ratio) or enzymatic oxidative potential, to extract and use the additional oxygen which is available [9, 25]. It is known that aerobic training is associated with increased capillarization, increased number and size of mitochondria, as well as increased concentration of oxidative enzymes in skeletal muscle [9, 25].

HEAT STRESS

During exercise, core temperature increases as a consequence of the metabolic intensity and is often independent of the environmental heat load [46]. To minimize these core temperature changes (reflecting body heat storage), vasomotor adjustments occur to increase skin blood flow and dilate superficial veins. These adjustments facilitate evaporative as well as radiative and convective heat loss, but also displace a portion of the central blood volume to the compliant cutaneous vasculature [42, 46]. Under conditions of combined exercise–heat stress, competition may exist between the circulatory requirements of metabolically active skeletal muscle and the cutaneous vasculature [42, 46]. Eventually this competition can compromise cardiac output as well as the ability to dissipate heat [42, 46]. Likewise, plasma provides the precursor fluid for the secreted sweat, which enables evaporative heat loss. Therefore, sweat secretion can reduce the blood volume and make it more difficult for the cardiovascular system to support the combined stress of exercise and heat [42, 44, 46].

There are several reasons why erythrocyte infusion could be beneficial to individuals performing exercise in the heat. Increased arterial oxygen content will improve muscle oxygenation at any level of muscle blood flow, and if blood volume increased, this would allow a higher stroke volume and cardiac output. Finally, some investigators believe that during exercise, core temperature responses are coupled to relative (percent of $\dot{V}O_2$max) exercise intensity [46]. Erythrocyte infusion will increase $\dot{V}O_2$max; therefore, the relative exercise intensity will be lower at a given level of submaximal oxygen uptake level, possibly resulting in lower core temperatures.

Two investigations have examined the influence of acute polycythemia on thermoregulation during exercise in the heat [43, 45]. In the first study [43] nine men, who were not heat acclimated, were infused with either 600 ml of a saline solution containing a 50% hematocrit ($n = 6$, infusion) or 600 ml of saline only ($n = 3$, control). Subjects attempted a heat–stress test while euhydrated at approximately 2 weeks preinfusion and 48 hours postinfusion. The heat stress test consisted of a 120-minute exposure (two repeats of 15-minute rest and 45-minute treadmill walking) in a hot (35°C, 45% relative humidity) environment. The erythrocyte

FIGURE 8.6

A typical local sweating response ($\dot{m}_s$) to esophageal temperature changes during the first exercise bout both pre- and posterythrocyte infusion for one non-heat-acclimated subject. (From Latzka WA, Sawka MN, Muza SR, Gonzalez RR, Young AJ, Pandolf KB, Dennis RC, Martin JW, Wenger CB, Valeri CR: Ergogenic influence of erythrocyte reinfusion: aerobic power and thermoregulation (Technical Report No. T28/87). Natick, MA, U.S. Army Research Institute of Environmental Medicine, 1987.)

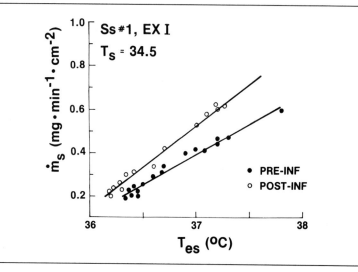

infusion group subjects tended to store less body heat during the postinfusion heat–stress test. For the control group, a tendency for a greater body heat storage was evident during the postinfusion heat–stress test (compared to preinfusion). The avenues of heat exchange responsible for the reduced body heat storage after erythrocyte infusion were inconclusive. For the erythrocyte infusion group, steady-state values for evaporative as well as radiative and convective heat exchange were not altered from pre-to postinfusion. However, the onset time for sweating and the local sweating transient response (Fig. 8.6) tended to improve postinfusion [20, 28]. It should be noted that these thermoregulatory advantages occurred despite the fact that erythrocyte infusion reduced plasma volume so that total blood volume was the same as during the preinfusion measurements [43]. These investigators [13] also reported that acute polycythemia reduced plasma levels of the stress hormone cortisol, but the infusion did not alter the fluid regulatory hormones of aldosterone and plasma renin activity during exercise in the heat.

This first study [43] raised several questions concerning the use of acute polycythemia as an ergogenic aid during exercise in the heat. First, would the small thermoregulatory advantage conferred by acute polycythemia still be present in heat-acclimated subjects? Heat acclimation enables an individual to perform exercise in the heat with reduced heat storage, and may elicit the optimal thermoregulatory benefits that acute polycythemia cannot improve upon. Therefore, acute polycythemia may not provide a thermoregulatory benefit in heat-acclimated (unlike unacclimated) subjects. Second, would acute polycythemia provide a thermoregulatory advantage or disadvantage in hypohydrated subjects during exercise in the heat? Hypohydration reduces plasma volume [44, 47], and this reduction may be accentuated by the acute polycythemia which could provide a thermoregulatory disadvantage during subsequent exercise in the heat. Therefore, acute polycythemia could potentially reduce exercise performance (below preinfusion levels) for hypohydrated subjects.

In the second study [19, 45], five heat-acclimated males attempted four heat–stress tests: two preinfusion and two postinfusion tests with autologous erythrocytes (product of two blood units) in saline solution (50% hematocrit). Both pre- and postinfusion, subjects attempted one heat–stress test while euhydrated and one heat–stress while hypohydrated (−5% of body weight). The protocol for the heat–stress tests was the same as in the previous investigation. During exercise, the subjects stored less body heat after erythrocyte infusion during both the euhydration and hypohydration heat stress tests (Fig. 8.7). In addition, the subjects demonstrated an improved sweating response to exercise–heat stress after erythrocyte infusion. Both total body sweating and steady-state local sweating were greater postinfusion, and the onset time for sweating tended to be more rapid. The slope of the local sweating response for a given core temperature was increased by about 68% after the infusion [19], and looks similar to the example presented in Figure 8.5. Unlike the previous study, erythrocyte infusion resulted in a slightly expanded plasma volume during rest and exercise in the heat-acclimated subjects (see Fig. 8.2). The slightly expanded plasma volume combined with the additional erythrocytes to result in an increased blood volume during both rest and exercise. Finally, the investigators found a reduced plasma hyperosmolality during the postinfusion hypohydration experiments.

The physiological mechanism responsible for improved thermoregulatory responses in the non-heat-acclimated subjects remains unclear [43], particularly since plasma volume was reduced below euhydration levels (although blood volume was unchanged). The tendency for improved sweat onset time may be due to a priming or initial filling of the sweat gland duct [8]. This response may reflect the changes seen in the

FIGURE 8.7

Individual data for the final exercise rectal temperature response to the pre-
and postinfusion heat stress test. (From Sawka MN, Gonzalez RR, Young AJ,
Muza SR, Pandolf KB, Latzka WA, Valeri CR, Dennis RC: Polycythemia
and hydration: effects on thermoregulation and blood volume during exercise—
heat stress. Am J Physiol (Reg Int Comp Physiol) *255:R456–R463,*
1988.)

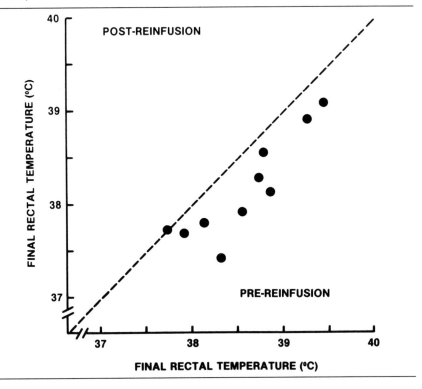

total circulating proteins after erythrocyte infusion. After infusion, the total circulating protein mass decreased rapidly, which may reflect a translocation of protein from the intravascular to the interstitial space. This increased interstitial protein could facilitate better hydration of these tissues. If proteins were partially translocated into the cutaneous interstitial space, the concomitant increase in interstitial fluid would provide more precursor fluid for sweat secretion and subsequently improve the sweating onset time.

For the heat-acclimated subjects, the physiological mechanisms responsible for the thermoregulatory advantage provided by acute polycythemia were probably different for the euhydration and hypohydration experiments. These mechanisms might include an increased blood volume and/or reduced plasma hyperosmolality. The expanded blood volume postinfusion would clearly mediate a thermoregulatory advantage in the hypohydration experiments. Hypohydration decreases an individual's blood volume, resulting in impaired evaporative as well as radiative and convective heat loss, thus elevating core temperature in comparison to euhydration [44, 47]. This thermoregulatory disadvantage due to hypohydration is somewhat related to the magnitude of hypovolemia [47] and can be reversed by the reestablishment of the normal blood volume during exercise in the heat [53]. Therefore, during the postinfusion hypohydration experiments, the maintenance of blood volume at essentially normovolemic levels (compared to preinfusion euhydration experiments) would mediate a thermoregulatory advantage compared to the preinfusion hypohydration heat stress test where hypovolemia occurred. Also, during the postinfusion euhydration experiments, the hypervolemia could have contributed to the thermoregulatory advantage compared to the preinfusion euhydration heat–stress test.

Plasma hyperosmolality has been shown to reduce thermoregulatory effector responses and thus elevate core temperature during exercise in the heat [44, 47]. During the euhydration experiments, plasma osmolality values were not different between the pre- and postinfusion heat–stress tests. During the hypohydration experiments, however, plasma osmolality values were significantly lower postinfusion [45]. These lower osmolality values might be explained by the larger blood volume enabling reduced activation (compared to the preinfusion hypohydration experiments) of the renin–angiotensin system by reducing stimulation of the juxtaglomerular cells. A blunted renin release and aldosterone secretion will cause a greater natriuresis, thus providing better regulation of plasma tonicity [58]. Regardless of the actual mechanism, maintenance of a lower plasma osmolality following reinfusion when hypohydrated provides a mechanism to mediate improved thermoregulatory effector responses.

Neither of the studies on polycythemia and thermoregulation directly quantified radiative and convective heat loss, but the selected environment kept radiative and convective heat exchange relatively low. As stated above, a smaller blood volume reduction and reduced hyperosmolality can each mediate improved thermoregulatory responses for evaporative as well as radiative and convective (dry) heat exchange [44]. An additional physiological mechanism for improved dry heat exchange after erythrocyte infusion can be hypothesized: A reduced skeletal muscle blood flow may allow increased cutaneous blood flow at a given cardiac output during submaximal exercise. Several human and animal studies report that hyperoxia reduces skeletal muscle blood flow during submaximal exercise [65, 66, 68].

HIGH ALTITUDE

At high terrestrial altitude, the decrease in barometric pressure results in a reduction in the partial pressure of inspired oxygen. Humans sojourning at high altitude increase ventilation, but alveolar and arterial oxygen pressures are still lower than at sea level. The resulting arterial desaturation reduces arterial oxygen content in the unacclimatized sojourner well below sea-level values. Therefore, the potential for erythrocyte infusion to have ergogenic effects might seem greatest at high altitude.

The cardiovascular responses of unacclimatized and acclimatized lowland residents exercising at high altitude have been reviewed in detail elsewhere [22, 70]. Briefly, with acute high-altitude exposure, tachycardia increases cardiac output during rest and submaximal exercise compared to at sea level, thereby offsetting the reduced arterial oxygen content and sustaining oxygen uptake (see Fick equation). Maximal cardiac output, however, is the same initially at high altitude as at sea level, but is achieved at a lower exercise intensity and oxygen uptake. The reduction in $\dot{V}O_2$max with acute high-altitude exposure is proportional to the reduction in arterial oxygen content. Eight to ten days of altitude acclimatization results in an increase in arterial oxygen content as a result of both increased hematocrit (hemoconcentration due to decreased plasma volume) and increased arterial saturation (ventilatory acclimatization raises alveolar and arterial O_2 pressure). $\dot{V}O_2$max remains reduced, however, because during the same time that arterial oxygen content is rising, maximal cardiac output declines; both the resting and submaximal cardiac output will fall. Total peripheral resistance increases during these early days of altitude acclimatization as a result of both an increased systemic vascular resistance (vasoconstriction) and increased blood viscosity. The fall in cardiac output with altitude acclimatization is due to a decrease in cardiac stroke volume at a given oxygen uptake. The reduced stroke volume can be attributed to the effects of decreased plasma and blood volume on ventricular filling (Frank-Starling relationship) as well as the increased total peripheral resistance. With acclimatization to moderate altitudes, tachycardia does not offset the falling stroke volume, so cardiac output declines. However, at very extreme altitudes (>6000 m) tachycardia does offset the reduced stroke volume, and cardiac output is maintained at sea-level values [36]. Whether or not erythrocyte infusion exerts an ergogenic effect at high altitude and the magnitude of any effect probably depends, among other things, on the elevation ascended and the acclimatization status of the subject.

The relationship between the decrement in $\dot{V}O_2$max and terrestrial elevation has been well studied [24, 55, 69]. There is little measurable decrement below 1000 m, a small and variable decrement between 1000 and 2000 m [24], and above 2000 m a linear decrease with altitude by about 10% for every additional 1000 m ascended [55]. Table 8.2 shows an idealized analysis of the separate effects of acute polycythemia and exposure to high altitude (4300 m) on each Fick equation component of the $\dot{V}O_2$max for a reasonably fit individual. Table 8.2 shows that prior to erythrocyte infusion, arterial desaturation from 97% to 70% would be expected to produce a 28% decrement upon arrival at 4300 m. This agrees well with actual measurements of the decrement in $\dot{V}O_2$max at 4300 m [70]. If ascent to high altitude were preceded by erythrocyte infusion, the predicted decrement would be smaller relative to the preinfusion sea-level value, 21% in this example. A 21% decrement in $\dot{V}O_2$max would normally be expected at an altitude of about 3200 m [24]. Note, however, that the percent decrement at high altitude is not smaller when expressed relative to the postinfusion, sea-level value.

Implicit in the analysis shown in Table 8.2 is the assumption that systemic oxygen transport is the limiting factor for $\dot{V}O_2$max. Although this is true at sea level, this may not be true at high altitude. Ventilation–perfusion inequalities and diffusion limitations are both greater during exercise under hypoxic as compared to normoxic conditions [63]. Thus, at altitude, $\dot{V}O_2$max may be limited by pulmonary gas exchange rather than systemic oxygen transport. If so, the decrements in maximal oxygen uptake calculated in Table 8.2 would underestimate the true decrement. Regardless of whether pulmonary gas exchange or systemic oxygen transport limits $\dot{V}O_2$max, the magnitude of the increase in $\dot{V}O_2$max due to erythrocyte infusion would be the same at altitude as sea level, unless some of the increase in $\dot{V}O_2$max resulted from an increase in maximal cardiac output. Any increase in $\dot{V}O_2$max due to an increased maximal cardiac output would probably be obviated at high altitude, since a decreased pulmonary capillary transit time for hemoglobin would exacerbate the effect of a limitation to pulmonary gas exchange.

The expected decrement in $\dot{V}O_2$max over a wide range of high altitudes and the theorized effect of erythrocyte infusion on the decrement is shown in Figure 8.8. The effect of erythrocyte infusion which is depicted must be considered theoretical since there have been no studies comparing effects of erythrocyte infusion at sea level and various high altitudes. However, Robertson et al. [38, 39] addressed this question using hypoxic breathing gas to simulate acute high-altitude exposure. Their results confirm the analysis shown in Table 8.2 and Figure 8.8. The $\dot{V}O_2$max while breathing hypoxic gas was greater postinfusion compared to preinfusion, but no more so than while breathing normoxic gas [39]. The decrement in $\dot{V}O_2$max with hypoxia was lessened by erythrocyte infusion due to the increased arterial O_2 content. However, the increased arterial O_2 content from infusion was insufficient to completely

TABLE 8.2
Effect of Erythrocyte Infusion on the Decrement in Maximal Oxygen Uptake ($\dot{V}O_2max$) with Acute High-Altitude Exposure

Altitude	Before Erythrocyte Infusion			After Erythrocyte Infusion		
	$\dot{V}O_2max$ (ml·min⁻¹)	= $\dot{Q}$ max × (l·min⁻¹)	(CaO₂ − Cv̄O₂) (ml·l⁻¹)	$\dot{V}O_2max$ (ml·min⁻¹)	= $\dot{Q}$ max × (l·min⁻¹)	(CaO₂ − Cv̄O₂) (ml·l⁻¹)
Sea level	5580	30	(197 − 11)	6120	30	(215 − 11)
	−28%			−28%		
	21%					
4300 m	4020	30	(145 − 11)	4410	30	(158 − 11)

The computations of $\dot{V}O_2max$ were based on the following assumptions: (*a*) maximal cardiac output ($\dot{Q}$ max) is unchanged by infusion or acute high altitude; (*b*) mixed venous O₂ content (Cv̄O₂) during maximal exercise is unchanged by infusion or acute high altitude; (*c*) preinfusion [Hb] equals 15.5g·dl⁻¹, is unchanged by acute high altitude, but is increased by 1.36g·dl⁻¹ following infusion of erythrocyte product of two units of blood; (*d*) arbitrary values were assigned to $\dot{Q}$ max (30l·min⁻¹), percent saturation of arterial blood at sea level (95%) and 4300 m (70%), percent saturation of mixed venous blood at sea level (50%) and 4300 m (50%).

FIGURE 8.8

The decrement in maximal oxygen uptake ($\dot{V}O_2max$) at high altitude expressed as a function of elevation. The solid line represents the decrement for subjects without additional erythrocytes infused [22], and the broken line depicts the theorized effect of erythrocyte infusion on this decrement. The increase in $\dot{V}O_2max$ due to the effect of erythrocyte infusion (line AB) results in a lowering (line BC) of an individual's physiological altitude.

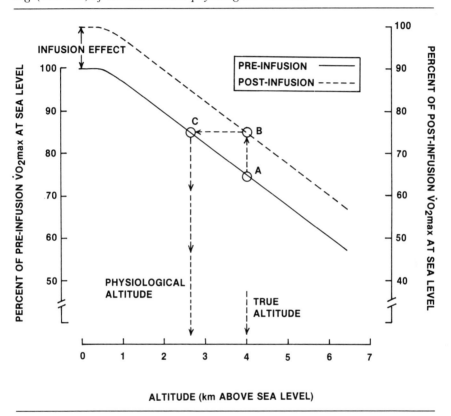

compensate for the fall in arterial O_2 saturation at that altitude (3600 m, simulated); thus arterial O_2 content and $\dot{V}O_2max$ were still lower than with normoxia [39]. It is possible, however, that erythrocyte infusion could fully offset the effects of hypoxia on maximal aerobic power at lower elevations. Recently, Robertson et al. [38] reported that the decrement in $\dot{V}O_2max$ produced by exposure to a simulated altitude of 2250 m was completely eliminated following erythrocyte infusion. This illustrates that there will be some threshold elevation below which the effect of erythrocyte infusion (increased arterial O_2 content) can entirely offset the effect of hypoxia (decreased arterial O_2 saturation), and the expected decrement in maximal aerobic power does not occur.

The improvement in hypoxic tolerance resulting from erythrocyte infusion was quantified by Pace et al. [35] by calculating the difference between the true altitude and physiological altitude. Physiological altitude is defined as the elevation at which a given exercise response observed following erythrocyte infusion would have been observed without infusion. For example, Pace et al. [35] found that the heart rate during a standardized exercise bout was the same for erythrocyte-infused subjects at 4712 m as for noninfused subjects at 3131 m. Thus, erythrocyte infusion provided a physiological advantage equal to a reduction of 1581 m. Figure 8.8 illustrates this concept of physiological altitude for the decrement in $\dot{V}o_2$max at high altitude. Obviously, the actual magnitude of the altitude-lowering effect from erythrocyte infusion (line BC in Fig. 8.8) will be determined by the magnitude of the infusion effect (line AB in Fig. 8.8), which was arbitrarily chosen for Figure 8.8.

Although erythrocyte infusion effects on maximal aerobic power are probably the same at altitude as at sea level, the effects of erythrocyte infusion on submaximal performance during acute high-altitude exposure may be of greater practical significance than at sea level. A given physical activity or exercise intensity (e.g., running at a given velocity and grade on a treadmill) elicits the same oxygen uptake at altitude as at sea level. However, this oxygen uptake represents a greater percentage of the reduced maximal aerobic power (increased relative exercise intensity) at altitude. Endurance during submaximal exercise is closely related to the relative exercise intensity [2, 17]. Furthermore, individuals working self-paced for prolonged (3–8 hours) periods will generally select a work pace corresponding to 30–40% of maximal aerobic power at sea level [29] as well as at high altitude [34]. Thus, just as at sea level, erythrocyte infusion will allow unacclimatized lowlanders at high altitude to sustain higher absolute intensities of exercise for longer periods of time.

No studies have been reported which investigated the effects of erythrocyte infusion at altitude for altitude-acclimatized humans. One altitude-acclimatization study [26], however, has implications regarding the efficacy of erythrocyte infusion as an ergogenic aid both at high altitude and at sea level. Remember, altitude acclimatization is associated with plasma volume reduction: Plasma volume can decrease by as much as 25% in 8–10 days at high altitude [22, 70]. Hematocrit values on the order of 54 divisions have been observed following 15 days of residence at 4300 m [26]. An experiment by Horstman et al. [26] provides evidence that when hematocrit becomes this high some of the effects of increased arterial oxygen content are negated by increased blood viscosity, at least during maximal exercise. In five altitude-acclimatized men whose hematocrits averaged 54 divisions, cardiac output during maximal exercise increased substantially following removal of 450 ml of blood to reduce hematocrit to 48 divisions. This observation was interpreted as indicating a viscosity impairment of blood flow, thereby limiting stroke volume, during maximal exercise [26]. However, maximal aerobic power decreased with phlebotomy despite the large increase in maximal cardiac output. Thus, the effect of decreased arterial oxygen content was greater than the effect of reduced blood viscosity. Whether by erythrocyte infusion or altitude acclimatization, it appears that an increase in hematocrit as high as 54 divisions will produce an increase in maximal aerobic power despite increased blood viscosity.

Earlier in this chapter the concept of optimal hematocrit was used in combination with observations of erythrocyte deformation when hematocrit exceeded 63 divisions to suggest that erythrocyte infusion from the product of two to three blood units would produce peak ergogenic effects. It is not known at what hematocrit above 54 divisions the reduction in maximal cardiac output due to increased viscosity would obviate the effects of increased arterial oxygen content. Another important but unresolved question is whether or not the reduction in plasma volume associated with altitude acclimatization is altered by erythrocyte infusion. For individuals sojourning at high altitude, the decision as to the optimal erythrocyte volume to be infused for peak ergogenic effects must be based on consideration for the effects of the expected plasma volume reduction, acclimatization level, and the individual's initial hematocrit and plasma volume. It appears that the study of erythrocyte infusion for individuals at high terrestrial altitude is an interesting area for research.

CONCLUSION

Acute polycythemia will increase an individual's maximal aerobic power and improve his or her ability to perform submaximal and maximal endurance exercise. In addition, acute polycythemia will usually reduce body heat storage and improve sweating responses during exercise in the heat. However, there is some evidence that erythrocyte infusion might reduce the exercise–heat performance of unacclimated subjects who become dehydrated. At high terrestrial altitude, the possible ergogenic effects of erythrocyte infusion are not well studied. In addition, it is becoming increasingly clear that the magnitude of the ergogenic effects and their mechanisms of action are modified by the subjects' acclimation state (e.g., heat or altitude) and physical fitness level. Finally, the interactive influences of environmental and exercise stress with erythrocyte infusion may produce extremely high hematocrits. The possible deleterious effects (to health as well as performance) of these high hematocrits which increase blood viscosity [30] need further evaluation. The interaction of increased blood viscosity with exercise and environmental stress may possibly have a potentiating effect on the clinical manifestations associated with hyperviscosity.

ACKNOWLEDGMENTS

The authors gratefully acknowledge Ms. Patricia DeMusis for preparing the manuscript.

The views, opinions, and findings contained in this report are those of the authors and should not be construed as an official Department of the Army position, policy, or decision, unless so designated by other official documentation. Approval for public release; distribution is unlimited.

REFERENCES

1. American College of Sports Medicine: Position stand on blood doping as an ergogenic aid. *Med Sci Sports Exer* 19:540–542, 1987.
2. Åstrand P-O: Quantification of exercise capability and evaluation of physical capacity in man. *Prog Cardiovasc Dis* 19:51–67, 1976.
3. Berglund B, Hemmingsson P: Effect of reinfusion of autologous blood on exercise performance in cross-country skiers. *Int J Sports Med* 8:231–233, 1987.
4. Berglund B, Hemmingsson P, Birgegard G: Detection of autologous blood transfusions in cross-country skiers. *Int J Sports Med* 8:66–70, 1987.
5. Burton AC: *Physiology and Biophysics of Circulation.* Chicago, Year Book Medical Publishers, 1972.
6. Brien AJ, Simon TL: The effects of red blood cells on 10-km race time. *JAMA* 257:2761–2769, 1987.
7. Buick FJ, Gledhill N, Froese AB, Spriet LL, Meyers EC: Effect of induced erythrocythemia on aerobic work capacity. *J Appl Physiol* 48:636–642, 1980.
8. Bullard RW: Studies on human sweat gland duct filling and skin hydration. *J Physiol (Paris)* 63:218–221, 1971.
9. Clausen JP: Circulatory adjustments to dynamic exercise and effects of physical training in normal subjects and in patients with coronary artery disease. *Prog Cardiovasc Dis* 18:459–495, 1976.
10. Dempsey JA, Hanson PG, Henderson KS: Exercise-induced arterial hypoxaemia in healthy human subjects at sea level. *J Physiol (Lond)* 355:161–175, 1984.
11. Ekblom B, Goldbarg AN, Gullbring B: Response to exercise after blood loss and reinfusion. *J Appl Physiol* 33:178–180, 1972.
12. Ekblom B, Wilson G, Åstrand P-O: Central circulation during exercise after venesection and reinfusion of red blood cells. *J Appl Physiol* 40:379–383, 1976.
13. Francesconi RP, Sawka MN, Dennis RC, Gonzalez RR, Young AJ, Valeri CR: Autologous red blood cell reinfusion: effects of stress and fluid regulatory hormones during exercise in the heat. *Aviat Space Environ Med* 59:133–137, 1988.
14. Gledhill N: Blood doping and related issues: a brief review. *Med Sci Sports Exerc* 14:183–189, 1982.
15. Gledhill N: The influence of altered blood volume and oxygen transport capacity on aerobic performance. In Terjung RL (ed): *Exercise and Sport Sciences Reviews.* New York, MacMillan, 1985, pp. 75–93.

16. Gledhill N, Spriet LL, Froese AB, Wilkes DL, Meyers EC: Acid–base status with induced erythrocythemia and its influence on arterial oxygenation during heavy exercise (abstract). *Med Sci Sports Exerc* 12:122, 1980.

17. Gleser MA, Vogel JA: Endurance capacity for prolonged exercise on the bicycle ergometer. *J Appl Physiol* 34:438–442, 1973.

18. Goforth HW, Campbell NL, Hodgdon JA, Sucec AA: Hematologic parameters of trained distance runners following induced erythrocythemia (abstract). *Med Sci Sports Exerc* 14:174, 1982.

19. Gonzalez RR, Sawka MN, Young AJ, Muza SR, Latzka WA, Dennis RC, Valeri CR, Pandolf KB: Erythrocyte reinfusion in heat acclimated males before and after 5% hypohydration improves sweating responses (abstract). *The Physiologist* 30:205, 1987.

20. Gonzalez RR, Sawka MN, Young AJ, Muza SR, Martin JW, Francesconi RP, Pandolf KB, Valeri CR: Influence of acute erythrocythemia on temperature regulation during exercise-heat stress (abstract). *Fed Proc* 45:529, 1986.

21. Gregersen MI, Rawson RA: Blood volume. *Physiol Rev* 39:307–342, 1959.

22. Grover RF, Weil JV, Reeves JT: Cardiovascular adaptations to exercise at high altitude. In Pandolf KB (ed): *Exercise and Sport Sciences Reviews*. New York, MacMillan, 1986, pp. 269–302.

23. Guyton AC, Jones CE, Coleman TG: *Circulatory Physiology: Cardiac Output and Its Regulation*. Philadelphia, WB Saunders, 1973.

24. Hartley LH: Effects of high altitude environment on the cardiovascular system of man. *JAMA* 215:242–244, 1971.

25. Holloszy JO: Biochemical adaptations to exercise aerobic metabolism. In Wilmore JH (ed): *Exercise and Sport Sciences Reviews*. New York, Academic Press, 1973, pp. 45–71.

26. Hortsman DH, Weiskopf R, Jackson RE: Work capacity during 3-week sojourn at 4300 m: effects of relative polycythemia. *J Appl Physiol* 49:311–318, 1980.

27. Kanstrup I, Ekblom B: Blood volume and hemoglobin concentration as determinants of maximal aerobic power. *Med Sci Sports Exerc* 16:256–262, 1984.

28. Latzka WA, Sawka MN, Muza SR, Gonzalez RR, Young AJ, Pandolf KB, Dennis RC, Martin JW, Wenger CB, Valeri CR: Ergogenic influence of erythrocyte reinfusion: aerobic power and thermoregulation (Technical Report No. T28/87). Natick, MA, U.S. Army Research Institute of Environmental Medicine, 1987.

29. Levine L, Evans WJ, Winsmann FR, Pandolf KB: Prolonged self-paced hard physical exercise comparing trained and untrained men. *Ergonomics* 25:393–400, 1982.

30. McGrath MA, Penny R: Paraproteinuria: blood hyperviscosity and clinical manifestations. *J Clin Invest* 58:1155–1162, 1976.

31. Mitchell JH, Blomquist G: Maximal oxygen uptake. *N Engl J Med* 284:1018–1022, 1971.

32. Morimoto T, Miki K, Nose H, Tanaka Y, Yamada S: Transvascular fluid shift after blood volume modification in relation to compliances of the total vascular bed and interstitial fluid space. *Jpn J Physiol* 31:869–878, 1981.

33. Muza SR, Sawka MN, Young AJ, Dennis RC, Gonzalez RR, Martin JW, Valeri CR: Elite Special Forces: physiological description and ergogenic influence of blood reinfusion. *Aviat Space Environ Med* 58:1001–1004, 1987.

34. Nag PK, Sen RN, Ray US: Optimal rate of work for mountaineers. *J Appl Physiol* 44:952–955, 1978.

35. Pace N, Lozner EI, Consolazio WV, Pitts GC, Pecora LJ: The increase in hypoxia tolerance of normal man accompanying the polycythemia induced by transfusion of erythrocytes. *Am J Physiol* 148:152–163, 1947.

36. Reeves JT, Grover BM, Sutton JR, Wagner PD, Cymerman A, Malconian MK, Rock PB, Young PM, Houston CS: Operation Everest II: preservation of cardiac function at extreme altitude. *J Appl Physiol* 63:531–539, 1987.

37. Robertson RJ, Gilcher R, Metz KF, Caspersen CJ, Allison TG, Abbott RA, Skrinar GS, Krause JR, Nixon PA: Hemoglobin concentration and aerobic work capacity in women following induced erythrocythemia. *J Appl Physiol* 57:568–575, 1984.
38. Robertson RJ, Gilcher R, Metz KF, Caspersen CJ, Allison TG, Abbott RA, Skrinar GS, Krause JR, Nixon PA: Effect of simulated altitude erythrocythemia in women on hemoglobin flow rate during exercise. *J Appl Physiol* 64:1644–1649, 1988.
39. Robertson RJ, Gilcher R, Metz KF, Skrinar GS, Allison TG, Bahnson HT, Abbott RA, Becker R, Falkel JE: Effect of induced erythrocythemia on hypoxia tolerance during physical exercise. *J Appl Physiol* 53:490–495, 1982.
40. Robinson BF, Epstein SE, Kahler RL, Braumwald E: Circulatory effect of acute expansion of blood volumes. *Circ Res* 19:26–32, 1966.
41. Rowell LB: Circulation. *Med Sci Sports Exerc* 1:15–22, 1969.
42. Rowell LB: Human cardiovascular adjustments to exercise and thermal stress. *Physiol Rev* 54:75–159, 1974.
43. Sawka MN, Dennis RC, Gonzalez RR, Young AJ, Muza SR, Martin JW, Wenger CB, Francesconi RP, Pandolf KB, Valeri CR: Influence of polycythemia on blood volume and thermoregulation during exercise–heat stress. *J Appl Physiol* 62:1165–1169, 1987.
44. Sawka MN, Francesconi RP, Young AJ, Pandolf KB: Influence of hydration level and body fluids on exercise performance in the heat. *JAMA* 252:1165–1169, 1984.
45. Sawka MN, Gonzalez RR, Young AJ, Muza SR, Pandolf KB, Latzka WA, Valeri CR, Dennis RC. Polycythemia and hydration: effects on thermoregulation and blood volume during exercise–heat stress. *Am J Physiol (Reg Int Comp Physiol)* 255:R456–R463, 1988.
46. Sawka MN, Wenger CB: Physiological responses to acute exercise-heat stress. In Pandolf KB, Sawka MN, Gonzalez RR (eds): *Human Performance Physiology and Environmental Medicine at Terrestrial Extremes.* Indianapolis, Benchmark Press, 1988, pp 97–151.
47. Sawka MN, Young AJ, Francesconi RP, Muza SR, Pandolf KB: Thermoregulatory and blood responses during exercise at graded hypohydration levels. *J Appl Physiol* 59:1394–1401, 1985.
48. Sawka MN, Young AJ, Muza SR, Gonzalez RR, Pandolf KB: Erythrocyte reinfusion and maximal aerobic power: an examination of modifying factors. *JAMA* 257:1496–1499, 1987.
49. Scatchard G, Batchelder AC, Brown A: Chemical, clinical and immunological studies on the products of human plasma fractionation. VI. The osmotic pressure of plasma and of serum albumin. *J Clin Invest* 23:458–464, 1944.
50. Senay LC Jr: Changes in plasma volume and protein content during exposures of working men to various temperatures before and after acclimation to heat: separation of the roles of cutaneous and skeletal muscle circulation. *J Physiol (Lond)* 224:61–81, 1972.
51. Senay LC, Mitchell D, Wyndham CH: Acclimatization in a hot, humid environment, body fluid adjustments. *J Appl Physiol* 40:786–796, 1976.
52. Spriet LL, Gledhill N, Froese AB, Wilkes DL: Effect of graded erythrocythemia on cardiovascular and metabolic responses to exercise. *J Appl Physiol* 61:1942–1948, 1986.
53. Stephenson LA, Wenger CB, Nadel ER: Acute plasma volume expansion during hypovolemic exercise. *Eur J Appl Physiol,* in revision.
54. Stone HO, Thompson HK, Schmidt-Nielsen K: Influence of erythrocytes on blood viscosity. *Am J Physiol* 214:913–918, 1968.
55. Squires RW, Buskirk ER: Aerobic capacity during acute exposure to simulated altitude, 914 to 2286 m. *Med Sci Sports Exerc* 14:36–40, 1982.

56. Taylor HL, Buskirk ER, Henschel A: Maximal oxygen intake as an objective measure of cardiorespiratory performance. *J Appl Physiol* 8:73–80, 1955.

57. Thomson JM, Stone JA, Ginsburg AD, Hamilton P: O_2 transport during exercise following blood reinfusion. *J Appl Physiol* 53:1213–1219, 1982.

58. Thrasher T, Wade CE, Keil LC, Ramsey DJ: Sodium balance and aldosterone during dehydration and rehydration in the dog. *Am J Physiol (Reg Int Comp Physiol)*: 247:R76–R83, 1984.

59. Valeri CR, Altschule MD: *Hypovolemic Anemia of Trauma: The Missing Blood Syndrome.* Boca Raton, FL, CRC Press, 1981.

60. Valeri CR, Donahue K, Feingold HM, Cassidy GP, Altschule MD: Increase in plasma volume after the transfusion of washed erythrocytes. *Surg Gynecol Obstet* 162:30–36, 1986.

61. Wagner PD: The lungs during exercise. *News Physiol Sci* 2:6–10, 1987.

62. Wagner PD, Gale GS, Moon RE, Torre-Bueno JR, Stolp BW, Saltzman HA: Pulmonary gas exchange in humans exercising at sea level and simulated altitude. *J Appl Physiol* 61:260–270, 1986.

63. Wagner PD, Sutton JR, Reeves JT, Cymerman A, Groves BM, Malconian MK: Operation Everest II: pulmonary gas exchange during a simulated ascent of Mt. Everest. *J Appl Physiol* 63:2348–2359, 1987.

64. Wasserman K, Mayerson HS: Mechanisms of plasma protein changes following saline infusion. *Am J Physiol* 170:1–10, 1952.

65. Welch HG, Mullin JP, Wilson GD, Lewis J: Effects of breathing O_2-enriched gas mixtures on metabolic rate during exercise. *Med Sci Sports Exerc* 6:26–32, 1974.

66. Welch HG, Petersen FB, Graham T, Klausen K, Secher N: Effects of hyperoxia on leg blood flow and metabolism during exercise. *J Appl Physiol* 42:385–390, 1977.

67. Williams MH, Wesseldine S, Somma T, Schuster R: The effect of induced erythrocythemia upon 5-mile treadmill run time. *Med Sci Sports Exerc* 13:169–175, 1981.

68. Wilson BA, Stainsby WN: Effect of O_2 breathing on RQ, blood flow and developed tension in *in situ* dog muscle. *Med Sci Sports Exerc* 10:167–170, 1978.

69. Young AJ, Cymerman A, Burse RL: Influence of cardiorespiratory fitness on the decrement in maximal aerobic power at high altitude. *Eur J Appl Physiol* 54:12–15, 1985.

70. Young AJ, Young PM: Human acclimatization to high terrestrial altitude. In Pandolf KB, Sawka MN, Gonzalez RR (eds): *Human Performance Physiology and Environmental Medicine at Terrestrial Extremes.* Indianapolis, Benchmark Press, 1988, pp 497–543.

9
Physiological Interactions between Pregnancy and Aerobic Exercise

LARRY A. WOLFE, Ph.D.
PATRICIA J. OHTAKE, M.Sc.
MICHELLE F. MOTTOLA, Ph.D.
MICHAEL J. McGRATH, M.D.

INTRODUCTION

Both pregnancy and aerobic conditioning are biological processes which involve striking physiological adaptations. Such adaptations may be in the same direction or in opposite directions, depending on the specific variable being studied (Table 9.1). For example, heart rate (HR) measured at rest or during submaximal exercise is augmented during pregnancy [29, 90] but is reduced as a result of physical conditioning [18, 146], whereas blood volume is increased by both stimuli [18, 98, 146]. Adaptations to pregnancy are mediated by endocrine factors. The physiological processes which lead to aerobic conditioning adaptations are poorly understood and have been loosely characterized in terms of recommended zones for exercise intensity, duration and frequency [4], and other basic training principles (e.g., overload and specificity).

Information on the interactive effects of pregnancy and physical conditioning is needed urgently because of the proliferation since the mid-1980s of physical conditioning programs for pregnant women [85]. In response to this popular trend, numerous medical and physical fitness authorities have formulated guidelines for prescription of exercise during pregnancy [3, 129, 163]. In the absence of a clear understanding of the physiology of exercise and physical conditioning during gestation, it is not surprising that significant disagreement exists among such authorities on issues such as the appropriate quantity and quality of exercise, methods for monitoring exercise intensity, and the validity of tests of aerobic fitness [25, 55, 163].

Of particular concern is that the purpose of most maternal adaptations during pregnancy is to accommodate the needs of the fetus and to preserve its well-being. On the other hand, adjustments to both acute and chronic exercise appear to be aimed at protecting maternal homeostasis. Thus, a real possibility exists of conflicting maternal and fetal demands for essential fuel substrates, blood flow, oxygen delivery, heat dissipation, etc. [102, 103]. This fear has been the basis for traditional

TABLE 9.1

Physiological Responses to Pregnancy and Physical Conditioning in the Resting State

Variable	First Trimester	Second Trimester	Late Gestation	Physical Conditioning (Nonpregnant Women)
$\dot{V}O_2$ (l/min)	↑	↑	↑↑	—
$\dot{V}O_2$ (ml/kg/min)	—	↓	↓	↑
$\dot{V}E:\dot{V}O_2$	↑	↑↑	↑↑	— or ↓
R	— or ↑	— or ↑	— or ↑	—
Heart rate (beats/min)	↑	↑↑	↑↑	↓↓
LVEDV (ml)	↑	↑↑	— or ↑	— or ↑
Stroke volume (ml/beat)	↑	↑↑	— or ↑	↑↑
Ejection fraction (%)	— or ↑	— or ↑	— or ↑	— or ↑
$\dot{Q}c$ (l/min)	↑	↑↑	— or ↑	— or ↓
Systolic blood pressure (mm Hg)	— or ↓	— or ↓	— or ↑	— or ↑
Diastolic blood pressure (mm Hg)	— or ↓	— or ↓	— or ↑	↓
Blood volume (l)	↑↑	↑↑↑	↑↑↑	↑
Cardiac mass (g)	↑	↑↑	↑↑	— or ↑

$\dot{V}O_2$ = oxygen uptake; $\dot{V}E:\dot{V}O_2$ = ventilatory equivalent for oxygen; R = respiratory exchange ratio; LVEDV = left ventricular end-diastolic volume; $\dot{Q}c$ = cardiac output. — = no change; single arrow = small increase or decrease; double arrow = moderate increase or decrease; triple arrow = substantial increase or decrease. (Changes are relative to nonpregnant, sedentary state.)

medical advice that pregnant women should rest. Again, without a clear knowledge of the limits of maternal and fetal physiological reserve, a conservative approach of obstetricians toward maternal exercise programs is the only justifiable course of action [3].

This review summarizes the current state of knowledge concerning maternal and fetal adaptations to both acute and chronic aerobic-type exertion. Particular emphasis is placed on maternal metabolic and cardiopulmonary adaptations and their implications for fetal well-being. This information can serve as a basis for development of guidelines for aerobic exercise in pregnancy and as a guide for future scientific investigation.

MATERNAL ADAPTATIONS TO PREGNANCY AT REST

Adaptations to pregnancy observed in the resting state are generally well documented and have been reviewed in detail by others [7, 66, 102, 103, 120]. Therefore this section is limited to an integrated overview of the basic metabolic and cardiorespiratory physiology of pregnancy.

Metabolic Rate

Metabolic rate, as reflected by resting oxygen uptake ($\dot{V}O_2$) increases gradually and reaches at term a value approximately 20–30% above that of the nonpregnant state [9, 16, 17, 90, 136, 161]. The absolute increase is approximately proportional to the change in fat-free body mass which results from fetal and uteroplacental growth and other anatomic adaptations [161]. However, as described below, increased pulmonary ventilation, cardiac work, and other factors are also of importance, particularly in early gestation. Fuel utilization as reflected by the respiratory exchange ratio ($R = \dot{V}CO_2:\dot{V}O_2$) indicates mixed utilization of fat and carbohydrate [9, 16, 17, 90, 137]. Two investigations [9, 90] reported moderately higher R values at rest in the pregnant versus nonpregnant state, suggesting augmented peripheral utilization of carbohydrate.

Cardiovascular Function

Cardiac output ($\dot{Q}c$) at rest becomes increasingly "hyperkinetic" during the first two pregnancy trimesters as a result of several interactive endocrine effects (Fig. 9.1). HR increased abruptly by approximately 7 beats/minute during the 1st 4 weeks of gestation, possibly due to the influence of human chorionic gonadotropin [29]. This is followed by a further gradual increase, reaching a plateau approximately 15 beats/ minute above resting HR in the nonpregnant state. This additional increase in HR may be a regulatory adjustment to the other hemodynamic and vascular changes of pregnancy, which are described below [29].

Stroke volume (SV) is also augmented during early and midgestation in association with an increase in venous return, increased aortic capacitance, and reduced peripheral vascular resistance [10, 147, 175, 176, 181]. There is a gradual expansion of maternal blood volume to approximately 40–50% above nonpregnant control levels [77, 140]. Red cell volume increases to a lesser extent, resulting in lower values for hematocrit and hemoglobin concentration and a relative state of anemia [105, 160]. The increase in maternal blood volume is partly offset by increased venous capacitance related to venous relaxation and enlargement of the pelvic veins. These effects are attributed to increased production of estrogen and progesterone [51, 64, 65].

Specific effects of pregnancy on the heart include an increase in left ventricular end-diastolic volume (LVEDV), only a moderate increase in left ventricular mass, and an increase in the left ventricular wall thick-

FIGURE 9.1

Cardiovascular adaptations to pregnancy in the resting state. Solid arrows *indicate positive effects;* dashed arrows *indicate negative effects. IVC = inferior vena cava; LVEDV = left ventricular end-diastolic volume. (Reproduced with permission from Hall P: Cardiovascular adaptations to physical conditioning during pregnancy. Unpublished master's thesis, Kingston, Canada, Queen's University, 1987.)*

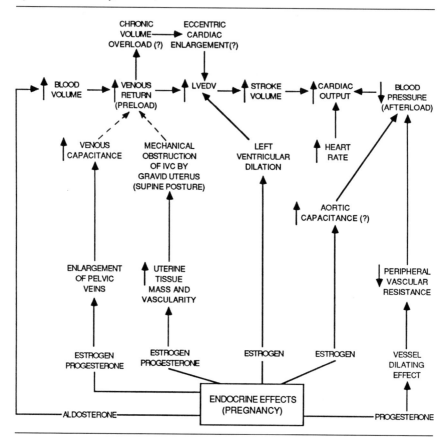

ness-to-radius (t:r) ratio [84, 93, 152]. Katz et al. [84] attributed left ventricular dilation in pregnancy to a state of chronic hemodynamic volume overload. However, data obtained by Morton et al. from guinea pigs [75, 118] suggested that the heart is "remodeled" in response to endocrine factors so that LVEDV increases without significantly altering ventricular elastic properties or filling pressure (preload). As summarized by Morton et al. [120], "a relatively thin ventricle delivers a larger stroke volume faster to a more compliant, low resistance arterial system." The expected increase in wall tension (afterload) associated with an increased t:r ratio is apparently avoided as a result of increased aortic capacitance [84] and reduced peripheral vascular resistance. The latter has been attributed to the vessel-dilating effects of reproductive hormones [175] and the vascular shunt created by growth of the uteroplacental unit. Measures of left ventricular performance are generally well preserved or slightly augmented [24, 84, 109, 111, 151, 152]. Slight improvement in indexes of resting left ventricular performance might be associated with increased circulating estrogen levels [88, 152, 181].

Since the increase in $\dot{Q}c$ is balanced by reduced peripheral vascular resistance, blood pressure is generally unchanged or moderately reduced in healthy pregnant women [152, 168]. Thus, myocardial work and oxygen demand are not greatly increased during pregnancy despite significant increases in both HR and $\dot{Q}c$.

The physiological scenario described above is applicable until the 3rd trimester, when blood flow in the inferior vena cava can be impeded by the enlarging uterus, resulting in venous pooling and a decline in venous return. This effect is most prominent in the supine posture, and is less pronounced in the sitting and left lateral decubitus positions [86, 87, 95, 176, 180]. As a result, both SV and $\dot{Q}c$ may be significantly reduced relative to values in the 2nd trimester, and some women may experience arterial hypotension (supine hypotensive syndrome). In order to compensate for the reduction in venous return, HR may be further augmented in the supine versus upright or left lateral postures [176].

Pulmonary Ventilation
Respiratory adaptations to pregnancy include modifications of resting lung volumes, capacities, and breathing mechanics (Fig. 9.2). As a result of uterine enlargement, diaphragmatic mid-position in the upright posture is raised by up to 4 cm [1, 144]. This is compensated by increases of approximately 2 cm in both the anteroposterior and transverse diameters of the thoracic cage. The substernal angle also increases from approximately 70° in the 1st trimester to 105° at term, and the circumference of the thoracic cage is increased by approximately 5–7 cm [1, 144]. These anatomic changes result in a reduction in functional residual capacity which is effectively offset by an increase in inspiratory capacity [1, 13, 37, 57, 90]. Therefore, there is little or no reduction in vital capacity, and only a modest decrease in total lung capacity [1, 144]. These anatomic changes tend to augment the oxygen cost of breathing because of a greater level of diaphragmatic work [11].

Changes to the airways include muscosal swelling related to capillary engorgement which can simulate inflammation, making talking and nose breathing difficult during late gestation [144]. However, lung compli-

FIGURE 9.2

Pulmonary adaptations to pregnancy in the resting state. FRC = functional residual capacity; IC = inspiratory capacity.

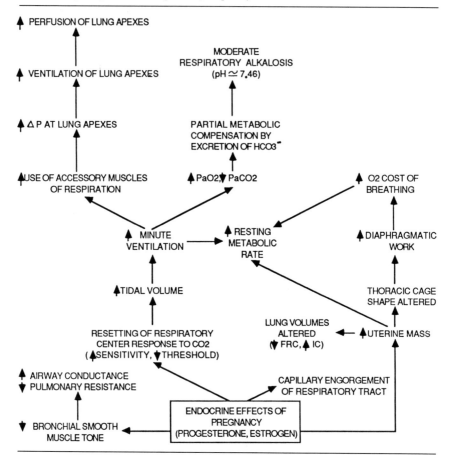

ance increases approximately 36% and airway resistance is reduced, apparently as a result of increased progesterone production leading to decreased smooth-muscle tone [57].

Pulmonary minute ventilation ($\dot{V}E$) increased progressively during pregnancy and reaches a peak in late gestation approximately 50% above nonpregnant values [21]. This is reported to be due to a larger tidal volume (VT) with little or no increase in breathing frequency [1, 9, 21, 90, 137]. Physiological dead space increases moderately and there is a substantial rise in alveolar ventilation [137]. The increase in $\dot{V}E$ is present early in pregnancy and is evident prior to significant changes in diaphragmatic function or thoracic cage dimensions. In this regard, several investigators have confirmed that increased circulating levels of progesterone augment pulmonary ventilation [20, 96, 107, 158]. Lyons and Antonio [107] hypothesized that during pregnancy the respiratory sensitivity to carbon dioxide was increased and the threshold for this response was also reduced.

The increase in $\dot{V}E$ during pregnancy is proportionately greater than that described above for $\dot{V}O_2$ [90, 137] resulting in an increased ventilatory equivalent for oxygen ($\dot{V}E:\dot{V}O_2$). The increased ventilatory response also leads to a reduction in arterial PCO_2 to approximately 30 mm Hg and an increase in arterial PO_2 to approximately 100 mm Hg. The resulting respiratory alkalosis is only partly compensated by excretion of bicarbonate, so that arterial pH remains moderately elevated to approximately 7.46 [9, 21, 78, 137]. The primary purpose of augmented ventilatory responses during pregnancy appears to be to reduce arterial PCO_2 rather than to increase PO_2. The resulting mild maternal alkalosis promotes placental gas exchange, especially during early pregnancy when the fetal cardiovascular system is not yet developed [99] and may also protect against fetal acidosis [96].

Consideration of body temperatures at rest and during exercise is essential for a correct assessment of the blood gases [103]. Blood analyzed for respiratory gases at a temperature below body temperature provides erroneously low arterial PO_2 and PCO_2 values and a high pH [162].

Pulmonary diffusing capacity is reported to be normal [14] or moderately reduced [56]. However, any impediment to oxygen diffusion will be partly offset by the increased efficiency of gas distribution in the lungs [37].

Closing capacity (CC) is the lung volume at which dependent lung zones cease to ventilate, presumably as a result of airway closure [94], and is the sum of closing volume (CV) measured during a vital capacity (VC) expiration and residual volume (RV). CC does not change during pregnancy, whereas CV increases [15, 35, 53]. Well-documented reductions in RV during pregnancy [1, 37] with an unchanged VC, lead to the observed increase in CV. The unchanged CC indicates that airway closure occurs at the same absolute lung volume during pregnancy [35]. A reduction of functional residual capacity (FRC) in the presence of an unchanged CC occasionally allows CC to exceed FRC [35, 150], suggesting that airway closure may influence ventilation–perfusion relationships, and subsequently arterial oxygenation. However, Russell and Chambers [150] found no correlation between arterial oxygenation and a CC greater than FRC, when patients were supine. In this regard, a marked redistribution of pulmonary blood flow in the apical direction has been reported [135] and has been attributed to reduced precapillary vascular resistance in the upper lung zones and to the increased $\dot{V}E$.

This increase requires activation of the accessory muscles of respiration leading to increased pressure changes in the upper thoracic zones and a redistribution of inspired air toward the lung apices. Neurohumoral mechanisms ensure accurate matching of pulmonary blood flow to maintain adequate ventilation–perfusion ratios.

MATERNAL RESPONSES TO SUBMAXIMAL EXERCISE

During standard submaximal non-weight-bearing exercise, the net oxygen cost of work is either unchanged or moderately increased [46, 69, 90, 136, 161], suggesting that mechanical efficiency and the contractile performance of skeletal muscle are not altered significantly during pregnancy.

Fuel utilization during submaximal exercise is a subject of much controversy and requires further study. Current knowledge is based primarily on comparisons of R values at similar power outputs in the pregnant versus nonpregnant state. The validity of such comparisons depends on subjects being in a physiological steady state during respiratory gas analyses. Furthermore, results may also be altered by variations in diet or by lactation [17, 89]. Finally, subjects should be compared at the same relative percentage of maximal $\dot{V}O_2$ ($\dot{V}O_2max$) since the ratio of fat to carbohydrate utilization in nonpregnant subjects is more closely related to relative (percentage of maximum) rather than absolute power output [18, 146].

Fuel utilization during submaximal exercise has been studied by several investigators. Knuttgen and Emerson [90] reported no difference in R at a standard power output of 60 W in late gestation compared to 6 weeks postpartum in 13 healthy women. Pernoll et al. [137] also observed consistent mean R values in a group of 12 healthy women studied during steady-state cycling at 50 W throughout pregnancy and at various intervals postpartum. These results suggest no important change in the ratio of fat to carbohydrate utilization at absolute levels of moderate submaximal exercise. However, as discussed below, HR is known to be higher during standard exercise in pregnancy. Consequently, subjects may have been working at a higher percentage of $\dot{V}O_2max$, suggesting a moderate shift toward fat metabolism. Since $\dot{V}O_2max$ was not measured in these studies, this hypothesis remains unsubstantiated.

In contrast to the results of the studies cited above, the findings of Clapp et al. [31] suggested enhanced utilization of carbohydrate versus fat during pregnancy. The authors reported a shift in the relationship between relative exercise intensity ($\dot{V}O_2$ expressed as percentage of preconception $\dot{V}O_2max$) during steady-state treadmill running in recreational runners studied at approximately 2 months preconception and 20 and 32 weeks' gestation. The mean steady-state R value was similar at each observation time, despite significantly lower relative exercise intensities at 20 and 32 weeks' gestation compared to preconception (57% [± 5] and 47% [± 2] vs. 74% [± 3]). These results implied that carbohydrate utilization by exercising muscle is increased during pregnancy. This viewpoint was further supported by pre- to postexercise changes in blood glucose levels. In the preconception assessment, mean blood glucose levels rose from 5.19 (± 0.14) to 6.63 (± 0.23) mmol/l. At 20 weeks' gestation, the mean preexercise level was lower (4.46 [± 0.16] mmol/l) and did not change after exercise (4.45 [± 0.08] mmol/l). Finally, at 32 weeks' gestation the mean blood glucose level fell from 5.30 (± 0.19) to 4.55 (± 0.15) mmol/l. Unfortunately, the design of this study did not permit firm conclusions regarding carbohydrate metabolism in exercising pregnant women since subjects' responses were not compared at the same absolute or relative exercise intensities and the relative exercise intensities during pregnancy were estimated as a fraction of $\dot{V}O_2max$ measured prior to conception rather than values obtained during pregnancy.

Resolution of this controversy is important in view of the potential effects of exercise-induced maternal hypoglycemia on fetal nutritional status. This will require actual measurement of maternal $\dot{V}O_2max$ and assessment of blood glucose levels before, during, and after maternal exercise of varying intensity and duration and at different time intervals during gestation.

Cardiovascular responses to light and moderate intensity exercise in the upright posture (Table 9.2) are parallel to those described above for the resting state. Guzman and Caplan [69] reported higher values for $\dot{Q}c$ and SV throughout gestation compared to the postpartum period during upright cycling at standard power outputs of 25, 41, and 57 W, with only a slight decrease near term at the highest power output. Ueland et al. [176] also reported a "hyperkinetic" circulation during upright cycling at power outputs representing mild (16 W) and moderate (33 W) levels of exertion. During mild exercise $\dot{Q}c$ and SV peaked at 20–24 weeks and remained elevated until term. During moderate exercise, $\dot{Q}c$ and SV also peaked at 20–24 weeks' gestation, but fell progressively until term. Values at 38–40 weeks were similar to postpartum reference measurements. In a later study, Ueland et al. [177] observed that the $\dot{Q}c$ and SV during mild intensity cycling peaked by 20–24 weeks and remained elevated above postpartum reference values until term. Ueland et al. [176] suggested that the tendency for $\dot{Q}c$ and SV to fall in late gestation during moderate exertion results from peripheral pooling of blood and mechanical obstruction of venous return by the gravid uterus.

Good agreement exists that HR during standard submaximal exercise rises progressively during pregnancy and is significantly higher than in

TABLE 9.2
Physiological Adaptations to Pregnancy and Physical Conditioning during Standard Weight-Supported Submaximal Exercise

Variable	First Trimester	Second Trimester	Late Gestation	Physical Conditioning (Nonpregnant Women)
$\dot{V}O_2$ (l/min)	— or ↑	— or ↑	— or ↑	—
$\dot{V}O_2$ (ml/kg/min)	↓	↓ ↓	↓ ↓ ↓	— or ↑
$\dot{V}E:\dot{V}O_2$	↑ ↑	↑ ↑	↑ ↑	— or ↓
R	— or ↑	— or ↑	— or ↑	↓
PA_{CO_2}	↓ ↓	↓ ↓	↓ ↓	—
Heart rate (beats/min)	↑	↑ ↑	↑ ↑	↓ ↓
Stroke volume (ml/beat)	↑	↑ ↑	— or ↑	↑ ↑
$\dot{Q}c$ (l/min)	↑	↑ ↑	— or ↑	— or ↓
Systolic blood pressure (mm Hg)	— or ↓	— or ↓	— or ↑	— or ↑
Diastolic blood pressure	— or ↓	— or ↓	— or ↑	↓
RPE	?	?	?	↓ ↓

$\dot{V}O_2$ = oxygen uptake; $\dot{V}E:\dot{V}O_2$ = ventilatory equivalent for oxygen; R = respiratory exchange ratio; PA_{CO_2} = partial pressure of alveolar carbon dioxide; $\dot{Q}c$ = cardiac output; RPE = rating of perceived exertion. — = no change; single arrow = small increase or decrease; double arrow = moderate increase or decrease; triple arrow = substantial increase or decrease; ? = no data availble. (Changes are relative to nonpregnant, sedentary state.)

the nonpregnant state [69, 90, 119, 177]. The greatest increase is reported to occur at low exercise levels [69] and may be most important during late gestation when the ability to augment SV may be limited [113]. In the absence of pregnancy-induced hypertension, values for arterial blood pressure during standard submaximal exercise are generally similar to those of the nonpregnant state due to the off-setting effects of a hyperkinetic $\dot{Q}c$ and reduced peripheral vascular resistance [5, 10, 43, 70, 167]. The effects of different exercising postures on HR–blood pressure relationships remain to be clarified, and additional research is needed on maternal cardiovascular responses to strenuous exercise.

Pulmonary adaptations to submaximal exercise during pregnancy are also similar to those described above for the resting state. Both minute $\dot{V}E$ and $\dot{V}E:\dot{V}O_2$ are increased relative to the nonpregnant state, resulting in lower partial pressures of alveolar and arterial carbon dioxide [9, 69, 90, 137]. The data of Guzman and Caplan [69] indicated that the greater ventilatory response was due to an increase in breathing frequency; however, results of other studies suggested that an augmented V_T is more important [90, 137].

Prowse and Gaensler [141] found that 60–70% of women experience dyspnea during pregnancy. This sensation of breathlessness occurs early in pregnancy and disappears by term [59, 60] and is not correlated with changes in lung function [37] or encroachment of the gravid uterus on the thorax. Dyspnea during pregnancy appears to be related to an individual's adaptation to the increase in ventilation which accompanies the pregnant state [116]. Dyspnea is experienced when a ventilatory response occurs that is inappropriate for the demand [26, 79] and is present in early pregnancy when the discrepancy between ventilation and $\dot{V}_{O_2}$ is the greatest [141]. The sensation of dyspnea appears to be related to alveolar P_{CO_2} (PA_{CO_2}) levels, being most prevalent when PA_{CO_2} is lowest [59]. This suggests that women with a more sensitive respiratory control system experience a low PA_{CO_2} and subsequent dyspnea more frequently [60].

Dyspnea occurs much less frequently during exercise than at rest [60], but when present is maximal when PA_{CO_2} is at its lowest point [59]. Rating of perceived exertion (RPE) has been suggested as a useful measure of exercise intensity and has been found to correlate better with $\dot{V}_E$ than with HR in nonpregnant individuals [128]. However, exertional dyspnea during pregnancy does not correlate well with $\dot{V}_E$ or dyspnea index [59], suggesting that RPE may be altered during pregnancy. RPE has been recommended as a method for monitoring and prescribing exercise intensity during pregnancy [25]. However, the usefulness of RPE in pregnant women remains to be substantiated due to the augmented ventilatory sensitivity and variability in dyspnea experienced during exercise.

MAXIMAL EXERCISE RESPONSES DURING PREGNANCY

Very little reliable information exists concerning the effects of pregnancy on $\dot{V}_{O_2}$max because of the potential risks involved and the need for a rapid and reliable method for the detection of fetal distress during strenuous maternal exertion (Table 9.3). To our knowledge, only one study [154] has attempted serial measurements of $\dot{V}_{O_2}$max during and following pregnancy. As discussed previously by Lotgering et al. [103], several studies have attempted to predict $\dot{V}_{O_2}$max from HR responses during submaximal exercise. Soiva et al. [167] and Sandström [155] reported a moderate reduction in physical working capacity (PWC^{170}), whereas others [39, 58] reported no significant change in this index. Using the Åstrand-Åstrand nomogram, Erkkola [48] observed values for predicted $\dot{V}_{O_2}$max (ml/kg/minute) for pregnant women which were similar to those of healthy

TABLE 9.3
Effects of Pregnancy on Maximal Aerobic Power (V̇O$_2$max) in Healthy Pregnant Women

Authors	Subjects	Index of V̇O$_2$ Max	Time of Assessments Pregnant	Time of Assessments Nonpregnant	Result
Gemzell et al. [58]	Healthy women (n = 20)	PWC[170] (W)	Approximately 14, 20, 30, and 36 weeks gestation	3 days and approximately 4.5 and 8.5 weeks postpartum	No difference pregnant vs. nonpregnant
Dahlström and Ihrman [39]	Healthy women (n = 46)	PWC[170] (W)	Approximately 20, 27, and 36 weeks gestation	2 months postpartum	No difference pregnant vs. nonpregnant
Sovia et al. [167]	Women with "normal pregnancy" (n = 13); pregnant controls (n = 19)	PWC[170] (W)	Late gestation	—	"Slightly" lower in pregnant group
Sandström [155]	Primigravidae (n = 10)	PWC[170] (W)	During first trimester	2 weeks after legal abortion	Values significantly lower in pregnancy
Erkkola [48]	Healthy primigravidae (n = 118)	Åstrand nomogram (predicted V̇O$_2$max, ml/kg/min)	Two weeks before term	—	Values similar to nonpregnant reference group
Dibblee and Graham [43]	"Unfit" women (n = 8)	CAFT (predicted V̇O$_2$max, l/min)	Last month of trimesters 1, 2, and 3	4 months postpartum	Gradual ↑ during gestation; ↓ postpartum
Sady et al. [154]	Healthy women (n = 8)	Measured V̇O$_2$ peak (l/min)	25 ± 3 weeks gestation	2 and 6 months postpartum	No differences V̇O$_2$max or heart rate max in pregnancy vs. postpartum

CAFT = Canadian Aerobic Fitness Test; PWC = physical working capacity.

nonpregnant women. Finally, the data of Dibblee and Graham [43] obtained using the Canadian Aerobic Fitness Test suggested that the absolute $\dot{V}O_2max$ (l/minute) of women of low initial physical fitness may actually increase as pregnancy progresses, perhaps as an adaptation to greater exertion during day-to-day weight-bearing activities. The authors also reported that predicted $\dot{V}O_2max$ values show an approximate average reduction of 2 ml/kg/minute during each pregnancy trimester.

The validity of the results cited above depends on the assumption used in submaximal predictions of $\dot{V}O_2max$ that HRmax is unchanged during pregnancy. Results obtained by Wiswell et al. [183] suggested that this assumption is not valid. The authors compared the responses of 9 pregnant women (mean gestational age-26 weeks) with those of 10 nonpregnant control subjects during exhaustive treadmill exercise. Values for peak $\dot{V}O_2$ were significantly lower (1.62 l/minute or 26.3 ml/kg/minute vs. 2.26 l/minute or 39.1 ml/kg/minute) in the pregnant group. Peak HR reached only 169 beats/minute, which was 23 beats/minute below age-predicted HRmax. The authors acknowledged that it was not possible to match the two groups for physical fitness and did not describe the criteria used to ensure that a true $\dot{V}O_2max$ was achieved. This may be a particularly important oversight since volitional fatigue may be achieved at a lower relative exercise level in pregnant subjects.

In contrast to the results of Wiswell et al., Sady et al. [154] reported no significant change in HRmax measured in eight women at approximately 25 weeks' gestation and at both 2 and 6 months postpartum. Mean values were 185 ($\pm$ 4), 188 ($\pm$ 6), and 188 ($\pm$ 7) beats/minute, respectively. Corresponding values for measured $\dot{V}O_2max$ were 1.99 ($\pm$ 0.42), 1.89 ($\pm$ 0.36), and 2.03 ($\pm$ 0.28) l/minute, suggesting no important effect of gestation on aerobic working capacity. Since measurements were not made during late gestation, the hypothesis that $\dot{V}O_2max$ and HRmax are reduced by pregnancy remains to be tested adequately. This will require a controlled longitudinal study design with serial measurements obtained throughout pregnancy and in the nonpregnant, nonlactating state. The criterion for achievement of a maximal response in such a study should be achievement of a plateau in $\dot{V}O_2$ during graded exercise testing. In this regard, variables such as peak HR, R values, and postexercise lactic acid values may be altered during pregnancy and may be unreliable criteria for achievement of a true maximal response.

Another controversial issue is whether maximal anaerobic power is affected by pregnancy. Artal et al. [9] reported significantly lower R values at the peak of exhaustive treadmill exercise in a group of 88 pregnant women (mean gestational age = 28.8 [$\pm$ 1.6] weeks) compared to a group of healthy nonpregnant women with a similar mean age. At rest, R was significantly higher in the pregnant group. Mean values for $\dot{V}CO_2$ and VT during peak exercise were also significantly lower and values for respiratory frequency and the $\dot{V}E:\dot{V}O_2$ equivalent also tended to be somewhat lower ($P > 0.05$). The authors concluded that pregnant women use less carbohydrate during strenuous exercise, and their ability to exercise anaerobically may be compromised. This may be a protective mechanism to maintain carbohydrate stores or to avoid production of respiratory alkalosis and associated reductions in fetal PCO_2 and PO_2 [115].

Avoidance of hypoglycemia during or following exercise may be particularly important because of fetal dependence on carbohydrate as an energy source. Clearly, further study is needed to determine the relative risks and benefits of strenuous versus moderate aerobic exercise during pregnancy.

FETAL WELL-BEING DURING ACUTE MATERNAL EXERCISE

A central issue related to exercise during pregnancy is whether fetal well-being is compromised as a result of blood flow redistribution, increased maternal core/fetal temperature, or increased maternal carbohydrate utilization [163]. The majority of existing studies of exercise and uterine blood flow have been conducted on laboratory animals rather than humans. The investigations of Lotgering et al. [100, 101] in sheep support the hypothesis that uterine blood flow decreases in proportion to both the intensity and duration of exercise and reaches approximately a 25% reduction during prolonged strenuous exercise (40 minutes at 70% of $\dot{V}O_2max$). Results from other laboratories suggested that myometrial blood flow in sheep may be compromised to a greater extent than cotyledonary flow, presumably due to a greater vascular sensitivity to circulating catecholamines [38, 68, 73]. The reduction in uterine blood flow, however, may not seriously compromise oxygen delivery to the uterus since it is at least partly offset by exercise-induced hemoconcentration [67, 102].

Fetal adaptability to increased maternal core temperature during exercise is not yet well understood [45, 102, 159]. In exercising sheep, Lotgering et al. [101] observed fetal temperatures which were approximately 0.5°C above maternal temperature changes. After strenuous exercise (40 minutes at 70% $\dot{V}O_2max$), fetal temperature required approximately 40 minutes to return to preexercise levels despite a substantial fetal–maternal temperature gradient. The authors pointed out that as augmented fetal temperature may increase metabolic rate via the Q_{10} effect causing rightward shifts in both the fetal and maternal oxyhemoglobin dissociation curves and perhaps reduced uterine blood flow [102]. In theory, these changes could contribute to fetal hypoxia by reducing fetal oxygen supply and increasing metabolic oxygen demand.

TABLE 9.4
Characteristics of Fetal Heart Rate (FHR) in a Healthy Unstressed Fetus

- FHR BASELINE: 120–160 beats/min
- BASELINE VARIABILITY > 5 beats/min
- FHR acceleration in association with fetal movement
- Absence or infequent occurrence of FHR decelerations > 15 beats/min.

As outlined above, strenuous exercise significantly increases use of carbohydrate by skeletal muscle. However, the data of Artal et al. [9] suggested that the ability of pregnant women to metabolize carbohydrate during strenuous exercise may be limited—perhaps as a protective adaptation to avoid compromising glucose availability to the fetus. In contrast, the recent findings of Clapp et al. [31] suggested that hypoglycemia may be observed after strenuous exercise in late gestation due to enhanced rather than reduced use of carbohydrate by skeletal muscle. The preliminary report of Treadway and Young [174] also indicated that fetal glucose uptake after strenuous exercise in pregnant rats was reduced by approximately 40% and that this effect was attributable to increased glucose uptake during exercise by maternal skeletal muscle. Clearly, more research will be needed to determine whether maternal exercise alters fetal glucose utilization at different stages of gestation.

From a practical viewpoint, uteroplacental oxygen delivery, fetal temperature, and fetal carbohydrate homeostasis are difficult or impossible to assess at this time in exercising human subjects. On the other hand, fetal heart rate (FHR) can be assessed noninvasively by auscultation, phonocardiography, external abdominal electrocardiogram (ECG), Doppler ultrasound, or two-dimensional ultrasound directed M-mode echocardiography [130, 131]. Under most circumstances, FHR is closely correlated with fetal cardiac output, since the Frank-Starling mechanism of the fetus does not operate as effectively as in the adult [148]. Characteristics of FHR in a healthy unstressed fetus are summarized in Table 9.4.

Of particular importance to the present discussion is fetal bradycardia (FHR baseline <120 beats/minute for >2 minutes). Bradycardia is the initial response of the normal fetus to acute hypoxia or asphyxia, but can also occur in response to other variables including heart block or congenital cardiac abnormalities, pharmacologic agents such as beta-blocking drugs, or hypothermia [131]. Profound bradycardia (FHR <100 beats/minute), especially if associated with normal baseline variability, may be seen in response to mild hypoxia and usually does not lead to fetal decompensation [131]. The mechanism leading to fetal bradycardia during hypoxia is not completely understood. It is usually also accompanied by hypertension and blood flow redistribution toward vital areas

TABLE 9.5
Fetal Heart Rate (FHR) Responses Associated with Varying Degrees of Hypoxia or Asphyxia

FHR Pattern	Measurement Criterion	Postulated Clinical Significance
Deceleration	Transient reduction of FHR >15 beats/min from previous FHR baseline	Normal FHR response to mild or transient hypoxia
Moderate bradycardia	FHR baseline 100–120 beats/min for more than 2 min	Initial response to hypoxia
Profound bradycardia	FHR baseline <100 beats/min for more than 2 min	Normal FHR adaptation to prolonged hypoxia
Tachycardia	FHR baseline >160 beats/min for more than 2 min	Compensatory adaptation during recovery from hypoxia
Reduced long-term variability	FHR baseline variability ≤6 beats/min	Probable cerebral tissue asphyxia

such as the brain, heart, adrenal gland, and placenta [32, 131]. These changes may be the result of increased vagal tone in response to peripheral and/or central chemoreceptor input.

As outlined in Table 9.5, several other FHR patterns are associated with different degrees of hypoxia or asphyxia. Tachycardia may be observed during recovery from hypoxia or asphyxia, presumably as a response to increased sympathoadrenal activity. Tachycardia may also result from maternal or fetal infection, beta-adrenergic angonist and parasympathetic blocking drugs, thyrotoxicosis, ectopic pacemaker activity, sinus arrhythmias, or extreme prematurity [131]. Fetal decelerations are transient reduction in FHR (>15 beats/minute for <2 minutes) which may occur in response to a mild or transient hypoxic stimulus. Finally, long-term variability refers to moderate changes in the FHR baseline which are thought to be caused by sporadic input from various cortical areas to the cardiovascular control center in the medulla oblongata, with subsequent effects on FHR via the vagus nerve. Loss of long-term variability of FHR suggests severe cerebral tissue asphyxia which can occur in association with severe or prolonged hypoxia but may also be due to other factors, including maternal drug ingestion or recording artifact [131].

In view of the hypothesis that exercise reduces uterine blood flow and the association of various FHR patterns with fetal hypoxia, several early investigations explored the use of a standard exercise test for the early detection of uteroplacental insufficiency or fetal distress. Hon and Wohlgemuth [74] observed the fetal ECG during the 3rd trimester in 26 obstetric patients before and after performance of a version of the Master's 2-step test. Ten of these women had normal pregnancies, 5 had preeclampsia, 2 exhibited chronic hypertension, and 2 exhibited mild diabetes. Seven additional patients (including one with essential hypertension) exhibited postmaturity with gestation times between 42 and 43 weeks. In 20 of the patients, no significant FHR abnormalities were observed. Three patients with fetal/umbilical cord difficulties had moderate preexercise FHR abnormalities that were accentuated by exercise. The fetuses of two additional patients who eventually required cesarian section exhibited moderate bradycardia, irregularity, and tachycardia following exercise. In a 3rd patient who required cesarian section, marked fetal bradycardia followed by prolonged tachycardia were observed after exercise.

Pomerance et al. [142] later studied FHR using auscultation immediately before and following an Åstrand-type cycle ergometer exercise test in 54 apparently healthy pregnant women (gestational age = 35–37 weeks). During labor–delivery, 11 of the fetuses of these women exhibited fetal distress, defined as one or more of the following: bradycardia with FHR <120 beats/minute, meconium-stained amniotic fluid, or 1-minute Apgar score <7. This was attributed to uteroplacental insufficiency in four cases, compromised umbilical cord circulation in six cases, and no apparent cause in one case. During testing, five fetuses showed changes in FHR >16 beats/minute, indicating a "positive" test. Four of those with positive tests were fetuses with distress at parturition attributable to uteroplacental insufficiency, while one fetus with no distress had a positive test result. Finally, none of the fetuses with distress due to compromised umbilical cord circulation exhibited positive responses to maternal exercise. These early studies demonstrated a greater incidence of FHR abnormalities in women with known obstetric problems. However, the usefulness of FHR monitoring during and following exercise depends on development of criteria for the identification of abnormal responses which are sufficiently sensitive and specific to allow the reliable detection of compromised uteroplacental function. Thus, it is extremely important to determine the FHR responses to material exercise which represent either the normal response or normal variants which are associated with normal birth outcomes.

A summary of recent investigations of FHR responses to exercise from apparently healthy women with varying levels of aerobic fitness is presented in Table 9.6. In the majority of these studies, exercise consisted of upright cycling, walking, or jogging at a submaximal intensity. Exceptions were the investigations of Artal et al. [6, 8], in which a progressive symptom-limited maximal treadmill test was employed, and those of Goodlin and Buckley [63] and Pijpers et al. [179], which used semi-

TABLE 9.6
Studies of Fetal Heart Rate (FHR) During and Following Maternal Exercise

Authors	No. of Subjects	Gestational Age (Weeks)	FHR Monitor Type	Exercise			FHR Response	
				Mode	Intensity	Duration	During	Following
Pernoll et al. [138]	16	24–30 31–35 36–term	Doppler Ultrasound	Cycling	Mild	6 min	NA	Slight → Slight → Slight ↑
Dale et al. [40]	4	31–37.5	Doppler Ultrasound	Treadmill	To 80% HR max	NA	↓ (3 subjects)	—
Hauth et al. [72]	7	28–38	Doppler Ultrasound	Jogging	NA	1.5 miles, 62 steps	NA	↑
Collings et al [33]	12	22.5–34.2	Doppler Ultrasound	Cycling	65–75% $\dot{V}o_2max$	25 min	Slight ↑	Slight ↑
Artal et al. [6]	19	34 ± 3	Doppler Ultrasound	Treadmill	To symptom-limited $\dot{V}o_2max$	7.5 min	↓ (3 subjects)	↑, ↓
Goodlin and Buckley [63]	5	3rd trimester	Doppler Ultrasound	Semirecumbent cycling	To HR, 150 beats/min	NA	↑	↑
Pijpers et al. [139]	28	35.6	Doppler Ultrasound	Semirecumbent cycling	30–40% $\dot{V}o_2max$	NA	NA	—

Study	N	$\dot{V}O_2$max	Method	Exercise	Intensity	Duration	FHR	HR
Clapp [30]	6	20 / 32	Doppler Ultrasound	Treadmill	36–79% $\dot{V}O_2$max	20 min	NA / NA	↑ / ↑
Collings and Curet [34]	25	28–38	Doppler Ultrasound	Walking, jogging, cycling	61–73% $\dot{V}O_2$max	30 min	NA	↑
Jovanovic et al. [83]	6	36.0–38.5	Doppler Ultrasound	Cycling	<50% $\dot{V}O_2$max	12.8 min	↓ (4 subjects)	Slight ↑
Veille et al. [178]	10	33±3	Doppler Ultrasound	Walking	70% HRmax	30 min	NA	↑
	10	37±1	Doppler Ultrasound	Cycling	50 W	10–15 min	NA	↑
Artal et al. [8]	15	35.1±1.4	Doppler Ultrasound	Treadmill	2.3–3.0 METs	15 min	↑	↑
	15	34.7±1.3	Doppler Ultrasound	Treadmill	5.0–6.0 METs	15 min	↑,↓ (2 subjects)	↑,↓
	15	34.1±2.0	Doppler Ultrasound	Treadmill	To symptom-limited $\dot{V}O_2$max	Average 7.5 min	↑,↓ (3 subjects)	↑,↓

HR = heart rate; $\dot{V}O_2$max = maximal aerobic power; MET = one resting metabolic rate ($\dot{V}O_2$ = 3.5 ml/kg/min). ↑ = increase relative to preexercise FHR baseline (mean responses); — = no significant change relative to preexercise FHR baseline (mean responses); ↓ = fetal bradycardia (FHR<120 beats/min) observed (some subjects); NA = data not available.

recumbent cycling as the exercise modality. In all cases, birth outcomes were successful and obstetric complications were either absent or of a mild nature. The pooled results of these studies support the generalization that the FHR baseline is moderately increased (approximately 5–15 beats/minute) immediately after exercise and recovers to the preexercise level within approximately 20 minutes depending on exercise intensity. Although only a few investigators were able to monitor FHR during exercise [6, 8, 33, 40, 83] it appears that the FHR baseline begins to increase soon after the start of maternal exercise and reaches peak values comparable to those of the immediate postexercise period. Values for the FHR baseline in late gestation appear to be systematically lower than those recorded in mid-gestation.

Hauth et al. [72] reported no difference in fetal reactivity (a reactive test involved at least two FHR accelerations ≥10 beats/minute in association with fetal movement) or time to achieve reactivity before compared to immediately following a 1.5-mile jog in 17 physically active pregnant women (gestational ages = 28–38 weeks). In this study, peak postexercise FHR exceeded 180 beats/minute in 9 of the 15 tests.

Transient fetal bradycardia during exercise has recently been reported by at least three investigative teams [6, 8, 40, 83]. Since the pregnant subjects in these studies had successful birth outcomes and no significant obstetric complications, these findings have been the subject of much controversy and speculation. Dale et al. [40] monitored FHR using an ultrasonic method in four pregnant distance runners (gestational ages = 31–37.5 weeks) before, during, and following a progressive submaximal treadmill test. Technically satisfactory data were obtained from three subjects. In each case, a moderate transient bradycardia (FHR of 100–115 beats/minute, lasting 2–3 minutes was observed beginning soon after the onset of exercise and returning to normal within the exercise bout.

Artal et al. [6, 8] measured FHR responses to treadmill exercise in a group of 45 healthy women (mean gestational age was approximately 35 weeks). Groups of 15 subjects performed mild (15 minutes, 2.3–3.0 resting metabolic rates [METs]), moderate (15 minutes, 5–6 METs), and strenuous (symptom-limited $\dot{V}O_2$max) exercise, respectively. FHR was monitored before (30 minutes, semisupine posture), during, and following (30 minutes, semisupine posture) the exercise bout. The FHR baseline increased moderately during all three exercise conditions and there was no apparent intensity effect. Following mild and moderate exercise, FHR recovered to preexercise baseline within approximately 15 minutes, but required a longer recovery period after strenuous exercise. Reactive FHR patterns were observed both before and after exercise in all conditions, and no difference was reported between the frequencies of FHR accelerations before and after exercise. Moderate bradycardia (FHR of

90–110 beats/minute for ≥2 minutes) was observed in three fetuses in association with strenuous exercise, and in two fetuses exposed to moderate maternal exertion. Bradycardia was not reported during or following mild maternal exercise. In each of the five cases, bradycardia occurred near the beginning of exercise and continued into the postexercise period.

Jovanovic et al. [83] studied FHR before upright cycle ergometer exercise (15 minutes), during exercise, and during recovery (15 minutes) in six healthy physically active pregnant women (gestational age = 36–38.5 weeks). Average steady-state exercise power output was 79 (± 0) W and mean exercise duration was 12.8 (± 1.7) minutes. Mean FHR baseline before exercise was 142 (± 4) beats/minute, 84 (± 34) beats/minute during exercise (range = 50–130 beats/minute) and 143 (± 8) beats/minute 1 minute postexercise. In addition, reactive FHR responses were documented before and after, but not during exercise. The exercise-induced reductions in FHR were reported to occur soon after the onset of exercise and returned to preexercise levels within 1 minute of exercise cessation.

The latter investigation in particular has been a subject of controversy in view of the fact that current Doppler ultrasound units such as the one used by Jovanovic et al. [83] employ autocorrelation circuits which may record artifacts related to rhythmic maternal movements during walking or cycling [8, 130, 131]. Specifically, FHR baseline values during exercise in this study corresponded either to the usual pedal rhythm used in most cycle ergometer tests (range = 50–55 beats/minute) or approximately double this value (range = 100–130 beats/minute). The fact that FHR reductions occurred soon after exercise onset and disappeared quickly after exercise cessation and the observation that FHR during exercise was not reactive to fetal movements further support the hypothesis that movement artifact rather than fetal bradycardia was recorded. However, the authors also observed a reduction in FHR from approximately 150 beats/minute to approximately 110 beats/minute in response to mild exercise in one woman who was tested using cineultrasonography.

In summary, good general agreement exists that the normal response to maternal aerobic exercise is a moderate increase in FHR baseline which usually recovers to preexercise control levels within approximately 20 minutes of exercise cessation. Fetal bradycardia has been reported by some investigators and may represent a normal adaptive response to moderate fetal hypoxia. Artal et al. [8] hypothesized that fetal hypoxia could result from catecholamine-mediated uterine vasoconstriction. Initially such hypoxia would induce FHR acceleration, but may in some instances progress to elicit fetal vagal activity and bradycardia. Further research involving different modalities, intensities, and durations will be needed to determine the true incidence and significance of exercise-induced fetal bradycardia during normal pregnancy. The value of exercise for the early detection of uteroplacental insufficiency or threats to fetal viability also remains to be clarified. Finally, future studies of FHR during exercise should pay particular attention to the prevention or proper interpretation of artifact related to maternal movement when modern Doppler ultrasound equipment is used.

MATERNAL ADAPTATIONS TO PHYSICAL CONDITIONING

Despite the proliferation of exercising guidelines for pregnant women published by various authorities, little information is available concerning the cardiopulmonary adaptations to physical conditioning during pregnancy. As a result of the many physiological changes, there exists a strong possibility that adaptations to such conditioning during pregnancy may differ from those of healthy nonpregnant subjects. In view of postulated risks of chronic exercise to the fetus, there is an urgent need for information on the interactions between pregnancy and exercise.

Published studies fall into the following general categories:

1. Case studies of active women,
2. Comparisons of exercise data from "fit" versus "unfit" pregnant women,
3. Longitudinal physical conditioning studies.

Case studies have been reported by several authors. Dressendorfer [44] observed sequential changes in $\dot{V}O_2$max (l/minute) during pregnancy and lactation which correlated closely with changes in running distance in one healthy woman. $\dot{V}O_2$max was lowest during the 1st trimester when the subject reduced training distance due to persistent nausea, and subsequently increased moderately with advancing gestation in response to increased running distance. The highest values were noted postpartum when running distance was highest. $\dot{V}O_2$max values were measured directly in the nonpregnant state and estimated by extrapolation from submaximal data during pregnancy. Ruhling et al. [149] observed no change in $\dot{V}O_2$ (ml/kg/minute) during treadmill exercise at a HR target of 148 beats/minute during the 3rd, 6th, and 9th months of gestation. The subject was a healthy 36-year-old woman who continued a jogging regimen (approximately 6 km/day, 6–7 days/week) started prior to becoming pregnant. During this time period, body weight increased from 59.0 to 63.7 kg. Finally, Hutchinson et al. [76] studied responses to treadmill running (6.0 mph, 0% grade) between the 3rd and 8th month of pregnancy in a 32-year-old recreational runner who continued to exercise during pregnancy. $\dot{V}O_2$ (l/minute) rose in proportion to increases in body weight with advancing gestation. However, HR, $\dot{V}_E$, $\dot{V}_E$:$\dot{V}O_2$, and R rose to a greater extent, suggesting that running speed should be reduced, especially in late gestation.

These reports are encouraging and suggest that aerobic fitness can be maintained by exercising during pregnancy without harm to the mother or child. Unfortunately, such studies lack statistical validity since conclusions were based on the observation of only one subject.

Two investigations have compared adaptations to acute exercise in women ($n = 16$) representing different levels of aerobic conditioning. Dibblee and Graham [43] reported serial changes in $\dot{V}O_2$max estimated from the Canadian Aerobic Fitness Test at the end of each pregnancy trimester and 4 weeks postpartum. Following initial testing at the end of the 1st trimester, subjects were divided into physically "fit" and "unfit" subgroups based on values for predicted $\dot{V}O_2$max. None of the subjects participated in organized exercise classes during the study period. The "fit" group had significantly higher mean values for predicted $\dot{V}O_2$max (l/minute) and lower values for resting and exercise HR and diastolic blood pressure than the "unfit" group during tests at the end of the 1st and 2nd trimesters. However, these differences were not present during the 3rd-trimester evaluation. In this regard, values for predicted $\dot{V}O_2$max (l/minute) did not change substantially in the "fit" group during the study period, whereas values in the "unfit" group increased between the 1st and 3rd trimesters and subsequently decreased postpartum. Since body weight increased during gestation, predicted $\dot{V}O_2$max decreased approximately 2 ml/kg/minute each trimester and increased postpartum for the group as a whole.

Morton et al. [119] studied cardiovascular responses to exercise in 23 pregnant women at 34 and 38 weeks' gestation and 12 weeks postpartum. Ten women were identified by questionnaire as being physically active for at least 2 years prior to the study and were classified as being "fit." The remaining subjects ($n = 13$) were classified as "nonfit." The entire group of women ($n = 23$) participated in a community-based exercise class between 16 weeks' gestation and term. The conditioning regimen included 30 minutes of aerobic-type exercise at 60–70% of age-predicted HRmax. The "fit" women also exercised outside of these classes for an average of 4.5 hours/week. $\dot{Q}c$ measured by impedance cardiography, HR, and SV were measured at rest in the sitting position, and both during and following upright cycling at a moderate power output (approximately 50 W). Pooled results from both subject groups suggested that $\dot{Q}c$ measured either at rest or during exercise in the sitting position is similar in late gestation and postpartum. However, HR was significantly higher at rest and SV lower during exercise and recovery in late gestation compared to postpartum. Also, the responses of "fit" women were similar to those of "nonfit" women in late gestation, but in the

TABLE 9.7
Studies of Aerobic Conditioning in Healthy Pregnant Women

Authors	Subjects	Conditioning Program					Exercise Test Protocol	Testing Times (weeks gestation)	Results
		Modality	HR Target (beats/min)	Duration	Frequency (sessions/week)	Gestational Age During Conditioning (weeks)			
Ihrman [80]	EG (n = 26) CG (n = 50)	"Full body movements"	140	35 min/session	2	20–30	Submaximal cycle ergometer	Approx 11 (pretraining), 20, 27, 36 weeks gestation, and 3–7 days and 2 months	Greater ↑ in heart volume, EG vs. CG; other circulatory adjustments to pregnancy not affected
Erkkola [50]	EG (n = 31) CG (n = 31)	"Independent" aerobic activities	140	50 min/session	3	12–36	Progressive cycle ergometer (to voluntary fatigue)	10–14 weeks (pretraining); EG monthly to term; CG end of 2nd, 3rd Tms	EG: ↑27% PWC CG: ↑10% PWC
Sibley et al. [164]	EG (n = 7) CG (n = 6)	Swimming	140 (approx)	20–43 min/week	3	22–34	Progressive submaximal treadmill (to 140 beats/min)	22 weeks (pretraining) 34 weeks (posttraining)	EG: ↑ 6% power output at 140 beats/min; CG: ↓ 21% power output at 140 beats/min; EG: ↓ 1% $\dot{V}o_2$ (ml/kg/min) at 140 beats/min; CG: ↓ 10% $\dot{V}o_2$ (ml/kg/min) at 140 beats/min
Collings et al. [33]	EG (n = 12) CG (n = 8)	Upright cycling	152	25 min/session	3	23–34	Progressive submaximal cycle ergometer (to 80% predicted HR max)	23 weeks (pretraining); 34 weeks (posttraining)	EG: ↑ 18% predicted $\dot{V}o_2max$ (l/min); CG: ↓ 4% predicted $\dot{V}o_2max$ (l/min); EG: ↑ 8% predicted $\dot{V}o_2max$ (ml/kg/min); CG: ↓ 10% predicted $\dot{V}o_2max$ (ml/kg/min)

Study	Subjects	Modality	Intensity	Duration	Frequency	Gestation (weeks)	Test	Test timing	Results
Kulpa et al. [92]	EG (n = 17 primigravid, n = 21 multigravid) CG (n = 20 primigravid, n = 27 multigravid)	Aerobic exercise (varying modalities)	75% HR-max	Not specified	Not specified	Not specified	Bruce test (Tm 1, PP); Åstrand cycle ergometer test (3rd Tm)	Tm 1, Tm 3, PP	EG vs. CG: greater ↑ in predicted $\dot{V}O_2$max (METs) Tm 1 vs. PP; conditioning effects "obscured" by pregnancy in primiparous EG vs. CG at Tm 3
Hall et al. [70, 184]	EG (n = 16) CG (n = 8)	Upright cycling	150	14–25 min/session	3	17–37	Three-stage submaximal cycle ergometer	Start Tm 2 (pretraining) end of Tm 2, Tm 3 (posttraining)	EG vs. CG: significant ↓ in HR, RPE during moderate and heavy steady state exercise.
Ohtake [127]	EG (n = 27) CG (n = 20)	Upright cycling	150	14–25 min/session	3	17–37	Three-stage submaximal cycle ergometer	Start Tm 2 (pretraining), end of Tm 2, Tm 3, (posttraining), 3 months PP (nonpregnant control)	EG vs. CG: pulmonary responses to exercise not changed substantially by physical conditioning
South-Paul et al. [165]	EG (n = 10) CG (n = 7)	Upright cycling	60–80% "HR max" (progressive ↑)	60 min/session (including warmup, muscular conditioning)	3	2nd Tm to 30 weeks gestation	"Maximal" progressive cycle ergometer	Start Tm 2 (pretraining), 20, 30 weeks gestation (posttraining)	EG: ↑ 0.23 l/min $\dot{V}O_2$max CG: ↑ 0.10 l/min $\dot{V}O_2$max

Values are means or ranges. EG = exercise group; CG = pregnant control group; Tm = trimester; PP = postpartum; HR = heart rate; $\dot{V}O_2$ = oxygen uptake; RPE = rating of perceived exertion (Borg scale); PWC = physical working capacity; MET = one resting metabolic rate (3.5 ml/kg/min).

postpartum period expected differences in the direction of a lower resting and exercise HR and higher SV were observed. The results suggested that exercise/training-induced increases in resting and exercise SV (and reductions in HR) are obscured during late pregnancy by interference with venous return by the gravid uterus.

The effects of physical conditioning during pregnancy can be determined most accurately by controlled longitudinal physical conditioning studies with reliable records of exercise actually performed by the subjects. Unfortunately, existing longitudinal conditioning studies are few in number, and vary considerably in both scope and experimental findings (Table 9.7). Exercise modalities employed for physical conditioning in longitudinal studies have included upright cycling [33, 70, 127, 165], swimming [164], and a variety of aerobic-type activities [50, 80, 92]. In the majority of studies, conditioning was conducted during the 2nd and 3rd trimesters. However, Ihrman [80] and South-Paul et al. [165] discontinued conditioning after the 30th week of gestation, while the subjects of Kulpa et al. [92] also exercised postpartum. Exercise intensity was prescribed using pulse rate targets of approximately 140–150 beats/minute except for the investigation of South-Paul et al. [165], where it appears that a lower HR range was employed (approximately 95–130 beats/minute, according to data provided). The duration of aerobic conditioning ranged from 14 to 60 minutes/session and the frequency of supervised exercise classes was usually 3 sessions/week. Ihrman [80] used only two formal conditioning sessions/week, but also instructed subjects to perform exercise for 10 minutes/day at home. The subjects of Erkkola [50] did not attend formal exercise classes but were asked to exercise on their own 3 days/week. Detailed records of actual exercise performed were kept either by the investigators [33, 70, 127] or the subjects themselves [92] in several studies. All investigations employed a sedentary nonpregnant control group for reference purposes, and postpartum measurements were available in the studies of Kulpa et al. [92] and Ohtake [127].

Of particular importance is the question whether or not $\dot{V}O_2$max expressed either on an absolute (l/minute) or relative (ml/kg/minute) basis can be maintained or increased as a result of aerobic conditioning in pregnancy. The data of Erkkola [50], Collings et al. [33], Hall et al. [70, 184], and Ohtake [127] suggested that absolute $\dot{V}O_2$max can be increased significantly, and relative $\dot{V}O_2$max can be maintained or moderately increased during the course of gestation despite significant maternal weight gain. These findings were based on significant reduction in HR during standard submaximal cycling [33, 70, 127] and an increase in the peak power output achieved during a progressive cycle ergometer test to volitional fatigue [50], respectively.

The investigations of Ihrman [80], Sibley et al. [164], and Kulpa et al. [92] resulted in findings which are less encouraging with respect to maternal "trainability" than those cited above. The aerobically conditioned subjects of Ihrman [80] exhibited moderately greater increases during gestation in heart volume measured at rest than control subjects. However, gestational effects on blood hematology, vital capacity, HR, blood pressure and orthostatic changes in blood pressure in the resting state, and HR and respiratory frequency during standard submaximal cycling were similar in the two groups and were apparently unaffected by physical conditioning. Absence of a significant reduction in HR during standard submaximal cycling during gestation in the exercised group suggested that absolute $\dot{V}O_2$max was not increased, perhaps as a result of the low frequency of formal exercise classes (2 sessions/week). In the investigation of Sibley et al. [164] a moderate (6%) increase in power output and only a slight (1%) decrease in $\dot{V}O_2$ (ml/kg/minute) were observed pre- to postconditioning at a standard HR of 140 beats/minute during treadmill exercise. Corresponding values in the control group were 21 and 10% reductions for power output and $\dot{V}O_2$, respectively, suggesting that swim conditioning prevented a significant reduction in maximal aerobic power during gestation. The reader should note that the results of this study may have differed from those of other investigators because the subjects were evaluated and conditioned using different exercise modalities (treadmill exercise vs. swimming).

Kulpa et al. [92] reported the effects of aerobic conditioning (varying modalities) on 38 subjects with low-risk pregnancies (17 primigravid and 21 multigravid women). A pregnant control group (20 primigravid and 27 multigravid women) was also studied. $\dot{V}O_2$max was evaluated during the 1st trimester and postpartum (exact time not specified) using a standard Bruce treadmill test. Subjects were also tested using a submaximal Åstrand-type cycle ergometer protocol during the 3rd trimester. The exercising subjects were given individual prescriptions for home exercise and kept logs of exercise during pregnancy and postpartum. An exercise intensity of 75% HRmax was employed, but mean exercise frequencies and durations were not specified. All subject groups had higher mean values for $\dot{V}O_2$max (METs) in postpartum versus 1st-trimester treadmill tests, but gains were greater in both the primigravid and multigravid exercisers compared to their respective control groups. During 3rd-trimester cycle ergometer tests, predicted $\dot{V}O_2$max was significantly higher in multiparous exercising subjects versus controls. However, mean values for exercising versus control primiparous subjects did not differ significantly. In this regard, the authors hypothesized that physiological changes during late gestation may have masked cardiovascular adaptations to aerobic conditioning.

The most detailed investigations of specific physiological adaptations to aerobic-type conditioning are the recent studies of Hall et al. [70, 184], Ohtake et al. [127], and South-Paul et al. [165]. The preliminary reports of Hall et al. [70, 184] and Ohtake et al. [127] summarize different aspects of a 2-year investigation at Queen's University (Kingston, Canada). The overall study design included a healthy pregnant experimental (exercising) group and control (nonexercising) group. Subjects were evaluated at the beginning of the 2nd trimester (preconditioning) and were reevaluated at the end of the 2nd and 3rd trimesters (postconditioning) and 3 months postpartum (nonpregnant control). The experimental group participated in physical conditioning during the 2nd and 3rd pregnancy trimesters and the majority of subjects deconditioned after delivery. The control group maintained their normal exercise habits. The physical conditioning regimen included both muscular and aerobic exercise components conducted during supervised sessions 3 days/week. Aerobic conditioning included upright cycling at 70% of maximal HR reserve (approximately 150 beats/minute). Exercise duration was increased gradually from 14 to 25 minutes/session during the course of the 2nd trimester and was maintained at 25 minutes/session during the 3rd trimester. Detailed logs of attendance and actual exercise performed were kept by the class instructors and subject adherence was very high. Serial measurements included basic physical characteristics (weight, skinfold thickness, static lung function), resting two-dimensional echocardiograms, resting HR, blood pressure, metabolic rate and pulmonary ventilation, metabolism, cardiorespiratory responses and RPE during a progressive submaximal cycle ergometer test, and pregnancy outcome. FHR before, during, and following a separate submaximal cycle ergometer test was evaluated at the end of the 2nd and 3rd trimesters.

Hall et al. [70, 184] reported cardiovascular responses to exercise, obtained during the 1st year of investigation. Data were available from 16 exercising subjects and 8 controls at the end of each pregnancy trimester (postpartum data not included). Resting HR and skinfold thicknesses did not change significantly during the course of gestation in either group, suggesting that these variables may be poor indicators of physical conditioning state in this population. Data were obtained at three absolute levels of steady-state cycle ergometer exercise (approximately 20, 45, and 65 W, respectively $\dot{V}O_2$ (l/minute) and at each standard submaximal power output did not change significantly in either group. However, HR and RPE (Borg Scale) decreased significantly at the two highest levels in the exercised group. Exercise $\dot{Q}c$ (CO_2 rebreathing method) and SV at each exercise level tended to increase at the end of the 2nd trimester and subsequently decreased at the end of the 3rd trimester in both groups. These effects were most pronounced at the two lowest exercise levels. The results supported the hypothesis previously advanced by Morton et al. [119] that $\dot{Q}c$ and SV responses to exercise are dominated by effects of pregnancy on blood volume and venous return regardless of physical conditioning status (Fig. 9.3). However, HR and RPE during moderate and heavy submaximal exertion are reduced following physical conditioning and appear to be useful indicators of exercise intensity during pregnancy.

The preliminary report of Ohtake et al. [127] summarizes metabolic and pulmonary findings obtained at rest and during the three-stage cycle ergometer test described above. Their completed 2-year study offers data from 27 exercising subjects and 20 controls at the start of the 2nd trimester (preconditioning), the end of the 2nd and 3rd trimesters (postconditioning), and 3 months postpartum (nonpregnant control). Findings for resting HR, skinfold thicknesses, and submaximal exercise $\dot{V}O_2$ and HR were essentially identical to those of Hall et al. [70, 184]. In both the exercising and nonexercising groups, $\dot{V}E$ and $\dot{V}E{:}\dot{V}O_2$ were augmented relative to postpartum. This was the result of a greater VT during gestation and resulted in significantly lower levels of end-tidal PCO_2 during gestation versus postpartum. The $VD{:}VT$ decreased with increasing exercise intensity, and this relationship was not altered by either pregnancy or aerobic conditioning. It was concluded that the magnitude and normal time course of ventilatory adaptations to steady state exercise during pregnancy are not changed substantially by aerobic conditioning.

South-Paul et al. [165] also recently reported the effects of physical conditioning on metabolic and pulmonary responses to exercise in pregnancy. Subjects included 10 exercising subjects and a control group ($n = 7$) who did not alter their physical activity levels during gestation. The exercise regimen was conducted 3 days/week between the 20th and 30th weeks of gestation and included both muscular and aerobic conditioning components. Aerobic conditioning consisted of upright cycling with a progressive increase in intensity during the 10-week program from 60 to 80% of measured peak HR during exercise tests (approximately 95–130 beats/minute; exercise duration not specified). In this regard, a progressive cycle ergometer test to volitional fatigue was conducted before and after the exercise program. Pre- and postconditioning comparisons of physiological data, including HR, $\dot{V}O_2$, R, $\dot{V}E$, f, VT and $\dot{V}E{:}\dot{V}O_2$, were made at a standard power output of 75 W and during "maximal" exercise. The only statistically significant change in either group was a moderate increase in VT at "maximal" exercise in the experimental group. The increase in absolute $\dot{V}O_2$ at peak exercise was only moderately higher in the exercising group compared to the control group (0.23 vs. 0.10 l/minute). Peak HR did not change in either group and mean values remained constant within a range of 155–160 beats/minute. Similarly, values for R at peak exercise did not change signifi-

FIGURE 9.3

Interactive effects of pregnancy and physical conditioning on cardiac output during standard submaximal exercise. HR = heart rate. Solid arrows indicate positive effects; dashed arrow *indicates a negative effect. (Adapted with permission from Hall P: Cardiovascular adaptations to physical conditioning during pregnancy. Unpublished master's thesis, Kingston, Canada, Queen's University, 1987.)*

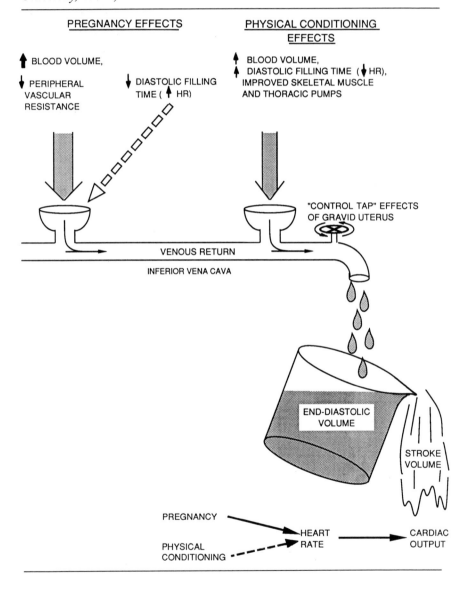

cantly and mean values remained within a range of 0.98–1.05. The lack of change in pulmonary ventilation during standard submaximal exercise is consistent with the findings of Ohtake et al. [127]. The failure to reduce submaximal exercise HR is not consistent with the data of Ohtake et al. [127] and other investigators [33, 50, 70, 184] probably relates to the lower exercise HR targets used and shorter duration of conditioning in this study.

In summary, available scientific evidence supports the hypothesis that absolute $\dot{V}O_2$max can be improved in previously sedentary pregnant women via regular, individually prescribed aerobic exercise. It also appears that values expressed in ml/kg/minute can be maintained or moderately increased despite increases in body weight during gestation. The magnitude of conditioning effects is probably proportional to exercise quantity and quality since Ihrman [80] and South-Paul et al. [165] reported negligible conditioning effects in association with mild conditioning stimuli. A major obstacle to acceptance of this hypothesis is that none of the available conditioning studies has evaluated maximal aerobic capacity with a plateau in measured $\dot{V}O_2$ as the criterion for a true maximal response. This is because of concerns for subject safety. It may also be difficult to motivate subjects to reach a true $\dot{V}O_2$max in late gestation because of a postulated reduction in the ability to exercise anaerobically [9]. Thus, fatigue may occur prior to reaching true maximal values for HR, $\dot{Q}c$, and $\dot{V}O_2$ since sufficient anaerobic energy sources may not be available to provide the supplementary metabolic power required for a supramaximal effort.

The investigations of Morton et al. [119] and Hall et al. [70, 184] suggested that the increase in SV usually observed during standard submaximal exercise may be obscured by the dominant effects of pregnancy on both HR and venous return (Fig. 9.3). Since these effects appear to be most prominent in the resting state and during mild exertion [70, 184], it may be necessary to employ a more intense exercise stimulus to detect cardiovascular conditioning adaptations in this population. Thus, aerobic conditioning effects may not be detectable in late gestation if submaximal tests involving only mild or moderate exertion are employed for the prediction of $\dot{V}O_2$max [43, 92, 119]. Further study is needed to clarify the normal cardiovascular adaptations to aerobic conditioning in pregnancy and devise reliable submaximal tests for the evaluation of $\dot{V}O_2$max in the population.

EFFECTS OF CHRONIC EXERCISE ON PREGNANCY OUTCOME

In general, studies of fetal responses during and following maternal exertion support the hypothesis that healthy women can perform acute bouts of upright submaximal exercise without compromising fetal well-being. The observed FHR patterns also suggest that such exercise may elicit mild transient hypoxia. If so, this appears to be well-tolerated by the fetus in the absence of uteroplacental insufficiency or other obstetric problems. Recovery of FHR to the preexercise baseline usually ensues within 10–20 minutes. However, the added physiological burden and possible complicating effects of various environmental stresses, advancing maternal age, maternal health problems (e.g., diabetes, hypertension, and heart diseases), pharmacological agents, nutritional interventions, different exercise postures, different exercise modes (e.g., static exercise and weight-bearing vs. not weight bearing) have not yet been clarified.

An additional concern is the effect of chronic exposure of the fetus to maternal exertion [66, 102]. If acute maternal exercise results in hypoxic, hypoglycemic, or thermal stress, repeated exposure to the exercise stimulus may eventually result in impaired fetal development. Potential ill effects could range from a moderate and benign reduction in birth weight to clinically significant intrauterine growth retardation or other serious developmental effects (Fig. 9.4). Alternatively, intermittent exposure to exercise stress which is within the adaptive capabilities of the mother and fetus may be beneficial to either or both. If the latter hypothesis is true, processes such as health screening and the accurate prescription of exercise may be critical to ensure the safety and efficacy of exercise programs during pregnancy.

Animal Studies
Studies of the effects of chronic exercise on pregnancy outcome in laboratory animals have resulted in varying experimental findings. Several explanations for the observed discrepancies may be suggested. Many animal studies reporting changes in "fetal" outcome may in fact be reporting on postnatal influences in combination with prenatal life, and these alterations may depend on when the offspring are assessed. In addition, studies finding fetal growth retardation may not include familiarization of the animals to the exercise protocol or exercise intensity prior to pregnancy. The stress of apparatus, new environment, etc., in addition to exercise may disturb the maternal system and lead to altered fetal development. Other factors such as the differences in species studied and the different intensities of maternal exercise used may also influence experimental results [103].

In rats familiarized to a running exercise protocol prior to pregnancy on a motorized treadmill using a mild (20 m/minute, 10° incline, 1 hour/day, 5 days/week) intensity exercise protocol [121], a moderate (30 m/minute, 10° incline, 1 hour/day, 5 days/week) intensity exercise protocol [12], or a severe (30 m/minute, 10° incline, 2 hours/day, 5 days/week) intensity exercise protocol [123], no significant differences were found in newborn body weight or number of fetuses/litter between the preg-

FIGURE 9.4

Hypothetical effects of aerobic exercise on fetal development.

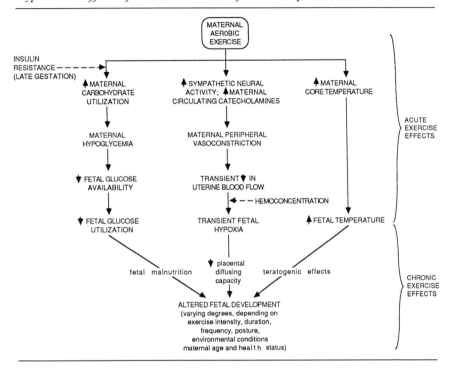

nant exercising groups and the nonexercising pregnant controls. In the severe maternal exercise intensity group, no significant differences were found in average newborn body weight or organ weights—brain, heart, liver, lung and kidney—or in cellular and histochemical characteristics of the newborn diaphragm, gastrocnemius, and sternomastoid muscles [123].

Although fetal outcome assessed at 1 day of age following different running intensities of maternal exercise in the rat was unaffected in the studies cited above [12, 121, 123], another series of earlier experiments [133, 134] using mild intensity (14–15 m/minute, 1 hour/day) maternal exercise (exercise began 2–3 days after mating, no familiarization) showed different results. Parizkova [133] reported that heart weight, the number of left ventricular muscle fibers, and the ratio of capillary to heart fibers of 50- and 100-day-old offspring of exercised maternal rats were significantly higher, and the diffusion distance in heart muscle significantly shorter, than in controls. In addition, Parizkova and Petrasek [134] reported that this mild aerobic maternal exercise significantly altered liver lipid metabolism in both male and female offspring of exercised rats when examined postnatally. Studies that report alterations to the offspring of exercised maternal animals past a few days after birth must be read with caution because these changes may be the results of not only the prenatal environment, but the combined effects of prenatal and postnatal conditions (lactational status, maternal and offspring care, etc.)

Wilson and Gisolfi [182] repeated the cardiovascular measurements of Parizkova (133) on the offspring (45–65 days postnatal) of trained maternal rats. The conditioning protocol of the Wilson and Gisolfi (182) exercised animals consisted of 7 weeks of prepregnancy exercise at 35 m/minute, 1% grade, 1 hour/day, 7 days/week (more intense than Parizkova, [133]), which continued throughout pregnancy. Wilson and Gisolfi [182] reported that in male offspring no significant difference occurred in body dimensions, organ weights (heart, kidney, spleen, and adrenals), cardiac muscle fibre:capillary ratio, and total capacity of myocardial capillaries between the trained maternal group and sedentary pregnant controls, which disagreed with the results of Parizkova [133]. Wilson and Gisolfi [182] also reported a significant increase in neonatal mortality in the offspring of the exercised maternal group and suggested this was due to maternal neglect and maternal cannibalism, both of which were observed in their study. Postnatal environment is a difficult factor to control and must be considered when "fetal" outcome is reported in chronic maternal exercise studies. An interesting example of reported "fetal" outcome changes due to maternal exercise [82] suggested that when littermates of control versus mild-exercise groups were assessed on a complex motor performance task at 21 days after birth (weaning), the offspring from the exercised dams performed significantly poorer on the motor performance test than controls.

Another variable to consider is the different maternal exercise protocols used. For example, Bonner et al. [22] swam pregnant rats (no prepregnancy familiarization) for 30–40 minutes/day and reported that in 5-day-old offspring of exercised maternal animals, primary cultures of myocardial cells beat at a slower rate and were larger than sedentary controls. They concluded that exercise of this type produced changes in the myocardium of the offspring.

When fetal assessment is actually performed in rats, usually between days 19 and 21 of gestation (term is approximately 21 days), during chronic maternal exercise studies, again discrepancies are reported in the literature. Garris et al. [54] found that rats exercised (28 m/minute, 0% grade, 1 hour/day) with no prepregnancy training or familiarization between days 12 and 21 of gestation (last part of pregnancy) showed a dramatic decrease in uteroplacental blood flow rates and a significant reduction in live births/litter when compared to controls. They concluded that maternal exercise performed only during the last half of gestation had the most severe consequences on gestational maintenance compared to sedentary controls. Treadway et al. [172] reported that in trained maternal rats (7 weeks prepregnancy conditioning, 27 m/minute, 5° incline, 1 hour/day) on day 19 of gestation, fetal number/litter was significantly lower and the number of fetal resorptions significantly higher than controls. Fetal body weight and body composition—body water, protein and lipid values—were not significantly different between the trained animals and controls. In contrast to the above problematic fetal analysis, Savard et al. [157] found no significant difference on day 21 of pregnancy for fetal number/litter, fetal body weight, and carcass lipid content in maternal rats trained to swim 3 hours/day, 6 days/week (14-day prepregnancy adaptation) when compared to sedentary controls. In addition, Treadway and Lederman [173] found no significant difference in fetal number/litter, or fetal body weight in maternal rats that swam 2 hours/day, 5 days/week, with a 3% tail weight when compared to nonexercised pregnant controls. Thus, even when fetal analysis is reported for maternal rats, not only is the gestational time at which exercise is performed important, but the intensity and differences in exercise protocols (running vs. swimming) also require consideration.

In many of the rat studies in which fetal outcome was maintained [12, 121, 123], alterations were noted in the maternal system. The exercised maternal rats gained significantly less weight during pregnancy than sedentary control animals. It was suggested that the decreased maternal body weight gain during pregnancy may be due to a diminished fat deposition in the pregnant running groups [122]. Craig and Treadway [36] reported that pregnant running rats (trained 8 weeks prepregnancy) exercising at an intensity of 27 m/minute, on a 5° incline, 1 hour/day, 5 days/week on day 19 of gestation, weighed significantly less and had 40% smaller adipocytes but the same number of adipocytes as control sedentary animals. The trained maternal rats also had adipocytes that were significantly more responsive to insulin, and at the maximal insulin concentration tested, these adipocytes took up and metabolized approximately twice as much glucose as the sedentary pregnant controls.

Effects of maternal exercise on fetal development have been examined in several other animal species. In mice, Terada [170] compared prepregnancy trained (4 weeks) runners on a motor driven treadmill (15 m/minutes, 1 hour/day, 6 days/week) that continued exercising throughout gestation to animals forced to run during midgestation (no prepregnancy training). The results indicated that forced exercise during midgestation (no prepregnancy training) caused an increase in fetal mortality (resorption and maceration) and a significant reduction in fetal body weight when compared to sedentary pregnant controls. The exercised maternal group also had smaller fetal body weight values but did not show an increased fetal mortality rate. However, both groups of exercised maternal animals showed a delay in fetal skeletal ossification when compared to controls. Terada [170] concluded that prepregnancy training may have reduced the effects of forced maternal exercise during mid-gestation. In a similar study. Boehnke et al. [19] observed that on day 19 of gestation (gestation is approximately 21 days) no significant differences were found in fetal number, fetal body weight, and number of resorptions when both maternal exercise groups were compared to sedentary controls. However, a significant number of the heavy maternal exercised fetuses showed a delay in bone ossification. Even though Boehnke et al. [19] showed a reduction in problematic fetal outcome, perhaps through increasing prepregnancy physical conditioning time (7 vs. 4 weeks) when compared to Terada [170], a delay in fetal bone ossification remained.

In guinea pigs, alterations in fetal body and organ weights with different intensities of acute repetitive maternal exercise (no prepregnancy conditioning) have been reported [61, 126]. The maternal exercise intensities consisted of a treadmill speed of 9.7 m/minute, 6.5% grade at one of four exercise levels, 5 days/week (exercise began between days 13 and 17 of gestation). The levels of exercise were increased by progressively increasing the total time run by 15 minutes (range = 15–60 minutes). The results demonstrated a significant decrease in fetal body weight and placental and fetal kidney weight values between days 62 and 64 of gestation (term is approximately 67 days) as the duration of maternal exercise increased. In addition, a decrease in placental weight and a reduction in placental diffusing capacity per kilogram of fetal weight was observed in the higher levels of maternal exercise. The authors concluded that problematic fetal outcome was dose dependent, since as intensity (level) increased so did the detrimental effects on fetal outcome [126]). Smith et al. [166], using the same exercise protocol, also demonstrated that placental diffusing capacity and maternal surface area in the placental peripheral labyrinth exchange area decreased as the level of maternal exercise increased. Not only is prepregnancy training important in reducing problematic fetal outcome, but these experiments involving the pregnant guinea pig suggest that the intensity of acute repetitive maternal exercise is necessary to consider, in addition to the difference in animal species.

Sheep and pygmy goats have been used extensively in acute maternal exercise studies. The fetuses of both species are large and both the pregnant mother and fetus have been used for invasive research which monitors uteroplacental blood flow, PO_2 levels, and fetal metabolism. Chronic maternal exercise studies in the pregnant sheep and goat are not as available, possibly because of problems with prepregnancy training or chronic catheter maintenance. As in the other species previously reported, discrepancies also exist in the literature reporting on sheep and goats.

Dhindsa et al. [42] found that pregnant pygmy goats accustomed to standing on a treadmill and walking at 1.5 mph up a 10° incline for 10 minutes 1–2 times/week produced significantly smaller twin birth weight values than matched controls. The singleton births of exercised mothers were of normal weight. However, before each study session the pregnant goats were kept from food for 20 hours but were allowed free access to water. Since maternal nutrition is an important element in fetal growth and development, perhaps the 20-hour food deprivation in these pregnant goats in combination with maternal exercise may have altered fetal outcome, especially in multiple pregnancies.

Hohimer et al. [73] measured uteroplacental blood flow in exercising pregnant pygmy goats and separated uteroplacental blood flow into myoendometrial and cotyledonary (placental) components of the uterine vasculature. Pregnant pygmy goats (of approximately 80 days' gestation; term is approximately 147 days) were taught to walk on a treadmill at a speed of 0.5 mph for 10 minutes, 3 times/week. The speed was gradually increased to between 1.5 and 2.0 mph up a grade of 10° or 15°, 3 times/week. This type of exercise did not affect birth weight values compared to controls, even in twin births. However, uterine artery blood flow was decreased by 32% from control values and total uterine blood flow decreased by 18%; cotyledonary (placental) blood flow decreased by 8%, while myoendometrial blood flow dropped by 52%. The authors concluded that the nonplacental portions of the uterus in pregnant pygmy goats showed significant alterations in blood flow as a result of acute repetitive maternal exercise. This redistribution of blood flow from the myoendometrium to the placental portions was also observed by Curet et al. [38] in pregnant sheep and may assist in maintaining fetal growth and development.

In contrast, Longo et al. [97] reported a significant decrease in fetal descending aortic Po_2 values which fell by 19% in nine chronically catheterized fetal lambs. The pregnant ewes exercised at a treadmill speed of 43 m/minute for 20–45 minutes on a 10° incline. Uterine blood flow (measured with an electromagnetic flow probe) significantly decreased by 59% during maternal exercise. In another group, four ewes were exercised for 15 minutes twice daily during the last 3–4 months of pregnancy. The fetal lambs of these animals weighed significantly less than controls. The authors concluded that "moderate" to "heavy" "sustained" maternal exercise resulted in significant fetal "hypoxia" and may cause intrauterine growth retardation.

Many of the animal studies cited above support the hypothesis that fetal development can be influenced by chronic maternal exercise. More

TABLE 9.8
Studies of Maternal Occupation and Pregnancy Outcome

Authors	Place/ Time	Subjects	Nature of Work	Evaluation Methods	Perinatal Outcome	Maternal Problems	Conclusions
Fox et al. [52]	U.S. Air Force 1974–76	Active-duty military personnel $n = 196$; nonactive duty $n = 196$; general population $n = 300$.	Not specified	Review of birth records	↑ midforceps rotation, bwt <2500 g, and mortality in active-duty group	↑ frequency toxemia anemia, abnormal Pap smears, premature c-sections in active-duty group	Lack of rest in active duty group may have contributed to poor obstetric outcome
Tafari et al. [169]	Ethiopia 1976–1977	Hard work, $n = 64$; Light work, $n = 66$	Carrying water long distances, grinding grain—hard work. Housewife with domestic help—light work.	Prospective	bwt significantly less (202 g) in hard work group	Less than optimum daily intake of calories and protein; ↓ in pregnancy weight gain in hard work group	Restricted diet effects on fetal growth increased by hard physical work.
Naeye and Peters [125]	U.S. working women (perinatal project)	$n = 7,722$: 1. Employment mostly standing 2. Employment mostly sitting 3. Did not work outside home	1. Retail sales, service workers, laborers 2. Clerical workers, students.	Review of birth records	↓ bwt (150–400 g) in underweight women, hypertensives, when outside work required standing	Length of gestation equal in all groups; large placental infarcts associated with late gestational standing work	No exertion levels measured; birth effects remain even after stratification of data for maternal race and class
Alegre et al. [2]	Spain 1979–1980	$n = 1,140$; paid work, $n = 731$; not employed $n = 720$	Not specified	Questionnaire	↓ bwt (200 g) in paid workers; bwt lower in working primigravid as in multigravids	Paid workers resting during last 6 weeks. Delivered normal bwt infants	↓ in bwt still evident after control of normal factors, e.g., smokers extreme height and weight; rest advisable during late gestation, especially when intrauterine growth

Study	Location/Years	n / Groups	Work categories	Method	Result (bwt)	Result (other)	Comments
Murphy et al. [124]	Great Britain 1965–1979	n = 69, 617: 1. Not employed 2. Work: sedentary 3. Work: not sedentary	2. Assembly line worker 3. Nurse.	Maternal interview and review of birth records	↓ bwt in not employed group	None	retardation suspected Adjusted for social class, but based on husband's occupation if married, father's occupation if unmarried
Meyer and Daling [114]	Washington State 1981	Control group is sitting group [2]	1. Housewife 2. Sitting ≥ 75% 3. Mixed; 25–75% sitting/standing 4. Standing ≥75% 5. Active strenuous work >25%	Review of birth records	No change in bwt due to maternal occupation	Not reported	Active work not associated with low bwt
Zuckerman et al. [188]	Boston 1977–1979	n = 1, 507. 1. No paid work outside home, n = 830 2. Paid work, standing into 3rd Tm, n = 112 3. Paid work, sitting or standing in 1st or 2nd Tm, n = 565	Standing; nurse, waitress, sales, cashier, housekeeper; Sitting; student, clerical	Maternal interview and review of birth record	No change in bwt, infant length, head circumference; group 2 delivered longer babies than group 1	No difference in length of gestation	Controlled for maternal factors, e.g., alcohol, smoking; population studied largely minority and low social class
Manshande et al. [108]	Central Zaire 1980–1982	n = 554: 1. Hard work 2. Light work 3. Rest–stay in maternity village.	1. Mining 2. Domestic work	Prospective	Rest >21 days in last Tm ↓'d rate of low bwt by 7.5-fold in female offspring	No difference reported	In developing countries, avoidance of heavy work in last Tm may ↑ bwt and ↓ perinatal mortality

bwt = birth weight; Tm = trimester.

animal research is necessary in order to explain some of the discrepancies and underlying mechanisms (Fig. 9.4) which may lead to changes in fetal outcome. In order to quantify stress and exercise intensity levels between studies, catecholamine values should be monitored in the future in both acute and chronic maternal exercise studies. One must always keep in mind the differences between species in anatomical features, physiology, and the endocrinology of pregnancy. It is difficult to mimic the upright posture of the pregnant human when studying animal models, and this represents one of the problems associated with applying the results seen in the animal model to predict findings in human subjects. Finally, the possible complicating influence of stress related to enforced versus voluntary exercise in laboratory animals must be considered. Unfortunately, controlled experiments which monitor maternal exercise intensity using human subjects are rather limited (especially at the higher intensities) for ethical reasons and thus controlled animal studies are a necessity.

Human Studies

Human observation is important in studies of chronic exertion and pregnancy outcome. Unfortunately, these studies are difficult to control and rely mainly on case study reports, and both retrospective and prospective studies of obstetrical outcomes. Many variables including lifestyle behaviors (smoking, alcohol, and stress), diet, exercise intensity, and type of exercise (weight bearing vs. notweight bearing) may influence the effects of chronic maternal exercise on fetal outcome.

Published studies of chronic exertion and pregnancy outcome in human subjects generally fall into the following categories:

1. Surveys of obstetrical outcomes in relation to maternal occupation;
2. Case studies or surveys of obstetrical outcomes in pregnant athletes;
3. Retrospective and prospective studies of obstetrical outcomes in women engaged in physical fitness programs.

Occupational Effects of Fetal Outcome

Studies of birth outcome in relation to maternal occupation have been conducted to determine the advisability of maternal confinement or rest, particularly during late gestation. The reader is directed to a historic overview written by Saurel-Cubizolles and Kaminski [156] on epidemiological studies relating to maternal work and perinatal outcome. The most recent and significant studies are presented in Table 9.8.

Epidemiological studies are difficult to compare because of differences in populations (number, geographic location), sample collection, control of maternal variables (smoking, alcohol, age, etc.), socioeconomic status, and statistical analysis, to name only a few. Many authors (Table 9.8) have reported that lack of rest in the 3rd trimester for women who perform hard physical work up until delivery may give birth to smaller infants [2, 52, 108, 125, 169] and suggested that this may be due to maternal upright posture (standing). In contrast, Murphy et al. [124] showed a decrease in birth weights in the group that was not employed and Meyer and Daling [114] and Zuckerman et al. [188] showed no change in birth weights due to maternal occupation and activity level when employed.

The majority of studies suggest that working (especially standing) until delivery results in a decrease in infant birth weight [23, 125]. This effect has been attributed to redistribution of blood flow away from the pregnant uterus during exertion in the upright posture [125]. However, maternal rest in the last few weeks prior to delivery may improve this problem [108]. However, not all complicating maternal variables have been controlled in existing studies, including psychosocial stress, social class, maternal nutrition, alcohol use, smoking, energy expenditure, environmental conditions during work, and the quality of perinatal medical care. The long-term health implications for the infants of working women have not been clarified and remain for future investigation.

Pregnancy Outcome in Athletic Women
A number of reports of successful obstetrical outcomes in athletic women who ran or jogged through pregnancy have appeared in various medical publications [44, 91]. Unfortunately, there reports are not reliable from a scientific viewpoint because of the small sample size and/or the anecdotal nature of the reports.

Other investigators have conducted retrospective surveys of pregnancy outcomes in elite athletes. Erdelyi [47] reported shorter mean labors and lower frequencies of toxemia, cesarian sections, and threatened abortions in 172 Hungarian athletes compared to 150 nonathletic controls. Two-thirds of the athletic women continued to exercise during the first 3–4 months of gestation, but the number who continued to exercise and the average level of exertion were not specified. Zaharieva [187] studied birth outcomes in women who participated in the Olympic Games between 1952 and 1972 ($n = 27$), women who were masters of sport ($n = 59$), and those who were "first grade" athletes ($n = 64$). Percentages who continued to train during pregnancy were 63, 76, and 77% for each group, respectively. The majority of Olympic athletes (70%) had no pregnancy complications and the remainder had only "mild complaints." Masters of sport had somewhat higher rates of birth complications such as rupture of membranes. The results of these two studies support the hypothesis that athletes who continue to train during pregnancy generally have a low incidence of pregnancy complications.

Aerobic Fitness and Pregnancy Outcome
The relationship between maternal "physical fitness" (i.e., $\dot{V}O_2max$) and pregnancy outcome has been examined in two studies. Erkkola [49]

TABLE 9.9
Retrospective and Prospective Studies of Birth Outcome in Physically Active Women

Authors	Subjects	Evaluation Methods	Findings
Retrospective Studies			
Dale et al. [40]	"Joggers" (*n* = 14) and "runners" (*n* = 7) who exercised during pregnancy	Written questionnaire; review of medical charts	Possible increase in incidence of failure to progress/cesarian section
Jarrett and Spellacy [81]	"Experienced runners" who jogged through pregnancy (*n* = 67)	Written questionnaire	Low incidence of obstetrical complications; no correlation between miles run during pregnancy and birth weight or gestational age
Lutter et al. [106]	"Low mileage" runners (*n* = 195)	Written questionnaire; follow-up	Obstetric outcomes usually normal; normal infant development in first year
Davis et al. [cited in 41]	Women who exercised regularly during pregnancy (*n* = 67); sedentary pregnant controls (*n* = 48); controls (*n* = 48)	Written questionnaire	No significant differences between groups for gestational age, birth weight, one-minute Apgar scores, length of labor
Prospective Studies			
Dale et al. [40]	Runners (*n* = 12) who ran during pregnancy; pregnant nonrunners (*n* = 11)	Written questionnaire, review of medical charts	Possible failure to progress/cesarian section in runners
Collings et al. [33]	Supervised exercise program (*n* = 12); controls (*n* = 8)	Review of medical charts; placental weight	No effect on fetal growth and placental weight or labor duration between groups

Clapp and Dickstein [28]	Pregnant exercisers who continued (n = 29) or discontinued exercise (n = 47) after 28th week; sedentary pregnant controls (n = 152)	Interviews, review of medical charts	Women who continued exercise gained less weight, delivered earlier, and had significantly lighter babies
Wong and McKenzie [185]	"Trained" (n = 10) and "untrained" (n = 10) classified HR response to submaximal cycling	Review of medical charts	No apparent positive or negative effects of maternal aerobic fitness on pregnancy outcome; improved fitness may shorten the active stage of labor
Kulpa et al. [92]	Women with low-risk pregnancies who performed regular aerobic exercise (n = 38); control group who exercised ≤ once/week during pregnancy (n = 47)	Detailed observation of labor and delivery; exercise logs; prediction of maximal aerobic power	No difference in neonatal morbidity or obstetric complications between groups
Hall and Kauffman [71]	Healthy pregnant women (n = 452) who performed strength/aerobic conditioning; pregnant control subjects (n = 393)	Review of medical charts; survey of patient perceptions	Shorter hospitalization, lower incidence of cesarian section and higher Apgar scores in exercising subjects vs controls; effects greatest in high-adherence exercise group (n = 61) vs. control group

reported that women with high scores on a cycle ergometer test of physical working capacity also tended to give birth to heavier babies. It was hypothesized that the fetuses of such women may have benefited from higher maternal circulatory and gas exchange capacities. Pomerance et al. [142] evaluated birth outcomes and $\dot{V}O_2$max (ml/kg/minute) predicted from the Åstrand-Åstrand nomogram in 54 women (gestational age = 35–37 weeks). No significant correlations were observed between physical fitness scores and length of gestation, pregnancy complications, length of labor in primiparas, 1-minute Apgar scores, birth weight, infant length, or infant head circumference. Physical fitness scores were inversely correlated ($p < 0.05$) with the length of labor in multiparas. Unfortunately, the authors in both of these studies did not evaluate the actual physical activity levels of their subjects so the effects of chronic exercise and genetic influences on "physical fitness" scores cannot be distinguished.

Existing retrospective studies of birth outcomes of women engaged in physical fitness regimens are summarized in Table 9.9. Three of the retrospective studies involved runners or joggers who continued to exercise during pregnancy [40, 81, 106], while one studied women who engaged in a wide range of physical activities [41]. With the exception of Dale et al. [40], who observed a high incidence failure to progress and subsequent cesarian section in a small group of runners/joggers, the results of these investigations suggested a low incidence of obstetric complications and normal fetal development in such women. Unfortunately, retrospective studies of this kind are prone to error because of the use of written questionnaires rather than medical records to evaluate pregnancy outcome; difficulties in the accurate determination of exercise quantity, quality, and adherence from questionnaire data; and a lack of an appropriate control group in studies of pregnant runners.

Prospective studies of physically active pregnant women are also summarized to Table 9.9. The investigation of Dale et al. [40] included both retrospective and prospective components which suggested a higher incidence of failure to progress/cesarian section in women who jogged or ran. The investigation of Wong and McKenzie [185] suggested that women representing higher levels of aerobic fitness may have shorter durations of labor than women with physically lower fitness levels. However, the usefulness of both of these studies is limited because of the small number of subjects studied.

Clapp and Dickstein [28] interviewed 336 antepartal obstetric patients to determine their exercise habits and plans to exercise during pregnancy. Subjects who participated in regular endurance exercise (varying combinations of running, aerobic dance and cross-country skiing) were reinterviewed between 28 and 34 weeks of gestation to determine actual exercise participation during pregnancy. Women with diabetes mellitus, early pregnancy wastage, multiple conception pregnancies, or home births and those who relocated were excluded from the study. Physically active subjects ($n = 76$) were divided into three groups in accordance with the level of exercise performance prior to pregnancy: minimal level ($n = 25$), moderate level ($n = 36$), and high level ($n = 15$). Approximately 60% of these subjects chose voluntarily for various reasons to discontinue exercise by the 28th week of gestation. Subjects who continued to exercise at or near pregnancy levels after the 28th week delivered significantly earlier (mean difference = 8 days), gained less weight (mean difference = 4.6 kg), and delivered lighter babies (mean difference = 500 g) than those who discontinued exercise. The active group who discontinued exercise gained more weight (mean difference = 2.2 kg) than sedentary control subjects. Gestational age and delivery and infant birthweight were similar in these two groups.

Kulpa et al. [92] examined pregnancy outcome over a 2½-year period in a group of 141 women with low-risk pregnancies. Following testing of aerobic working capacity in the 1st trimester, all subjects were given an individualized prescription for aerobic exercise (walking, jogging, cycling, swimming, cross-country skiing, racquetball, or aerobic exercise) and target pulse rate for exercise (75% of HRmax). Logs of exercise performed were kept by the subjects. Noncompliant subjects ($n = 2$), dropouts ($n = 20$), and spontaneous abortions ($n = 8$) were excluded from the study results. Those with serious perinatal complications ($n = 26$) were assigned to a separate "nonqualifying group." The remaining 85 "qualifying" subjects were divided into an exercising group ($n = 38$) and a control group ($n = 47$). The criteria for inclusion in the exercising group were not specified, but control subjects were those who exercised no more than once/week for 15–20 minutes at the target HR. Exercising subjects had significantly greater gains between 1st trimester and postpartum for aerobic working capacity (METs). There was no increase in the incidence of neonatal morbidity or obstetric complications in exercising versus control groups for either primiparous or multiparous subjects. Multigravid controls gained significantly more weight than multigravid exercising subjects (33.9 vs. 27.5 lb), but the level of weight gain was greater than accepted standards for all groups. Primigravid exercising subjects appeared to have a shorter second (active) stage of labor than primigravid controls. No significant difference existed for gestational age at delivery, birth weight, or Apgar scores. A unique aspect of this investigation was that all subjects received nutritional counseling aimed at ensuring that nutritional intake was sufficient to satisfy caloric needs, including energy expenditure related to aerobic exercise.

Hall and Kauffman [71] studied a group of 845 women receiving obstetric care in private practice settings in Florida. Subjects without exercise contraindications were offered the opportunity to participate in an individually prescribed exercise regimen during the course of gestation. This consisted of a 5-minute warm-up on a cycle ergometer or treadmill; approximately 45 minutes of muscular conditioning for the trunk, arms, and legs; and an aerobic workout on a cycle ergometer (HR $\leq$ 140 beats/minute, power output approximately 50 W, duration not specified). Supervised exercise sessions were conducted 3 days/week and logs of exercise sessions were kept by qualified instructors. Physical fitness was evaluated on entry to the study and at 10-week intervals to modify individual exercise prescriptions. Birth outcome was evaluated from medical records. Subjective responses to the exercise program including self-image, effects on pregnancy discomforts, relief of tension, and recovery time relative to earlier pregnancies were surveyed at 6 weeks postpartum. Subjects were divided into the following groups based on the total number of exercise sessions attended: control group (n = 393, 0–10 sessions), low-exercise group (n = 82, 11–20 sessions), medium-exercise group (n = 309, 21–59 sessions), and high-exercise group (n = 61, 60–99 sessions). No significant differences existed for length of labor for primigravid women among the groups. Birth weight was moderately lower (65–151 g, $p < 0.05$) in the control group compared to the exercised groups. The rate of cesarian section decreased with increasing exercise participation. One- and 5-minute Apgar scores did not differ greatly across groups, but mean values were highest in the high-exercise group. The mean length of hospital stay was highest in the control group (2.9 days) and lowest in the high exercise group (2.2 days) despite somewhat higher mean parity in the former group (0.9 vs. 0.7). All exercising subjects reported in the postpartum survey that the conditioning program improved self-image, decreased pregnancy discomforts, and relieved tension. Multiparous exercising patients also felt that recovery from childbirth was more rapid than in earlier pregnancies.

In summary, results of animal studies suggest generally that forced exercise can affect variables such as maternal weight gain, placental size and surface area, number of surviving fetuses/litter, fetal weight, and fetal organ development. Data obtained from guinea pigs [61, 126, 166] further suggested that the degree of fetal compromise depends on the duration of exercise. Similarly, it appears that women who work outside the home during late gestation may deliver lighter babies and may have a greater incidence of perinatal complications. Variables such as undernutrition [125, 169] or prolonged standing at work [23, 125] may exacerbate the effects of increased maternal caloric expenditure.

Studies of elite athletes who continued conditioning during pregnancy [47, 187] have generally reported favorable pregnancy outcomes. However, these women may represent a selected population with a greater physiological reserve and tolerance for exertion. The relationship between material physical fitness and pregnancy outcome also remains to be clarified. Retrospective studies of pregnancy outcome in physically active women have also reported generally that pregnancy outcome is not compromised by regular exercise. Unfortunately, such investigations are weak from a methodologic viewpoint due to the use of post-hoc questionnaires for data collection and lack of appropriate control groups in some studies.

A major difficulty with all three existing prospective studies is that subjects were classified as sedentary or active based on a post-hoc analysis of exercise adherence. Thus, results may be biased in one direction or another by selection factors. The optimal study design would involve random assignment of a large number of subjects to groups which would participate in different amounts of prescribed exercise in a closely monitored setting or act as inactive control subjects. The groups should be matched for age, parity, socioeconomic status, aerobic fitness, body fatness, and other relevant characteristics. Unfortunately, such a study may not be feasible due to probable difficulties in maintaining exercise adherence or the high cost of ensuring such adherence. Thus, the question of whether or not chronic exercise alters pregnancy outcome may not be answerable in the immediate future.

CONCLUSIONS

On the basis of results of completed scientific studies, the following conclusions appear to be warranted with respect to maternal/fetal adaptations to aerobic exercise:

1. The metabolic cost of standard submaximal exercise is not greatly affected by pregnancy, but HR and pulmonary ventilation are significantly increased. Effects of pregnancy on RPE are not well documented.
2. During mild or moderate submaximal exertion SV and $\dot{Q}c$ are augmented progressively until late gestation. Depending on maternal posture, venous return, SV, and $\dot{Q}c$ are reduced to varying degrees in late gestation as a result of compression of the inferior vena cava by the gravid uterus. Cardiovascular adaptations to more strenuous exertion may differ from mild or moderate exercise and remain for future investigation.
3. Physical conditioning appears to reduce both HR and RPE during strenuous steady-state exercise. The usual increase in submaximal exercise SV may be obscured since pregnancy effects on venous return appear to dominate the influences of aerobic conditioning, particularly at low exercise intensities.
4. Effects of pregnancy on $\dot{V}O_2max$ are poorly documented because of concerns related to the safety of maximal exercise testing during gestation. Reductions in both HRmax and $\dot{V}O_2max$ have been pos-

tulated, but have yet to be confirmed by serial studies of maximal exercise performance. Effects of physical conditioning on both maximal aerobic and anaerobic power also remain for clarification.

5. Studies of FHR during acute maternal exertion suggest that the fetus may be exposed to moderate transient hypoxia. Apparently, this is well tolerated by the fetus in the absence of uteraplacental insufficiency, maternal metabolic and cardiovascular diseases, environmental stresses, or other complicating factors. Further research concerning fetal adaptability to maternal exercise is definitely needed.

6. Studies of laboratory animals and human epidemiological studies suggest that pregnancy outcome can be altered by chronic exertion, especially if exercise is excessively strenuous or accompanied by occupational, nutritional, or other environmental stresses. On the other hand, the bulk of available evidence suggests that carefully prescribed fitness training promotes maternal physical and psychological health without compromising fetal well-being. Additional research is needed urgently to properly test this hypothesis.

The purpose of this communication was to review available information on the interactions between pregnancy and aerobic-type physical conditioning and to identify specific problems for future scientific study. Of particular concern is the recent proliferation of exercising guidelines and exercise programs from pregnant women in the absence of scientific information from controlled physical conditioning studies involving adequate subject samples. Medical authorities, exercise scientists and biomedical research granting agencies are urged to consider the importance of such investigations so that scientifically validated guidelines for exercise in pregnancy can be formulated.

ACKNOWLEDGMENTS

We have received financial support for exercise/pregnancy research from the Advisory Research Committee of Queen's University, Fitness Canada, Canadian Fitness and Lifestyle Research Institute, Ministry of Health (Ontario), National Science and Engineering Research Council of Canada, Ministry of Tourism and Recreation (Ontario), Ontario Respiratory Diseases Foundation, and Health and Welfare (Canada). Patricia J. Ohtake holds a Canadian Heart Foundation Traineeship.

We wish to thank Mrs. Barbara Vale for expertise and patience in typing of the final manuscript.

REFERENCES

1. Alaily AB, Carroll KB: Pulmonary ventilation in pregnancy. *Br J Obstet Gynecol* 85:518–524, 1978.

2. Alegre A, Rodriguez-Essudero F, Cruz E, Prada M: Influence of work during pregnancy on fetal weight. *J Reprod Med* 29:334–336, 1984.
3. American College of Obstetricians and Gynecologists: Pregnancy and the postnatal period. In *ACOG Home Exercise Programs.* Washington, DC, American College of Obstetricians and Gynecologists, 1985, pp 1–5.
4. American College of Sports Medicine: *Guidelines for Graded Exercise Testing and Prescription,* ed 3. Philadelphia, Lea and Febiger, 1986, pp 82–83.
5. Artal R, Platt LD, Sperling M, Kammula RK, Jilek J, Nakamma R: Exercise in pregnancy I. Maternal cardiovascular and metabolic responses in normal pregnancy. *Am J Obstet Gynecol* 140:123–127, 1981.
6. Artal R, Romem Y, Paul RH, Wiswell R: Fetal bradycardia induced by maternal exercise. *Lancet* 2:258–260, 1984.
7. Artal R, Wiswell RA (eds): *Exercise in Pregnancy.* Baltimore, Williams & Wilkins, 1985.
8. Artal R, Rutherford S, Romem T, Kammula RK, Dorey FJ, Wiswell RA: Fetal heart rate responses to maternal exercise. *Am J Obstet Gynecol* 155:729–733, 1986.
9. Artal R, Wiswell R, Romem Y, Dorey F: Pulmonary responses to exercise in pregnancy. *Am J Obstet Gynecol* 154:378–383, 1986.
10. Bader RA, Bader ME, Rose DJ, Braunwald E: Hemodynamics at rest and during exercise in normal pregnancy as studied by cardiac catheterization. *J Clin Invest* 34:1524–1535, 1956.
11. Bader RA, Bader ME, Rose DJ: The oxygen cost of breathing in dyspneic subjects as studied in normal pregnant women. *Clin Sci* 18: 223–235, 1959.
12. Bagnall KM, Mottola MF, McFadden KD: The effects of strenuous exercise on maternal rats and their developing fetuses. *Can J Appl Sport Sci* 8:254–259, 1983.
13. Baldwin GR, Moorthl DS, Whelton JA, MacDonnell KF: New lung functions and pregnancy. *Am J Obstet Gynecol* 127:235–239, 1977.
14. Bedell GN, Adams RW: Pulmonary diffusing capacity during rest and exercise. A study of normal persons with atrial septal defect, pregnancy and pulmonary disease. *J Clin Invest* 41:1908–1914, 1962.
15. Bevan DR, Holdcroft A, Loh L, MacGregor WG, O'Sullivan JC, Sykes MK: Closing volume and pregnancy. *Br Med J* 1:13–15, 1974.
16. Blackburn MW, Calloway DH: Basal metabolic rate and work energy expenditure of mature pregnant women. *J Am Diet Assoc* 69:24–28, 1976.
17. Blackburn MW, Calloway DH: Energy expenditure and consumption of mature, pregnant and lactating women. *J Am Diet Assoc* 69:29–37, 1976.
18. Blomqvist G, Saltin B: Cardiovascular adaptations to physical training. *Annu Rev Physiol* 45:169–189, 1983.
19. Boehnke WH, Chernoff GF, Finnell RH: Investigation of the teratogenic effects of exercise on pregnancy outcome in mice. *Teratog Carcinog Mutagen* 7:391–397, 1987.
20. Bonekat HW, Dombovy ML, Staats BA: Progesterone-induced changes in exercise performance and ventilatory response *Med Sci Sports Exerc* 19:118–123, 1987.
21. Bonica JJ: Maternal respiratory changes during pregnancy and parturition. *Clin Anesth* 10:1–19, 1974.
22. Bonner HW, Buffington CK, Newman JJ, Farrar RP, Acosta D: Contractile activity of neonatal heart cells in culture derived from offspring of exercised pregnant rats. *Eur J Appl Physiol* 39:1–6, 1978.
23. Briend A: Maternal physical activity, birthweight and perinatal mortality. *Med Hypotheses* 6:1157–1170, 1980.
24. Burg JR, Dodek A, Kloster FE, Metcalfe J: Alterations of systolic time intervals during pregnancy. *Circulation* 49:560–564, 1974.

25. Caldwell F, Jopke T: Questions and answers: ACSM 1985. *Physician Sportsmed* 13:146–147, 1985.

26. Campbell EJM, Howell JBL: The sensation of breathlessness. *Br Med Bull* 19:36–40, 1963.

27. Chandler KD, Bell AW: Effects of maternal exercise on fetal and maternal respiration and nutrient metabolism in the pregnant ewe. *J Dev Physiol (Oxf)* 3:161–176, 1981.

28. Clapp JF III, Dickstein S: Endurance exercise and pregnancy outcome. *Med Sci Sports Exerc* 16:556–562, 1984.

29. Clapp JF III: Maternal heart rate in pregnancy. *Am J Obstet Gynecol* 152:659–660, 1985.

30. Clapp JF III: Fetal heart rate response to running in midpregnancy and late pregnancy. *Am J Obstet Gynecol* 153:251–252, 1985.

31. Clapp JF III, Wesley M, Sleamaker RH: Thermoregulatory and metabolic responses prior to and during pregnancy. *Med Sci Sports Exerc* 19:124–130, 1987.

32. Cohn HE, Sacks EJ, Heyman MA, Rudolph AM: Cardiovascular responses to hypoxemia and acidemia in fetal lambs. *Am J Obstet Gynecol* 120:817–824, 1974.

33. Collings CA, Curet LB, Mullin JP: Maternal and fetal responses to a maternal aerobic exercise program. *Am J Obstet Gynecol* 145:702–707, 1983.

34. Collings CA, Curet LB: Fetal heart rate responses to maternal exercise. *Am J Obstet Gynecol* 151:498–501, 1985.

35. Craig DB, Toole MA: Airway closure in pregnancy. *Can Anaesth Soc J* 22:665-672, 1975.

36 Craig BW, Treadway JL: Glucose uptake and oxidation in fat cells of trained and sedentary pregnant rats. *J Appl Physiol: Respir Environ Exerc Physiol* 60:1704–1709, 1986.

37. Cugell DW, Frank NR, Gaensler EA, Badger TL: Pulmonary function in pregnancy. I. Serial observations in normal women. *Am Rev Tuberc Pulm Dis* 67:568–597, 1953.

38. Curet LB, Orr JA, Rankin JHG, Ungerer T: Effect of exercise on cardiac output and distribution of uterine blood flow in pregnant ewes. *J Appl Physiol: Respir Environ Exerc Physiol* 55:834–841, 1976.

39. Dahlström H, Ihrman K: Clinical and physiological study of pregnancy in a material from northern Sweden. V. The results of work tests during and after pregnancy. *Acta Soc Med Upsal* 65:305–314, 1960.

40. Dale E, Mullinax KM, Bryan DH: Exercise during pregnancy: effects on the fetus. *Can J Appl Sport Sci* 7:98–103, 1982.

41. Work J: Study: exercise okay in normal pregnancy. *Physician Sportsmed* 15:51, 1987.

42. Dhindsa DS, Metcalfe J, Hummels DH: Responses to exercise in the pigmy goat. *Respir Physiol* 32:299–311, 1978.

43. Dibblee L, Graham TE: A longitudinal study of changes in aerobic fitness, body composition, and energy intake in primigravid women. *Am J Obstet Gynecol* 147:908–914, 1983.

44. Dressendorfer RH: Physical training during pregnancy and lactation. *Physician Sportsmed* 6:74–80, 1978.

45. Edwards MJ: Congenital defects in guinea pigs following induced hyperthermia during gestation. *Arch Pathol* 84:42–48, 1967.

46. Edwards MJ, Metcalfe J, Dunham MJ, Paul MS: Accelerated respiratory response to moderate exercise in late pregnancy. *Respir Physiol* 45:229–241, 1981.

47. Erdelyi GJ: Gynecological survey of female athletes. *J Sports Med Phys Fitness* 2:174–179, 1962.

48. Erkkola R: The physical fitness of Finnish primigravidae. *Ann Chir Gynaecol* 64:394–400, 1975.

49. Erkkola R: The physical work capacity of the expectant mother and its effect on pregnancy, labor, and the newborn. *Int J Gynaecol Obstet* 14:153–159, 1976.

50. Erkkola R: The influence of physical training during pregnancy on physical work capacity and circulatory parameters. *Scand J Clin Lab Invest* 36:747–754, 1976.

51. Fawer R, Dettling A, Weihs D, Welti H, Schelling JL: Effect of the menstrual cycle, oral contraception, and pregnancy on forearm blood flow, venous distensibility and clotting factors. *Eur J Clin Pharmacol* 13:251–257, 1978.

52. Fox ME, Harris RE, Brekken AL: The active-duty military pregnancy: a new high-risk category. *Am J Obstet Gynecol* 129:705–707, 1977.

53. Garrard GS, Littler WA, Regman CWG: Closing volume during normal pregnancy. *Thorax* 33:488–492, 1978.

54. Garris DR, Kasperck GJ, Overton SV, Alligood GR: Effects of exercise on fetal-placental growth and uteroplacental blood flow in the rat. *Biol Neonate* 47:223–229, 1985.

55. Gauthier MM: Guidelines for exercise during pregnancy: too little or too much? *Physician Sportsmed* 14:162–169, 1986.

56. Gazioglu K, Kaltreider NL, Rosen M, Yu PN: Pulmonary function during pregnancy in normal women and in patients with cardiopulmonary disease. *Thorax* 25:445–450, 1970.

57. Gee JGL, Packer BS, Millen JE, Robin ED: Pulmonary mechanics during pregnancy. *J Clin Invest* 46:945–952, 1967.

58. Gemzell CA, Robbe H, Stromme G: Total amount of hemoglobin and physical working capacity in normal pregnancy and puerperium (with iron medication). *Acta Obstet Gynecol Scand* 36:93–136, 1957.

59. Gilbert R, Epifano L, Auchincloss HJ: Dyspnea of pregnancy. A syndrome of altered respiratory control. *JAMA* 182:97–101, 1962.

60. Gilbert R, Auchincloss HJ: Dyspnea of pregnancy. Clinical and physiological observations. *Am J Med Sci* 252:270–276, 1966.

61. Gilbert RD, Cummings LA, Juchau MR, Longo LD: Placental diffusing capacity and fetal development in exercising or hypoxic guinea pigs. *J Appl Physiol: Respir Environ Exerc Physiol* 46:828–834, 1979.

62. Gimovski, ML, Caritis SN: Diagnosis and management of hypoxic fetal heart rate patterns. *Clin Perinatol* 9:313–324, 1982.

63. Goodlin RC, Buckley KK: Maternal exercise. *Clin Sports Med* 3:881–894, 1984.

64. Goodrich SM, Wood JE: Peripheral venous distensibility and velocity of venous blood flow during pregnancy or during oral contraceptive therapy. *Am J Obstet Gynecol* 90:740–744, 1964.

65. Goodrich SM, Wood JE: The effect of estradiol-17 beta on peripheral venous distensibility and velocity of venous blood flow. *Am J Obstet Gynecol* 96:407–412, 1966.

66. Gorski J: Exercise during pregnancy: maternal and fetal responses. A brief review. *Med Sci Sports Exerc* 17:407–416, 1985.

67. Greenleaf JE, Convertino VA, Stremel RW, Bernauer EM, Adams WC, Vignau SR, Brock PJ: Plasma (Na+), (Ca2+), and volume shifts and thermoregulation during exercise in man. *J Appl Physiol* 43:1026–1032, 1977.

68. Greiss FC Jr: Differential reactivity of the myoendometrial and placental vasculatures: adrenergic responses. *Am J Obstet Gynecol* 112:20–30, 1972.

69. Guzman CA, Caplan R: Cardiorespiratory response to exercise during pregnancy. *Am J Obstet Gynecol* 108:600–605, 1970.

70. Hall P: Cardiovascular adaptations to physical conditioning during pregnancy. Unpublished master's thesis. Kingston, Canada, Queen's University, 1987.

71. Hall DC, Kaufman DA: Effects of aerobic and strength conditioning on pregnancy outcomes. *Am J Obstet Gynecol* 157:1199–1203, 1987.

72. Hauth JC, Gilstrap LC, Widmer K: Fetal heart rate reactivity before and after maternal jogging during the third trimester. *Am J Obstet Gynecol* 142:545–547, 1982.
73. Hohimer AR, McKean TA, Bissonette JM, Metcalfe J: Maternal exercise reduces myometrical blood flow in the pregnant goat (abstract). *Fed Proc* 41:4190, 1982.
74. Hon EH, Wohlegemuth R: The electronic evaluation of fetal heart rate. IV. The effect of maternal exercise. *Am J Obstet Gynecol* 81:361–371, 1961.
75. Hosenpud JD, Hart MV, Morton MJ, Hominer AR: Chronic estrogen administration increases left ventricular size and stroke volume (abstract). *Clin Res* 192A, 1983.
76. Hutchinson PL, Cureton KJ, Sparling PB: Metabolic and circulatory responses to running during pregnancy. *Physician Sportsmed* 9:55–58, 61, 1981.
77. Hytten FE, Paintin DB: Increase in plasma volume during normal pregnancy. *J Obstet Gynaecol Br Commonw* 70:402–407, 1963.
78. Hytten FE: Physiological changes in early pregnancy. *J Obstet Gynaecol Br Commonw* 75:1193–1197, 1968.
79. Hytten FE, Chamberlain G: *Clinical Physiology in Obstetrics*. Boston, Blackwell Scientific Publications, 1980.
80. Ihrman K: A clinical and physiological study of pregnancy in a material from northern Sweden. VIII. The effect of physical training during pregnancy on the circulatory adjustment. *Acta Soc Upsal* 65:335–347, 1960.
81. Jarrett JC, Spellacy WN: Jogging during pregnancy: an improved outcome? *Obstet Gynecol* 61:705–709, 1983.
82. Jenkins RR, Ciconne C: Exercise effect during pregnancy on brain nucleic acids of offspring in rats. *Arch Phys Med Rehabil* 61:124–127, 1980.
83. Jovanovic L, Kessler A, Peterson CM: Human maternal and fetal responses to graded exercise. *J Appl Physiol* 58:1719–1722, 1985.
84. Katz R, Karliner JS, Resnik R: Effects of a natural volume overload state (pregnancy) on left ventricular performance in normal human subjects. *Circulation* 58:434–441, 1978.
85. Keerdoja E, DeQuine J, Albow K, Keene S, Bailey E: Now the pregnancy workout. *Newsweek* July 23, 1984, p. 70.
86. Kerr MG, Scott DB, Samuel E: Studies of the inferior vena cava in pregnancy. *Br Med J* 1:532–533, 1964.
87. Kerr MG: Cardiovascular dynamics in pregnancy and labour. *Br Med Bull* 24:19–24, 1968.
88. King TM, Whitehorn WV, Reeves B, Kubota R: Effects of estrogen on composition of cardiac muscle. *Am J Physiol* 196:1282–1285, 1959.
89. Knopp RH: Fuel metabolism in pregnancy. *Contemp Obstet Gynecol* 12 (July):83–90, 1978.
90. Knuttgen HG, Emerson K Jr: Physiological response to pregnancy at rest and during exercise. *J Appl Physiol* 36:549–553, 1974.
91. Korcok M: Pregnant jogger: what a record! *JAMA* 246:201, 1981.
92. Kulpa PJ, White BM, Visscher R: Aerobic exercise in pregnancy. *Am J Obstet Gynecol* 156:1395–1403, 1987.
93. Laird-Meeter K, Van De Ley G, Bom TH, Wladimiroff JW, Roelandt J: Cardiocirculatory adjustments during pregnancy: an echocardiographic study. *Clin Cardiol* 2:328–332, 1979.
94. LeBlanc P, Ruff R, Milic-Emili J: Effects of age and body position on "airway closure" in man. *J Appl Physiol* 28:448–451, 1970.
95. Lees MM, Scott DB, Kerr MG, Taylor SH: The circulatory effects of recumbent postural change in late pregnancy. *Clin Sci* 32:453–465, 1967.
96. Liberatore SM, Pistelli R, Patalano F, Moneta E, Incalzi RA, Ciappi G: Respiratory function during pregnancy. *Respiration* 46:145–150, 1984.

97. Longo LD, Hewitt CW, Lorijn RHW, Gilbert RD: To what extent does maternal exercise affect fetal oxygenation and uterine blood flow? *Fed Proc* 37:905, 1978.

98. Longo LD: Maternal blood volume and cardiac output during pregnancy: a hypothesis of endocrinologic control. *Am J Physiol* 245:R720–R729, 1983.

99. Lopatin VA: Some mechanisms of changes in external respiration during the menstrual cycle and pregnancy. *Hum Physiol* 5:134–143, 1979.

100. Lotgering FK, Gilbert RD, Longo LD: Exercise responses in pregnant sheep: oxygen consumption, uterine blood flow and blood volume. *J Appl Physiol: Respir Environ Exerc Physiol* 55:834–841, 1983.

101. Lotgering FK, Gilbert RD, Longo LD: Exercise responses in pregnant sheep: blood gases, temperatures, and fetal cardiovascular system. *J Appl Physiol: Respir Environ Exerc Physiol* 55:842–850, 1983.

102. Lotgering FK, Gilbert RD, Longo LD: The interactions of exercise and pregnancy: a review. *Am J Obstet Gynecol* 149:560–568, 1984.

103. Lotgering FK, Gilbert RD, Longo LD: Maternal and fetal responses to exercise during pregnancy. *Physiol Rev* 61:1–36, 1985.

104. Lucius H, Gahlenbeck H, Kleine H-O, Fabel H, Bartels H: Respiratory functions, buffer system and electrolyte concentrations of blood during human pregnancy. *Respir Physiol* 9:311–317, 1970.

105. Lund CJ, Donovan JC: Blood volume during pregnancy. Significance of plasma and red cell volumes. *Am J Obstet Gynecol* 98:393–403, 1967.

106. Lutter JM, Lee V, Cushman S: Fetal outcomes of women who ran while pregnant, A preliminary report. *The Melopomene Report* 3 (October):6–8, 1984.

107. Lyons HA, Antonio R: The sensitivity of the respiratory center in pregnancy and after administration of progesterone. *Trans Assoc Am Physicians* 72:173–180, 1959.

108. Manshande JP, Eckels R, Manshande-Desmet V, Vlietinck R: Rest versus heavy work during the last weeks of pregnancy: influence on fetal growth. *Br J Obstet Gynaecol* 94:1059–1067, 1987.

109. Martin CM, Combs DT, Unzelmon RF: Systolic time intervals in normal pregnant women. *Milit Med* 141:396–400, 1976.

110. Martin CB Jr: Physiology and clinical use of fetal heart rate variability. *Clin Perinatol* 9:339–352, 1982.

111. Mashini IS, Albazzaz SJ, Fadel HE, Abdulla AM, Hadi HA, Harp R, Devoe LD: Serial noninvasive evaluation of cardiovascular hemodynamics during pregnancy. *Am J Obstet Gynecol* 156:1208–1213, 1987.

112. Metcalfe J, Ueland K: Cardiovascular adjustments to pregnancy. *Prog Cardiovasc Dis* 40:363–374, 1974.

113. Metcalfe J, McAnulty JH, Ueland K: Cardiovascular physiology. *Clin Obstet Gynecol* 24:693–710, 1981.

114. Meyer BA, Daling JR: Activity level of mothers' usual occupation and low infant birth weight. *J Occup Med* 27:841–845, 1985.

115. Miller FC, Petrie RH, Arce JJ, Paul RH, Hon EH: Hyperventilation during labor. *Am J Obstet Gynecol* 120:489, 1974.

116. Milne JA, Howie AD, Pack AI: Dyspnoea during normal pregnancy. *Br J Obstet Gynecol* 85:260–263, 1978.

117. Moore LG, McCullough RE, Weil JV: Increased HVR in pregnancy: relationship to hormonal and metabolic changes. *J Appl Physiol: Respir Environ Exerc Physiol* 62:158–163, 1987.

118. Morton M, Tsang H, Hohimer R, Ross D, Thornburg K, Faber J, Metcalfe J: Left ventricular size, output, and structure during guinea-pig pregnancy. *Am J Physiol* 246:R40–R48, 1984.

119. Morton MJ, Paul NS, Compos GR, Hartz MV, Metcalfe J: Exercise dynamics in late gestation: effects of physical training. *Am J Obstet Gynecol* 152:91–97, 1985.
120. Morton MJ, Paul MS, Metcalfe J: Exercise during pregnancy. *Med Clin N Am* 69:97–108, 1985.
121. Mottola M, Bagnall KM, McFadden KD: The effects of maternal exercise on developing rat fetuses. *Br J Sports Med* 17:117–121, 1983.
122. Mottola MF, Bagnall KM, Belcastro AN, Foster J, Secord D: The effects of strenuous maternal exercise on maternal body components in rats. *J Anat* 148:65–75, 1986.
123. Mottola MF, Bagnall KM, Belcastro AN: Effects of strenuous maternal exercise on fetal organ weights and skeletal muscle development in rats. *J Dev Physiol*, in press.
124. Murphy JE, Dauncey M, Newcombe R, Garcia J, Elbourne D: Employment in pregnancy: prevalence, maternal characteristics, perinatal outcomes. *Lancet* 1:1163–1166, 1984.
125. Naeye RL, Peters EC: Working during pregnancy: effects on the fetus. *Pediatrics* 69:724–727, 1982.
126. Nelson PS, Gilbert RD, Longo LD: Fetal growth and placental diffusing capacity in guinea pigs following long-term maternal exercise. *J Dev Physiol* 5:1–10, 1983.
127. Ohtake PJ, Wolfe LA, Hall P, McGrath M: Ventilatory responses to physical conditioning during pregnancy. *FASEB J* 31:A158, 1988.
128. Pandolf KB: Advances in the study and application of perceived exertion. In Terjung RL (ed): *Exercise and Sport Sciences Reviews*. Philadelphia, Franklin Institute Press, 1983, pp. 118–158.
129. Paolone AM, Worthington S: Cautions and advice on exercise during pregnancy. *Contemp Obstet Gynecol* 25 (May):150–158, 1985.
130. Paolone AM, Shangold M, Paul D, Minnitti J, Weiner S: Fetal heart rate measurement during maternal exercise—avoidance of artifact. *Med Sci Sports Exerc* 19:605–609, 1987.
131. Parer JT: Fetal heart rate. In Creasy RK, Resnick RI (eds): *Maternal-Fetal Medicine: Principles and Practice*. Philadelphia, W.B. Saunders, 1984, pp 285–319.
132. Parizkova J, Watchtlova M, Soukupova M: The impact of different motor activity on body composition, density of capillaries and fibers in the heart and soleus muscles, and cell's migration in vitro in male rats. *Int Agnew Physiol Einschl Arbeitsphysiol* 30:207–216, 1972.
133. Parizkova J: Impact of daily workload during pregnancy on the microstructure of the rat heart in male offspring. *Eur J Appl Physiol* 34:323–326, 1975.
134. Parizkova J, Petrasek R: The impact of daily workload during pregnancy on lipid metabolism in the liver of the offspring. *Eur J Appl Physiol* 39:81–87, 1978.
135. Perel'man YUM, Lutsenko MT, Noresko BV: Regional lung function in the last stages of physiological pregnancy. *Hum Physiol* 9:120–126, 1983.
136. Pernoll ML, Metcalfe J, Schlenker TL, Welch JE, Matsumoto JA: Oxygen consumption at rest and during exercise in pregnancy. *Respir Physiol* 25:285–293, 1975.
137. Pernoll ML, Metcalfe J, Kovach PA, Wachtel R, Durham MJ: Ventilation during rest and exercise in pregnancy and postpartum. *Respir Physiol* 25:295–310, 1975.
138. Pernoll ML, Metcalfe J, Paul M: Fetal cardiac response to maternal exercise. In Lange LD, Reneau DD, (eds): *Fetal and Newborn Cardiovascular Physiology: Fetal and Newborn Circulation* New York, Garland, 1978, pp 389–398.
139. Pijpers L, Wladimiroff JW, McGhie J: Effect of short-term maternal exercise on maternal and fetal cardiovascular dynamics. *Br J Obstet Gynaecol* 91:1081–1086, 1984.
140. Pritchard JA: Changes in the blood volume during pregnancy and delivery. *Anesthesiology* 26:393–399, 1965.
141. Prowse CM, Gaensler EA: Respiratory and acid–base changes during pregnancy. *Anesthesiology* 26:381–392, 1965.

142. Pomerance JJ, Gluck L, Lynch VA: Maternal exercise as a screening test for utero-placental insufficiency. *Obstet Gynecol* 44:383–387, 1974.
143. Pritchard JA, MacDonald PC, Grant NF: William's Obstetrics, ed 17. Norwalk, CT, Appleton-Century-Crofts, 1985.
144. Ratigan TR: Anatomic and physiologic changes of pregnancy: anesthetic considerations. *J Am Assoc Nurse Anesth* 51:38–42, 1983.
145. Rochard F, Schifrin BS, Goupil F, Legrande H, Blattiere J, Sureau C: Nonstressed fetal heart rate monitoring in the antepartal period. *Am J Obstet Gynecol* 126:699–706, 1976.
146. Rowell LB: Human cardiovascular adjustments to exercise and thermal stress. *Physiol Rev* 54:75–159, 1974.
147. Roy SB, Malkani PK, Ranjit V, Bhatia ML: Circulatory effects of pregnancy. *Am J Obstet Gynecol* 96:221–225, 1966.
148. Rudolph AM, Heymann MA: Cardiac output in the fetal lamb: the effects of spontaneous and induced changes of heart rate on right and left ventricular output. *Am J Obstet Gynecol* 124:183–192, 1976.
149. Ruhling RO, Cameron J, Sibley L: Maintaining aerobic fitness while jogging through a pregnancy: a case study (abstract). *Med Sci Sports Exerc* 13:93, 1981.
150. Russell IF, Chambers WA: Closing volume in normal pregnancy. *Br J Anaesth* 53:1043–1047, 1981.
151. Rubler S, Schneebaum R, Hammer N: Systolic time intervals in pregnancy and the postpartum period. *Am Heart J* 86:182–188, 1973.
152. Rubler S, Damani PM, Pinto ER: Cardiac size and performance during pregnancy estimated with echocardiography. *Am J Cardiol* 40:534–540, 1977.
153. Sady S, Carpenter M, Sady M, Haydon B, Thompson P, Coustan D: Cardiovascular response to exercise during pregnancy (abstract). *Med Sci Sports Exerc* 20:511, 1988.
154. Sady M, Haydon B, Sady S, Carpenter M, Coustan D, Thompson P. Maximal exercise during pregnancy and postpartum (abstract). *Med Sci Sports Exerc* 20:511, 1988.
155. Sandström B: Adjustments of the circulation to orthostatic reaction and physical exercise during the first trimester of primipregnancy. *Acta Obstet Gynecol Scand* 53:1–5, 1974.
156. Saurel-Cubizolles MJ, Kaminski M: Work in pregnancy: its evolving relationship with perinatal outcome (a review). *Soc Sci Med* 22:431–442, 1986.
157. Savard R, Palmer JE, Greenwood MRC: Effects of exercise training on regional adipose tissue metabolism in pregnant rats. *Am J Physiol: Regul Integrat Comp Physiol* 250:R837–R844, 1986.
158. Schoene RB, Robertson HT, Pierson DJ, Peterson, AP: Respiratory drives and exercise in menstrual cycles of athletic and non-athletic women. *J Appl Physiol: Respir Environ Exerc Physiol* 50:1300–1305, 1981.
159. Schröder H, Gilbert RD, Power GG: Fetal heat dissipation: a computer model and preliminary experimental results from fetal sheep. In *Scientific Abstracts of the 29th Annual Meeting of the Society for Gynecological Investigation.* 1982, 113.
160. Scott DE: Anemia in pregnancy. *Obstet Gynecol Annu* 1:219, 1972.
161. Seitchik J: Body composition and energy expenditure during rest and work in pregnancy. *Am J Obstet Gynecol* 97:701–713, 1967.
162. Severinghaus JW: Blood gas calculator. *J Appl Physiol* 21:1108–1116, 1966.
163. Shangold MM, Metcalfe J, Longo LD, Clapp JF III: Symposium: Exercise during pregnancy—state of the art (abstract). *Med Sci Sports Exerc* 17:218, 1985.
164. Sibley L, Ruhling RO, Cameron-Foster J, Christensen C, Bolen T: Swimming and physical fitness during pregnancy. *J Nurse-Midwifery* 26:3–12, 1981.

165. South-Paul JE, Rajagopal KR, Tenholder MS: The effect of participation in a regular exercise program upon aerobic capacity during pregnancy. *Obstet Gynecol* 71:175–179, 1988.

166. Smith AD, Gilbert RD, Lammers RJ, Longo LD: Placental exchange area in guinea-pigs following long-term maternal exercise: a stereological analysis. *J Dev Physiol* 5:11–21, 1983.

167. Soiva K, Salmi A, Grönros M, Peltonen T: Physical working capacity during pregnancy and effect of physical work tests on foetal heart rate. *Ann Chir Gynaecol Fenn* 53:187–196, 1963.

168. Sullivan JM, Ramanathan KB: Management of medical problems in pregnancy—severe cardiac disease. *N Engl J Med* 313:304–309, 1985.

169. Tafari N, Naeye RL, Gobeze A: Effects of maternal undernutrition and heavy physical work during pregnancy on birth weight. *Br J Obstet Gynecol* 87:222–226, 1980.

170. Terada M: Effect of physical activity before pregnancy on fetuses of mice exercised forcibly during pregnancy. *Teratology* 10:141–144, 1974.

171. Templeton A, Kelman GR: Maternal blood gases (Pao_2-Pao_2), physiological shunt and VD/VT in normal pregnancy. *Br J Anaesth* 48:1001–1004, 1976.

172. Treadway J, Dover EV, Morse W, Newcomer L, Craig BW: Influence of exercise training on maternal and fetal morphological characteristics in the rat. *J Appl Physiol: Respir Environ Exerc Physiol* 60:1700–1703, 1986.

173. Treadway JL, Lederman SA: The effects of exercise on milk yield, milk composition and offspring growth in rats. *Am J Clin Nutr* 44:481–488, 1986.

174. Treadway JL, Young JC: Decreased glucose uptake in the fetus after exercise (abstract). *Med Sci Sports Exerc* 19:55, 1987.

175. Ueland K, Parer JT: Effect of estrogen on the cardiovascular system of the ewe. *Am J Obstet Gynecol* 96:400–406, 1966.

176. Ueland K, Novy MJ, Peterson EN, Metcalfe J: Maternal cardiovascular dynamics IV. The influence of gestational age on the maternal cardiovascular response to posture and exercise. *Am J Obstet Gynecol* 104:856–864, 1969.

177. Ueland K, Novy MJ, Peterson EN, Metcalfe J: Cardiorespiratory responses to pregnancy and exercise in normal women and patients with heart disease. *Am J Obstet Gynecol* 115:4–10, 1973.

178. Veille JC, Hohimer AR, Burry K, Speroff L: The effect of exercise on uterine activity in the last eight weeks of pregnancy. *Am J Obstet Gynecol* 151:727–730, 1985.

179. Villarosa L: Running and pregnancy. Having it all. *The Runner* 7:24–31, 1985.

180. Vorys N, Ullery JC, Hanusek GE: The cardiac output changes in various positions in pregnancy. *Am J Obstet Gynecol* 82:1312–1321, 1961.

181. Walters WA, Lim YL: Cardiovascular dynamics in women receiving oral contraceptive therapy. *Lancet* 2:879–881, 1969.

182. Wilson NC, Gisolfi CV: Effects of exercising rats during pregnancy. *J Appl Physiol: Respir Environ Exerc Physiol* 48:34–40, 1980.

183. Wiswell RA, Artal R, Romem Y, Kammula R, Dorey FJ: Hormonal and metabolic response to exercise in pregnancy (abstract). *Med Sci Sports Exerc* 17:206, 1985.

184. Wolfe LA, Hall P, McGrath MJ, Burggraf GW, Tranmer JE: Cardiovascular responses to physical conditioning during pregnancy (abstract). *Can J Sport Sci* 12:27, 1987.

185. Wong SC, McKenzie DC: Cardiorespiratory fitness during pregnancy and its effects on outcome. *Int J Sports Med* 8:79–83, 1987.

186. Woodward SL: How does strenuous maternal exercise affect the fetus? A review. *Birth Fam J* 8:17–24, 1981.

187. Zaharieva E: Olympic participation by women. *JAMA* 221:992–995, 1972.
188. Zuckerman BF, Frank DA, Hingson R, Marelock S, Kayne HL: Impact of maternal work outside the home during pregnancy on neonatal outcome. *Pediatrics* 77:459–464, 1986.

10
Growth Hormone: Physiology, Therapeutic Use, and Potential for Abuse
ALAN D. ROGOL, M.D., Ph.D.

NEUROENDOCRINOLOGY OF GROWTH HORMONE SECRETION

The complex system that encompasses the release and action of growth hormone (GH) includes many neurotransmitters, hormones, and organs. Among these are biogenic amines such as dopamine and serotonin in the brain; growth-hormone-releasing hormone (GHRH) and somatostatin or somatotropin-release-inhibiting hormone (SRIH) in the hypothalamus; somatotropin or GH in the pituitary; and insulin-like growth factors I (IGF-I or somatomedin C) and possibly II (IGF-II) in the liver and other organs [35, 38, 77, 78]. The mechanisms by which this complex system generates growth as a result of GH production and release from the pituitary are rapidly being elucidated.

Growth hormone is secreted in an intermittent, pulsatile, burst-like pattern. Hormone concentrations are usually below the level of detectability between the secretory episodes in the usual radioimmuno- or immunoradiometric assays employed. A number of phasic changes in GH secretion are mediated by brain centers under the stimulus of biogenic amines. For example, dopamine augments GH secretion. The arcuate nucleus, in particular, and possibly the ventromedial nucleus as well, respond by releasing GHRH and SRIH [13]. Both are transported from the hypothalamus via the portal system to the pituitary, where they attach to their respective receptors on the somatotropes [88, 102]. Somatostatin is present in organ systems other than the brain (for example, the pancreas and gut). Three approximately equipotent forms of GHRH have been identified—one with 44, one with 40, and one with 37 amino acids [38, 79]. The first two have been identified in the hypothalamus [14, 61]. Although disappearance rates for GHRH 1-40 or 1-44 were previously considered to be 50 minutes [28], GHRH is rapidly degraded by cleavage of the intact molecule by a plasma depeptidylaminopeptidase producing the biologically much less active peptide GHRH 3-44 (and 3-40) [29]. The synthesis and release of GH from the somatotropes are under the control of the adenosine 3':5'-cyclic phosphate (cAMP) second messenger system. Both synthesis and release are sensitive to calcium ion fluxes and diacylglycerol. Protein kinase-C, the putative phorbol ester receptor, also plays an important role in the stimulated secretory pathway for GH, as indicated by marked increases in GH release from anterior pituitary cells of rats following stimulation with the phorbol ester, phorbol-12-myristate-13-acetate [92]. Growth-hormone-releasing hormone, cholera toxin, and forskolin lead to cAMP accumulation in somatotropes and stimulate growth hormone release [21]; somatostatin inhibits both effects of these secretagogues, and thus its action is also closely related to the cAMP system [20]. As pituitary portal blood concentrations of GHRH and SRIH change, serum levels of GH rise and fall in an intermittent, pulsatile fashion [72, 97].

The feedback mechanisms that control GH release are multiple and complex. For example, GHRH can diminish its own secretion, as shown by Tannenbaum [95], who injected GHRH in graded doses into the cerebral ventricles of rats. Increasing doses given in this manner led to a dose-dependent inhibition of GH secretion. This profound effect was not due to SRIH secretion, as shown by the inability of an antiserum to SRIH to reverse the suppression of GH release. Thus, GHRH can affect its own secretion by means of an ultra-short loop negative feedback mechanism. In addition, GHRH produces negative feedback at the somatotrope after lengthy exposure to the peptide. Pretreatment of anterior pituitary cells cultured with GHRH results in decreased cAMP and GH concentrations in these cells when they are reexposed to GHRH [12]. However, evidence from in vivo studies in humans indicates that GHRH stimulates GH secretion in an intermittent pulsatile manner even after continuous infusion to normal subjects for up to 2 weeks. Indeed, there was even a marked increase in nocturnal GH secretion and an overall increase in IGF-I levels [100]. The interaction with somatostatin probably differentiates the in vivo from the in vitro experimental paradigm. Recent data suggest that GHRH and somatostatin may regulate their own secretion. In vitro GHRH inhibits its own secretion in hypothalamic fragments, but increases somatostatin release [3, 4]. Similarly, somatostatin inhibits its own release [70]. Intracerebroventricular administration of somatostatin increases and similar administration of GHRH reduces circulating GH levels [56, 57].

Insulin-like growth factors also are involved in the feedback control of GH secretion. An inhibitory effect probably occurs at both hypothalamic (increased somatostatin and decreased GHRH release) and pituitary levels [9, 62, 90]. When placed in the cerebral ventricles, IGF-I causes a profound decrease in the spontaneous, intermittent secretion of GH in rats [96]. This action may be mediated by SRIH, since it has been demonstrated that IGF-I directly stimulates the acute release of SRIH from rat hypothalamic fragments in culture [89].

Growth hormone also plays a feedback role in its own secretion. Growth hormone acts on the hypothalamus to stimulate both the synthesis and release of SRIH. Abrams et al. [1] had previously demonstrated that GH injections given daily for 6 days in humans diminished GH release by the pituitary when insulin was given 8 hours after the last GH injection. It was not ascertained, however, whether this was a direct effect of the GH or an indirect effect through somatomedin generation [1]. More recently Rosenthal et al. [83] have shown that exogenous GH inhibits GHRH-induced GH secretion as well. The mechanism is probably that of increased somatostatin secretion [83, 84]. In summary, there is a complex, hierarchical series of negative feedback loops that control the tonic and phasic secretion of GH mediated through the release of GHRH and SRIH.

After GH is released into the circulation, it is attached to a GH binding protein. The GH binding protein, like the cell membrane bound GH receptor, specifically binds GH. This binding protein, in fact, is the extracellular domain of the GH receptor. Children with Laron-type dwarfism are very short despite high circulating levels of GH. They are deficient in both the GH receptor and its binding protein [6, 22] thus demonstrating the physiological relevance of these proteins. The GH-bound complex travels to the liver and other tissues, including chondrocytes in growing cartilage. In the liver and cells of other tissues, GH stimulates the production of IGF-I and probably IGF-II. These growth factors, homologues of the proinsulin molecule, have biologic effects that are qualitatively similar to those of insulin.

Nutritional status also influences levels of IGF-I. Despite very high levels of GH in severely malnourished infants, circulating concentrations of IGF-I (and IGF-II) are very low [91]. Nutritional rehabilitation leads to a marked diminution of the excessive GH levels and an increase in IGF-I concentrations to age-appropriate levels [91]. In adult volunteers fasting quickly causes an increase in GH concentrations and a decrease in IGF-I levels [17, 39]. Both return toward normal with refeeding [19].

To determine the dietary components required to maintain normal plasma IGF-I concentrations, Isley et al. [44] fasted normal-weight volunteers for 5 days, and then refed them with one of three test diets: (*a*) normal energy and protein, (*b*) low protein and normal energy, or (*c*) low protein and low energy. There was an average decline in IGF-I levels of 64% after fasting. The normal energy/normal protein (control) diet was associated with a 72% restoration of circulating IGF-I levels by the 5th day. The low protein/normal energy diet resulted in an increase to 55% of the control values, whereas the diet deficient in both nitrogen and energy led to a further decline in IGF-I levels. Thus, both nitrogen and energy contents of the diet influence circulating IGF-I levels; however, caloric content appears to be the more important variable (see Fig. 10.1).

FIGURE 10.1

Change in plasma somatomedin C/insulin-like growth factor I levels in response to test diets of defined composition. Five normal-weight volunteers were fasted for 5-day intervals, then refed one of three test diets. The dietary compositions are indicated in the text. The results represent the mean ± 1 SE. (Reproduced with permission from Isley WL, Underwood LE, Clemmons DR: Dietary components that regulate serum somatomedin C concentrations in humans. J Clin Invest 71:175–182, 1983.)

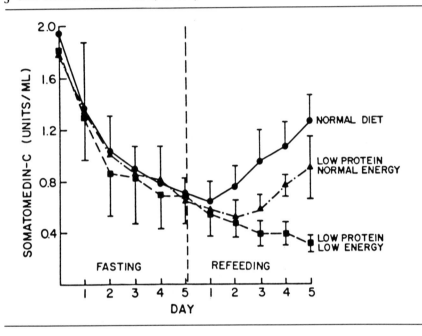

Molecular weights of the IGFs are approximately 7,500 daltons, and the factors resemble proinsulin in that about 50% of the amino acid residues in the A and B chains are identical with the corresponding sequences in human proinsulin. Radioimmunoassays specific for each of the peptides and a radioreceptor assay of IGF-II have been developed.

Both IGF-I and IGF-II are under GH control, since concentrations of both have been reported to fall with GH deficiency. There is no question that IGF-I uniformly falls with GH deficiency; however, IGF-II levels are normal in most patients with GH deficiency (15). Only IGF-I rises above adult values with GH excess (acromegaly) [18]. Moreover, the concentration of IGF-I rises slowly throughout childhood and peaks during adolescence at levels that are two to three times higher than preadolescent values. IGF-II increases sharply after birth and normally remains constant throughout life. The insulin-like growth factors also differ in their growth-promoting activity: IGF-I is a potent promoter of the synthesis of sulfated proteoglycans in cartilage but IGF-II is a weak promoter.

IGF-I itself is probably essential to growth, although the possibility that GH may act directly on chondrocytes has not been totally excluded. Recent studies have suggested a direct effect of GH administration to the epiphyseal cartilage growth plate of hypophysectomized rats on longitudinal bone growth [43]. The locally administered hormone increased longitudinal bone growth of only the treated but not the untreated contralateral leg, suggesting a direct interaction with cells of the epiphyseal growth plate [85]. Chondrocytes within the epiphyseal cartilage show marked spatial asymmetry. The proximal zone close to the bony epiphysis consists of a narrow band of germinal or stem cell chondrocytes [49, 50]. These cells differentiate to enter the proliferative layer (divided into intermediate and distal zones) where the cells undergo *limited* clonal expansion. Growth hormone preferentially stimulates the stem cell chondrocytes (prechondrocytes) that border the bony epiphysis, while IGF-I stimulates mainly those cells in the more distal proliferative zones [42]. These data suggest that GH stimulates the differentiation of progenitor cells while the action of IGF-I is related to the clonal expansion of these more differentiated cells. The data are also consistent with the hypothesis that locally produced IGF-I is critical to the process of bone growth in length. Schlechter et al. [87] have shown that local infusion of neutralizing antibodies to IGF-I blocks the stimulatory effect of infused GH, providing direct evidence for a physiologic role for locally produced IGF-I.

Together, these observations of the local effects of GH and IGF-I are similar to the "dual effector theory" of GH action proposed by Green et al. [34]. Thus, GH directly stimulates the differentiation of prechondrocytes or young differentiating chondrocytes. These cells attain responsiveness to IGF-I and increase the local production of IGF-I in the differentiating cells themselves. Locally produced IGF-I supports the clonal growth of IGF-I responsive proliferating chondrocytes by autocrine or paracrine mechanisms [43] (see Fig. 10.2). Even the generation of IGF-I, however, does not guarantee normal growth. In certain individuals with a GH-deficient-like phenotype, GH and IGF-I concentrations are normal or elevated, but growth does not occur normally, implicating an IGF-I receptor or postreceptor defect [86]. Therefore, the cell must be able to bind IGF-I and translate its presence into action by synthesis of DNA, leading to cell multiplication.

Levels of circulating IGF-I are low in infancy, rise precipitiously in adolescence, fall to adult levels by the end of adolescence, and decline in men to prepubertal and hypopituitary levels after age 50 years. Gonadal steroid hormone levels also increase at adolescence. In boys, peak height velocity occurs in the latter stages of puberty when testosterone

FIGURE 10.2

A proposed model for growth hormone (GH) and insulin-like growth factor I (IGF-I) interaction in chondrocytes of epiphyseal growth plate. (Reproduced with permission from Isaksson OGP, Isgaard J, Nilsson A, Lindahl A: Direct action of GH. In Bercu BB (ed): Basic and Clinical Aspects of Growth Hormone. *New York, Plenum Press, 1988, pp 199–211.)*

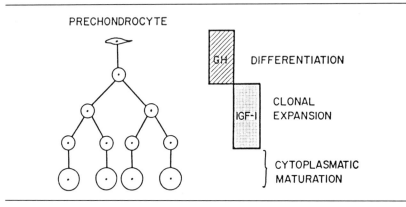

concentrations have risen to adult levels. It is at this time that IGF-I levels reach their zenith. The rise in IGF-I concentration, like the growth spurt, occurs approximately 2 years earlier in girls than boys. Peak height velocity and peak IGF-I concentration are coincident at approximately age 12 years in girls and 14 years in boys.

What are the underlying mechanisms that subserve both the increase in IGF-I levels and accelerated growth? If gonadal steroid hormones play a role in the pubertal generation of IGF-I, they might exert their effects in any of four different ways: (*a*) They may have a direct effect on IGF-I production, (*b*) they may act by augmenting or potentiating the effect of GH on IGF-I generation, (*c*) they may act synergistically with hormones other than GH, or (*d*) they may increase IGF-I levels by augmenting pituitary GH secretion. The fourth mechanism has been tested in prepubertal children and adolescents. Testosterone administration increased GH and IGF-I levels in normal prepubertal boys, but has no effect on IGF-I concentrations in prepubertal, GH-deficient boys [68]. The levels of IGF-I after treatment with GH and testosterone alone did not differ from those after combined therapy with GH and testosterone in GH-deficient subjects. In contrast, GH-sufficient, prepubertal boys who received testosterone had significant increases in IGF-I concentrations after testosterone therapy alone [68]. In a complementary study, Link et al. found [55] not only an increase in the 24-hour mean GH concentration after testosterone therapy in prepubertal, GH-sufficient children, but also increased number of large GH pulsations (amplitudes greater than 10 ng/ml) and level of IGF-I.

In a concurrent group treated with the nonaromatizable androgen oxandrolone, 0.1 mg/kg/day, no increase in mean GH concentrations nor IGF-I levels were noted. The growth rates of both groups of prepubertal boys were accelerated; however, those for the oxandrolone-treated group were only one-half those for the testosterone-treated group (55). This effect of testosterone on GH levels may reflect an exaggeration of the physiologic process occurring in males during spontaneous puberty and suggests that aromatization of the steroid nucleus may be important. However, the data also suggest that androgenic compounds can increase growth by a mechanism that does not involve the augmented secretion of GH and raised IGF-I levels. Whether the direct stimulus is the androgen, testosterone, or one of its aromatization products, for example, estradiol, cannot be determined from the data. In young and old adults, secretion of GH more closely follows the circulating estradiol concentration than that for testosterone [40].

As boys proceed through adolescence, the mode of secretion is altered to permit the release of greater quantities of GH. The frequency of spontaneous GH pulsations in late puberty remains virtually constant (compared to prepubertal boys), but the amount of GH released per pulse is markedly augmented ("amplitude modulation") [60]. This study has been extended to a larger group of adolescent boys and shows that the amount of GH secreted closely parallels the growth velocity chart and IGF-I levels with a peak in late mid-puberty and a decrease to adult levels at the time of bony epiphyseal fusion (Martha, Blizzard, and Rogol, unpublished data, 1988).

In adolescent girls, there is a biphasic effect of estrogens on IGF-I levels. Low doses are stimulatory and higher doses inhibitory. The earlier growth spurt in girls during puberty and the earlier rise and subsequent fall in IGF-I levels may reflect the biological action of estradiol on the hypothalamic–pituitary axis for GH secretion.

Growth Hormone Action
What does growth hormone do in the whole organism? The general metabolic effects are to reduce glucose and protein metabolism by shifting oxidative metabolism toward the utilization of fatty acids while sparing glucose and amino acids [51]. Peripheral adipose stores are diminished following GH administration, the plasma levels of fatty acids increase, and more lipid is transported and stored in the liver [51, 59].

What are the effects of GH on muscle tissue? Muscle growth depends on an adequate supply of amino acids given the required changes in nucleic acid (DNA and RNA) synthesis and metabolism. Following an initial lag phase, amino acid uptake is increased. Nucleic acid and protein synthesis peak after a considerable lag. The control of GH-mediated growth differs from work-induced growth [31, 104]. The synthesis of new RNA is required for exercise-induced muscle growth [33], whereas

GH enhances the rate and translation of existing RNA [51]. Does GH augment the strength of the newly synthesized muscle? This question has been addressed in normal, hypertrophied, and atrophied muscle [5, 11, 32]. Although GH-treated normal rats were 20% heavier, had a quadraceps weight 26% greater, and an increase in muscle fiber cross-sectional diameter 6–12% greater than did control rats, the quadraceps did not develop any greater tension. When expressed per weight of muscle the quadraceps of the GH-treated animals did not perform as well as that from control animals. Either the added muscle bulk did not consist of contractile elements or a defect in neuromuscular transmission or propagation of the contractile impulse had been induced [11, 59].

In a study of the effect of GH on atrophied muscle [5], growth hormone increased the weight of the atrophied gastrocnemius in the rat by 19% from the basal value of 62% of control. Twitch and tetanic tensions increased by approximately 60% compared to non-GH-treated control animals with atrophied muscle; however, as shown in the study described above there was no increase in the tension developed in the nonatrophied, contralateral control muscle.

In a study of hypertrophied muscle all GH-treated muscles increased in size compared to the non-GH-treated controls [32]. The investigators concluded that GH increased the basal rate of muscle protein synthesis, which in turn was determined by the amount of work performed [59]. From these data it is difficult to give a precise reason for lack of increased strength within the GH-treated muscle whether initially normal, atrophied, or hypertrophied.

STIMULATING GROWTH IN SHORT, NON-GROWTH-HORMONE-DEFICIENT CHILDREN

Human GH is a proved efficacious pharmacological agent to accelerate linear growth in GH-deficient children [2, 26, 27, 45, 47, 63, 73, 74, 103]. Pituitary-derived and recombinant-DNA-manufactured human GH are approximately equally potent [45, 47] irrespective of whether the methionyl GH or the natural-sequence recombinant DNA hormones are employed. Detailed dose-response relationships of GH therapy in GH-deficient children have been described [26].

With the recent availability of the recombinant human GH, there is a potentially limitless supply of human GH. Might this proved effective agent in hypopituitary patients be useful to promote accelerated growth in non-GH-deficient but short children? There has been an explosion of interest in this subject within the past few years. Several longitudinal, well-controlled studies have been conducted in (*a*) girls with Turner syndrome [58, 75, 76, 82, 94]; (*b*) children with short stature, normal responses of circulating GH to provocative (pharmacologic) stimuli, delayed bone age, and a decreased growth rate for age [46]; (*c*) children

TABLE 10.1
Annual Growth Rate (cm/year)[a]

Phase	1. Control	2. Oxandrolone	3. Methionyl Growth Hormone	4. Combination
			Group	
Prerandomization				
Mean	4.2	4.1	4.5	4.3
SD	1.1	1.0	0.8	0.9
n	18	18	17	17
Year 1				
Mean	3.8	7.6	6.6	9.8
SD	1.1	1.5[b]	1.2[b]	1.4[b]
n	16	18	17	17
Year 2[c]				
Mean	8.3	7.1	5.4	7.4
SD	1.2[b]	1.6[b]	1.1[b]	1.4[b]
n	16	17	17	16
Year 3				
Mean	6.7	5.3	4.6	6.1
SD	1.4[b]	2.4[b]	1.4[b]	1.5[b]
n	16	16	17	16

[a] Reproduced with permission from Rosenfeld RG, Hintz RL, Johanson AJ, Sherman B, Brasel JA, Burstein S, Chernausek S, Compton P, Frane J, Gotlin RW, Kuntze J, Lippe BM, Mahoney PC, Moore WV, New MI, Saenger P, Sybert V: Three-year results of a randomized prospective trial of methionyl human growth hormone and oxandrolone in Turner syndrome. *J Pediatr* 113:393–399, 1988.
[b] Significantly greater than annual growth rate for control group in year 1 ($p < 0.05$). Annual growth rate for group 4 is significantly greater than that for group 3 for each of 3 years ($p < 0.05$).
[c] First year of phase 2 for groups 1 and 2. This phase began 12–months after beginning of phase 1.

with constitutional delay of growth and adolescence [10]; and (*d*) short children with intrauterine growth retardation, glucocorticoid-induced stunting of growth, osteochondrodystrophies, and other disorders [81].

Turner Syndrome
Girls with Turner syndrome have ovarian failure, short stature, and considerable individual variability in a large number of other dysmorphic features with cardiac or renal malformations [67]. Rosenfeld et al. [82] evaluated a large group of girls with Turner syndrome to determine if GH, oxandrolone (a weak nonaromatizable androgen), or a combination of the two agents could augment growth rate. Patients were divided into four groups during the first phase of the trial, which lasted from 12 to 20 months. Group 1 received no treatment; group 2 received oxandrolone, 0.125 mg/kg/day; group 3 received methionyl hGH, 0.125 mg/kg, three times a week; and group 4 received oxandrolone and methionyl hGH in the amounts listed for group 2 and 3 (Table 10.1). During phase 2 all

subjects were given combination methionyl hGH and oxandrolone therapy with the exception of the group originally receiving methionyl hGH alone (group 3), who continued to receive only methionyl hGH. The original oxandrolone dosage was reduced by 50%, to 0.0625 mg/kg/day because of mild androgenization in 20% of the oxandrolone recipients.

Table 10.1 shows mean annual growth rates for the girls in each group. Combination therapy (group 4) resulted in significant increases in annual growth rate for each of the 3 years, compared with either prerandomization growth rate or the control group growth rate in the 1st year. Growth rates of those receiving methionyl hGH alone (group 3), compared with prerandomization growth rate or control group growth rate in year 1, increased significantly in years 1 and 2. Mean growth rate in year 3 of methionyl hGH alone was 4.6 (± 1.4) cm/year compared, with the mean control group growth rate for year 1 of 3.8 (± 1.1) cm/year, which did not quite reach statistical significance. Growth rates for combination therapy were significantly higher than for methionyl hGH alone in all 3 years. The growth velocity data are summarized in Figure 10.3, which depicts the mean, and two standard deviations from the mean, growth velocity for girls with (untreated) Turner syndrome.

Will these short-term accelerations in growth velocity alter the ultimate (adult) stature in these young women? A definitive answer cannot be determined from the data; however, one may obtain a preview by esti-

---

FIGURE 10.3

Growth velocity in four study groups: methionyl growth hormone (met-hGH; group 3); combination met-hGH and oxandrolone (group 4); control–combination (Ctrl→Comb); group 1, no therapy for treatment period 1, followed by combination met-hGH and oxandrolone for treatment period 2. Closed circle = group 2, oxandrolone for treatment period 1, followed by combination met-hGH and oxandrolone for treatment period 2. Open circle = *pretreatment; oxandrolone–combination (Oxan→Comb); met-hGH alone;* asterisk = *combination met-hGH and oxandrolone;* plus sign = *oxandrolone alone.* Heavy line *represents mean growth velocity for patients with untreated Turner syndrome;* light lines *are ± 1 and ± 2 SD. Numbers in upper right-hand corner of each box represent mean Z score ± 1 SD for each group. For groups 3 (met-hGH) and 4 (original combination) study data are presented as sequential years 1, 2, and 3. For group 1 (control–combination) and group 2 (oxandrolone–combination), data are divided into periods 1 and 2. Period 1 lasted 12–20 months for each individual subject. Period 2 (when subjects received combination therapy) is divided into years 1 and 2. (Reproduced with permission from Rosenfeld RG, Hintz RL, Johanson AJ, Sherman B, Brasel JA, Burstein S, Chernausek S, Compton P, Frane J, Gotlin RW, Kuntze J, Lippe BM, Mahoney PC, Moore WV, New MI, Saenger P, Sybert V: Three-year results of a randomized prospective trial of methionyl human growth hormone and oxandrolone in Turner syndrome.* J Pediatr *113:393–399, 1988.)*

mating the "predicted" adult height using stature attained, bone age, and the Bayley-Pinneau method [7], although the last is neither based on nor intended for girls with Turner syndrome. At the end of 3 years of therapy, mean increases in predicted adult stature were all positive, and the maximal increment (8.2 ± 1.4 cm) was achieved in patients receiving combination therapy (group 4). The data for all groups are summarized in Figure 10.4 and show significant augmentation in all groups except for the control group in year 1.

The data from this and several other studies [75, 93, 94] support the conclusion that methionyl hGH, both alone and in combination with oxandrolone, stimulates linear growth in girls with Turner syndrome. The data also support the conclusion that linear growth in girls with

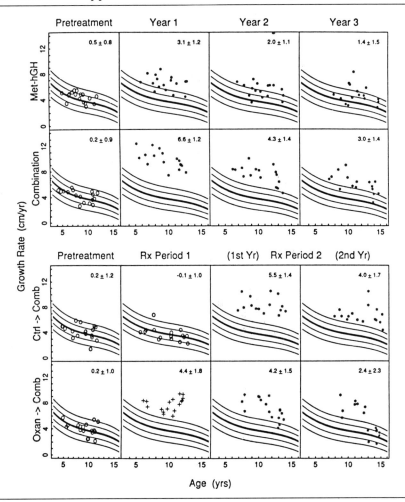

FIGURE 10.3

FIGURE 10.4

Cumulative change in predicted adult height, according to method of Bayley and Pinneau. Error bars *represent ± SEM. met-hGH = methionyl growth hormone. (Reproduced with permission from Rosenfeld RG, Hintz RL, Johanson AJ, Sherman B, Brasel JA, Burstein S, Chernausek S, Compton P, Frane J, Gotlin RW, Kuntze J, Lippe BM, Mahoney PC, Moore WV, New MI, Saenger P, Sybert V: Three-year results of a randomized prospective trial of methionyl human growth hormone and oxandrolone in Turner syndrome.* J Pediatr *113:393–399, 1988.)*

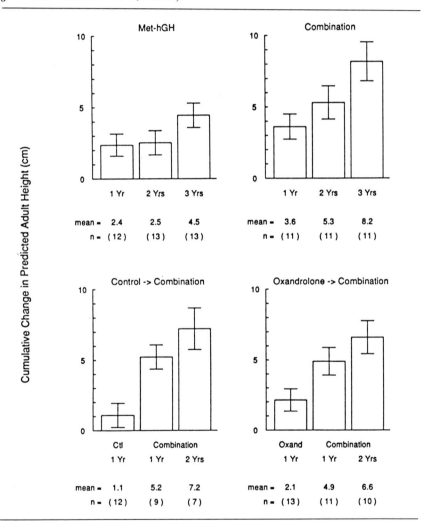

Turner syndrome can be augmented without compromising final stature [82]. The latter conclusion is critical since these girls and young adolescent women can gain stature during the years that their peers are entering their growth spurts.

Short Children with Subnormal Growth Velocities and Normal Growth Hormone Responses to Pharmacologic Stimuli
Children within this category include a wide variety of individuals within the normal range or with minimally or mildly pathologic conditions. Generally, no specific diagnoses can be made, and nutritional or psychologic factors may be prominent. Children and adolescents can have slow growth rates permanently, or they may be transient, making evaluation and response to any type of therapy difficult to monitor. It is not surprising, therefore, that quantification of results in groups of such children has large variance. For example, in an evaluation of the response of 34 children with these characteristics, Kaplan [46] found that 24 had an acceleration of growth rate of 2 cm or more above baseline after 6 months of treatment. Most of those who responded with accelerated growth showed a similar, but quantitatively smaller response upon reinitiation of GH therapy following 6 months without therapy. These recent results are similar to others obtained in similar or slightly different patient groups [8, 30, 37, 71, 101]. It is important to note that very few of these children have attained adult stature; therefore, it is premature to validate the observed advancement in predicted adult stature.

None of the current GH secretory patterns or stimulatory tests provides a reliable discriminatory index of selection of patients for an accelerated growth response to GH therapy [46]. Growth hormone treatment represents a therapeutic trial which may merely replace normally secreted quantities of GH or supplement them. More careful selection of patients (i.e., defined subgroups) and detailed dose–response relationships must be obtained before such therapy can be considered efficacious and appropriate.

Constitutional Delay of Growth and Adolescence
Children with this condition are short and have a low-normal or slightly subnormal growth velocity, a delay in bone age (physiologic age), and a consistent family history. The condition is seen predominantly in boys, but this may be due to an ascertainment bias given the greater psychosocial dysfunction in short, sexually underdeveloped boys. The condition probably represents a physiological alteration in growth rate and tempo of adolescent sexual development and is thus not a disease. However, there may be moderate to severe psychologic dysfunction based on the short stature so that many have advocated short-term growth-promoting therapy (see below).

Do these children secrete normal amounts of GH? Might they benefit from GH therapy (either "replacement" or pharmacologic)? A large number of studies of the amounts and patterns of GH secretion in children with constitutional delay of growth and adolescence (CDGA) were reviewed by Bierich [10]. Although not all studies demonstrated diminished GH secretion, Bierich noted a significant decrease (47%) in total integrated GH secretion in boys with CDGA. However, there was a large overlap with integrated GH results obtained in normally growing boys of the same stage of sexual development. Maximal GH concentrations were also diminished compared to controls; however, there were no differences between the delayed and normally growing boys when responses to pharmacologic stimuli were quantitated. The discrepancy between the diminished spontaneous and the stimulated secretion is noteworthy in that hypothalamic (GHRH and somatostatin) rather than pituitary dysfunction is suggested.

Theoretically, two types of therapy are possible. The first is to use low-dose androgen treatment, which increases spontaneous GH secretion [55, 60] and begins to virilize the boys, and GH therapy. If the former is used, small doses of oxandrolone (0.1 mg/kg/day) or long-acting testosterone esters are indicated and 50 mg once a month of the heptanoate or cypionate esters is a usual starting dose. These doses will promote sexual maturation without impairing ultimate stature and are indicated for 3–6 months before increasing to 100 mg per month. When testicular enlargement occurs, the medication may be stopped, since the individual's own pubertal mechanisms have become operative. Growth hormone has been tried in "replacement" doses. The results depicted in Figure 10.5 are promising in that they show short-term augmentation of growth velocity. Preliminary observations [10] suggest that the adult stature may increase by 4 or 5 cm, depending on the age at which treatment was begun.

Before such results can be considered as fact, a large, long-term longitudinal study of the efficacy of androgen, GH, and no therapy must be completed. At present there are no convincing data that any mode of therapy in constitutionally delayed boys will increase their adult stature. It is incontrovertible, however, that augmentation of growth velocity and acceleration of sexual development can favorably affect the psychological well-being of constitutionally delayed adolescent boys.

Other Causes of Short Stature

Growth hormone therapy has been tried in almost every category of children with short stature [81]. Virtually none of the children with various osteochondrodystrophies have responded. However, some children within the broad category of intrauterine growth retardation (IUGR) (birth weight and/or length 2 SD or more below the mean for gestational age, sex, maternal size, or birth order) have responded to GH therapy. For example, Tanner et al. [98] reported that in 17 children with IUGR,

FIGURE 10.5

Treatment with growth hormone over 4 years in 16 children with constitutional delay of growth and adolescence. Ordinate: height velocity, standard deviation score. (Reproduced with permission from Bierich JR: Constitutional delay of growth and adolescent development. In Bercu BB (ed): Basic and Clinical Aspects of Growth Hormone. *New York, Plenum Press, 1988, pp 289–302.)*

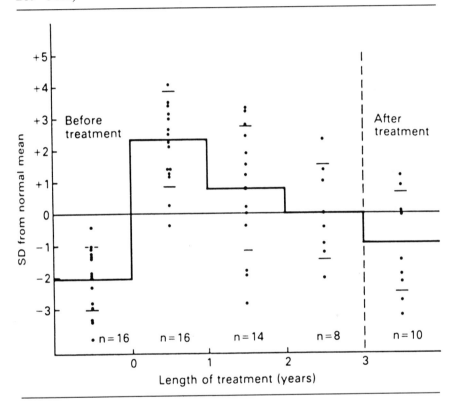

a small number without Russell-Silver syndrome displayed significant hGH-associated acceleration in growth rate that was maintained for the 3 years of treatment. Several more recent studies have shown small increments in growth with usual [52, 53] or markedly increased amounts of GH [23]. In the latter study there was an indication of a dose–response relationship up to five times the amount used for the treatment of GH deficiency. Children with Russell-Silver syndrome, which is characterized by low birth weight and IUGR, facial asymmetry, and hemihypertrophy of the trunk and limbs, have not in general had favorable response to GH therapy [98].

Children with Cushing's syndrome of any cause do not grow well since glucocorticoids diminish linear growth by inhibiting GH secretion and (primarily) by antagonizing the anabolic effects of GH mediated by somatomedins at the cellular level [48]. The majority of children with glucocorticoid-induced growth retardation will be receiving therapy for diseases other than adrenocortical deficiency (asthma, nephrotic syndrome, juvenile rheumatoid arthritis, inflammatory bowel disease, and chronic active hepatitis) [41] as little as 45 mg/m²/day of cortisone can diminish growth rate and skeletal maturation in otherwise normal children. Osteopenia especially of trabecular bone is a frequent concomitant of glucocorticoid therapy in children [41]. The pharmacologic doses needed cannot easily be stopped to permit full expression of the patient's growth potential.

Is GH therapy effective in these generally catabolic patients to increase their linear growth rate? Significant numbers of children with juvenile rheumatoid arthritis treated with large doses of prednisone experience increased growth rates over 2 years of hGH therapy [16]. However, these children received alternate-day treatment in contrast to large numbers of children who received daily glucocorticoid treatment. Similar studies in large numbers of patients have not been reported. Data for a small series of patients indicate that daily administration of glucocorticoids is not as promising as alternate-day therapy [81]. Even if IGF-I levels are increased by long-term GH therapy in glucocorticoid-treated children, there is the possibility that inhibitors of the biological activity of the induced growth factor ("peripheral resistance") will not permit the expression of its activity [81]. Inhibitors of IGF-I have been detected in growth-retarded children receiving long-term glucocorticoid therapy and in those with chronic renal or other metabolic diseases. The mechanism of the growth retardation may involve many of the steps of collagen biosynthesis since linear growth requires the formation of new bone, a process dependent upon the synthesis of Type 1 collagen [41].

Daily corticosteroid therapy, at least in children with inflammatory bowel disease, leads to markedly lower concentrations of the C-terminal propeptide of Type I collagen. Alternate-day corticosteroid therapy is much less suppressive [41]. More complete and extensive studies have been undertaken in adults with malnutrition, diabetes, and uremia [81].

Although short-term growth increments in some of these children may be promising, there are no data to indicate long-term alterations in growth rate or adult stature. Alternate-day treatment at the smallest possible dose is clearly preferable to daily therapy if the underlying disease process can be managed in this manner. However, systematic prospective long-term dose–response studies can now be undertaken since there is an abundant supply of biosynthetic GH. These considerations make it unlikely that GH or IGF-I therapy will be effective in the long term for children with growth suppression due to glucocorticoid therapy except for that group that receives lower dose treatment on alternate days.

CAN GROWTH HORMONE THERAPY BE EFFECTIVE TO INCREASE ADULT STATURE IN NORMALLY GROWING CHILDREN?

This question might be considered a crucial issue to prepubertal children (and their parents) who consider that success in athletics and in many other activities is dependent on ultimate stature. I am at present unaware of any prospective long-term studies that are relevant to this issue. In my opinion it is highly unethical to perform such studies that fall under the title of "cosmetic endocrinology." If hormonal treatment were efficacious, it would be necessary to give more than the daily amount secreted since there would undoubtedly be inhibition of endogenous GH secretion mediated by the nueroendocrine feedback loops outlined in the first section of this chapter. What are the possible outcomes? First, the child–adolescent might grow at an accelerated rate and be taller as an adult than his or her genetic potential. This would be considered a successful outcome of therapy. At what cost? Aside from the considerable monetary cost of the hormone, the chance of untoward side effects must increase with escalation of the dose. Alterations in intermediary metabolism, especially carbohydrate tolerance, would be expected to be magnified as the dose of GH increased, Deleterious effects of skeletal muscle, the heart, and soft tissues as noted in acromegalic patients are more likely with greater doses and longer duration of treatment. Such side effects are not inevitable, but are more and more likely, and are entirely unacceptable in otherwise normally growing humans.

The development of hypothyroidism during hGH therapy has been observed in a number of GH-deficient patients [25], although this condition may simply be a reflection of the natural history of hypopituitarism [80].

The development of growth-attenuating antibodies to hGH has always been of theoretical interest. In the early history of hGH therapy, many patients developed antibodies to hGH, but only a minority had attenuation of growth rate. As more highly purified preparations of pituitary and biosynthetic hormone have become available, this particular problem has diminished, but has not disappeared [64, 69]. It may be that increased doses of hGH may lead to an increased incidence of both problems.

GROWTH HORMONE SUPPLEMENTATION IN THE MATURE HUMAN

Given that human GH is anabolic, nonadrogenic, and lipolytic in the human, why should virtually all athletes who depend on strength and power not use it to augment performance? The following statements are either anecdotal or personal opinion, since there are no well-controlled, double-blind studies to evaluate the efficacy of hormonal treat-

ment on parameters of strength and endurance let alone sport performance.

How might one increase the amount of circulating hGH? Considering
the physiologic precepts outlined in the first section of this review, one
might take neurotransmitters or their antagonists (e.g., clonidine) or
specific amino acids (e.g., arginine, ornithine) to augment GH secretion.
Although such agents are efficacious in the short term (e.g., diagnostic
tests), there are no data which indicate any long-term increase in hGH
secretion. Given the multiple and complex feedback mechanisms, one
could reason that the hierarchical negative feedback loops would conspire to reduce GH secretion to normal levels. One might also argue
that the potentially altered pulsatile secretion of GH would diminish the
effects of the same amounts of GH if secreted in the intermittent physiological manner. Growth-hormone-releasing factor given in the physiological manner, or once or twice daily, to GH-deficient children augments growth rates to levels indistinguishable from those of similar children
treated with GH [99]. Might the releasing hormone also be safe and
effective in augmenting GH secretion over the long term in non-GH-
deficient athletes? For the same physiological reasons listed above for
neurotransmitters and amino acids, one would expect that the physiologic negative feedback regulatory loops would regulate GH secretion
to approximately the proper physiological amounts. The expense and
virtual unavailability of GHRH will not permit an answer to the question
of its effectiveness in athletes.

Injecting growth hormone itself in an undetermined dosage schedule
and amount would be the most likely way that athletes would augment
the daily amount of circulating GH. Undoubtedly, the concentration of
GH would rise. In fact there are mounting anecdotal reports of massive
increases in muscle bulk and weight in strength and power athletes who
take GH. How one might factor gains due to the anabolic agent or to
alterations in training, as for the many years of anabolic steroid misuse,
are indeterminate. One can obtain glowing reports (as also with anabolic
steroid hormones). The side effects, however, are quite distant to the
purported salutary effects. This situation is similar to that for anabolic
steroids. Many years of misuse have left us with indeterminant knowledge of their efficacy.

Theoretically, one might consider use of the insulin-like growth factors
(somatomedins). There simply are not enough data for humans to determine if there might be any anabolic benefit in non-GH-deficient subjects.

How does one summarize the anecdotal "evidence" and theoretical
objections to GH usage in children and adolescents on the one hand
and adult athletes on the other? As a pediatric endocrinologist it is my
firm conviction that the practice of cosmetic endocrinology to augment

stature (if possible) is entirely unacceptable. The potential and actual side effects would preclude any blinded scientific evaluation in normally growing, immature humans. As stated in the second section of this chapter, there are a large number of studies in progress for therapeutic trials of GH and other anabolic agents in abnormally short children. The small doses used and the potential benefits to be accrued outweigh the potential harmful effects. My consideration here does not include trials of massively supraphysiologic doses until such doses have been shown to be nontoxic in adults.

Adult athletes have been taking anabolic and ergogenic aids since time immemorial. Despite frequent moral objections and toxic effects, such compounds continue to be ingested and injected. Virtually no pleas for their proscription have been or will be heeded. Will the use of hGH follow the pattern of anabolic steroid abuse, that is, if a little (replacement doses) is good, then a lot (massive pharmacological doses) is better? Clearly the side effects, including hepatocellular carcinoma, have settled the issue with very large doses of anabolic steroid hormones [67]. For the present, the very high cost of biosynthetic growth hormone will not permit athletes to take massive doses. The side effects expected from the usual doses as presently prescribed for hypopituitary children are mild and probably will occur only after long-term usage since these amounts merely suppress endogenous GH secretion.

The use of much larger doses may result in conditions similar to acromegaly with its disfiguring potential and not inconsequential mortality—50% or more by age 50 years. Complications of this condition include diabetes mellitus; atherosclerotic cardiovascular disease, often with heart failure and poor ejection fraction (cardiomyopathy); neuropathy; and myopathy (especially proximal) in apparently hypertrophied muscles [54, 65].

One should not forget the real possibility for the transmission of the human immunodeficiency virus with shared needles. Although not likely in the immature human, there is danger of this occurrence in those who inject GH or anabolic steroid. This danger is obviously magnified in those groups of athletes whose social behavior puts them at high risk for the acquired immune deficiency syndrome.

REFERENCES

1. Abrams RL, Grumbach MM, Kaplan SL: The effect of administration of human growth hormone, cortisol, glucose and free fatty acid response to insulin: evidence for growth hormone autoregulation in man. *J Clin Invest* 50:940–950, 1971.
2. Aceto T, Frasier SD, Hayles AB, Meyer-Bahlburg HFL, Parker ML, Munschauer R, Di Chiro G: Collaborative study of effects of human growth hormone in growth hormone deficiency. I. First year of therapy. *J Clin Endocrinol Metab* 35:483–496, 1972.

3. Aguila MC: GRF stimulation of somatostatin release in vitro via opioids (abstract). Presented at the 67th Annual Meeting of the Endocrine Society, Baltimore, 1985.

4. Aguila MC, McCann SM: Stimulation of somatostatin release in vitro by synthetic growth hormone-releasing factor by a non-dopaminergic mechanism. *Endocrinology* 117:762–765, 1985.

5. Apostolakis M, Deligiannis A, Madena-Pyrgaki A: The effects of human growth hormone administration on the functional status of rat atrophied muscle following immobilization. *Physiologist* 23(suppl):S111–112, 1980.

6. Baumann G, Shaw MA, Winter RJ: Absence of plasma growth hormone-binding protein in Laron-type dwarfism. *J Clin Endocrinol Metab* 65:814–816, 1987.

7. Bayley N, Pinneau SR: Tables for predicting adult height from skeletal age: revised for use with the Greulich-Pyle hand standards. *J Pediatr* 40:423–441, 1952.

8. Bercu BB, Shulman D, Root AW, Spiliotis BE: Growth hormone provocative testing frequently does not reflect endogenous growth hormone secretion. *J Clin Endocrinol Metab* 63:709–716, 1986.

9. Berelowitz M, Szabo M, Frohman LA: Somatomedin-C mediates GH negative feedback by effects on both the hypothalamus and the pituitary. *Science* 212:1279–1281, 1981.

10. Bierich JR: Constitutional delay of growth and adolescent development. In Bercu BB (eds): *Basic and Clinical Aspects of Growth Hormone.* Plenum Press, New York, 1988, pp 289–302.

11. Bigland B, Jehring B: Muscle performance in rats, normal, and treated with growth hormone. *J Physiol* 116:129–136, 1952.

12. Bilezikjian LM, Vale WW: Chronic exposure of cultured rat anterior pituitary cells to GRF causes partial loss of responsiveness to GRF. *Endocrinology* 115:2032–2034, 1984.

13. Bloch B, Gaillard RC, Brazeau P, Lin HD, Ling N:Topographical and ontogenetic study of the neurons producing growth hormone-releasing factor in human hypothalamus. *Regul Pept* 8:21–31, 1984.

14. Bohlen P, Brazeau P, Bloch B, Ling N, Gaillard R, Guillemin R: Human hypothalamic growth hormone-releasing factor (GRF): evidence for two forms identical to tumor derived GRF-44-NH$_2$ and GRF-40. *Biochem Biophys Res Commun* 114:930–936, 1983.

15. Bucher H, Zapf J, Torresani T, Prader A, Frosch ER, Illig R: Insulin-like growth factors I and II, prolactin and insulin in 19 growth hormone deficient children with excessive, normal or decreased longitudinal growth after operation for craniopharygioma. *N Engl J Med* 309:1142–1146, 1983.

16. Butenandt O: Rheumatoid arthritis and growth retardation in children: treatment with human growth hormone. *Eur J Pediatr* 130:15–28, 1979.

17. Clemmons DR, Klibanski A, Underwood LR, Ridgeway EC, MacArthur JW, Bietens IZ, Van Wyk JJ: Reduction in plasma immunoreactive somatomedin-C during fasting in humans. *J Clin Endocrinol Metab* 53:1247–1250, 1981.

18. Clemmons DR, Van Wyk JJ, Ridgeway EC, Klineman B, Kjellberg RN, Underwood LE: Evaluation of acromegaly by radioimmunoassay of somatomedin-C. *N Engl J Med* 301:1138–1142, 1979.

19. Clemmons DR, Seek MM, Underwood LE: Supplemental essential amino acids augment the somatomedin-C/IGF-I response to refeeding after fasting. *Metabolism* 34:391–395, 1985.

20. Cronin MJ, Rogol AD, Myers GA, Hewlett EL: Pertussis toxin blocks the inhibition of growth hormone release and cyclic AMP accumulation by somatostatin. *Endocrinology* 113:209–215, 1983.

21. Cronin MJ, Hewlett EL, Evans WS, Thorner MO, Rogol AD: hpGRF and cyclic AMP

evoke GH release from anterior pituitary cells: the effects of pertussin toxin, cholera toxin, forskolin and cycloheximide. *Endocrinology* 114:904–913, 1984.

22. Daughaday WH, Trivedi B: Absence of serum growth hormone binding protein in patients with growth hormone receptor deficiency (Laron dwarfism). *Proc Natl Acad Sci USA* 84:4636–4640, 1987.

23. Foley TP Jr, Thompson RG, Shaw M, Baghdassariam A, Nissley SP, Blizzard RM: Growth responses to human growth hormone in patients with intrauterine growth retardation. *J Pediatr* 84:635–641, 1974.

24. Frasier SD: Dose-response relationship of growth hormone therapy. In Bercu BB (ed): *Basic and Clinical Aspects of Growth Hormone.* Plenum Press, New York, 1988, pp 303–309.

25. Frasier SD: Side effects of pituitary growth hormone therapy. In Laron Z (ed): *Pediatric and Adolescent Endocrinology.* Karger, Basel, 1987, vol 16, pp 155–163.

26. Frasier SD, Costin G, Lippe BM, Aceto T, Bunger PF: A dose–response curve for human growth hormone. *J Clin Endocrinol Metab* 53:1213–1217, 1981.

27. Frasier SD, Aceto T, Hayles AB, Mikity VG: Collaborative study of the effects of human growth hormone in growth hormone deficiency: IV. Treatment with low doses of human growth hormone based on body weight. *J Clin Endocrinol Metab* 44:22–31, 1977.

28. Frohman LA, Thominett JL, Webb CB, Vance ML, Uderman H, Rivier J, Vale W, Thorner MO: Metabolic clearance and plasma disappearance rates of human pancreatic tumor growth hormone releasing factor in man. *J Clin Invest* 73:1304–1311, 1984.

29. Frohman LA, Downs TR, Williams TC, Heimer EP, Pan YCE, Felix AM: Rapid enzymatic degradation of growth hormone-releasing hormone by plasma *in vitro* and *in vivo* to a biologically inactive product cleaved at the NH_2 terminus. *J Clin Invest* 78:906–913, 1986.

30. Gertner JM, Genel M, Gianfredi SP, Hintz RL, Rosenfeld RG, Tamborlane WV, Wilson DM: Prospective clinical trial of human growth hormone in short children without growth hormone deficiency. *J Pediatr* 104:172–176, 1984.

31. Goldberg AL: The role of insulin in work-induced growth of skeletal muscle. *Endocrinology* 83:1071–1073, 1968.

32. Goldberg AL, Goodman HM: Relationship between growth hormone and muscle work in determining muscle size. *J Physiol* 200:655–666, 1969.

33. Goldberg AL, Etlinger JD, Goldsink DF, Jablecki C: Mechanism of work-induced hypertrophy of skeletal muscle. *Med Sci Sports* 7:248–261, 1975.

34. Green H, Morikawa M, Nixon T: A dual effector theory of growth hormone action. *Differentiation* 29:195–198, 1985.

35. Green JD, Harris GW: The neurovascular link between the neurohypophysis and adenohypophysis. *J Endocrinol* 5:136–146, 1947.

36. Grossman A, Savage MO, Lytras N, Preece MA, Suerias-Diaz J, Coy DH, Rees LH, Besser GM: Responses to analogues of growth hormone-releasing hormone in normal subjects and in growth hormone deficient children and young adults. *Clin Endocrinol* 21:321–330, 1984.

37. Grunt JA, Howard C, Daughaday WH: Comparison of growth and somatomedin responses following growth hormone treatment in children with small-for-date short stature, significant idiopathic short stature, and hypopituitarism. *Acta Endocrinol (Copenh)* 106:168–174, 1984.

38. Guillemin R, Brazeau P, Bohlen P, Esch F, Ling N, Wehrenberg WB: Growth hormone releasing factor from a human pancreatic tumor that caused acromegaly. *Science* 218:585–587, 1982.

39. Ho KY, Veldhuis JD, Johnson ML, Furlanetto R, Evans WS, Alberti KGMM, Thorner MO: Fasting enhances growth hormone secretion and amplifies the complex rhythms of growth hormone secretion in man. *J Clin Invest* 81:968–975, 1988.

40. Ho KY, Evans WS, Blizzard RM, Veldhuis JD, Merriam GR, Samojlik E, Furlanetto R, Rogol AD, Kaiser DL, Thorner MO: Effects of sex and age on the 24-hr secretory profile of GH secretion in man: importance of endogenous estradiol concentrations. *J Clin Endocrinol Metab* 64:51–58, 1987.

41. Hyams JS, Carey DE: Corticosteroids and growth. *J Pediatr* 113:249–254, 1988.

42. Isaksson OGP, Janssen J-O, Gause IAM: Growth hormone stimulates longitudinal bone growth directly. *Science* 216:1237–1239, 1982.

43. Isaksson OGP, Isgaard J, Nilsson A, Lindahl A: Direct action of GH. In Bercu BB (ed): *Basic and Clinical Aspects of Growth Hormone*. Plenum Press, New York, 1988, pp 199–211.

44. Isley WL, Underwood LE, Clemmons DR: Dietary components that regulate serum somatomedin C concentrations in humans. *J Clin Invest* 71:175–182, 1983.

45. Kaplan SL: Clinical trial of protropin. Presented at a meeting of the Endocrinologic and Metabolic Drug Advisory Committee Food and Drug Administration, Bethesda, MD, September, 1984.

46. Kaplan SL: Improvement in growth rate and mean predicted height during long-term treatment with growth hormone in children with non-growth-hormone deficient short stature. In Bercu BB (ed): *Basic and Clinical Aspects of Growth Hormone*. Plenum Press, New York, 1988, pp 285–288, 1988.

47. Kaplan SL, Underwood LE, August GP, Bell JJ, Glethen SL, Blizzard RM, Brown DR, Foley TP, Hintz RL, Hopwood NJ, Johansen A, Kirkland RT, Plotnick LP, Rosenfeld RG, Van Wyk JJ: Clinical studies with recombinant-DNA-derived methionyl human growth hormone in growth hormone deficient children. *Lancet* 1:697–700, 1986.

48. Kappy MS: Regulation of growth in children with chronic illness. Therapeutic implications for the year 2000. *Am J Dis Child* 141:489–493, 1987.

49. Kember NF, Sissons HA: A quantitative histology of the human growth plate. *J Bone Joint Surg* 58B:426–435, 1976.

50. Kember NF: Cell kinetics and the control of growth in long bones. *Cell Tissue Kinet* 11:477–485, 1978.

51. Kostyo JR, Reagan CR: The biology of growth hormone. *Pharmacol Ther* 2:591–604, 1976.

52. Lanes R, Plotnick LP, Lee PA: Sustained effect of human growth hormone therapy on children with intrauterine growth retardation. *Pediatrics* 63:731–735, 1979.

53. Lee PA, Blizzard RM, Cheek DB, Holt AB: Growth and body composition in intrauterine growth retardation (IUGR) before and during human growth hormone administration. *Metabolism* 23:913–919, 1974.

54. Linfoot JA: Acromegaly and giantism. In Daughaday WH (ed): *Endocrine Control of Growth*. New York, Elsevier North Holland, 1981, pp 207–267.

55. Link K, Blizzard RM, Evans WS, Kaiser DL, Parker MW, Rogol AD: The effect of androgens on the pulsatile release and the twenty-four-hour mean concentration of growth hormone in peripubertal males. *J Clin Endocrinol Metab* 62:159–164, 1986.

56. Lumpkin MD, Negro-Vilar A, McCann SM: Paradoxical elevation of growth hormone by intraventricular somatostatin: possible ultrashort-loop feedback. *Science* 211:1072–1074, 1981.

57. Lumpkin MD, Samson WK, McCann SM: Effects of intraventricular growth hormone-releasing factor on growth hormone release: further evidence for ultrashort loop feedback. *Endocrinology* 116:2070–2074, 1985.

58. Lyon AJ, Preece MA, Grant DB: Growth curve for girls with Turner syndrome. *Arch Dis Child* 60:932–935, 1985.

59. MacIntyre JG: Growth hormone and athletes. *Sports Med* 4:129–142, 1987.

60. Mauras N, Blizzard RM, Link K, Johnson ML, Rogol AD, Veldhuis JD: Augmentation of growth hormone secretion during puberty: evidence for a pulse amplitude-modulated phenomenon. *J Clin Endocrinol Metab* 64:596–601, 1987.

61. Mayo KE, Vale W, Rivier J, Rosenfeld MG, Evans RM: Expression cloning and sequence of cDNA encoding human growth hormone-releasing factor. *Nature* 306:86–88, 1983.

62. Melmed S, Yamashita S: Insulin-like growth factor-I action on hypothyroid rat pituitary cells: suppression of triiodothyronine-induced growth hormone secretion and messenger ribonucleic acid levels. *Endocrinology* 118:1483–1490, 1986.

63. Milner RDG, Rusell-Fraser T, Brook CGD, Coates PM, Farguhar JW, Parker JM, Preece MA, Snodgrass GJAI, Mason AS, Tanner JM, Vince FP: Experience with human growth hormone in Great Britain: the report of the MRC working party. *Clin Endocrinol (Oxf)* 11:15–38, 1979.

64. Moore WV, Leppert P: Role of aggregated human growth hormone (hGH) in development of antibodies to hGH. *J Clin Endocrinol Metab* 51:691–697, 1980.

65. Naugelsparen M, Trickey R, Davies MJ, Jenkins JS: Muscle changes in acromegaly. *Br Med J* 2:914–915, 1976.

66. Overly WL, Dankoff JA, Wang BK, Singh UD: Androgens and hepatocellular carcinoma in an athlete. *Ann Intern Med* 100:158–159, 1984.

67. Palmer CG, Reichmann A: Chromosomal and clinical findings in 110 females with Turner syndrome. *Hum Genet* 35:35–49, 1976.

68. Parker MM, Johanson AJ, Rogol AD, Kaiser DL, Blizzard RM: Effect of testosterone on somatomedin C concentrations in prepubertal boys. *J Clin Endocrinol Metab* 59:87–90, 1984.

69. Perez AR, Pena C, Poskus E, Paladini AC, Domene HM, Martinez AS, Heinrich JJ: Antibodies against animal growth hormones appearing in patients treated with human growth hormone: their specificities and influence on growth velocity. *Acta Endocrinol (Copenh)* 110:24–31, 1985.

70. Peterfreund RA, Vale WW: Somatostatin analogs inhibit somatostatin secretion from cultured hypothalamus cells. *Neuroendocrinology* 39:397–402, 1984.

71. Plotnick LP, Van Meter QL, Kowarski AA: Human growth hormone treatment of children with growth failure and normal growth hormone levels by immunoassay. *Pediatrics* 71:324–327, 1983.

72. Plotsky PM, Vale W: Patterns of growth hormone-releasing factor and somatostatin secretion into the hypophysial-portal circulation of the rat. *Science* 230:461–463, 1985.

73. Preece MA, Tanner JM, Whitehouse RH, Cameron N: Dose dependence of growth response to human growth hormone in growth hormone deficiency. *J Clin Endocrinol Metab* 42:477–483, 1976.

74. Raben MS: Treatment of a pituitary dwarf with human growth hormone. *J Clin Endocrinol Metab* 18:901–903, 1958.

75. Raiti S, Moore, WV, Van Vliet G, Kaplan SL: The National Hormone and Pituitary Program. Growth-stimulating effects of human growth hormone therapy in patients with Turner syndrome. *J Pediatr* 109:944–949, 1986.

76. Ranke MB, Pfluger H, Rosendahl W, Stubbe P, Enders H, Bierich JR, Majewski F: Turner syndrome: spontaneous growth in 150 cases and review of the literature. *Eur J Pediatr* 141:81–88, 1983.

77. Reichlin S: Growth hormone content of pituitaries from rats with hypothalamic lesions. *Endocrinology* 69:225–230, 1961.

78. Rivier J, Spiess J, Thorner M, Vale W: Characterization of a growth hormone releasing factor from a human pancreatic islet tumour. *Nature* 300:276–278, 1982.

79. Rivier J, Spiess J, Thorner M, Vale W: Sequence analysis of a growth hormone

releasing factor from a human pancreatic islet tumor. *Biochemistry* 21:6037–6040, 1982.

80. Root AW, Bongiovanni AM, Eberlein WR: Diagnosis and management of growth retardation with special reference to the problem of hypopituitarism. *J Pediatr* 78:737–753, 1971.

81. Root AW, Diamond F: Effects of human growth hormone in normal short children and in patients with intrauterine growth retardation, glucocorticoid-induced stunting of growth, osteochondrodystrophies and other disorders. In Bercu BB (ed): *Basic and Clinical Aspects of Growth Hormone*. Plenum Press, New York, 1988, pp 311–326.

82. Rosenfeld RG, Hintz RL, Johanson AJ, Sherman B, Brasel JA, Burstein S, Chernausek S, Compton P, Frane J, Gotlin RW, Kuntze J, Lippe BM, Mahoney PC, Moore WV, New MI, Saenger P, Sybert V: Three-year results of a randomized prospective trial of methionyl human growth hormone and oxandrolone in Turner syndrome. *J Pediatr* 113:393–399, 1988.

83. Rosenthal SM, Hulse JA, Kaplan SL, Grumbach MM: Exogenous growth hormone inhibits growth hormone-releasing factor-induced growth hormone secretion in normal men. *J Clin Invest* 77:176–180, 1986.

84. Ross RJM, Borges F, Grossman A, Smith R, Ngahjoong L, Rees LH, Savage MO, Besser GM: Growth hormone pretreatment in man blocks the response to growth hormone-releasing hormone: evidence for a direct effect of growth hormone. *Clin Endocrinol* 26:117–123, 1987.

85. Rusell SM, Spencer EM: Local injections of human or rat growth hormone or of purified human somatomedin C stimulate unilateral tibial epiphyseal growth in hypophysectomized rats. *Endocrinology* 116:2563–2567, 1985.

86. Schaff-Blass E, Burstein S, Rosenfield RL: Advances in diagnosis and treatment of short stature with special reference to the role of growth hormone. *J Pediatr* 104:801–813, 1984.

87. Schlechter NL, Russell SM, Spencer EM, Nicoll CS: Evidence suggesting that the direct growth-promoting effect of growth hormone on cartilage *in vivo* is mediated by local production of somatomedin. *Proc Natl Acad Sci USA* 83:7932–7934, 1986.

88. Seifert H, Perrin M, Rivier J, Vale W: Binding sites for growth hormone releasing factor on rat anterior pituitary cells. *Nature* 313:487–489, 1985.

89. Sheppard MC, Kronheim S, Pimstone BL: Stimulation by growth hormone of somatostatin release from the rat hypothalamus, *in vitro*. *Clin Endocrinol* 9:583–586, 1978.

90. Shibisaki T, Yamaguchi N, Hotta M, Masuda A, Imaki T, Demura H, Ling N, Shizume K: *In vitro* release of growth hormone releasing factor from rat hypothalamus: effect of insulin-like growth factor-1. *Regul Pept* 15:47–53, 1986.

91. Soliman AT, Hassan AEHI, Aref MK, Hintz RL, Rosenfeld RG, Rogol AD: Serum insulin-like growth factors (IGF) I and II concentrations and growth hormone and insulin responses to arginine infusion in children with protein-energy malnutrition before and after nutritional rehabilitation. *Pediatr Res* 20:1122–1130, 1986.

92. Summers ST, Canonico PL, MacLeod RM, Rogol AD, Cronin MJ: Phorbol esters affect pituitary growth hormone (GH) and prolactin release: the interaction with GH releasing factor, somatostatin and bromocriptine. *Eur J Pharm* 111:371–376, 1985.

93. Takano K, Hizuka N, Shizume K: Growth hormone treatment in Turner's syndrome. *Acta Paediatr Scand Suppl* 325:58–63, 1986.

94. Takano K, Hizuka N, Shizume K: Treatment of Turner's syndrome with methionyl human growth hormone for six months. *Acta Endocrinol (Copenh)* 112:130–137, 1986.

95. Tannenbaum GS: Growth hormone-releasing factor: direct effects on growth hormone, glucose and behavior via the brain. *Science* 226:464–466, 1984.

96. Tannenbaum GS, Guyda HJ, Posner BI: Insulin-like growth factors: a role in growth

hormone negative feedback and body weight regulation via the brain. *Science* 220:77–79, 1983.

97. Tannenbaum GS, Ling N: The interrelationship of growth hormone (GH)-releasing factor and somatostatin in the generation of the ultradian rhythm of GH secretion. *Endocrinology* 115:1952–1957, 1984.

98. Tanner JM, Whitehouse RH, Hughes PRC, Vince FP: Effect of human growth hormone for 1 to 7 years on growth of 100 children, with growth hormone deficiency, low birth weight, inherited smallness, Turner's syndrome, other complaints. *Arch Dis Child* 46:745–782, 1971.

99. Thorner MO, Rogol AD, Blizzard RM, Klingesmith GJ, Najjar J, Misra R, Burr I, Chas G, Martha P, McDonald J, Pezzoli S, Chitwood J, Furlanetto R, River J, Vale W, Smith P, Brook S. Acceleration of growth rate in growth hormone-deficient children treated with human growth-hormone releasing hormone. *Pediatr Res* 24:145–151, 1988.

100. Thorner MO, Vance ML, Evans WS, Blizzard RM, Rogol AD, Ho K, Leong DA, Borges JLC, Cronin MJ, MacLeod RM, Kovacs K, Asa S, Horvath E, Frohman L, Furlanetto R, Klingensmith GJ, Brook C, Smith P, Reichlin S, Rivier J, Vale W: Physiological and clinical studies of GRF and GH. *Recent Prog Horm Res* 42:589–640, 1986.

101. Van Vliet G, Styne DM, Kaplan SL, Grumbach MM: Growth hormone treatment for short stature. *N Engl J Med* 309:1016–1022, 1983.

102. Velicelebi G, Santacroce TM, Harpold MM: Specific binding of synthetic human pancreatic growth hormone releasing factor (1- 40-OH) to bovine anterior pituitaries. *Biochem Biophys Res Commun* 126:33–39, 1985.

103. Vicens-Calvet E, Vendrell JM, Albisu M, Potau N, Audi L, Gusine M: The dosage dependency of growth and the maturity in growth hormone deficiency treated with human growth hormone. *Acta Paediatr Scand* 73:120–126, 1984.

104. Zachmann M, Prader A: Interactions of growth hormone with other hormones. In Mason AS (ed): *Human Growth Hormone.* London, William Heinemann Medical Books, 1972.

11
Exercise-Induced Stress Fractures and Stress Reactions of Bone: Epidemiology, Etiology, and Classification

BRUCE H. JONES, M.D.
JOHN McA. HARRIS, M.D.
TUYETHOA N. VINH, M.D.
CLINT RUBIN, Ph.D.

"Stress fractures" are a common overuse injury of bone attributed to the repetitive trauma associated with vigorous, usually weight-bearing activities such as running, jogging, walking, and marching. Stress fractures are not only one of the most common overuse injuries suffered by athletes and other physically active individuals, but also one of the more potentially serious injuries of this type. Despite the frequency with which "stress fractures" are seen in orthopedic, sports medicine, and military clinics, the actual incidence with which they occur is not well documented, especially for nonmilitary populations. Thus, it is not surprising that few risk factors for "stress fractures" have been clearly identified by either experimental or epidemiologic studies. The pathophysiology of stress fractures is somewhat better understood, but even their etiology has been and continues to be a subject of debate. Evidence of this debate is the number of hypothetical etiologies [18, 46, 48, 50. 69, 77] and the variety of schemes of classification and nomenclatures employed or suggested by different authors [1, 25, 34, 36, 46, 50, 77, 78].

The term "stress fracture" is itself somewhat of a misnomer and potentially misleading. Most of the injuries diagnosed and classified under the rubric of stress fractures show no evidence of a fracture line or break in the continuity of bone. The continued use of the term "stress fracture" to describe a broad range of bone pathology, from asymptomatic lesions evident only on bone scan to exquisitely painful lesions with simultaneous radiographic evidence of a fracture of remodeling bone, has led to confusion in regard to both the incidence and the etiology of these reactions of bone to unaccustomed stress.

It has been postulated that even when gross radiologic evidence of a fracture does not exist, microfractures of the bone have preceded the radiographic findings of periosteal new bone and/or scintigraphic findings of intense focal uptake of radioisotope which are required to make

the diagnosis of "stress fracture" [37, 51]. This postulation of microfractures may merely be an attempt to rationalize or force a consistency
between the pathophysiology and the accepted nomenclature. In any
case, it is clear from human histopathologic specimens [39; Harris unpublished data, 1983], and recent animal models [32, 75] that it is possible
to observe radiographic findings such as exuberant periosteal new bone
formation with no associated histologic evidence of fractures or microfractures.

In order to gain a better understanding of the broad spectrum of
osseous reactions to "stress" currently referred to as stress fractures the
remainder of this chapter is devoted to a discussion of what is known
of the epidemiology, etiology, and evolution of these injuries. We will
discuss the problems and ambiguities that arise in the literature as a
result of the currently unrefined and sometimes indiscriminant classification of what are called stress fractures. Several schemes for classifying
clinically significant stress reactions of bone will be described, along with
recent proposals for grading radiographic and scintigraphic signs of
these reactions. Finally, we will propose a system of classification that
we feel reflects the underlying etiologic process evolving from normal
response of bone to unaccustomed stress to the catastrophic failure of
bone. The proposed classification will also take into consideration recent
methods for grading x-rays and bone scans. We will argue that the term
"stress fracture" should be reserved for only the catastrophic failures of
bone detected radiographically by a fracture line since this is ultimately
what we hope to prevent by earlier detection of the underlying imbalance
in the usual antecedent remodeling response. Furthermore, the term
"stress fracture" implies a fracture, although in most cases no fracture
is evident. "Stress reaction" is a more appropriate term for the majority
of what are now called "stress fractures" but which do not involve disruption in the structural continuity of bone.

BACKGROUND

Since 1855 when Breithaupt [5] is first credited with describing the
syndrome of painful swollen feet associated with marching in Prussian
Army soldiers [1, 34, 68, 69], the majority of reports on stress reactions
of bone have come from military authorities. In the last 15 years, however, increasing numbers of reports describing stress reactions in civilian
runners and other exercise and sports populations have appeared in the
orthopedic and sports medicine literature. The sudden increase in the
level of interest on the part of nonmilitary physicians is probably the
result of an increased frequency of complaints of injuries diagnosed as
stress fractures seen in their practices. By the 1980s up to 10% of the
injuries seen in civilian sports medicine practices were stress fractures

[51]. This trend of more frequent complaints of stress reactions of bone has been attributed to the increasing societal preoccupation with health and emphasis on leisure time physical activity, especially running [1, 51, 69].

Ironically, despite the increased interest in so-called stress fractures, the actual rate of occurrence of the condition has not been documented among runners or most other athletic populations. For this reason it is not certain whether the greater frequency of complaints consistent with the diagnostic criteria for stress reaction of bone is due to an increased rate (incidence) of occurrence among those who are active or simply to an increase in the number of runners and exercise participants exposed to heightened risk. Our suspicion is the latter. Most civilian and military reports have been from clinical case series which do not allow for the calculation of risks or rates of injury occurrence. As a result of this weakness the majority of the military and the civilian literature provides no grounds to conclusively identify risk factors for injury. Most of our beliefs about the causation of stress reactions and associated risk factors are based on opinion and anecdotal evidence. Although there are now a few epidemiologically sound military studies which have confirmed some of the early suspicions concerning potential risk factors, others have been refuted. The next section discusses the epidemiology of "stress fractures" and risk factors for their occurrence. This discussion will rely heavily on a few recent military studies and the limited inferences that can be drawn from the civilian sports medicine literature and past military case series.

EPIDEMIOLOGY OF STRESS FRACTURES AND REACTIONS OF BONE

Epidemiologically it is important to determine what exposures or characteristics of subgroups within a population place them at increased risk for a particular adverse health event such as stress fractures. To do this one of two approaches is usually taken. One approach is to identify otherwise similar populations with different levels of exposure to a suspected risk factor. These populations or subpopulations are then followed and the eventual incidence or risk of the adverse event, in this case a stress fracture, is quantified and contrasted to determine whether the exposure or level of exposure made a difference. The other approach is to collect a sizeable number of cases of the adverse event, that is, those with stress fractures, and establish a control group of individuals who have not experienced the outcome. Then the percent of those exposed to a risk factor among the cases is contrasted with that among the controls to see whether it differs. If the percent exposed is significantly greater among controls, then the factor may in fact be a risk factor for the adverse outcome, in this instance a stress fracture. Neither of these approaches has been taken in most studies of stress fracture causation, yet it is presumed that the primary risk or exposure is repetitive vigorous physical activity or a change in activity level.

It is probably not a coincidence that the majority of early reports of stress fractures, or march fractures as they were called then, came from military physicians. Military populations, until the recent fitness boom, were the only large populations routinely engaged in the type of activity presumably most likely to cause significant stress reactions of bone. Although stress fractures have been reported in almost all athletic populations, including wrestlers and swimmers [1, 41], the frequency of reports on soldiers and runners suggests that there is something unique about their activities that predisposes them to suffer stress injuries of bone. Also, reports of the distribution of stress fractures by sport from general orthopedic and sports medicine practices indicate that by far the greatest percent of stress fractures among civilians occurs in runners (See Fig. 11.1). In fact, in those series reporting a cross section of sports, more stress fractures occur in runners than all other sports and fitness activities combined. We suspect that something about the combination of continuous, repetitive muscular activity and the weight bearing of marching and running exposes military recruits and runners to excessive skeletal stress which exceeds the body's ability to adapt. Whether compressive gravitational forces or contractile muscular forces are most responsible for adaptive failure of bone has not been demonstrated. What seems clear, however, is that stress reactions and fractures occur predominantly in association with vigorous physical activity usually of a weight-bearing nature in relative young otherwise healthy individuals.

Despite their frequent occurrence, the incidence of stress fractures outside of military populations is not well established. Even within the military the incidence of stress fractures is only relatively firmly established for initial entry basic training populations, but not for trained troops. Despite the limited focus of these studies of military trainees, they are quite informative. There are at least six published reports of the incidence of stress fractures and reactions occurring in United States military trainees [6, 27, 43, 58, 60, 68]. In the last 10 years the incidence of stress fractures among male Army and Marine Corp trainees has varied between 0.9% and 2% (see Table 11.1). Scully [68] reported that an Army-wide survey of basic training posts revealed an incidence of stress injuries of bone of 4.8%, however, the criteria for inclusion as a case (i.e., a stress fracture) in this survey were not reported. The incidence of stress reactions and fractures among female trainees has generally ranged between 10 and 20% (see Table 11.1). Although Brudvig [6] reported an incidence among female trainees of 3.4% in the population, she observed the rate for white females was 11.8%. Even in Brud-

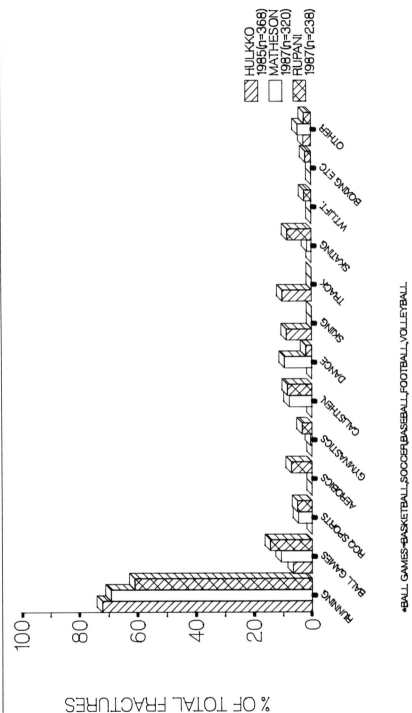

FIGURE 11.1
Distribution of stress fractures by sport or physical activity. Data are from civilian sports medicine and orthopedic clinics.

vig's study the relative risk of this type injury for all females compared to males was more than 3.5 times higher (3.4% vs 0.9%). The relative risks of incurring a stress injury of bone for females versus males in studies observing both genders have ranged between 3.5 to 1 and 10 to 1 (see Table 11.1).

A recent series of articles reporting an unusually high incidence of stress fractures among male Israeli Defense Forces trainees has alarmed their military authorities [16, 29, 53, 54]. Milgrom et al. [54] reported an incidence of stress fractures among Israeli trainees of 31% in 1985. Their concern was heightened because this rate was more than six times higher than the highest incidence (4.8%) reported for male U.S. military trainees in recent years. However, the Israelis used different diagnostic techniques to establish the ultimate diagnosis of a stress fracture. Whereas the U.S. studies [6, 43, 58, 60, 68] reporting incidence data all relied on x-ray criteria to establish the definitive diagnosis, the Israelis used a combination of more sensitive bone scan criteria and x-rays. In their report [54], the Israelis stated that only 20% of bone scan confirmed stress fractures were x-ray positive. Thus, if we correct for the difference between bone scan criteria and x-ray information on stress fractures, only 6.2% of the trainees they observed would have been positive by the criteria employed in the U.S. studies. Although still high, this is more compatible with the percent at risk reported among U.S. military trainees, and is consistent with the 5% incidence of x-ray positive stress fractures reported by Hallel et al. [33] on another population of Israeli soldiers.

In regard to gender, it is apparent from the preceding discussion that women are at greater risk of suffering stress injuries of bone than men in U.S. military training populations (see Table 11.1). This is also true when the risks for females versus males are separated by age and race (see Tables 11.2 and 11.3). Besides gender, other potential risk factors for stress injuries of bone that epidemiologic studies of U.S. military trainees have examined are age, race, physical fitness history, and footwear.

Two studies have examined the influence of age on the likelihood of incurring a stress fracture [6, 27]. Brudvig et al. [6] reported that risk of a stress fracture increased from 1.27% for 17- to 22-year-old Army trainees, to 2.32% of 23- to 28-year-olds, to 5.01% for 29- to 34-year-olds (see Table 11.2). The risk for those over the age of 35 was reported as 2.36%, but the number of women and men of this age was so small that these data were unreliable. The same trends of increasing risk with increasing age were observed when men and women were examined separately (see Table 11.2). Gardner et al. [27] found that the risk of suffering a stress fracture among male Marine recruits was almost twice as high for those age 21 or older as for those age 20 or younger (risk

TABLE 11.1
Cumulative Incidence (Risk, %) of Stress Fractures for Male and Female Military Trainees Reported by Different Authors over the Last 15 Years and Calculated Relative Risk of Females (F) versus Males (M)

| Study | Year | Population | Observation Period | Cumulative Incidence | | Relative Risk F/M |
				Females	Males	
				%	%	
Protzman (58)	1977	Cadets, West Point (n = 1330; M = 1228, F = 102)	8 wks	10.0	1.0	10.0
Reinker (60)	1979	Army trainees	8 wks	12.0	2.0	6.0
Kowal (43)	1980	Army trainees (n = 347; all females)	8 wks	21.0	—	—
Scully (68)	1982	Army trainees (n = 6677; all males)	8 wks	—	1.3	—
Brudvig (6)	1983	Army trainees (n = 20422; M = 16000, F = 4422)	8 wks	3.4	0.9	3.8
Gardner (27)	1988	Marine recruits (n = 3025; all males)	12 wks	—	1.3	—
Jones	Unpublished data 1984	Army trainees (n = 310; M = 124, F = 186)	8 wks	13.9	3.2	4.3
Jones	Unpublished data 1987	Army trainees (n = 323; all males)	13 wks	—	2.2	—

TABLE 11.2
Cumulative Incidence (Risk, %) of Stress Fractures over 8-Week Army Basic Training Cycle for Males and Females by Age Group with Calculated Relative Risks for Females (F) Versus Males (M) and for Each Other Age Group Versus the Youngest

Sex	Group 1 (17–22 years)		Group 2 (23–28 years)		Group 3 (29–34 years)		Group 4 (> 34 years)	
	Cumulative Incidence	Relative Risk (G1/G1)	Cumulative Incidence	Relative Risk (G2/G1)	Cumulative Incidence	Relative Risk (G3/G1)	Cumulative Incidence	Relative Risk (G4/G1)
	%		%		%		%	
Females	2.7	1.0	4.7	1.7	8.2	3.0	7.7	2.9
Males	0.9	1.0	1.3	1.4	3.0	3.3	0.0	—
Relative Risk (F/M)	3.0		3.6		2.7		—	

TABLE 11.3
Cumulative Incidence (Risk, %) of Stress Fracture during 8-Week Army Basic Training Cycle for Males and Females by Racial Group with Calculated Relative Risks for Females (F) Versus Males (M) and Blacks Versus Whites

Sex	White (W)		Black (B)	
	Cumulative Incidence	Relative Risk (W/W)	Cumulative Incidence	Relative Risk (B/W)
	%		%	
Females	11.8	1.00	1.4	0.12
Males	1.1	1.00	0.2	0.18
Relative risk (F/M)	10.7	—	7.0	—

ratio = 1.82%/1.01% = 1.8). However, because fitness test scores tend to be lower and percent body fat higher in older trainees (Jones, personal data, 1984), it may be that the real risk factor in these training populations may not be age per se, but declining fitness with age. On the other hand, Carter et al. [14] and others [42] have demonstrated that the bone of older individuals is less resistant to fatigue fractures when examined in a purely material sense.

A few anecdotal reports from military sources since the beginning of World War II have implicated race as a risk factor for stress fractures [3, 55, 57]. However, as with age there are only a few papers in the literature that report the actual incidence of stress fractures by race [6, 27]. Brudvig et al. [6] reported risks for white males of 1.07% versus 0.23% for black males, a risk ratio of 4.7 (see Table 11.3). For white females versus black the risks were 11.83% and 1.39%, respectively, a risk ratio of 8.5. Brudvig et al. also found that all other racial groups combined had lower risks than whites. Similar results are reported by Gardner et al. [27], who found the risks for white male Marine recruits to be 2.5 times higher than for all other races combined. Risk for white Marines was 1.56% versus 0.6% and 0.67%, respectively, for blacks and hispanics. Thus these more recent studies where risks have been calculated tend to confirm the earlier impressions that for some reason blacks are less likely to develop stress fractures. The lower risk for stress fractures among blacks may be related to findings of higher bone densities reported for blacks [40, 72]. If it is bone density that makes a difference in these risks, it may be a difference in activity levels between whites and blacks and/or inherited racial traits that underlie the finding.

Several other risk factors for stress fractures were also examined by Gardner et al. [27]. Among these was physical activity level of recruits prior to entering the Marine Corp, which was assessed by means of a survey questionnaire. The risks of a stress fracture that they reported declined from 12.0% for those marines who assessed themselves as inactive, to 2.2% for those below average, to 1.6% for those who reported average activity levels, to 0.9% for those above average, to 0.6% for those who assessed themselves as very active. These results tend to support earlier suspicions that the most sedentary and least fit individuals entering the armed services and sports programs were the most likely to suffer stress fractures [1, 8, 36]. The least active individuals may be at greater risk because the relative increase in activity associated with military or other training is much greater for them.

Another significant finding of Gardner et al. [27] was in regard to footwear. The primary reason for their survey of 3000 Marines was to test the efficacy of a shock-absorbent boot insole to prevent stress fractures in a randomized trial. At the time of their study the Marines wore running shoes for calisthenics and running, but boots for all other training activities that required footwear. Also, in general Marine recruits at that time marched two to three times as many miles as they ran over the 12 weeks of initial training. What Gardner et al. found was that shock-absorbent insoles made no difference in stress fracture incidence (incidence in shock-absorbent insole group versus control 1.35% vs. 1.13%, respectively). This finding was similar to results of a randomized trial of several hundred female Army trainees testing three types of shock-absorbant insoles versus a control reported in an Army Technical memorandum by Dr. Carolyn Bensel of the U.S. Army Natick Research and Development Center in Massachusetts in 1985.

Gardner et al. [27] also examined the effect of different running shoe characteristics on the likelihood of suffering a stress fracture. Using price as a surrogate for the quality of running shoes worn by Marine recruits, they found that wearing expensive shoes (price greater than $40) versus inexpensive shoes (price less than $25) made no difference in the incidence of injury. In regard to footwear, Gardner's group did identify one factor that had a significant impact on risk of incurring a stress fracture during recruit training—running shoe age. They found that those recruits wearing newer shoes were less likely to suffer stress fractures.

Most of the remaining data on military populations are derived from a number of large case series. It is dangerous to give too much credence to generalizations about risk factors based on case series data. However, since World War II there appear to be several trends or changes in the distribution of the location at which stress fractures occur and also the point in time in the military training cycle when they occur that may provide fruitful hints of what to examine in future studies.

Military reports of stress fractures from World War II and before describe primarily injuries of the foot [2, 3, 8, 34, 36]. Several early case series report the frequency of all stress fractures seen by the reporting physicians (see Fig. 11.2 for relative distributions by site). In these early series 83–96% of all diagnosed stress fractures occurred in the foot, primarily the metatarsals. By the 1960s reports from U.S. Army populations indicate a slight shift toward greater relative number of stress fractures occurring in the leg [20, 55, 76]. Nevertheless, 63–82% of reported stress fractures still involved the foot (metatarsals and calcaneus), while only 13–27% involved the leg (tibia and fibula), and 3–4% the femur (see Fig. 11.3). By the 1980s a more radical shift in the distribution had taken place within U.S. military populations where only 42–65% of stress fractures reportedly occurred in the foot, while 24–39% involved the leg, and 5–19% in the femur [6, 28, 30] (see Fig. 11.4).

Physicians of the Israeli Defense Forces have recently reported an even more radical departure from the classically expected military distribution of stress fractures which would be expected to occur primarily in the metatarsal and calcaneus. Two of these authors, Milgrom [53, 54] and Giladi [29], have reported that 56–72% of the stress fractures in the Israeli troops that they have followed were in the leg, primarily the tibia, with another 26–34% occurring in the thigh (shaft and neck of the femur), while only 2–9% reportedly involved the foot (see Fig. 11.5). These authors went to great lengths to account for the unexpectedly low frequency of metatarsal and calcaneal stress fractures which they observed, as well as the previously mentioned overall high incidence of stress fractures.

One of the Israeli publications [29] points out the trend observed in the military literature toward an increasing percent of stress fractures occurring in the legs (tibia) rather than the feet of soldiers since World War II. They speculate that changes in the nature of training, equipment, and selection of military personnel over time probably account for this trend. Specifically comparing the "unusual distribution" of stress fractures that they observed to those reported for recent U.S. military trainees, they speculated that differences in training and the more sensitive screening process employed by them, that is, use of bone scans, probably contributed to the apparent discrepancies. They stated that in the basic training population studied by them more emphasis was placed on running and marching than in U.S. populations and significantly less on drill and ceremony. For this reason they felt the distribution they observed more closely resembled one that might be expected for a civilian population of athletes. However, most civilian studies report that 20% or more of stress fractures, and as many as 38%, occur in the feet among runners and other athletes (see Fig. 11.6). Thus, while training factors

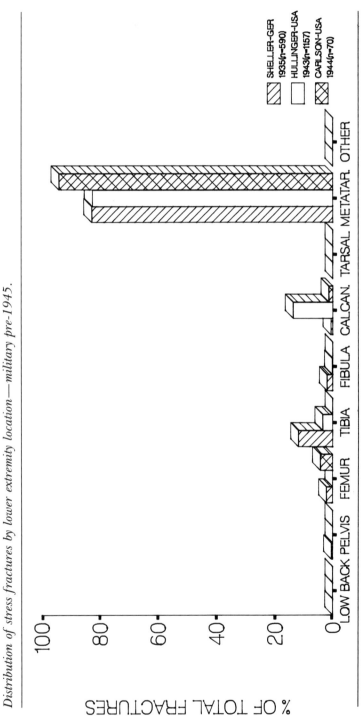

FIGURE 11.2
Distribution of stress fractures by lower extremity location—military pre-1945.

FIGURE 11.3
Distribution of stress fractures by lower extremity location—U.S. Army, 1960–1970.

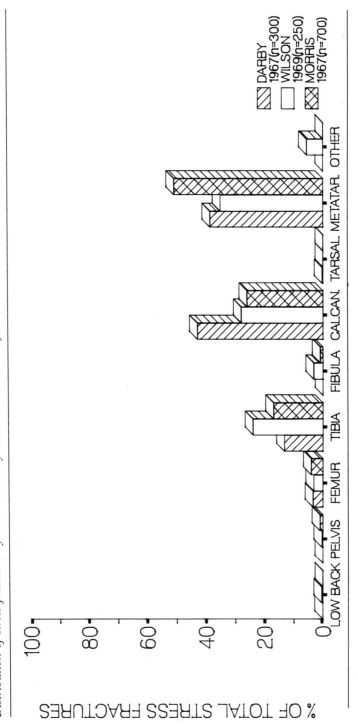

FIGURE 11.4
Distribution of stress fractures by lower extremity location—U.S. Army, post-1970.

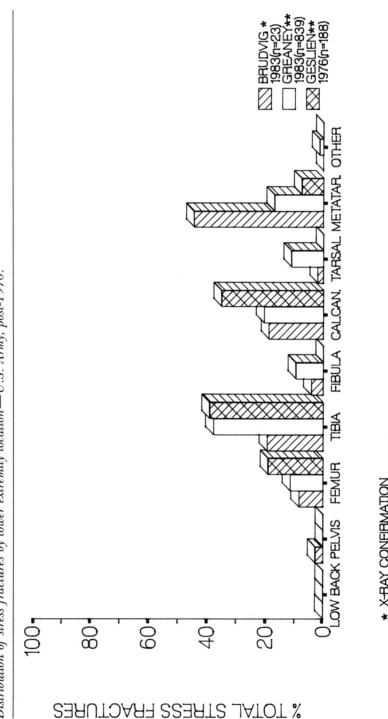

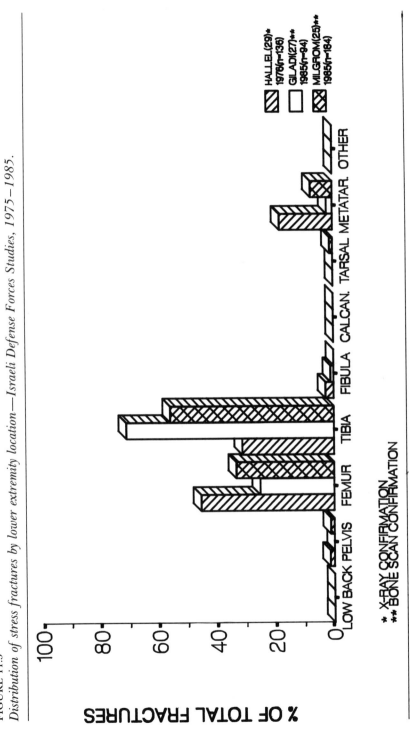

FIGURE 11.5
Distribution of stress fractures by lower extremity location—Israeli Defense Forces Studies, 1975–1985.

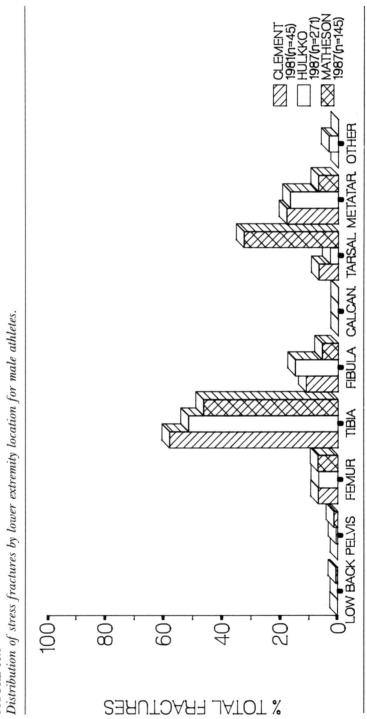

FIGURE 11.6
Distribution of stress fractures by lower extremity location for male athletes.

such as less drill and ceremony and "fewer parades on pavement" may contribute to the decreased frequency of stress fractures of the foot among Israeli trainees compared to ones of the U.S. military, some other factors must also be operating.

As an aside, the Israelis also speculated that their increased use of bone scans might also have contributed to the disparities they observed in the distribution of stress fractures. This probably accounted for some of the discrepancy, since most of the U.S. military studies have relied on x-rays to establish the diagnosis of stress fractures. However, active case finding methodologies in the prospective Israeli studies certainly must have contributed as well. Giladi et al. [29] reported that 33% of femoral stress fractures were asymptomatic, and Milgrom et al. [54] reported that 69% of the femoral stress fractures they observed were asymptomatic. Presumably, since the U.S. military data were based on clinical populations, most of those with stress fractures reported on "sick call" because of symptoms of discomfort and therefore asymptomatic stress fractures would not have been noted. The intent of this discussion is not to criticize the Israeli studies in question, but rather to emphasize the dangers of making direct comparisons between the results of studies which have employed different operational definitions of injury or disease (i.e., stress fractures diagnosed on the basis of bones scans versus x-rays) and which have employed different means of identifying cases (i.e., active versus passive). As pointed out, these differences in diagnostic criteria and case selection can bias not only the distribution of injury but also the rates of occurrence.

In regard to the time of occurrence of stress fractures during the training cycle, reports from World War II indicate that the frequency of stress fractures peaked usually somewhere between 2–4 months of training [2, 3, 44, 46] (see Fig. 11.7). More recent military studies that have documented the point in time in the training cycle that stress fractures have been reported clinically demonstrate peaks in frequency among trainees occurring in any of the first 10 weeks, usually before 8 weeks. In a recent study of U.S. Marines a peak occurrence in the 1st week of training was reported [30]. This peak in the first week accounted for 46% of all the stress fractures observed (see Fig. 11.8). In another population of Marines we observed a peak frequency accounting for 18% of the observed stress fractures in the 9th week of training (unpublished data) (see Fig. 11.8). Protzman and Griffis [58] reported a peak in the 5th and 6th weeks of an initial 8-week training period for male and female West Point cadets that accounted for 46% of all the stress fractures reported (see Fig. 11.9). Two separate Israeli studies reported disparate peaks (see Fig. 11.10). One by Milgrom et al. reported an early peak with 51% of all stress fractures occurring in the 3rd to 4th weeks, while

FIGURE 11.7

Distribution of stress fractures by week of training for U.S. Army trainees—World War II.

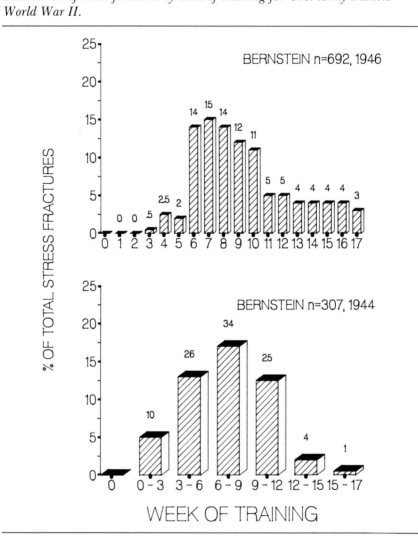

the other group, Giladi et al. [29] reported a peak of 40% in the 7th and 8th weeks (see Fig. 11.10).

Clearly the peak occurrence of stress fractures from one population to another is highly variable, but it is not clear what factors determine when trainees will be most susceptible to stress injuries of bone. Certainly one must suspect that the rate of progression of training volume and

FIGURE 11.8
Distribution of stress fractures by week of training of U.S. Marine recruits—1980s.

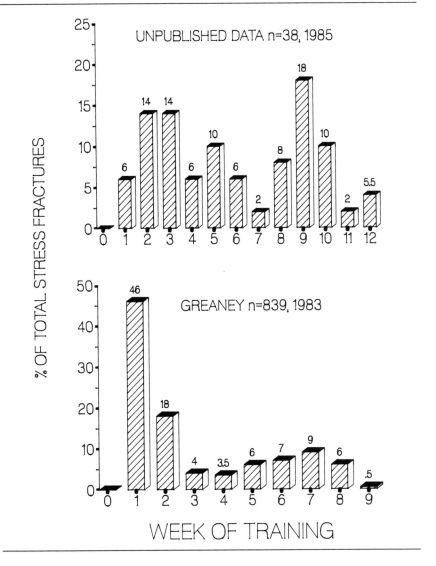

FIGURE 11.9

Distribution of stress fractures by week of training in male and female West Point cadets—1977.

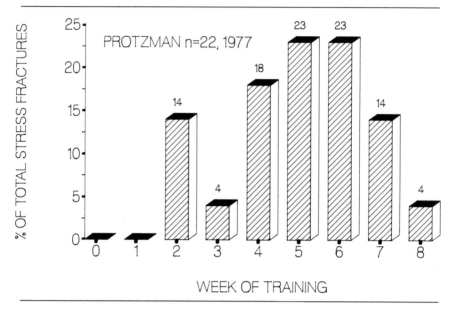

intensity and the average initial fitness of troops would influence how high and how soon the peak stress fracture rates would be. Thus, it could be that the increased emphasis on running to enhance the fitness of soldiers since 1970 and the relative decrease in emphasis on marching since World War II have contributed to the earlier peak occurrence of stress fractures in recent years. It may also be that youth entering the military services in recent years have lower levels of muscular and skeletal conditioning prior to entry than those joining during World War II. While it may be argued that factors such as increased emphasis in running and/or lower levels of fitness may have shifted the peak incidence of stress injuries of bone toward earlier periods in the training cycle, it is not possible to conclusively explain the shift toward earlier occurrence or the high degree of variability in peak occurrence of stress fractures with the little information provided.

To some extent the recent variability observed between military populations may be due to methodological differences. For instance, Greaney et al. [30] relied on bone scans to make their diagnoses, whereas in our study of Marines (unpublished data) we relied on x-ray confirmation which probably delayed diagnosis 2–3 weeks. Even this could not ac-

FIGURE 11.10

Distribution of stress fractures by week of training of Israeli Defense Force recruits—1985.

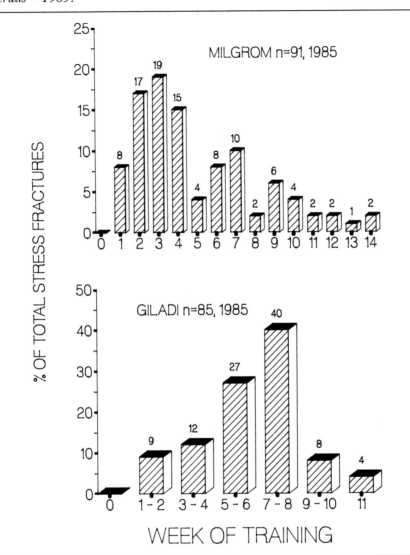

count for our respective observations of peaks in the 1st and 9th weeks (see Fig. 11.8). If we are going to credibly explain such divergent observations, more information on contributing factors such as the volume and type of training in different populations, changes in activity, and the average levels of fitness and other characteristics of individuals will be needed.

SUMMARY OF EPIDEMIOLOGY AND REQUIREMENTS FOR FUTURE STUDY

It is evident from the preceding discussion that one of the great weaknesses of the existing literature on stress reactions and fractures is the paucity of studies that quantify the incidence or risk of suffering a stress fracture in a population exposed to risk. This naturally has not only limited the ability of those publishing results to compare their findings with those of other authors, but it has also prohibited the identification of risk factors for stress injuries to bone in such deficient studies. Although there is an abundance of clinical opinion regarding causative or risk factors for stress injuries of bone, most of it is unsubstantiated. As such these opinions must be viewed as hypotheses in need of testing.

Even in those studies that do quantify incidence or risk, most have not systematically attempted to identify modifiable risk factors or exposures such as the amount or intensity of training, or changes in training that may lead to increased risk. Most of the studies that have quantified population risks have been primarily descriptive in nature. From these, however, it does appear that gender ([6, 58, 60], Jones, unpublished data, 1984), age [6, 27], and race [6, 27] are either directly associated with risk or with some other factor that is associated with ultimate risk. Because these inherent characteristics of individuals are associated with different degrees of risk, they must be accounted for and controlled for in any study purporting to identify other perhaps modifiable risk factors, such as type or amount of training or sporting activity. So far the only potentially modifiable risk factors identified as being associated with an increased risk of stress fractures are low levels of past physical activity [27] and the older, more worn-out training shoes used by some recruits [27].

There is, however, abundant circumstantial evidence and conjecture that certain types of physical activity, such as running and marching, and parameters of training, such as the intensity, duration, and frequency of an activity, are likely to be associated with stress injuries of bone [1, 19, 29, 48, 51]. Also, it seems intuitively reasonable to expect that there might be a dose–response relationship between the amount of training or exposure and the likelihood of injury at least for individuals of comparable fitness level. It is also felt that specific activities are associated with stress injuries of specific bones, for example, stress reactions of the metatarsal shaft with marching and ballet, the tibia with running, the hamate with golfing, tennis, and batting, etc. [18]. Nevertheless, such conjectures are of little practical value unless the types of activities that place an individual at risk are clearly identified and the volume or level of activity associated with an increase in risk are established and quantified. This quantification of exposure and level of risk would appear to be one of the main priorities of "stress fracture" research in the near future. In addition, it will be important to document changes in the type or level of training activity, since the common denominator for all stress injuries is with little doubt a change in activity to which the bone is unaccustomed. It will also be important to quantify the degree of disability as measured by time to recovery and the degree of intervention, for example, rest only or cast plus rest, for different categories or grades of stress injury to bone.

Another urgent need is to establish standardized, widely accepted schemes for grading bone scans and x-rays, and diagnostic criteria for stress reactions, that allow for relative consistency of interpretation and comparability of results between studies. Furthermore, there is a great need for a system of classification and nomenclature for stress injuries of bone that distinguishes between lesions of different degrees of severity or pathology. Standardized grading of bone scans in particular would be helpful since it has not only been shown that increasing grade of bone scan is associated with increased likelihood of positive x-rays [78], but also with more prolonged periods of recovery [16, 78]. Also, it would be beneficial to at least distinguish between stress injuries of bone diagnosed on the basis of x-rays demonstrating cortical lucency, those demonstrating periosteal new bone formation, and those with evidence of frank fracture, since these and combinations of these findings must certainly reflect different stages of response and degrees of pathology. Some agreement would also seem necessary regarding the assessment of positive bone scans associated with symptomatic and asymptomatic lesions, since inclusion of asymptomatic lesions in study results will not only increase the apparent incidence of stress fractures, but will also effect the distribution of stress reactions by location. Among other things, femoral lesions are more likely to be asymptomatic [29, 31, 54]. If nothing else it would be helpful if future studies documented and reported different operationally defined stress reactions separately instead of assuming that one "stress fracture" is like another regardless of the diagnostic tools (e.g., bone scan vs. x-ray) and other criteria (e.g., symptomatic vs. asymptomatic) employed to identify them. Such naivete can have profound epidemiologic and prognostic repercussions.

In regard to the nomenclature for stress injuries of bone, a number of recent authors have expressed dissatisfaction with the use of the term "stress fracture" to describe these lesions [25, 50, 78]. Zwas [78] stated, "A true fracture occurs only when the removal of cortex is accelerated beyond the capacity of the periosteal reaction to offer adequate reinforcement. Thus, it seems that the term stress or fatigue 'fracture' limits the meaning of the full range of stress bone injuries appearing in the evolution of dynamic osteogenic bone response." In a similar vein, Floyd et al. [25] state, "It is our opinion . . . that the term stress fracture should be reserved for those lesions that have a positive bone scan and roentgenographic evidence of fracture." They also warn that "bone scan alone should not be used to diagnosis fractures." They suggest a nomenclature that might be more descriptive along with associated clinical and radiographic findings (see Table 11.4). A richer more precisely descriptive nomenclature not only would be of value from an epidemiologic perspective but would likely be clinically beneficial from the standpoint of prognostic value.

The remainder of the chapter will summarize our current understanding of the etiology of stress injuries of bone from a histologic and clinical perspective. We will then present a graded system of classification and a parallel nomenclature that is consistent with our current understanding of the etiology and clinical evolution of stress injuries to bone.

ETIOLOGY OF STRESS FRACTURES AND STRESS REACTIONS OF BONE

Ever since Breithaupt's description in 1855 of the syndrome of pain and swelling of the feet associated with prolonged marching [5], the nature and etiology of the condition have been subjects of controversy. The etiology of the syndrome became less of a mystery after Stechow [70], another German military surgeon, published a review of foot swelling associated with x-ray findings which demonstrated that at least some of the events were fractures.

The first histologic evidence of a "march fracture" leading to callus formation and local evidence of fracture healing in the absence of a frankly visible fracture line was published by Strauss in 1932. His case was one of a "big, healthy and rather obese woman of 30 years" who worked in a cafeteria on her feet all day and had a slowly progressive painful mass develop in her foot. This mass was palpable on examination, and x-ray showed a growth of new bone at the site with hazy and indistinct margins and erosions. A diagnosis of tumor was made and the metatarsal was excised to confirm the diagnosis prior to amputation. Examination of the "tumor" mass revealed "well developed and partially calcified osteoid tissue." In addition, on gross examination a narrow fracture line across the old metatarsal was found; however, the surrounding mass of callus (new bone) was not involved. Findings such as these fueled the assumption that all these injuries represented fractures at some level, gross or microscopic, which were followed by healing and callous formation which accounted for the radiographic signs commonly associated with the condition.

Since the first descriptions, a variety of both experimental models and analyses of clinical specimens have led to a fairly full appreciation of the histologic process underlying these lesions. One of the authors (John M. Harris) has reviewed 60 cases from the files of the Armed Forces Institute of Pathology, for which there was sufficient x-ray, historical, and histologic evidence to draw conclusions about the location of the lesions, their time sequence, and pathology.

In this case series, the earliest lesions in terms of history of local symptoms showed evidence of a process that had been going on longer than the symptoms. In the earliest specimens tunneling or excavation of the cortex of the bone and periosteal new bone was evident, and in addition, there was evidence of early primary haversian system in filling of the periosteal new bone and excavated cortex with osteoid. From these human materials it was apparent that the histologic and roentgenographic presentation in each instance were one piece of a spectrum of presentation. Changes ranged from minor ones, barely detectable by standard roentgenographic techniques and visible histologically only as minimal cortical tunneling with minimal new bone formation, to massive remodeling associated with tremendous reduction in cortical mass secondary to tunneling and exuberant callus formation clearly visible on roentgenographs. In the latter instance the callus cannot be distinguished from reparative callus about an acute fracture except by historic means such as serial x-rays. However, in this series, though all displayed radiographic evidence of new bone formation, there was no radiographic or histologic evidence of a fracture initially, and only one case exhibited a fracture after serial x-rays.

In addition to clinical specimens, various animal models have been developed to study the effect of overload to various bones and the subsequent reactions of bone to the imposed "stress." These methods include excision of a portion of the dog radius to overload the ulna after which the animal is exercised [56, 66, 67, 73, 74]. Also, such innovations as cages with electric floors that elicit repetitive jumping behavior in rabbits have been used to induce stress reactions and fractures [32]. Direct 3-point mechanical bending of the ulna in various animals using external loading devices [7] and external compressive loading of the avian ulna using permanently affixed metal caps are other techniques used to generate "stress fracture"-like lesions [63, 64]. Another technique involves actual preweakening of the bone by immobilization and then release the limb, after which the animal is exercised [75]. All of these models have in common the ability to sample an area of damaged bone at a prede-

TABLE 11.4
Comparison of Proposed Graded System of Classification and Nomenclature with Systems Proposed by Other Authors (21, 25, 62, 78) and Schemes for Grading Bone Scans (16, 25, 62, 78) and X-rays (25, 62)

	←GRADE 0→	←GRADE I→	←GRADE II→	←GRADE III→	←GRADE IV→
Proposed Stress reaction grade Nomenclature	Normal remodeling	Mild stress reaction	Moderate stress reaction	Severe stress reaction	Stress fracture
Elton (1968) Nomenclature	Normal bone	←——————Stress reaction——————→			←——Stress fracture→
Zwas (1987) Nomenclature		(?)—"Mild stress fracture"—(?)		(?)—Stress fracture—(?)	
Bone scan grade Description		←Grade I→ "Small ill defined cortical area of mild increased uptake"	←Grade II→ "Larger well defined elongated area of moderately increased activity"	←Grade III→ "Wide fusiform corticomedullary area of highly increased activity"	←Grade IV→ "Extensive transcortical area of intensely increased activity"
Chisin (1987) Bone scan grade Description	←Grade 1→ "Irregular uptake and/or a poorly defined area of increased activity compared with contralateral side"	←Grade 2→ "Similar to Grade 1 but more intense"	←——————Grade 3→ "Sharply marginated area of increased activity compared with the contralateral side, usually focal or fusiform shape"	←——————Grade 4 "Similar to Grade 3 but more intense uptake comparable to that of iliac crest"——————→	
Symptoms	←——————Less painful——————			——————More painful——————→	

Floyd (1987)				
Nomenclature	←"Occult stress reaction"→	←"Stress reaction"→	←"Occult stress fracture"→	←Stress fracture→
Bone scan appearance	←Normal bone scan—	"Hot spot" on bone scan→		
Early x-ray	Normal →	Early x-ray (+/−)→	Fracture→	
Late x-ray		←Healing fracture or fracture→	Fracture→	
Symptoms		←"Pain"→		
Roub (1979)				
Bone scan		←Bone scan (+/−)→	←Bone scan (+)—	
Description		"Nondescript poorly defined area of slightly increased uptake"	"Focal fusiform, sharply marginated area of increased activity"	
X-ray			X-rays (+)	
Description of x-ray			Vague lucent cortical areas	Periosteal and endosteal thickening / Cortical fracture
Nomenclature	Unstressed Bone	Normal remodeling / Accelerated remodeling	Fatigue	Exhaustion
Scale/grade	----	5. / 4. / 3.	2.	1.
Pathology	Resorp./Replace.	Resorp. > Replace.	Resorp. >> Replace. Cortex weakened by resorp. cavities	Resorp. >>> Replace. Cortex buttressed by periosteal and endosteal bone

termined time that coincides with a specified amount of repetitive stress rather than on the basis of symptoms. In all of these models it is possible, therefore, to observe and document early changes that occur in bone as a result of these artificial but quantifiable "stresses."

What is seen on the histologic level early in the process is a brisk intracortical remodeling by excavation or tunneling and the production of periosteal and occasionally endosteal new bone. Once the initial lesion is established, the progression of the healing parallels that seen in the human specimens with conversion of the periosteal new bone and the markedly excavated cortical areas to primary haversian bone with subsequent further remodeling to a secondary haversian type of architecture. In addition to providing a more complete histologic picture of the process, these models give some insight into the question of etiology.

The simplest and most naive approach treats bone as an inert substance and fractures as the outcome of the cumulative effect of repetitive deformations of the bone. Failure of bone specimens used in these models resulted from the purely mechanical loss of structural integrity in the same manner as any composite material which will eventually fail when the number of cycles of loading in combination with the amount of force exceeds the fatigue life of the substance, like a wire that is bent too frequently. The fatigue life of bone has been described by testing small segments of cadaver bone which have been machined and treated as purely material substances [9–14, 22–24, 42, 45, 71]. Evidence from these purely mechanical models employing cadaver bone suggests that the strain (i.e., relative deformation of the bone or change in length per unit length) rather than the stress (i.e., the absolute load per unit area) is most important in determining the fatigue life of bone. From these mechanical tests of cadaver bone, it has been estimated that in the physiologic strain range, that is, levels up to 3000 microstrain, the maximum fatigue life of cortical bone should be in the range of 10,000–100,000 cycles.

Although there are probably certain circumstances, such as "insufficiency" fractures which occur in individuals with underlying bone disease or elderly persons with reduced bone mass, where mechanical failure occurs as a result of the purely mechanical effects of repetitive loading [26, 38], this is probably not the case with stress fractures in young athletes and soldiers. Bone is a dynamic substance which responds to changes in load frequency and magnitude; it will adapt especially if the new strain is spread out over enough time. Certainly the animal model of Uhtoff and Javorski [75] shows that even after reducing the stock of bone available through immobilization, it is possible to create a circumstance where the classic findings of a stress reaction are present, but no evidence of mechanical failure of bone or associated fracture or microfracture is discernible.

As stated earlier, pure mechanical or fatigue failure is not the likely etiology for the more common stress reactions which are found in military recruits or in vigorously active young and usually healthy sports enthusiasts who can overload their bones far in excess of the 10,000–100,000 cycles estimated from the purely mechanical model. It has been calculated that an individual will take between 500 and 1000 foot strikes per foot per mile of running or walking, respectively [47]. Studies by one of the authors following recruits through basic training have documented marching and running mileage of 200 miles (70 marching and 130 running) over the course of 12 weeks of infantry training, which is in addition to the walking required for normal daily activities. Even the least enthusiastic recruit under these circumstances would have traveled at least 200 miles and experienced the impact of 140,000 foot strikes. If purely mechanical principals prevailed, this would certainly put a significant proportion of the recruit population into the range where frank fracture should have occurred. The previous epidemiologic evidence in this chapter clearly indicates that the frequency of actual stress reactions in bone, let alone catastrophic failure, does not approach a number that would suggest that pure fatigue damage on the basis of material failure alone is the cause of the problem.

It seems much more likely that the process leading to stress reaction and stress fractures is in fact a physiologic process of the bone adapting to a change in mechanical environment. This imperative for adaptation is commonly known as "Wolf's law," after Julius Wolf who annunciated it in a series of articles between 1869 and 1892 [61]. Certainly the generalized process of bone remodeling, irrespective of the signal to start the process, fits with what is found histologically. The remodeling process involves both removal of bone which has become extraneous to the requirements of the new loading environment and the addition of new bone in an array that is best suited to withstand the new mechanical strain. Under ordinary circumstances this process is well modulated and does not cause symptoms. What is crucial in the situation leading to stress fractures is not the physiologic process but rather the magnitude of stimulus relative to the status of the exposed individual's skeletal system.

Individuals incurring such stress reactions and fractures characteristically have been exposed to some marked change in the overall mechanical environment which may be an "overload," in terms of the magnitude of loading and/or the frequency with which that load is applied. The result is a variable but clearly excessive load to which the bone must respond. If the response is moderate and the amount of bone removed is not sufficient to unduly weaken structure, and the addition of new bone occurs sufficiently rapidly to correct any weakness prior to failure, the process will successfully lead to a bone with appropriate material strength and architecture to withstand the new load environment. Should this balance between removal and reconstruction be marginal, symptoms may occur and eventually lead to signs detectable by x-ray or other tests. In these circumstances, evidence of the process may be grossly visible by x-ray studies. Such was certainly the case for the majority of patients who had biopsies that were sent to the Armed Forces Institute of Pathology. In these cases, with one exception, there was no evidence of frank fractures, but all of them had evidence of removal in the form of cortical tunneling and of new bone formation, in terms of periosteal on-lay of new bone and of in-filling of the new bone and of the tunneled cortises with primary haversian bone. Within the human biopsy material, evidence of frank fracture was unusual. Although the sample is biased because a catastrophic end result or fracture would have led to a clear diagnosis obviating the need for a biopsy being sent to the Institute of Pathology, it is clear that it is not necessary to have a fracture or microfracture to develop the clinical symptoms and radiologic signs of a "stress fracture."

As the process of a bone's adaptation to a new stress becomes more out of balance and the more resorption occurs prior to efficient addition of new bone, the possibility of fracture or catastrophic failure increases. There is no question that such fractures are a significant problem in any population, such as military recruits, which is subjected to a marked change of mechanical loading. Such frank fractures represent a tremendous clinical problem in individual cases since they are often difficult to treat, especially those of the femur [4, 59]. However, while there is a significant risk of stress injuries of bone associated with military and other vigorous weight-bearing training, most do not go on to become frank fractures even after symptoms have appeared.

From the point of view of etiology, the effect of fatigue damage of bone as a material cannot be completely discounted. It is quite possible that the ultimate failure of bone that has been weakened by excessive acute loads or by imbalanced remodeling does result from mechanical overload. The work of multiple authors shows microscopic damage to bone structure in areas where the overall process of stress reaction of bone is at its peak [7, 15, 32, 66, 73–75). Most recently Burr et al. [7], using a 3-point bending model in the dog, found marked increases in microdamage to bone in areas loaded well within the physiologic range both in terms of microstrain deformity and of cycles of load. These artificial 3-point bending studies are not evidence, however, that such microdamage is necessary to elicit the original response to "stress" leading to intracortical tunneling and remodeling. It is also evident from the work of Guoping et al. [32] and Uhtoff et al. [75], using a physiologic or more "natural" model, that microcracks are not always present even though there is evidence of radiologic and histologic remodeling. This clearly needs more investigation.

Parenthetically, another unresolved issue is how or whether the process of remodeling actually leads to improved bone resistance to the repetitive loading which seems to excite the response. Specifically, it is unclear why the bone reorganizes to eventually have a complex secondary haversian structure in response to "stress" when, as a material, bone with such structure is in fact less resistant to fatigue and to tensile damage than bone with a circumferential lamellar structure [10, 14, 42].

The physiologic process underlying stress reactions and fractures of bone may progress to pathologic extremes under some circumstances which lead to problems with both diagnosis and definition of the condition. Both the physiologic process and the pathologic process may be characterized by the production of new bone as well as removal of old bone which adds to the confusion. A location in a bone where the remodeling process is going on to a significant degree will be evident on studies such as bone scans which highlight areas of new bone production. The result of this is that the physiologic process may be detected before it reaches the pathologic extreme. The matter of defining pathology is further complicated by the fact that symptomatology is not uniform even if the process in two bones has reached the same level of intensity. In experimental situations where a large number of recruits had bone scans performed as a screening process rather than in response to symptoms, it was apparent that the femoral neck does not develop symptoms until the process is quite advanced by bone scan. On the other hand, in the tibia and the foot, the bone scan and x-ray findings develop early and seem to parallel the degree of symptomatology in most cases [31, 78]. Furthermore, there can be a discordance between the bone scan findings and x-ray findings, with the former preceding not only positive x-ray findings, but also symptoms in some cases. Thus, it seems that bone scans can detect the physiologic process even when it is not likely to have reached pathologic intensity.

By assessment of the intensity of uptake of the radioisotope and distribution of isotope, it is possible to refine the bone-scanning techniques to yield more informative interpretations, reflecting reactions that range from physiologic to pathologic. However, if the bone scan is used as the only criteria for making the diagnosis, it is theoretically possible that very early stress reactions characterized only by cortical tunneling in the absence of new bone formation may appear as unremarkable cold spots [52]. This may occur at a time when the process of cortical excavation may place the bone in its greatest jeopardy of fracture. Furthermore, bone scans cannot distinguish reliably between exuberant remodeling and actual frank fracture secondary to remodeling. Thus, to thoroughly describe stress reactions and injuries of bone, a combination of clinical symptoms plus scintigraphic and roentgenographic signs is necessary.

CLASSIFICATION AND GRADING OF STRESS FRACTURES AND REACTIONS

Since the first descriptions of stress injuries of bone in the 19th century, there has been debate over their etiology and dissatisfaction with their nomenclature and classification. One of the earliest terms ascribed to them as "march fracture," because of the clear association between marching and the incidence of classical stress reactions. However, as it was gradually discovered that other vigorously active groups of individuals could incur these lesions from a variety of activities, new terms arose. Some of the terms used for varying periods of time have been "fatigue fracture," "crack fracture," "insufficiency fracture," "pseudofracture," and "exhaustion fracture" [1, 77]. Virtually all of these terms have been intended to describe some etiologic attribute of the stress injuries of bone. In recent years the most commonly used term has been "stress fracture." However, there is currently dissatisfaction with this term [25, 50, 78].

At a bare minimum it would seen necessary to have terms to distinguish between stress injuries that result in ultimate failure of the involved bone, that is, stress fractures and those which merely exhibit various degrees of remodeling, that is, stress reactions.

From both a clinical and an epidemiologic standpoint it would be of benefit to have a system of classification and nomenclature that differentiated between physiologic remodeling and various degrees of the pathologic process using readily available methods and technology. In addition, it would be helpful to distinguish the true fracture or catastrophic failure of structural support from the underlying process which may weaken bone or may simply be physiologic remodeling. Our epidemiologic, clinical, and histologic experience and review of the literature suggest that most stress fractures can, in fact, be more appropriately classified as stress reactions of bone. These stress reactions can be further subdivided into those which have resulted in catastrophic failure, that is, true stress fractures; those that are clinically significant in that they represent a significant weakening of the bone; and those that are in fact not pathologic but simply local efforts of remodeling of appropriate degree to adapt to a new physical loading exposure. Accordingly, we suggest the following graded classification system to characterize stress injuries to bone along a five-grade scale from grade 0 to IV (see Table 11.4):

Grade 0 would be used to characterize physiologic responses of bone to a change in mechanical environment with relation to either load or repetitions of loads. These responses would be detectable by bone scan techniques since they entail the production of new bone, but would not be symptomatic, would probably not represent any immediate danger to the bone in terms of failure, and would not result in detectable changes on x-rays.

Grade I would be employed to describe clinically significant stress reactions of bone in that symptoms would be present and the bone scan would be positive. Symptoms would include local pain exacerbated by activity and a history of recently increased activity or onset of a new activity. Tenderness of the area would be minimal or absent. There would not be sufficient change in the bone to be either visible by x-ray or to notably endanger the structural integrity of the bone.

Grade II would be used to characterize clinically significant stress reactions with positive bone scans, symptoms, and barely detectable changes using standard radiographic techniques. Symptoms most likely would include localized pain associated with mild localized tenderness to palpation, but no palpable mass. Also, the onset of pain would be expected to have been associated with a recent change in activity.

Grade III would represent stress reactions of bone with potential structural significance characterized not only by symptoms and positive bone scans, but also positive x-rays suggesting sufficient change in the bone to place its structural integrity in jeopardy. These lesions are characterized by localized pain that may not completely abate with the cessation of exercise. Marked local tenderness and possibly a palpable fullness or mass would be common with these lesions. A history of increased amount or intensity of activity associated with the onset of pain would be expected, followed by insidious increase in level and duration of discomfort if activity were not terminated.

Grade IV would characterize clinically significant stress reactions of bone which have failed structurally, resulting in a frank fracture. These we would refer to as stress fracture. Such stress fractures would be evident as an area of increased uptake on bone scans associated with marked symptoms and positive x-ray. On x-ray there would be evidence of a frank fracture and simultaneous evidence of changes consistent with a chronic process of remodeling and new bone formation—healing— rather than a single acute catastrophic traumatic overloading of the bone. These lesions are extremely painful and may make even minimal weight bearing difficult. Other characteristics and history are similar.

The histologic basis of this grading schema can be found within the materials of the Armed Forces Institute of Pathology, with the exception of Grade 0. There is, however, histopathologic material available from various animal models of repetitive loading which would appear to match the setting of a Grade 0 lesion which would probably correspond to the asymptomatic lesion of military recruits detected in some studies [29,

FIGURE 11.11
Grade 0. Section of avian ulna showing thin layer of periosteal new bone.
Five days load, high physiologic strain. (× 150)

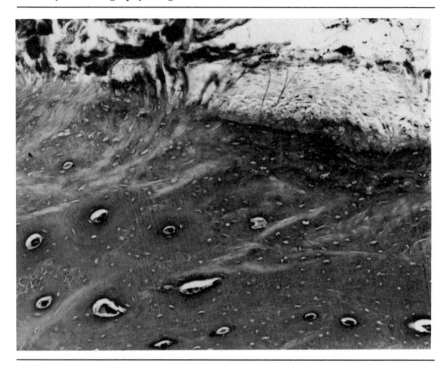

54]. Figure 11.11 represents such a lesion from a sectioned avian ulna bone that was loaded well within the physiologic range of strain for a brief period of time prior to sacrifice of the animal. It shows a thin rim of periosteal new bone in the absence of any notable cortical tunneling or other changes. This rim of cortical bone would be sufficient to generate a localized eccentric area of increased isotope uptake in the cortex of the bone visible on the bone scan. In the absence of any ability to assess symptoms it would appear, therefore, to be a physiologic representation of the minimal lesion that can be detected by any means.

Grade I lesions on occasion have been biopsied in humans. Figure 11.12 is a biopsy of such a lesion from the right fibula in a 47-year-old female with a history of calf pain after taking a tour of Europe which involved some increased walking. The biopsy from which the illustrations are taken was performed on the basis of localized symptomatology and displays both extensive cortical tunneling and some periosteal reaction. This is clearly a lesion with some possible implications to the strength

FIGURE 11.12

Grade 1. Biopsy of painful fibula lesion in 47-year-old female after extended walking. Extensive cortical tunneling and periosteal new bone are evident. (×30)

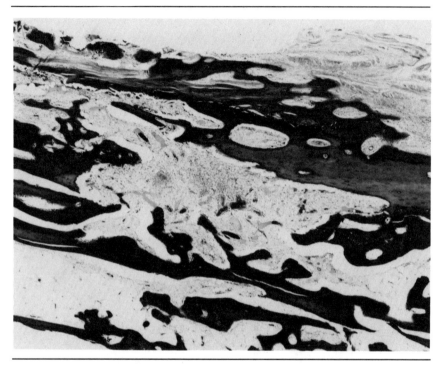

of the fibula, but neither the x-ray evidence nor symptoms suggest that this is of impending significance.

Figure 11.13 represents a lesion in the Grade II category. The patient had an approximate 4-week history of right tibial pain with no specifically defined change in activities. The pain was sufficiently persistent that x-rays, which had been normal when initially taken, were repeated 9 days later showing localized periosteal reaction. The biopsy was taken from this area and shows marked cortical resorption with some periosteal reaction. This is a Grade II lesion which is visible by x-ray and again has some implications in terms of strength of the bone, but does not appear to represent an immediate threat to structural integrity.

Figure 11.14 shows a Grade III lesion. This lesion occurred in an 18-year-old male recruit with a sedentary life-style prior to induction. He developed pain in the right femur following 2 weeks of training. X-rays at the time of presentation showed cortical tunneling and periosteal

FIGURE 11.13
Grade 2. Biopsy right tibial lesion with periosteal new bone—marked cortical tunneling and scant periosteal new bone. (×15)

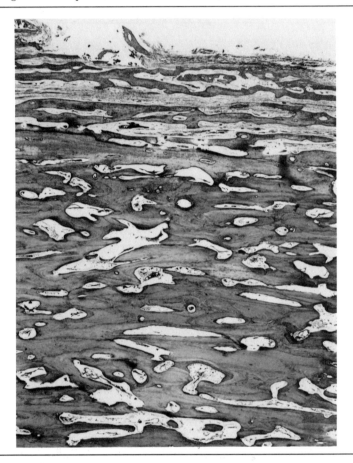

reaction. A biopsy was performed, and the material in the illustration shows extensive periosteal and reactive bone formation resorption. This is a lesion which would be extensive by bone scan, is clearly visible by x-ray, and clearly has implications for structural integrity of the femur which was undoubtedly weakened in the remodeling process.

A Grade IV lesion, synonymous with a "stress fracture," is shown in Figure 11.15. This is from the left distal fibula of a vigorous 54-year-old female gardener who had increased her activities over the preceding 5 weeks as a result of the onset of spring. The histology shows trabecular fragmentation with necrosis and fibrovascular reaction which is consist-

FIGURE 11.14
Grade 3. Right femoral lesion in previously sedentary recruit. Marked cortical tunneling and extensive periosteal new bone. (×15)

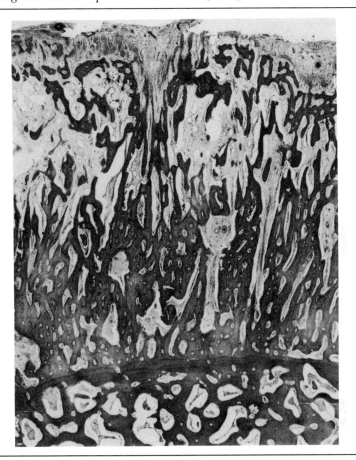

ent with repair of a fracture, and the x-rays show both fractures and periosteal reaction immediately prior to the biopsy.

Our graded system of classification is compatible with the various schemes for grading bone scans suggested by other authors [16, 78], as shown in Table 11.4. It is also compatible with the nomenclature, the pathophysiology, and the scintigraphic and radiologic schemes suggested by other recent authors [25, 62], as shown in Table 11.4. It would be helpful from both a clinical and an epidemiologic standpoint if a scheme for grading bone scans and x-rays could be universally accepted that would parallel a system of graded classification of stress reactions such

FIGURE 11.15

Grade 4. Left fibula biopsy fracture in area of 5 weeks' pain. Resorption and new bone with trabecular fragmentation, necrosis, and fibrovascular reaction compatible with callus formation. (×75)

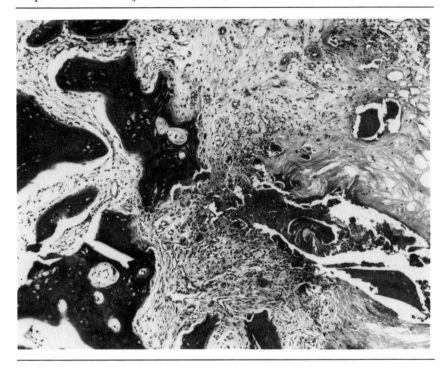

as that proposed here. An associated nomenclature is easily derived for such a classification system. We suggest that grade 0 stress reactions be referred to as normal remolding, grade I as mild stress reactions, grade II as moderate stress reactions, grade III as severe stress reactions, and grade IV as stress fractures. An advantage of this nomenclature is that it employs terms already used in the literature.

Such a parallel system of nomenclature and graded classification of injury, bone scans, and x-rays is imperative if the diagnosis of stress injuries of bone is to have any predictive or prognostic value. It should be kept in mind that from both a clinical and an epidemiologic standpoint it is unlikely that all individual cases will be perfectly categorized by such a scheme. However, it should provide for much greater discrimination than the current term "stress fracture" provides and should minimize gross misclassification. Also, if, as is suspected, the different degrees of scintigraphic and radiologic findings are of prognostic value, such a scheme should assist clinicians and epidemiologists in studying and quantifying the degree of disability associated with different levels of pathology and grades of classification. It would also help to more meaningfully quantify the degree of risk associated with various factors such as sex, age, race, and activity level.

Among other reasons, we have proposed this system of classification and nomenclature because we feel that there is a clear need to distinguish between lesions such as the stress fracture seen on the right in Figure 11.16 and the stress reaction seen on the left of Figure 11.16. Both these lesions occurred in the same Marine recruit, and the underlying process of remodeling with cortical excavation and some periosteal new bone formation must have been similar in both legs, yet the consequences of the pathology evident on x-rays were radically different. In fact, on the day the two x-rays were taken after the recruit collapsed during a routine run with severe left leg pain, his right leg had become asymptomatic. The catastrophic failure of the bone of his left tibia, a stress fracture, clearly had more serious implications for this recruit's health and treatment than the periosteal reaction taking place in his right leg. Although he had reported the right leg pain a week earlier, x-rays at that time were negative, and while the x-rays were positive at the time he fractured his left leg, the injury to the right had become asymptomatic.

CONCLUSION

Stress injuries of bone are very commonly associated with military training, vigorous sports, and recreational and some occupational activities. Recommended treatment of these injuries is usually 2–12 or more weeks of rest of the injured limb. Despite the frequency with which these injuries are treated we do not have any clear idea of what their actual incidence is in different military and civilian populations. Also, while there is still debate regarding the exact etiology of stress injuries of bone, there is good evidence that many do not occur in association with either fractures or microfractures of the involved bone.

In order to develop preventive strategies and more scientific treatment protocols for stress injuries of bone, it will be necessary to establish and contrast their incidence in different populations. In future studies factors known to be associated with risk for these injuries, such as age, race, and physical activity levels, must be documented and controlled for in a systematic way. A system for grading the clinical symptoms and signs of these injuries which reflects what is know of their etiology and clinical severity will make epidemiologic data more meaningful. A nomenclature that parallels the clinical grading of symptoms, bone scans, and x-rays will contribute to the utility of both future clinical and epidemiologic studies. Such a system of classification should also impart greater prog-

FIGURE 11.16

A 19-year-old male Marine recruit presented with an acute fracture of the mid-shaft left tibia sustained while running on level surface. There were no prodromal symptoms on the left, but 1 week before he had presented to the Branch Medical Center with mid-shaft right tibial pain and negative x-ray. The film labeled R *was taken at the time of his acute fracture and shows periosteal new bone formation with underlining cortical tunneling* (black arrow). *At the time of the left tibial fracture, the right leg had become asymptomatic.*

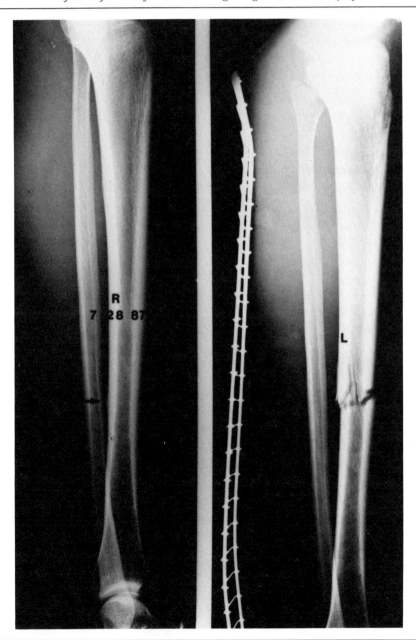

nostic value to the individual clinician's diagnoses of stress fractures and various degrees of stress reactions.

The ultimate objective of both epidemiologic and clinical research is to prevent structural failure of bone (stress fractures) by identification and modification of risk factors and by early recognition of unbalanced remodeling (stress reactions). Early identification of stress reactions should not only help prevent stress fractures but also shorten the recovery period.

REFERENCES

1. Belkin SC: Stress fractures in athletes. *Orthop Clin North Am* 11:735–741, 1980.
2. Bernstein A, Childers MA, Fox KW, Archer MC, Stone JR: March fractures of the foot: care and management of 692 patients. *Am J Surg* 71:355–362, 1946.
3. Bernstein A, Stone JR: March fracture: a report of 307 cases and a new method of treatment. *J Bone Joint Surg* 26:743–750, 1944.
4. Blickenstaff LD, Morris JM: Fatigue fracture of the femoral neck. *J Bone Joint Surg* 48A:1031–1047, 1966.
5. Breithaupt: Zur Pathologie des menschlichen fusses. *Medicishche Zeitung* Berlin 1855; 36:169–171, and 37:175–177.
6. Brudvig TJS, Gudger TD, Obermeyer L: Stress fractures in 295 trainees: a one-year study of incidence as related to age, sex, and race. *Mil Med* 148:666–667, 1983.
7. Burr DB, Mortin RB, Schaffner MB, Radin EL: Bone remodeling in response to *in vivo* fatigue micro damage. *J Biomech* 1B:189–200, 1985.
8. Carlson GD, Wertz RF: March fractures, including others than those of the foot. *Radiology* 43:45–53, 1944.
9. Carter, DR, Spengler DM, Frankel VH: Bone fatigue in uniaxial loading at physiologic strain rate. *IRCS J Med Sci* 5:592, 1977.
10. Carter DR, Hayes WC: Compact bone fatigue damage. I. Residual strength and stiffness. *J Biomech* 10:325–337, 1977.
11. Carter DR, Hayes WC: Compact bone fatigue damage. A microscopic examination. *Clin Orthop Relat Res* 127:265–274, 1977.
12. Carter DR, Calder WE, Spengler DM, Frankel VH: Fatigue behavior of adult cortical bone. The influence of mean strain and strain range. *Acta Orthop Scand* 52:481–490, 1981.
13. Carter DR, Calder WE, Spengler DM, Frankel VH: Uniaxial fatigue of human cortical bone. The influence of tissue physical characteristics. *J Biomech* 14:461–470, 1980.
14. Carter DR, Hayes WC: Fatigue life of compact bone: effects of stress amplitude, temperature and density. *J Biomech* 9:27–34, 1976.
15. Chamay A: Mechanical and morphological aspects of experimental overloading and fatigue of bone. *J Biomech* 3:263–270, 1970.
16. Chisin R, Milgrom C, Giladi M, Stein M, Margulies J, Kashtan H: Clinical significance of nonfocal scintigraphic findings in suspected tibial stress fractures. *Clin Orthop Relat Res* 220:200–205, 1987.
17. Clement DB, Taunton JE, Smart GW, McNicol KL: A survey of overuse injuries. *Physician Sportsmed* 9:47–58, 1981.
18. Daffner RH: Stress fractures: current concepts. *Skeletal Radiol* 2:221–229, 1978.
19. Daffner RH, Martinez S, Gehweiler JA: Stress fractures in runners. *JAMA* 247:1039–1041, 1982.
20. Darby RE: Stress fractures of the os calcis. *JAMA* 200:131–132, 1967.
21. Elton RC: Stress reactions of bone in army trainees. *JAMA* 204:104–106, 1968.

22. Evans FG: The fatigue strength of human compact bone. *Anat Rec* 112:327, 1952.
23. Evans FG, Rioli ML: Relations between the fatigue life and histology of adult cortical bone. *J Bone Joint Surg* 52A:1579–1586, 1970.
24. Evans FG, Lebow M: Strength of human compact bone under repetitive loading. *J Appl Physiol* 10:127–130, 1957.
25. Floyd WN, Butler JE, Clanton T, Kim EE, Pjura G: Roentgenologic diagnosis of stress fractures and stress reactions. *South Med J* 80:433–439, 1987.
26. Freeman MAR, Todd RC, Pirie CJ: The role of fatigue in the pathogenesis of senile femoral neck fractures. *J Bone Joint Surg* 56B:698–702, 1974.
27. Gardner L, Dziados JE, Jones BH, Brundage JF, Harris JM, Sullivan R, Grill R: Prevention of lower extremity stress fractures: a controlled trial of a shock absorbent insole. *Am J Public Health* 78:1563–1567, 1988.
28. Geslien GE, Thrall JH, Espinosa JL, Older RA: Early detection of stress fractures using 99m Tc-polyphosphate. *Radiology* 121:683–687, 1976.
29. Giladi M, Ahronson Z, Stein M, Danon YL, Milgrom C: Unusual distribution and onset of stress fractures in soldiers. *Clin Orthop Relat Res* 192:142–146, 1985.
30. Greaney RB, Gerber FH, Laughlin RL, Kmet JP, Metz CD, Kilcheski TS, Rau BR, Silverman ED: Distribution and natural history of stress fractures in U.S. marine recruits. *Radiology* 146:339–346, 1983.
31. Groshar D, Lam M, Evan-Sapir E, Israel O, Front D: Stress fractures and bone pain: are they closely associated? *Injury* 526–528, 1985.
32. Guoping L, Zhang S, Chen G, Chen H, Wang A: Radiographic and histologic analyses of stress fractures in rabbit tibias. *Am J Sports Med* 13:285–294, 1985.
33. Hallel T, Amit S, Segal D: Fatigue fractures of the tibial and femoral shaft in soldiers. *Clin Orthop Relat Res* 118:35–43, 1976.
34. Hartley JB: "Stress" or "fatigue" fractures of bone. *Br J Radiol* 16:255–262, 1943.
35. Hulkko A, Orava S: Stress fracture in athletes. *Int J Sports Med* 8:221–226, 1987.
36. Hullinger CW: Insufficiency fracture of the calcaneus. *J Bone Joint Surg* 26:751–757, 1944.
37. Jackson DW, Striazak AM: Stress fractures in runners, excluding the foot. In Mack RP (ed): *Symposium on the Foot and Leg in Running Sports.* St Louis, C.V. Mosby, 1982, pp 109–122.
38. Jeffery CC: Spontaneous fracture of the femoral neck. *J Bone Joint Surg* 44B:543–549, 1962.
39. Johnson LC, Stradford HT, Geis RW, Dineen JR, Kerley E: Histiogenesis of stress fractures (abstract). *J Bone Joint Surg* 45-A:1542, 1963.
40. Johnston CC, Smith DM, Yu P, Deiss WP: In vivo measurement of bone mass in the radius. *Metabolism* 17:1140–1153, 1968.
41. Keating TW: Stress fracture in the sternum of a wrestler. *Am J Sports Med* 15:92–93, 1987.
42. Keller TS, Lovin JD, Spengler DM, Carter DR: Fatigue of immature baboon cortical bone. *J Biomech* 18:297–304, 1985.
43. Kowal DM: Nature and causes of injuries in women resulting from an endurance training program. *Am J Sports Med* 8:265–268, 1980.
44. Krause GR, Thompson JR: March fracture: an analysis of two hundred cases. *Am J Roentgenol* 52:281–290, 1944.
45. Lafferty JF: Analytic model of fatigue characteristics of bone. *Aviat Space Environ Med* 49:170–174, 1978.
46. Leveton AL: March (fatigue) fractures of the long bones of the lower extremities and pelvis. *Am J Surg* 71:222–232, 1946.
47. Mann RA: Biomechanics of running. In Mack PP (ed): *Symposium on the Foot and Leg in Running Sports.* St. Louis, C.V. Mosby, 1982, pp 1–29.

48. Markey KL: Stress fractures. *Clin Sports Med* 6:405–425, 1987.
49. Matheson GO, Clement DB, McKenzie DC, Taunton JE, Lloyd-Smith DR, Macintyre JG: Stress fractures in athletes: a study of 320 cases. *Am J Sports Med* 15:46–58, 1987.
50. Matheson GO, Clement DB, McKenzie DC, Tauton JE, Loyd-Smith DR, Macintyre JG: Scintigraphic uptake of 99m Tc at non-painful sites in athletes with stress fractures. *Sports Med* 4:65–75, 1987.
51. McBryde AM: Stress fractures in runners, *Clin Sports Med* 4:737–752, 1985.
52. Milgrom C, Chisin R, Giladi M, Stein M, Kashtan H, Margulies J, Altan H: Negative bone scans in impending tibial stress fractures. A report of three cases. *Am J Sports Med* 12:488–491, 1984.
53. Milgrom C, Giladi M, Chisin R, Dizian R: The long term follow-up of soldiers with stress fractures. *Am J Sports Med* 13:398–400, 1985.
54. Milgrom C, Giladi M, Stein H, Kashton H, Margulies J, Chisin R, Steinberg R, Aharonson Z: Stress fractures in military recruits: a prospective study showing an unusually high incidence. *J Bone Joint Surg* 67-B:732–735, 1985.
55. Morris JM, Blickenstaff LD: Fatigue fractures. A clinical study. Springfield, IL, Charles C Thomas, 1967.
56. Muller W: Experimental Unteosuchungen uber mechanisch bedingte Umbildungs progresse am wachsenden und fertigen knocken undihre Bedeutung fur die Pathologie des knockens, besondere die Epiphyenstorung bei rachitisahnlichen Erkrankungen. *Bruns' Beitr Klin Chir* 127:251–290, 1922.
57. Prather JL, Nusynowitz ML, Snowdy HA, Hughes AD, McCartney WH, Raymond JB: Scintigraphic findings in stress fractures. *J Bone Joint Surg* 59A:869–874, 1977.
58. Protzman RR, Griffis CC: Comparative stress fracture incidence in males and females in and equal training environment. *Athletic Training* 12:126–130, 1977.
59. Provost RA, Morris JM: Fatigue fractures of the femoral shaft. *J Bone Joint Surg* 51A:487–498, 1969.
60. Reinker KA, Ozburne S: A comparison of male and female orthopedic pathology in basic training. *Mil Med* 144:532–536, 1979.
61. Roesler H: Some historical remarks on the theory of cancellous bone structure (Wolff's Law). In Cowin SC (ed): *Mechanical Properties of Bone*. New York, American Society Mechanical Engineers, 1981, pp 27–42.
62. Roub LW, Gumerman LW, Hanley EN, Clark MW, Goodman M, Herbert DL: Bone stress: a radionuclide imaging perspective. *Radiology* 132:431–483, 1979.
63. Rubin CT, Lanyon LE: Regulation of bone mass by peak strain magnitude. *Trans Orthop Res Soc* 8:70, 1983.
64. Rubin CT, Lanyon LE: Bone remodeling in response to applied dynamic loads. *Trans Orthop Res Soc* 6:64, 1981.
65. Rupani HD, Holder LE, Espinola DA, Semra IE: Three-phase radionuclide bone imaging in sports medicine. *Radiology* 156:187–196, 1985.
66. Rutishauser E, Majino G: Lesions osseues par surchange dans le squelette normal et pathologique. *Bull Schweiz Akad Med Wiss* 6:333–342, 1950.
67. Rutishauser E, Majino G: Les lesions osseues par surchange dans le squelette normal. *Schweiz Med Wochenschr* 79:281–288, 1949.
68. Scully TJ, Besterman G: Stress fracture—a preventable injury. *Mil Med* 147:285–287, 1982.
69. Stanitski CL, McMaster JH, Scranton PE: On the nature of stress fractures. *Am J Sports Med* 6:391–396, 1978.
70. Stechow. Fussoden und Rontgensfrahlen. *Militararztliche Z* 26:30–47, 1897.
71. Swanson AAV, Freeman MAR, Day WH: The fatigue properties of human cortical bone. *Med Biol Eng* 9:23–32, 1971.

72. Trutter M, Broman GE, Peterson RR: Densities of white and Negro skeletons. *J Bone Joint Surg* 42A:50–58, 1960.
73. Tschantz P, Reiner M, Candardjis G: Consideration experimentales et cliniques sur la physio-pathologie des lesion osseuse par surcharge Symposium Ossium—London. London, E and S Livingstone, 1970, pp 247–251.
74. Tschnatz P, Rutishauser E: La surchange mechanique de l'os vivant: let deformation plastique initiales et l'hypertrophic d'adaption. *Ann Anat Pathol* 12:223–248, 1967.
75. Uhtoff HK, Jaworski ZFG: Periosteal stress-induced reactions resembling stress fractures. *Clin Orthop Relat Res* 199:284–291, 1985.
76. Wilson ES, Katz FN: Stress fractures. *Radiology* 92:481–486, 1969.
77. Worthen BM, Yanklowitz BAD: The pathophysiology and treatment of stress fractures in military personnel. *J Am Podiatry Assoc* 68:317–325, 1978.
78. Zwas ST, Elkanovitch R, Frank G: Interpretation and classification of bone scintigraphic findings in stress fractures. *J Nucl Med* 28:452–457, 1987.

12
Physical Activity Epidemiology: Concepts, Methods, and Applications to Exercise Science

CARL J. CASPERSEN, Ph.D., M.P.H.

Physical activity as a health-related behavior has been studied as part of other disease-specific epidemiologic research, most commonly for coronary heart disease [145, 157]. However, epidemiologic principles have also been applied in studying how physical activity relates to various chronic diseases such as hypertension [162], stroke [122], certain cancers [233], and conditions such as musculoskeletal injuries [20]. A grasp of how physical activity research has included epidemiologic principles will provide an understanding of how we have now reached an area of study that can be termed "physical activity epidemiology."

This chapter provides some definitions of physical activity, exercise, and epidemiology; an overview of epidemiology and epidemiological methods and concepts; an outline of the breadth and scope of physical activity epidemiology; and examples of previous and potential applications of physical activity epidemiology as part of exercise science.

DEFINITIONS

Epidemiology
Last defined epidemiology as "the study of the distribution and determinants of health-related states and events in populations, and the application of this study to the control of health problems" [125]. This basic definition can be extended to include the study of intervention activities designed to improve health [246].

Traditionally, the uses of epidemiology are to (*a*) establish the magnitude of a health problem; (*b*) identify the factor(s) that causes the health problem as well as the mode(s) by which the factor is transmitted; (*c*) develop the scientific basis for preventive activities or the allocation of health resources; and (*d*) evaluate the effectiveness of preventive or therapeutic maneuvers [246]. When applied in such a comprehensive way, epidemiology is very useful in establishing sound health policies [248].

The science of epidemiology is concerned with carefully quantifying the rate of health-related states or events that occur within the population being studied. Epidemiology has the ultimate goal of generalizing this information to larger populations [174]. However, the events of interest are only a small part of the focus in epidemiologic research. For the science of epidemiology to be most appropriate, the epidemiologist is concerned with the population to which the individual events can be made relative. In epidemiology's simplest conceptualization the events serve as the numerator and the population serves as the denominator for the calculation of rates. Rates will be discussed later in this chapter.

Descriptive epidemiology, which is concerned with establishing the rates of a disease or health-related event, is traditionally begun by providing those rates according to age, sex, race, occupation, social class, and geographic location [247]. Providing rates according to age categories helps to reflect those characteristics of the person (or host) that pertain to developmental factors (for infants, children, youth, and young, middle-aged, and older adults), to the potential length of exposure to a particular etiologic factor over time (particularly for cancer epidemiology), or to the ability of the person to survive a condition (such as pneumonia or influenza). Gender and race can each pertain to biological and social factors. Occupation, social class, and geographic factors can relate to socioeconomic status and environmental factors. As such, the rates provided in a descriptive epidemiologic study should fully reflect persons of a specified population who have a well-defined disease, event, or condition within a specified place and time [125].

Analytic epidemiology is concerned with trying to identify potential causative factors that may be associated with a disease or health-related event [125]. In such investigations persons are typically classified by whether or not they have the disease (or by whether or not the health-related event occurred). At the same time, each person or situation is also labeled by potentially causative factors such as gender, race, age, other disease(s), biochemical or physiological characteristics, socioeconomic status, occupation, residence, other aspects of the environment, or behavioral characteristics [125]. One such behavioral characteristic, physical activity, is central to the scope of this chapter.

Physical Activity
In an epidemiologic investigation, as in any scientific study, the health-related state or event being investigated must be defined and measured [174]. To this end, Caspersen et al. have offered definitions of "physical activity," "exercise," and "physical fitness" that are useful for epidemiologic and other health-related research and that make particular note of physical activity as a behavior [40]. Physical activity is basically defined as any bodily movement produced by skeletal muscles that results in caloric expenditure. The total amount of this energy expenditure is governed by force generated by the total muscle mass producing the

movement(s) and by the duration and frequency of these muscle contractions [225].

The term "exercise" is often thought to be identical to the term "physical activity." Caspersen et al. [40] have interpreted exercise to be a subcategory of physical activity. In this context, exercise was defined as physical activity that is planned, structured, repetitive, and results in the improvement or maintenance of one or more facets of physical fitness. Further, Caspersen et al. classified physical activity and exercise as behaviors and physical fitness as a set of outcomes or traits that relate to the ability to perform physical activity. That is, physical fitness was seen as something that people possess or achieve, such as aerobic power, muscular endurance, muscular strength, body composition, and flexibility [40].

The behaviorally oriented definitions offered by Caspersen et al. are quite different from the definitions that Knuttgen [112] offered for work, force, power, and exercise, and their intent. Although his definitions are useful in quantifying the precise amount of physical work done in a laboratory setting, their utility in epidemiologic and health-related research is limited because they were not intended to characterize behavioral patterns.

Physical Activity Epidemiology
When the definitions of epidemiology and epidemiologic concepts are linked with the definition of physical activity as a health-related behavior, the concept of physical activity epidemiology begins to emerge.

As such, physical activity epidemiology can be defined as a two-part process. First, it studies (*a*) the association of physical activity, as a health-related behavior, with disease and other health outcomes; (*b*) the distribution and the determinants of physical activity behavior(s); and (*c*) the interrelationship of physical activity with other behaviors. Second, it applies that knowledge to the prevention and control of disease and the promotion of health. An underlying methodologic concern in physical activity epidemiology is the development and application of reliable and valid measures of physical activity for (*a*) the study of disease and health outcomes, (*b*) the surveillance of physical activity patterns, (*c*) the evaluation of interventions, and (*d*) use as a dependent variable in the study of physical activity determinants.

BREADTH AND SCOPE OF PHYSICAL ACTIVITY EPIDEMIOLOGY

Physical activity epidemiology encompasses a substantial breadth and scope (Fig. 12.1). As with traditional forms of disease-specific epidemiology, physical activity can be studied as an exposure variable to ex-

FIGURE 12.1
Schematic of the breadth and scope of physical activity epidemiologic research.

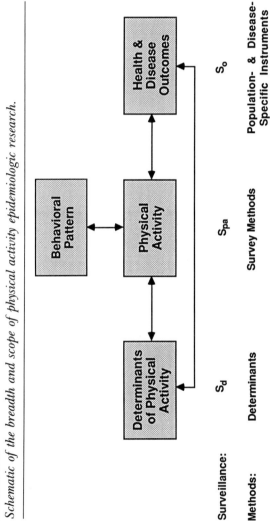

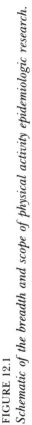

S_d = Surveillance systems for determinants.

S_{pa} = Surveillance systems for physical activity prevalence.

S_o = Surveillance systems for health and disease outcomes affected by physical activity.

amine its association with disease or health states. For example, increased levels of physical activity can be studied for their beneficial and detrimental effect on sudden death [207], their deterimental association with musculoskeletal injuries [113], or their beneficial association with improved mental health and functioning [67, 183, 215].

Epidemiologic methods have been used in the study of physical activity and coronary heart disease (see Table 12.1) [7, 8, 28, 29, 32, 34, 35, 43, 50, 51, 58, 68, 69, 71, 74, 89, 90, 93, 101, 103, 104, 106, 124, 127, 128, 133, 136, 137, 146–149, 158, 161, 163, 167, 169, 172, 177, 181, 182, 190, 191, 200, 201, 206, 207, 209, 213, 223, 226, 232, 242, 249, 252], stroke (see Table 12.2) [91, 104, 124, 135, 138, 172, 190], and certain cancers [73, 80, 96, 159, 168, 226, 232, 233, 245]. In this context physical activity has played a role in disease-specific epidemiologic research. However, physical activity epidemiology has also been applied to conditions such as musculoskeletal injuries that are induced by running [20, 41, 98, 113, 134, 135, 171, 234], ice hockey [13, 88, 94, 130, 164, 218, 220], aerobic dance [75, 184], martial arts [14], football [2, 23, 24, 77, 79, 82, 151, 156, 229], rugby [154, 185], soccer [1, 62–65, 92, 155, 180, 217], gymnastics [76, 132, 170], cycling [107], tennis [84], and other exercises [114, 116, 235].

The descriptive epidemiology of physical activity as an individual behavior provides insights into the types and amounts of physical activity performed by members of a population and into how such patterns might inform the development, implementation, and evaluation of a public health policy designed to promote an active society (214). Generally, to achieve national estimates, survey research procedures are necessary to sample and survey the physical activity patterns of large, representative segments of the population.

Physical activity is rarely performed in the absence of other beneficial or detrimental health-related behaviors [19]. The study of the interrelationship of physical activity with other health- and non-health-related behaviors is essential to explaining how multiple risk factors affect various health and disease outcomes, and to determining what independent contribution physical activity might have on such outcomes. This interrelationship becomes especially important in epidemiologic investigations of chronic disease, where multicausation is the norm rather than the exception. Such information has scientific value not only in explaining etiologic factors or applying statistical control to potential confounding variables, but is also helpful to the intervention specialist, who must decide how much effort should be spent on changing a single behavior. It is in this latter context that physical activity epidemiology takes on an applied form and ultimately has policy implications.

The study of physical activity determinants is also an important part of physical activity epidemiology, albeit a new, and far from resolved,

TABLE 12.1
Results of Epidemiologic Studies of Coronary Heart Disease Yielding Statistically Significant and Nonsignificant Associations

Type of Design	Significant Inverse Association	Nonsignificant Association
Occupational cohort	London postal workers/civil servants [118][a] London Transport busmen [118] U.S. railroad workers [181] North Dakota residents [207] Washington, DC, postal workers [78] Yugoslavia residents [27, 28] Italy residents [55, 56] Greek islands residents [4, 5] Italian railroad employees [109] Israeli kibbutzim male residents [25] Israeli kibbutzim female residents [25] West Finland residents [142] San Francisco, CA, longshoremen [21, 128]	London Transport busmen [69] London Transport busmen [117] Los Angeles, CA, civil servants [42] Bell Telephone employees [120] U.S. railroad workers [183] Chicago utility company employees [173] Evans County, GA, residents [36, 107] East Finland residents [142]
Cohorts with various types of physical activity measures	Chicago Western Electric employees [133] Harvard alumni [129, 130] British civil servants [43, 119] Framingham, MA, male residents [80, 81] Framingham, MA, female residents [80, 81] Los Angeles, CA, firemen and policemen [135] Gothenberg, Sweden, residents [196] New York health insurance subscribers [161]	Gothenberg, Sweden, residents [187] Gothenberg, Sweden, residents [196] Gothenberg, Sweden, female residents [99] San Francisco corporate employees [146] Oslo, Norway, residents (leisure) [72] North Karelia, Finland, female residents [152] Belgian male factory workers (leisure) [170] Framingham, MA, male residents (work) [82]

San Francisco, CA, federal employees [145]
Oslo, Norway, residents (work) [72]
North Karelia, Finland, male residents [152]
Oslo, Norway, workers [103]
Belgian male factory workers (fitness) [170]
MRFIT men [102]
Honolulu, HI, residents [50, 204]
Puerto Rico residents [61]
Finnish men and women [151]

Mortality study
Great Britain residents [118]
California residents [22]
Iowa residents [137]

San Francisco, CA, coroner's cases [58]
Florida residents [70]

Case-control study
Seattle, WA, residents [166, 167]
Netherlands, male residents [104]
Netherlands, female residents [104]
Auckland, New Zealand men [160]
Auckland, New Zealand women [160]

a Reference number.

TABLE 12.2
Results of Epidemiologic Studies of Stroke Yielding Statistically Significant and Nonsignificant Associations

Type of Design	Significant Inverse Association	Nonsignificant Association
Occupational cohort	San Francisco longshoremen [106][a] Italian railroad workers [108]	Framingham male residents (81)
Cohorts with varying types of physical activity measures	Gothenberg, Sweden female residents [99] North Karelia, Finland, male residents [152] North Karelia, Finland, female residents [152] Iowa male residents [137] Iowa female residents [137] Dutch men [71] Dutch women [71]	

[a] Reference number.

area of inquiry [57]. Not only is it important to identify those factors that generally promote or impede the adoption of a physically active life-style, but more specific detail is also desirable in identifying what factors predict the adoption of individual activities such as running, team sports, or walking. Although such information is of tremendous empirical value to the behavioral sciences, it is also critical and perhaps even rate limiting in the development of cost-effective intervention strategies that result in enduring physical activity behavior change.

The next sections of this chapter will provide an overview of methodological issues and epidemiological concepts that are important in physical activity epidemiology.

METHODOLOGIC ISSUES IN PHYSICAL ACTIVITY EPIDEMIOLOGY

Denominators and Rates
Central to the broad spectrum of research done in physical activity epidemiology is the need for a well-specified denominator and the calculation of precise rates [174]. A rate is the number of persons with a health problem or event (the numerator) divided by the population at risk for the problem (the denominator). For instance, in epidemiologic studies of coronary heart disease (CHD), a rate might be determined whereby the numerator was the number of persons experiencing a fatal CHD event and the denominator was all persons originally free of CHD at the beginning of the study.

Physical activity epidemiologic studies that focus on a disease outcome compare rates between active and inactive persons. For example, in the classic London Busmen Study, Morris et al. found that the age-standardized, 5-year incidence rate of ischemic heart disease for the active conductors was 4.7 per 100 men, whereas that for less active drivers was 8.5 per 100 men [147].

Statistical comparisons between active and inactive groups can be made via the rate difference or the rate ratio [125]. The rate difference provides an estimate of the absolute magnitude of the two rates while the rate ratio provides a relative comparison of the two rates. When a rate difference is calculated, the rate is expressed in the same units as calculated. With the rate ratio, the ratio is dimensionless. From the London Busmen Study data we would find a rate difference of a 3.8 per 100 men (8.5—4.7) during the 5-year period [147]. On the other hand, the rate ratio of ischemic heart disease incidence for the less active drivers compared with that of the more active conductors would be 1.81 (8.5/4.7). This ratio can also be thought of as an 81% greater risk of ischemic heart disease for less active drivers relative to the active conductors.

The term "incidence rate," as used above, relates to the number of new disease cases or health-related events that develop within a given population during a specified period of time [247]. Such a rate is found by dividing the number of new cases or events by the population "at risk" during that period of time. For the 5-year incidence rates of Morris et al. to be correct, those persons with evidence of preexisting ischemic heart disease were excluded from the rate calculation [147]. The excluded persons would not be at risk for developing ischemic heart disease because they already had it.

The term "prevalence rate" pertains to the total number of cases or health-related events that exist at a specified time [247]. This rate differs from an incidence rate, a more dynamic concept that pertains only to new cases or events developing within the time period specified. A prevalence rate is found by dividing the total cases or events by the total population in which they exist or occur. The relationship between prevalence and incidence rates is dependent on the duration of the disease or health-related event under study. The relationship is given by:

$$\text{Prevalence rate} = \text{Incidence rate} \times \text{Duration (time)}.$$

The calculated incidence rates can be expressed relative to a denominator such as total persons at risk during a given time frame or to a denominator that includes the specific time of exposure (e.g., person-years). In either case the denominator is selected to provide the best conceptualization of the population. For example, the reader would have difficulty envisioning the rate of an occurrence relative to a population of 10,000 when the sample dealt with was less than 100. The trade-off comes when one is trying to express the rate relative to conventional scientific notation, so that a one- or two-digit number is followed by a one- or two-digit decimal form which is raised to a multiple of 10 (5.3×10^{-2} instead of 53×10^{-3}, $.53 \times 10^{-1}$, or .053).

An example of this trade-off is to express the risk of an event and its rate of occurrence. For example, Koplan et al. [113] indicated that the risk of musculoskeletal injury was slightly more than 35% for male runners 1 year following the Peachtree Road Race. That is, each male runner had about a one in three risk of suffering an injury during the observational period. Koplan actually expressed the incidence rate as 0.37 injuries per person-year. The concept of a third of an injury per person per year is cumbersome; hence, one could express the incidence rate as 37 injuries per 100 persons per 1 year (which expression incidentally also matched the time frame employed in that survey) [41]. Although the same information is offered by both the decimal and whole number data, the latter's meaning is somewhat different and perhaps easier to convey to the reader.

One should also avoid implying a level of precision greater than that actually available when one made the measure. This caution has to be weighed against what previous authors used in reporting similar rates, lest the rates one is reporting seem by comparison exaggerated or underestimated. Care is likewise required in comparing rates where the denominator varies. For example, in the Peachtree Road Race injury data, the rate of musculoskeletal injury in male runners was 37 per 100 person-years, whereas the rate of hazardous events was 11 per 1000 person-years [41]. If one simply compared the numbers 35 and 11, the rates of these two events would appear to differ by a factor of about 3, when they actually differed by a factor of 30. Careful selection of the appropriate denominator not only reflects the need for selecting the best units but also helps highlight the importance of denominators in physical activity epidemiology.

Physical Activity Measures for Epidemiologic Research
PROBLEMS IN PHYSICAL ACTIVITY ASSESSMENT. Historically, methodologic problems have impeded research in physical activity epidemiology [42, 122]. In part, these problems stem from (*a*) the diverse definitions of physical activity and exercise employed in some studies; (*b*) the absence of valid, reliable, and standardized assessment instruments that can be used across studies; (*c*) the large measurement error of the instruments; (*d*) the inappropriate use of a physical activity measure as part of a research design; and (*e*) the failure to select an instrument that reflects the health-related components of physical activity. Even when precise measures are available, they are usually impractical or too costly for epidemiologic research.

Because physical activity is a complex behavior, problems arise when making operational definitions of it [40]. Physical activity can be done as part of occupational activity, or as leisure-time pursuits (e.g., sports, conditioning, yardwork, household cleaning, or home repair). Physiologically, it may not matter where or when the activity is done; however, different categories of physical activity may relate to specific aspects of health [122]. For example, cigarette smoking has a negative association with leisure activity but a positive association with work activity [19]. Because different types of physical activity may have entirely different determinants [57], it may be important to consider them separately in epidemiologic research—especially when such data are being interpreted for public health interventions [97].

It is also important to note that the physical activity measurement methods used depend on the desired precision required by investigators and evaluators in the research they perform [40]. For example, although the great precision of measures made in a laboratory is desirable in bench research, such extremely precise measures are generally infeasible in large-scale epidemiologic research. Epidemiologic research is most concerned with analyzing a representative sample from which generalizations can be drawn. Therefore, physical activity epidemiology tends to rely on less costly and precise measures that will more crudely classify individuals or groups of individuals according to a level of physical activity. Hence, the cost, precision, and accuracy of the measures used for physical activity will decrease from laboratory research to epidemiologic research [40].

TYPES OF PHYSICAL ACTIVITY MEASURES. A number of review articles have discussed the various ways to assess physical activity for epidemiologic research [6, 66, 105, 122, 141, 193, 239, 243]. As noted above, physical activity has been measured in a variety of ways [122]. For example, calorimetry, job classification, survey procedures, physical fitness, doubly labeled water, behavioral observation, heart rate monitors, mechanical monitors, electronic monitors, heart rate/motion sensors, and dietary measures all have been used as methods to assess physical activity in epidemiologic and laboratory settings. Hence, the operational definition of physical activity is known to vary as well.

Table 12.3, a modification of a table prepared by LaPorte et al. [122], lists each of these physical activity assessment procedures according to several factors relevant to large-scale, population-based, epidemiologic research. Those factors relate to whether the instrument or procedure is (*a*) practical relative to its costs in either money or time to the investigator or the subject; (*b*) socially and personally acceptable; (*c*) compatible with normal daily activities; and (*d*) able to measure some of the specifics of the activity performed [122]. Table 12.3 is arranged so that the reader can quickly determine, from the shade of each row, the overall suitability of the instrument or procedure for epidemiologic research.

The various instruments or procedures vary in their applicability for epidemiologic research. For example, although calorimetry [54, 55, 59–61, 165] provides very precise detail about the energy expended during the time frame of measurement and for specific activities performed, it is not suitable for epidemiologic research: It cannot be applied to large populations, it is costly, it either limits or otherwise affects the types of physical activity performed, and it is generally unacceptable to the subject [122, 141].

Perhaps the most convenient and most commonly used measure of physical activity in CHD research has been job classification [7, 8, 32, 34, 35, 68, 69, 73, 80, 102, 124, 137, 138, 145, 147, 148, 157, 177, 190, 212, 213, 223, 226, 232, 233, 252]. Job classification identifies levels or classes of physical activity according to particular job tasks or occupational titles [122, 141]. The procedure has several advantages: It can easily be employed in large, representative, employed populations or cohorts; it is not costly; it does not affect the physical activity being

TABLE 12.3
Physical Activity Assessment Procedures and Their Potential Utility for Large-Scale, Population-Based Epidemiologic Research[a]

Assessment Instrument or Procedure	Can Be Used with These Age Groups[b]						Can Measure Large Groups	Small Study Money Cost	Small Study Time Cost	Small Subject Time Cost	Small Subject Effort Cost	Unlikely to Affect Activity Behavior	Acceptability		Activity specifics
	I	C	A	Y	M	E							Self	Social	
Calorimetry															
Direct	*	•	*	*	*	*	•	•	•	•	•	•	•	•	++
Indirect	•	•	*	*	*	*	•	•	•	•	•	•	•	•	++
Job Classification	•	•	*	•	*	•	++	++	++	++	++	++	++	++	+
Surveys															
Indirect calorimetry-diary	•	•	*	*	*	*	•	+	+	•	•	•	−	•	++
Task-specific diary	•	*	*	*	*	*	++	+	+	+	+	++	++	++	++
Recall questionnaire	•	*	*	*	*	*	++	+	+	++	+	++	++	++	++
Quantitative history	•	•	*	*	*	*	++	+	•	++	++	++	++	++	++
Global self-report of activity	•	*	*	*	*	*	++	++	++	++	++	++	++	++	•
Physiologic markers															
Cardiorespiratory fitness	•	*	*	*	*	*	++	•	•	•	++	++	−	−	•
Doubly labeled water	•	*	*	*	*	*	+	•	•	++	++	+	−	++	•
Behavioral observation	•	*	*	*	*	*	++	•	•	•	++	++	++	−	++
Mechanical/electronic monitors															
Accelerometers	*	*	*	*	*	*	+	+	+	+	+	++	++	++	•
Electronic motion sensor	•	*	*	*	*	*	++	•	++	++	++	++	++	++	•
Pedometers	•	•	*	*	*	*	+	+	++	++	++	++	++	++	•
Heart rate	*	*	*	*	*	*	•	•	•	++	+	++	++	++	•
Heart rate and motion sensor	*	*	*	*	*	*	•	•	•	+	++	+	−	++	•
Gait assessment	•	•	*	*	•	*	•	+	++	•	•	•	−	++	•
Horizontal time monitor	•	*	*	*	*	•	•	•	+	++	++	++	++	++	•
Stabilometers	*	•	*	*	*	*	•	•	•	•	•	•	++	++	•
Dietary measures	*	•	*	*	*	*	++	+	+	•	•	++	++	++	•

[a] Modified from LaPorte RE, Montoye HJ, Caspersen CJ: Assessment of physical activity in epidemiologic research: problems and prospects. *Pub Health Rep* 100:131–146, 1985.

[b] I = infant, C = child, A = adolescent, Y = young adult, M = middle age, E = elderly.
* = fully meets the criterion; • = doesn't meet the criterion; − = may meet the criterion; + = may meet the criterion; ++ = fully meets the criterion; = = cannot be determined.

measured; and is acceptable to the subject. The principal disadvantages are that many job classifications have (*a*) considerable variability in either the volume or intensity of physical work done, (*b*) changes in physical activity either seasonally or over time, (*c*) self-selection bias, (*d*) an inability to account for leisure time physical activity, and (*e*) limited utility for populations of children, homemakers, the unemployed, and retirees. Because few jobs today require sustained physical activity, the use of job classification as a measure of physical activity has declined in CHD epidemiologic research [122, 141, 176]. For example, Powell et al. noted in a review of studies on physical activity and CHD that 20 of the 25 studies conducted prior to 1970 used job classification [176]. After 1970, an increasing number of studies based their measurements on leisure-time physical activity [176]. It is very important to note that the use of job classification was very useful in generating hypotheses about the relationship of physical activity and CHD. Further, at the time job classifications were used, traditional work weeks were long and leisure time tended to be inactive. The use of job classification to generate hypotheses can also be noted for some current studies on physical activity and cancer [73, 80, 159, 226, 232, 233]. However, even though job classification has been, and can continue to be, useful in providing epidemiologic insights into the etiology of CHD, cancer, and other chronic diseases, measures of leisure time physical activity will continue to be necessary for applied epidemiologic studies on ways to prevent CHD or cancer.

Surveys, which are based on self-reports, are the most practical for measuring physical activity in large-scale epidemiologic studies [122]. Physical activity surveys can easily measure large populations at a relatively low cost to the study and the subject and provide considerable detail about specific physical activity (if queried and scored accordingly) (Table 12.3).

Physical activity surveys can be prospective diaries or records, retrospective recall questionnaires, and quantitative histories [9, 18, 26, 43, 86, 90, 104, 143, 163, 179, 187, 189, 201, 225, 250, 251]. Each of these three types of surveys has been employed in epidemiologic research [122, 189]. Diaries tend to require more effort from the subject and may result in changes in the physical activities performed during recording. When used with the process of indirect calorimetry, the diary procedure is even more burdensome to the subject and may not be socially acceptable [122]. For those reasons the diary tends to be the least desirable of the survey procedures. Because of the work involved, diaries tend to be suitable only for short time periods of 1–3 days [141], which leads to questions regarding the representativeness of the individual's physical activity pattern [122, 141].

Recall surveys do not influence the physical activity behavior and also tend to be less effort for the subject than do diaries. However, a degree of effort is required to carefully remember details from previous events [12]. Recall surveys have been used for periods of 1 day, 1 week, 1 year, and, most recently, even for lifetime activity [117]. Recall surveys can be either self- or interviewer-administered and can query for specific details of, or general perceptions of, usual physical activity participation that occurs during a given time frame.

The retrospective quantitative history, a more rigorous form of survey procedure, tends to cover a 1-year time frame and asks for details of specific activities [122, 189]. As a result, although the quantitative history provides an enormous amount of data, and tends to account for seasonal variation, the subject is burdened with having to recall so much detail. The history also results in greater study costs due to increased survey administration and data processing costs [122].

Another form of survey, the global self-report of physical activity, appears to have some validity even for such rapid measures as it can provide [39, 86, 208, 237]. Usually, global self-reports have used a self-assessed comparison of an individual's physical activity relative to other people in general. However, Caspersen and Pollard have noted that even though these measures appear to be valid, researchers should employ caution when comparing diverse groups that vary by age or gender because the general self-report tends to obscure the very different physical activities performed by those groups [39].

Several physiological markers have been employed in assessing physical activity, in particular in assessing cardiorespiratory fitness [10, 15–17, 21, 53, 85, 100, 101, 144, 153, 169, 203–205, 209, 210, 241, 242] and in the doubly labeled water technique [18, 109, 196–198]. The well-known direct association between cardiorespiratory fitness and frequency and duration of vigorous physical activity has led to the use of cardiorespiratory fitness as a surrogate physical activity measure [122]. Although the correlation between measures of physical activity and cardiorespiratory fitness are modest in populations where a considerable amount of vigorous activity was likely to be performed [225], the correlation has been weak when an all-inclusive summary score, such as the kilocalorie score, has been the index of physical activity in populations that do not perform much vigorous physical activity [56, 201]. For populations that are likely to perform vigorous physical activity, estimates of cardiorespiratory fitness have been successfully employed [15–17, 21]. The major disadvantages to the use of cardiorespiratory fitness are its costs to the study and the subject, its safety, and its inability to provide detail on specific activity participation [122, 141]. Further, there is some genetic contribution to cardiorespiratory fitness [25].

The doubly labeled water technique, another physiologic marker, requires a subject to ingest water with isotopically labeled hydrogen and oxygen atoms [18, 109, 196–198]. Energy expenditure is estimated by comparing the amount of unmetabolized water with that of water that has passed through the energy cycle. The subject tolerates the measurement procedure well, and there is no problem with social acceptability [122]. Although the measurement error with this technique is quite small, the study costs are high and the subject must be seen at least three times. Further, there is no detail regarding specific activities performed, unless the subject is burdened with keeping an activity diary. In total, the utility in large, population-based studies is not good relative to survey procedures because the doubly labeled water technique has much higher study costs than survey procedures.

Behavioral observation [11, 33, 110] has also been employed as a means to assess physical activity and has incorporated either direct observation or that made available via photography [33]. This technique has been most commonly used in studying the activity patterns of children [11, 110]. Behavioral observation requires little effort from the subject but entails vast study time and expense and can influence the physical activity under observation (Table 12.3) [122]. Although this technique can provide specific detail of physical activity, its utility in large population studies is poor.

Heart rate monitors [27, 52, 54, 81, 236] and mechanical [13, 78, 83, 111, 231, 238, 244] and electronic monitoring devices [44–46, 70, 111, 118–122, 142] have been used to measure physical activity. As a group these instruments are superior to surveys because they avoid the bias of self-report and require little or no effort on the part of the subject [122, 141]. Although the wearing of the monitor may influence the behavior being measured, most subjects tend to ignore the monitor after an initial adjustment period [141]. At present, motion sensors such as pedometers and accelerometers are less costly than heart rate monitors or combined heart rate and motion sensors [152, 166, 206, 221, 222]. That the subject must be seen at least twice, however, reduces the utility of such monitors in epidemiologic research. Also, these monitoring devices do not provide detail regarding specific activities performed unless a concurrent diary is kept.

Dietary measures have been used as surrogates of physical activity assessment [211]. Although dietary measures that result in kilocalorie scores of energy intake can be thought of as equaling energy expenditure if caloric balance is assumed, there is no specific reference to actual activities performed, and the cost to the subject is not negligible.

In summary, Table 12.3 reveals that surveys are the most convenient procedure for assessing physical activity in large, population-based studies because they are economical, acceptable, and can provide activity-specific information. Unfortunately, very little is known about the reliability and validity of most physical activity surveys. The use of objective monitoring through heart rate, motion sensors, mechanical devices, and

TABLE 12.4
Dimensions of Physical Activity with Proposed Mechanism of Effect,
Validation Criteria, and Diseases Affected

Physical Activity Dimension	Possible Mechanism(s)	Possible Validation Criteria	Disease(s) Affected
Caloric expenditure	Energy utilization	Dietary survey; doubly labeled water	CHD[a]; NIDDM; obesity; cancer
Aerobic intensity	Enhanced cardiac function	Maximal oxygen uptake; historical records	CHD; NIDDM
Weight bearing	Gravitational force	Motion sensor; pedometer	Osteoporosis
Flexibility	Range of motion	Flexometer; historical records; goniometer	Disability
Muscular strength	Muscle force generation	Strength measure; historical records	Disability

[a] CHD = coronary heart disease; NIDDM = non-insulin-dependent diabetes mellitus.

doubly labeled water procedures appears promising. However, these methods are still evolving and are too costly to implement in large-scale studies, although they may be useful in validating physical activity surveys.

HEALTH-RELATED COMPONENTS OF PHYSICAL ACTIVITY. It is difficult to determine what characteristics of physical activity will produce health benefits, because there are many, potentially interrelated dimensions of physical activity [122]. For the purposes of physical activity epidemiologic studies, the dimensions of interest are mainly health- or disease-related and are at least five in number: caloric expenditure, aerobic intensity, weight bearing, flexibility, and strength. Epidemiologic investigations should employ physical activity measures that correspond to the dimension or dimensions that relate to the disease or health outcome under investigation.

Table 12.4 lists those five dimensions of physical activity as they may relate to various health and disease states or outcomes. Table 12.4 also offers physiologic mechanisms through which each dimension may exert its health-related effect. For example, caloric expenditure relates to the amount of energy used by the skeletal muscles during physical activity and is a direct consequence of the types of muscles contracted, the force these muscles generate, the rate at which they contract, and the total duration and frequency of movements [40, 225]. The dimension associated with caloric expenditure results in the physiological effect of energy utilization and thereby enhances weight loss or control [19, 40].

This effect, in turn, may be useful in preventing or managing CHD, diabetes mellitus, and obesity [19, 176].

The dimension of physical activity that corresponds to aerobic intensity is concerned with the rate that the circulatory and respiratory systems supply oxygen and fuel during sustained physical activity as well as the associated elimination rate of fatigue products after fuel is supplied [40]. Increased aerobic intensity enhances the ability of the cardiorespiratory as well as other systems to perform a given workload and may have a beneficial influence on cardiovascular disease [133, 146, 163, 200, 207]. There is also suspicion that increased aerobic intensity may serve as a marker for increased rate and force of muscular activity that, in turn, may be related to the rate of musculoskeletal injuries [174]. The amount of aerobic intensity that may be associated with musculoskeletal injury is perhaps best determined relative to the maximal capacity of the individual's cardiorespiratory system.

The dimension of physical activity that relates to weight bearing is mediated by the muscular activity needed to overcome the effects of gravity to either maintain an upright posture or perform movements while on one's feet. It is the force generally associated with overcoming the effects of gravity. Weight-bearing activity is thought to be useful in the prevention and treatment of osteoporosis [3–5].

The dimension of flexibility relates to the range of motion available at a joint [40]. Flexibility is important because it may help protect against disability and may enhance regular physical activity participation, which may in turn deter other diseases. The dimension of muscular strength relates to the amount of external force that a muscle can exert, whether through repeated dynamic movements or through a single isometric contraction. Muscular strength, like flexibility, may be important in protecting against disability. Insufficient flexibility and muscular strength are more likely to adversely affect the health of older individuals than of younger individuals because of the relative decline in the maximal amounts of these two factors with increasing age.

Few of the physical activity dimensions are exclusive to only one type of activity or to each other [122]. For example, activities that promote cardiorespiratory endurance also require considerable energy expenditure. Furthermore, any weight-bearing activity will also produce some caloric expenditure and if done vigorously may require increased aerobic intensity.

It should be readily apparent that the physical activity dimension that is measured in an epidemiologic investigation should pertain to the disease of interest or the suspected physiologic mechanism(s) that may be operating [122].

SUMMARY SCORES. An important issue that has recently emerged is how to formulate a summary score of physical activity data that is useful in epidemiologic research. Historically, the kilocalorie score has been used as a method of adjusting, by kilocalorie-weighting factors, the time spent in various physical activities according to the relative intensity of energy expenditure [225]. The resulting score can be made relative to daily, weekly, monthly, seasonal, or yearly time frames. This kilocalorie score can be used to rank populations from low to high, according to the total amount of activity performed. The score has the added advantage of being scaled on units that have very clear meaning to the physical sciences [231]. The principal disadvantage of the kilocalorie score is that someone who performs 1000 kcal/week can do so in 1 day of intensive activity or in 7 days of moderate activity. These differences may lead to different health benefits and may have different risks associated with them [40].

Recently, Caspersen et al. have introduced a different method that prepares a category score that yields four groups for leisure-time physical activity participation: sedentary; irregularly active; regularly active, but nonintensive and not using large, rhythmically contracting muscle groups; and regularly active, but intensive ($\geq 60\%$ of maximal cardiorespiratory capacity) and requiring rhythmically contracting muscle groups [36]. Both the category score and the kilocalorie score have been used in reporting population prevalence of physical activity in the 1985 National Health Interview Survey–Health Promotion/Disease Prevention supplement [36, 199]. Caspersen et al. [37] have compared the prevalences, by age, of men expending the highest level of a kilocalorie score (≥ 3.0 $\text{kcal·kg}^{-1}\text{·day}^{-1}$) with the prevalence of those men in the most active category and found that each score may represent a different physical activity status (see Fig. 12.2) [37]. Those authors also found that those men who expend the greatest number of kilocalories also reported a large amount of time in lawn and garden/home repair activities. Because such activities were more likely to be performed less frequently, those respondents were less likely to be in the highest, most regular category of physical activity used by Caspersen et al. [37]. This comparison helps to highlight the need to select a summary score for physical activity measures that will have the greatest meaning for the health or disease event under investigation.

LIFETIME PHYSICAL ACTIVITY ASSESSMENT. Even if issues such as measurement error, cost, the ability to measure appropriate dimensions of physical activity, reliability and validity, and summary scores can be suitably dealt with, it will still be important to clarify lifetime physical activity exposures [122]. Lifetime physical activity assessment, which has been attempted recently in a study of postmenopausal bone density [117], is also necessary for cancer epidemiologic research (which must allow for long latency periods and may have to account for physical activity done early in youth, as Frisch maintains might be the case in

FIGURE 12.2

Percentage of men performing appropriate physical activity and ≥ 3.0 kcal ·
kg⁻¹ · day⁻¹, by age. (From Caspersen CJ, Pollard RA, Pratt SO: Scoring
physical activity data with special consideration for elderly populations. In
Proceedings of the 21st National Meeting of the Public Health Conference on Records and Statistics: Data for an Aging Population, July
13–15, 1987 *(DHHS Pub. No. (PHS) 88-1214). Washington, DC, U.S.*
Department of Health, and Human Services, 1987, pp 30–34).

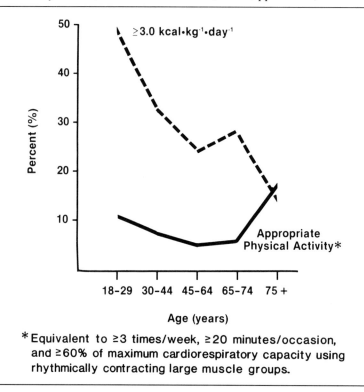

*Equivalent to ≥3 times/week, ≥20 minutes/occasion,
and ≥60% of maximum cardiorespiratory capacity using
rhythmically contracting large muscle groups.

breast cancer) [72]. A survey procedure that can address the dimensions
of physical activity over a lifetime will be of considerable utility in case-
control and even cohort studies [122]. These epidemiologic designs will
be described in the next major section.

THE NEED FOR QUALITY PHYSICAL ACTIVITY MEASURES. In their
critique of physical activity and CHD epidemiologic studies Powell et al.
[176] indicated that physical activity measures should (*a*) use operational
definitions that are clearly stated and interpretable; (*b*) have established
reliability and validity; (*c*) measure individually reported activities rather

than group assignments (e.g., job classification); (*d*) include information about the frequency, duration, and intensity of the activities; (*e*) account for physical activity during earlier periods of life; (*f*) establish the adherence to physical activity classification for cohort studies; and (*g*) be systematically collected by using specified standard methods. These are reasonable criteria; however, very few studies of physical activity and CHD were able to account for lifetime physical activity or for adherence to activity classification in cohort studies [176]. Further, few studies employed measures of physical activity exposure that had reasonably established reliability and validity.

The need for quality physical activity measures should not be understated. For example, it has been presumed that physical activity measures vary both in type and quality, thereby obscuring their association with CHD [42, 126]. Powell et al.'s [176] methodologic critique evaluated the quality of measures of physical activity exposure, of the CHD outcome measures, and of the epidemiologic design methodologies. Using criteria to establish quality, they judged that 40% of the measures of physical activity exposure measures were unsatisfactory, 40% were satisfactory, and only 20% were good (see Fig. 12.3). In contrast, they judged that 2% of the CHD outcome measures were unsatisfactory, 58% were satisfactory, and only 40% were good. Hence, when compared with the quality of the CHD outcome measure, the physical activity measure was considerably poorer [42, 176]. That critique also revealed that as the quality of the physical activity measurement increased from unsatisfactory to good, the proportion of studies revealing a statistically significant association increased from about 50% to 88% (see also Fig. 12.3). Poorer measures of physical activity exposure, which have been quite prevalent in physical activity and CHD studies, appear more likely to limit the ability to detect a significant association than are CHD outcome measures or epidemiologic design factors.

The poorer quality of physical activity measures helps explain why researchers have been unable to fully appreciate the importance of physical inactivity as a CHD risk factor [42]. The difficulty in measuring the specific dimensions of physical activity may also limit researcher's ability to detect significant associations between physical activity and other disease outcomes such as hypertension, osteoporosis, or diabetes [42].

EPIDEMIOLOGIC DESIGN METHODOLOGY

Types of Epidemiologic Designs

Although many research designs must be considered in physical activity epidemiology [139], they can be classified into two major categories: experimental and observational studies [175]. In experimental studies the researchers assign individuals to different treatment or exposure

FIGURE 12.3
Percentages of 43 epidemiologic studies of physical activity and coronary heart disease having specified quality of measures and methodology and percentages of 47 comparisons from those studies reporting statistically significant associations. (Data derived from Powell KE, Thompson PD, Caspersen CJ, Kendrick JS: Physical activity and the incidence of coronary heart disease. Ann Rev Public Health 8:253–287, 1987.)

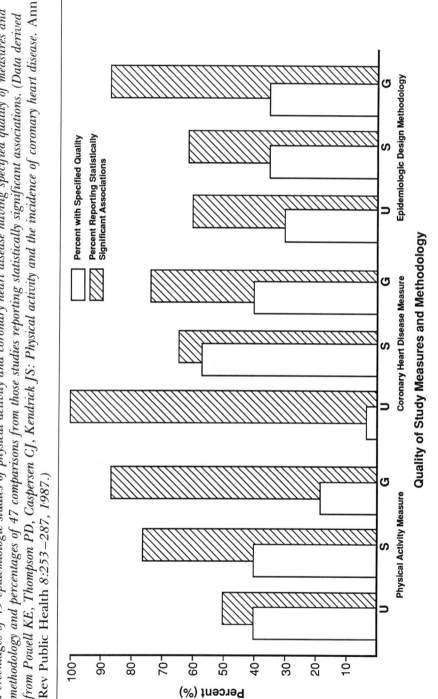

groups and follow them for some particular outcome of interest. In some studies the groups are randomly assigned. The principal advantage of experimental studies is that they exert great control over the factor of interest. Further, they are more commonly accepted by clinical researchers, who almost exclusively incorporate such designs on a much smaller scale. Unfortunately, experimental studies are very expensive and cannot be used to study rare diseases or health events [139]. Hence, experimental studies have been rare in physical activity epidemiologic research. Taylor et al. [223, 224] noted that randomized trials for the study of physical activity and CHD suffer from the need for a very large sample size and from problems associated with persons dropping out of the trial or crossing over from active to inactive assignment and vice versa.

Observational studies are also of interest to physical activity epidemiology and include case series, cross-sectional, ecologic, case-control, and cohort studies [139, 175, 234]. In observational studies persons are not assigned to treatment groups or to groups that have specified exposure to an etiologic factor; this assignment is left to occur by choice or by chance [139]. Perhaps the greatest advantage of such studies is the relative ease with which populations can be identified, sampled, and measured according to exposure to etiologic factor(s) and to the outcome of interest. The principal disadvantage is that certain predisposing variables may cause subjects to expose themselves to a presumed etiologic factor.

Case series studies, commonly reported by practitioners, may form the basis of a clinical hypothesis [139]. Case series reports are useful in giving a crude impression of factors that may be associated with morbidity or mortality, in providing insights into efficacious modes of therapy and the amount of health care resources required for such therapy, and in providing insights into the natural history of the given condition for the population under examination. The principal use of case series data for the physical activity epidemiologist has been in injury epidemiology studies, where the method has been useful in gleaning ideas of suspected risk factors for a given outcome that can be tested in studies having better research designs and more representative samples [174, 235]. The major advantage of case series data for injury epidemiology is that the data are already collected, making this observational approach relatively inexpensive. The major disadvantage is that there is no denominator on which to calculate rates. For example, more injuries may be seen in runners at one orthopedic clinic because it attracts more clients, it is more conveniently located than another clinic, or the treatment rates are cheaper. Another problem is a referral bias [235]. For example, if a podiatrist were to report high rates of foot problems and an orthopedic surgeon were to report high rates of knee problems in runners that they see, we would not know which anatomic site was truly injured most often in runners. Moreover, because a denominator is lacking, it is impossible to establish the true importance of suspected risk factors for injury [174, 235].

Cross-sectional studies, which are often termed "survey or prevalence studies," attempt to identify associations between an outcome and a potential etiologic factor(s) by studying a population at one point in time [139]. An advantage of this type of study is that it is possible to compare changing rates in appropriately sampled cross-sectional populations over time [30, 216]. A cross-sectional study was employed in national- and state-based population surveys of physical activity prevalence [40, 199]. The most unfortunate problem with the cross-sectional study is that it cannot establish the temporal or causal sequence connecting the suspected etiologic factor(s) and the outcome. For example, persons with CHD may reduce their physical activity level. Hence, if such persons are included as part of a cross-sectional study, then the association between decreased physical activity and CHD will be spuriously large.

An ecologic study uses data that are regularly gathered for separate purposes and compares the occurrence of an outcome in one data base with the distribution of a suspected risk factor(s) among similar groups in another data base [139]. The principal advantage of ecologic studies is that they tend to use available data bases and, therefore, are relatively inexpensive. The principal disadvantage is that because groups of people are being compared, it is impossible to link the exposure to a risk factor to the actual outcome experience of a given individual. As a result, the link between the risk factor exposure and the outcome can only be inferred. When false conclusions arise from this limitation it is termed "an ecologic fallacy." An ecologic study was conducted by Thompson et al. when they estimated the rates of sudden death in men attributed to jogging in Rhode Island [230]. The rate of jogging-related sudden death was calculated by dividing the total number of deaths that occurred during jogging by the estimated number of male joggers (determined via a random telephone survey).

Case-control studies, also known as "case-referent" studies, start with the identification of an individual who has the outcome of interest (the case) and then compare the exposures to presumed risk factors of that individual with the exposures of another individual in the same population. That latter individual is termed the "control" or "referent." When cases are found to have greater exposure to a suspected risk factor, that factor is suspected to have caused the disease [139]. The case-control study is an extension of the case-series study and seeks to overcome the problem of not having a comparison population for analyzing the exposure to suspected risk factors. This study design is especially useful and quite efficient in studying rare health events. Siscovick et al. used a case-control study to examine the association of physical activity relative to the rare occurrence of primary cardiac arrest [207]. Although matching can improve the efficiency of the study design, there are some dangers with the matching process. Overmatching occurs when one ultimately matches for a variable that is only linked with the exposure variable and not with the outcome. For example, overmatching might be encountered in a case-control study of the determinants of physical activity where those running daily for 30 minutes (cases) would be compared to sedentary persons (controls) by matching on the census tract of the home as an adjustment for socioeconomic status. If the determinant under investigation was the proximity to local facilities, analyses would not yield any significant association because the form of matching ruled out any difference between cases and controls on exposure to available facilities.

Another observational study is the cohort study, which is also termed the "longitudinal" or "prospective" study [115, 139, 219]. In this type of study the epidemiologist selects a group of persons (a cohort) that can be readily identified relative to their exposure to a risk factor of interest and thereafter follows them to determine their status for some health outcome [139]. The cohort study is similar to the experimental study, except that the subjects are not assigned to groups. Paffenbarger et al. [157] employed a cohort study by establishing the activity status of longshoremen at the beginning of the study and following them for 22 years to compare rates of CHD in those with greater and lesser amounts of physical activity. Some cohort studies establish exposure to suspected risk factors via past records and assess outcome that has occurred prior to the time the study is conducted. Such studies are termed "historical prospective," "historical cohort," or "retrospective cohort" studies.

Quality Criteria for Epidemiologic Design Methodology
In their critique of physical activity and CHD epidemiologic studies, Powell et al. [176] indicated that epidemiologic design methodology should (*a*) assure that the physical activity measurement should precede the onset of the CHD ascertainment; (*b*) adjust for relevant variables known to be related to the risk of CHD (e.g., blood pressure, smoking, and cholesterol) that may confound an observed relationship between physical activity and CHD; (*c*) use either the entire population or a random sample of the entire population to assure representativeness; (*d*) assure that those subjects who are lost to follow-up in cohort studies have similar physical activity behavior and other relevant variables as those who remain a part of the sample; and (*e*) randomize to active and inactive groups in cohort studies. In addition, they recommended that case-control studies specifically should (*a*) use predetermined protocols for the selection of cases and controls, (*b*) equally apply any constraint to cases and controls, and (*c*) assure that data collectors and respondents are blind to the experimental hypothesis under consideration [176]. Each of those cri-

teria is helpful in assuring that the quality of any epidemiologic investigation is maintained and in assessing the quality of investigations that have been performed.

EPIDEMIOLOGIC CONCEPTS

Agent, Host, and Environment

Another set of important concepts in physical activity epidemiology is the notion of agent, host, and environment that has traditionally applied to infectious disease epidemiology [125]. Each concept has been portrayed by Koplan et al. in a review of exercise and sports injury epidemiology (see Table 12.5) [114].

The agent in injury epidemiology pertains to that facet of the behavior that results in the injury. In the case of aerobic dance this might be the duration and frequency of workouts, how percussive the movements are, how high one jumps in certain movements, warm-up (and perhaps even cool-down) time, etc. Host factors are such things as age, gender, body somatotype or composition, genetic factors, prior health and injury status, level of physical fitness (muscular strength and endurance, aerobic power, flexibility, etc.), and other risk factors (perhaps smoking). Environmental factors would be climate (outdoor or indoor as applicable), footwear, surface, or even social factors such as how peers perform their movements. The interrelationship of these three factors governs the nature and severity of injury in this particular context or in other health outcomes when events other than injury are studied (e.g., CHD, cancer).

Surveillance

An important part of physical activity epidemiology is surveillance. As defined by Langmuir [123], surveillance is "the continued watchfulness over the distribution and trends of incidence through the systematic collection, consolidation and evaluation of morbidity and mortality reports and other relevant data."

The following extension of Langmuir's definition was adopted by the Centers for Disease Control (CDC):

> Epidemiologic surveillance is the ongoing systematic collection, analysis, and interpretation of health data essential to the planning, implementation, and evaluation of public health practice, closely integrated with the timely dissemination of these data to those who need to know. The final link in the surveillance chain is the application of these data to prevention and control. A surveillance system includes a functional capacity for data collection, analysis, and dissemination linked to public health programs. [49]

TABLE 12.5

Factors That May Influence the Occurrence of Injuries in Several Types of Physical Activities Commonly Done in Exercise Programs[a]

Type of Physical Activity Performed	Factors		
	Agent	*Host*	*Environment*
Aerobic dance	Frequency Duration Preexercises or postexercises Percussive movement Jumping height	Age Sex Habitus (weight, height; varus/valgus)	Air temperature Humidity Shoes Flooring Social factors Instructor
Calisthenics	Frequency Duration Preexercises or postexercises Type of exercise	Age Sex Habitus (flexibility)	Surface
Cycling	Frequency Duration Preexercises or postexercises Speed Distance	Age Sex Habitus	Air temperature Humidity Bicycle (toe clips; ratios of parts) Wind Road surface Inclines/declines Type road Helmet use
Swimming	Frequency Duration Preexercises or postexercises Stroke Technique Distance Speed	Age Sex Habitus (ear canal anatomy)	Temperature Body of water (pool, lake, ocean) Water quality (pH, purity, chlorine)
Running, walking	Gait Frequency Speed Distance Duration Preexercises or postexercises	Age Sex Habitus, (weight, height; varus/valgus)	Air temperature Humidity Shoes Surface (composition; slant) Location

[a] Modified from Koplan JP, Siscovick DS, Goldbaum G: The risk of exercise: a public health view of injuries and hazards. *Public Health Rep* 100:189–195, 1985.

The CDC definition indicates that surveillance must be ongoing to be considered a surveillance system. Further, as implied in the CDC definition of surveillance, a surveillance system is most useful when it is applied to the planning, implementation, and evaluation of public health practices and programs, with the ultimate intent of leading to disease prevention and control [228]. In this context a surveillance system that is linked to public health activities qualifies as public health surveillance [228]. Even an ongoing and systematic surveillance system that collects data and analyzes the results would not qualify as public health surveillance unless it were applied to public health programs and practices. For example, the surveillance of all cases of CHD among London busmen that was part of the epidemiologic investigation used by Morris et al. [145] would not qualify as public health surveillance system according to the CDC definition because it was not continually collected and interpreted for public health planning, implementation, and evaluation.

The definition of surveillance proposed by Langmuir was for the detection and reporting of communicable diseases. As the CDC definition stipulates, a surveillance system can also include other forms of health data. This stipulation is important in physical activity epidemiology, which is rarely concerned with communicable diseases. Figure 12.1 illustrates how surveillance can be extended within the realm of physical activity epidemiology to monitor chronic diseases or health events such as musculoskeletal injuries (S_o), the prevalence of physical activity patterns (S_{pa}), and certain behavioral determinants of physical activity (S_d).

Several chronic diseases are of interest to physical activity epidemiology. For example, physical activity is apparently associated with CHD [176] and perhaps with colon cancer [73, 80, 96, 159, 168, 226, 232, 233, 245]. Understanding the incidence of CHD and its distribution according to selected demographic and certain geographic variables can suggest to the physical activity epidemiologist the magnitude of the disease burden and the potential for disease prevention when physical activity is employed as a public health intervention.

Recreational and sports injuries are health events that are also associated with certain physical activity patterns [114, 116, 235]. Surveillance systems that monitor such events are of interest to the physical activity epidemiologist. For example, since 1931 football fatality data have been collected by groups such as the American Football Coaches Association, the National Collegiate Athletic Association, and the National Federation of State High School Associations, and by investigators at the University of North Carolina [150]. This system has been able to track football fatalities by acquiring information from a variety of sources such as coaches, athletic directors and trainers, administrators, state and national athletic organizations, sporting goods companies, and a national news clipping service [150]. This system is a good example of using a variety of sources to track down these relatively rare fatalities. Further, the surveillance system has been extended to include catastrophic events such as cervical and spinal cord injuries. Because this system also contacts the coach or athletic director and administers a standardized questionnaire to query such information as the football player's personal habits or health history, details about the accident, emergency treatment, and equipment, it is possible to get a crude sense of certain etiologic factors. Unfortunately, this system has a drawback: Because the denominator of "at-risk" players must be estimated, precise rates cannot be directly ascertained. Nonetheless, the system is useful for monitoring such fatalities and trying to precipitate preventive activities.

Physical activity epidemiologists are also interested in the surveillance of physical activity patterns themselves. A prominent example is the Behavioral Risk Factor Surveillance system, which includes annual measures of physical activity and other disease risk factors for participating states [47]. Recently the CDC reported age-, sex-, and region-specific prevalence estimates of states where low reported levels of leisure-time physical activity defined their respondents at risk for a sedentary lifestyle (see Figs. 12.4, 12.5, and 12.6). At present, relatively few surveillance systems monitor state or national patterns of physical activity. There are, however, data from the National Health Interview Survey–Health Promotion/Disease Prevention [HPDP] supplement [36, 199]. In addition, Brooks has used data from market-based research groups to help identify physical activity patterns [31]. The HPDP survey will have to be replicated in future years to qualify as a true surveillance system, just as the more available market-based research data will have to include analyses of additional years.

Surveillance of physical activity prevalence is important for several reasons. First, the analysis of the data can be linked with data on disease surveillance. Comparing patterns of physical activity over the same time period where disease rates are monitored could link the results of two surveillance systems in a form of ecologic study. From this linkage one might infer the role that physical activity plays when rates of disease change. Second, such prevalence data are useful in determining whether national initiatives are helping to promote physical activity.

Finally, surveillance can be applied to the determinants of physical activity, such as when one catalogs the existence of available facilities for physical activity promotion [188], daily physical education requirements for states [178], or attitudes towards exercise [140]. These are unique examples of how surveillance in physical activity can be applied to events that are not immediately linked to a disease outcome. In such instances, it is assumed that the facilities and legislation are important links to the promotion and maintenance of physical activity levels that will ultimately

FIGURE 12.4

Box-plot summaries of the age-specific distribution of sedentary life-style preva-
lences from 22 states participating in the 1985 Behavioral Risk Factor Sur-
veillance System. (From Centers for Disease Control: Sex-, age-, and region-
specific prevalence in selected states—the Behavioral Risk Factor Surveillance
System. MMWR *36:195–204, 1987.)*

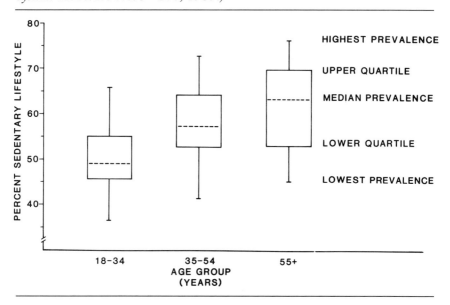

have beneficial links to disease prevention and health promotion. This assumption qualifies stable surveillance systems as public health surveillance in that the data collected and their interpretation are integrally linked with the formulation of public health policies that govern physical activity promotion.

Biases in Physical Activity Epidemiologic Research
Many biases can arise in epidemiologic research. Biases can vary with the type of epidemiologic design, the type of disease or health outcome, the risk factor of interest, or the population being investigated, as well as with combination of these. These biases are treated extensively in other sources [95, 125, 186]; however, several are worth noting in physical activity epidemiology.

Self-selection is a particularly disturbing possibility in cross-sectional, cohort, and case-control studies that rely on observational data. Considerable care must be taken to limit self-selection in the study design (by the selection of exposure and outcome variables) and in the analyses.

FIGURE 12.5

Box-plot summaries of the sex-specific distribution of sedentary life-style preva-
lences from 22 states participating in the 1985 Behavioral Risk Factor Sur-
veillance System. (From Centers for Disease Control: Sex-, age-, and region-
specific prevalence in selected states—the Behavioral Risk Factor Surveillance
System. MMWR 36:195–204, 1987.)

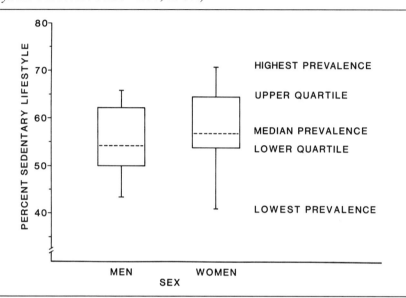

For example, if individuals having CHD symptoms such as angina would self-select to lesser amounts or forms of physical activity at about the time that the study was measuring physical activity exposure, a spurious beneficial association between physical activity and CHD may arise. Paffenbarger et al. indicated that an advantage of studying physical activity and CHD in San Francisco longshoremen was that union rules required entry-level employees to begin in physically demanding job assignments and return to that level even following periods of sickness [157]. That study's design ensured that decedents were ascribed a job category for the June prior to their demise to reduce the likelihood that the final job category held was a result of a recent job transfer. In addition, an extension of the study's original analysis found that the strength of the association between physical activity and CHD remained about the same in those subgroups of longshoremen whose job categories were chosen from different time periods prior to the fatal outcome. This finding was observed up to about 4.5 years prior to the fatal outcome [28]. Also, during statistical analyses, the researchers carefully considered self-se-

FIGURE 12.6

Box-plot summaries of the region-specific distribution of sedentary life-style prevalences from 22 states participating in the 1985 Behavioral Risk Factor Surveillance System. (From Centers for Disease Control: Sex-, age-, and region-specific prevalence in selected states—the Behavioral Risk Factor Surveillance System. MMWR 36:195–204, 1987.)

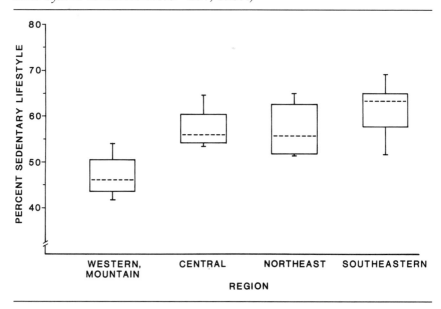

lection bias by showing that the time periods for a transfer from heavy to lighter work assignments were similar for those with and without fatal outcome [157]. Finally, the researchers separately analyzed non-sudden and sudden death, because the latter would be less likely to have been associated with recent transfers in work categories. This separation also revealed that 65% of vigorous workers and 67% of more sedentary workers had no prior evidence of hypertensive–arteriosclerotic abnormalities. As can be seen, carefully considering population selection, the defined variables of exposure and outcome, and analyses can all help discount the influence of selection bias in interpreting epidemiologic findings.

The healthy exerciser effect is a form of self-selection bias that often appears in epidemiologic studies that sample from a unique population, such as subjects from a certain occupation or a cohort of exercisers. For example, in a study of runners injuries for 10-km race registrants, Jacobs and Berson indicated that a "healthy runner" effect may be operating in that runners who were injured and could not enter the race would not be a part of the sample of race registrants that were studied for training-related injuries [98]. Walter et al. made note of this bias and took precautions to limit its effect by using all entrants to a 16-km race as the denominator, whether or not they ran that race [234].

Selection bias can result when the final study sample is different from the population it is meant to represent or a comparison group that is being used as a contrast [139]. Avoiding this bias is critical to epidemiologic research, which relies heavily on the identification of an appropriate denominator for the calculation of rates [176]. Koplan et al. took efforts to identify the nature and extent of selection bias by sampling nonrespondents to their mail survey and administering a telephone questionnaire to them [113]. The researchers detected differences between the nonrespondents and respondents to their mail survey and indicated that those differences should be considered in interpreting their results.

Whereas selection bias is concerned with who might respond to a survey, response bias pertains to a subtle tendency in how subjects respond to survey questions in a differential manner [139]. Response bias is difficult to reveal. For example, in a case-control study, patients with CHD might be more likely than their control comparison subjects to try harder to find reasons for having had a heart attack and might thereby falsely overstate their sedentary habits. To help reduce the likelihood of response bias in case-control studies of physical activity and CHD, one would have to ensure that not only the cases and controls but also the data collectors were unaware of the hypothesis under investigation [176].

A confounding factor bias would arise when an observed statistically significant association might actually be due to a factor or factor(s) not currently taken into consideration [139]. For example, Caspersen found that when data were pooled across mile-per-week running strata, persons reporting fewer years of running experience had higher injury rates [41]. However, in logistic regression analyses that adjusted for age, gender, body mass index, a running speed index, and past injury history, the years of previous running experience was no longer a statistically significant risk factor for running injury [41]. This finding indicates that the association was explained by a combination of confounding factors rather than by years of running experience.

One must be judicious with confounders so as not to control for a variable that is not only known to be independently associated with the outcome but also mediates the effect between physical activity and some outcome. For example, when one studies the independent influence of physical activity on CHD, the statistical control of high-density lipoprotein levels might yield a nonsignificant association, and lead to an erroneous conclusion that there was no effect due to physical activity at all [108].

A positive paper bias may result from the fact that epidemiologic investigations that report statistically significant associations are more likely to be published [195]. This is an important bias when one is trying to establish a causal association that is based on interpretation of the available published literature. It has been proposed that a journal for nonsignificant results be established to overcome this bias [195]. However, until such countermeasures occur, the reviewer of epidemiologic findings must be aware of this potential bias when interpreting the consistency of an association between physical activity and a given health or disease outcome across studies. At the same time, physical activity epidemiologists must explore all relevant hypotheses and report all findings of their analyses that pertain to the associations they are investigating.

Population Attributable Risk
The concept of population attributable risk has been used to help provide a balanced view between the need to act on relatively strong risk factors that affect fewer people and the need to act on relatively weaker risk factors that are more prevalent in a population [125]. For example, to grasp the relative importance of changing each of five risk factors in a population of Harvard alumni, given the respective prevalences of each factor, Paffenbarger et al. calculated what they called a "community attributable risk," or what is often simply called a population attributable risk [125].

Paffenbarger et al. indicated that for Harvard alumni the relative risk (RR) of all-cause mortality for the 62% of that group who expended less than 2000 kcal/week was 1.31 relative to the other 38% who expended more than 2000 kcal/week [160]. This relative risk can be thought of as a 31% increased risk of death for the sedentary group. Paffenbarger also reported relative risks for those Harvard alumni for the following conditions: 1.73 for those having physician-diagnosed hypertension, 1.76 for cigarette smokers, 1.33 for those who gained ≥15 pounds during the follow-up period, and 1.15 for those whose parents died before age 65 years. Corresponding prevalences for the respondents were 9.4%, 38.2%, 35.1%, and 33.3%, respectively. Hence, although several of the risk factors (RF) had somewhat stronger relative risk values than did sedentary life-style, their prevalences were not nearly as great.

The following formula is for calculating the population attributable risk:

$$\text{Population attributable risk} = \frac{(\text{Prevalence}_{RF}) \cdot (RR_{RF} - 1)}{((\text{Prevalence}_{RF}) \cdot (RR_{RF} - 1)) + 1}.$$

This formula can be treated as a percent by multiplying the result by 100.

FIGURE 12.7

Percentages of U.S. population at risk for recognized risk factors related to coronary heart disease and risk ratio for each risk factor. (From Caspersen CJ: Physical inactivity and coronary heart disease (guest editorial). Physician Sportsmed *15:43–44, 1987.)*

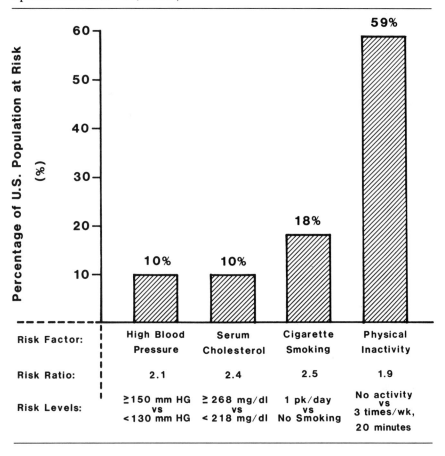

Paffenbarger et al. calculated the following population attributable risks: sedentary lifestyle = 16.1%, hypertension = 6.4%, cigarette smoking = 22.5%, weight gain = 10.3%, and parental death (<65 years) = 4.8%. These population attributable risk percentages indicate that for those alumni, sedentary life-style was second only to cigarette smoking in its potential relative impact on all-cause mortality if each risk factor were eliminated.

The same concept of population attributable risk was recently portrayed visually for a comparison of CHD risk factors (see Fig. 12.7) [42,

48]. Pooling the results of 43 epidemiologic investigations revealed that the median relative risk between physical activity and CHD was 1.9 [141]. That median relative risk was similar to the median values of the following risk factors previously reported in the Coronary Pooling Project for five studies [138]: 2.1 for high systolic blood pressure ($\geq$150 mm Hg vs. <130 mm Hg), 2.4 for serum cholesterol ($\geq$268 mg% vs. < 218 mg%), and 2.5 for smoking ($\geq$1 pack of cigarettes/day vs. no smoking). Because the relative risks for those four CHD risk factors were very similar, the prevalence of each risk factor in the United States was thought to help express the population attributable risk without mathematical analyses [48]. The prevalence of those at risk for the three other CHD risk factors was small compared with the prevalence of those failing to perform regular physical activity [42, 48]. With its potential population impact, physical activity thus appeared to be a more important concern than the other three CHD risk factors.

CAUSAL INFERENCE IN PHYSICAL ACTIVITY EPIDEMIOLOGY

Schlesselman has indicated the importance of carefully appraising the following means of assessing direct or indirect causal associations: epidemiologic designs, biases, the influence of confounding factors, and even chance. He has indicated that criteria for causality set forth by the U.S. Surgeon General may help guide the process [195]. Criteria should be established when interpreting scientific data because virtually no experiment can provide definitive proof of causation. In most instances, establishing the causal nature of a risk factor, such as cigarette smoking on lung cancer, will be provided by observational data because data may not be economically or ethically gathered in a randomized controlled clinical trial. Observational data must be carefully interpreted to help direct public policy and/or to establish treatment guidelines in the absence of definitive experimental proof.

We can follow the logic behind causal inference by examining the evaluation conducted by Powell et al. [176]. As was true with the association between cigarette smoking and lung cancer, there are no randomized controlled clinical trials on the association between physical activity and coronary heart disease. Therefore, those reviewers used six criteria to examine the potential causal association between physical activity and CHD. The reviewers found that (*a*) the results were *consistent* in that more than two-thirds of the studies reported statistically significant associations between physical activity and CHD; (*b*) the *strength* of the association between physical activity and CHD was reasonably strong, having a median value of 1.9 for the studies reviewed and being of similar strength as those relative risks observed for the commonly ac-

cepted CHD risk factors of high systolic blood pressure, serum cholesterol, and cigarette smoking [173]; (c) an *appropriate temporal sequence* was
observed in most of the studies; (d) more than two-thirds of the studies
having suitable data could demonstrate a *dose–response* effect, whereby
lower levels of physical activity were associated with greater likelihood
of CHD (see Fig. 12.8); (e) a thorough review of other scientific literature
revealed a number of *plausible and coherent* physiologic mechanisms,
whereby increased physical activity could induce a favorable effect on
CHD; and (f) better studies were more likely to report a statistically
significant inverse association even if there was no *experimental evidence*
to more firmly establish the association between physical activity and
CHD. From these criteria the authors concluded that a causal, statistically
significant, inverse association exists between physical activity and CHD
[176]. Moreover, the authors were able to discount the influences of
confounding and selection bias as likely factors explaining the consistency and strength of the observed association.

When the association between physical inactivity and CHD is compared
with that observed between cigarette smoking and lung cancer, some
useful parallels can be identified. Most important is that the strength of
the association was much weaker between physical activity and CHD
(RR = 1.5 to 2.5) than between smoking and lung cancer (RR = 5 to
15). However, such weaker associations are commonly found in CHD
epidemiology [173]. Also, the consistency of the association is greater in
the case of smoking and cancer. Because only about two-thirds of the
studies showed a significant association between physical activity and
CHD, other reviewers concluded that a causal association was quite unlikely [126]. However, by conducting a very thorough methodologic critique, Powell et al. found that improvements in the measures of physical
activity and heart disease, as well as in the quality of the epidemiologic
design, increased the strength and magnitude of the association [42,
176]. This finding helped assure those reviewers that although the consistency among the studies was not greater than two-thirds, it might well
have been higher if there had been fewer vagaries of physical activity
assessment. The finding also suggests that in making causal inferences,
we should differentially focus on the results of the objectively established
"better" studies.

APPLICATION OF PHYSICAL ACTIVITY EPIDEMIOLOGY TO POLICY ISSUES

One of the principal objectives of physical activity epidemiologic studies
is to try to establish, as clearly as possible, whether a causal association
exists between physical activity, as a behavior, and a particular disease
or health outcome. However, even though a causal association may exist,

FIGURE 12.8

Relative risk of first heart attack by physical activity index for strenuous sports and other activities in a 6- to 10-year follow-up of Harvard male alumni (first-order multiple logistic model). (From Paffenbarger RS Jr, Wing AL, Hyde RT: Physical activity as an index of heart attack risk in college alumni. Am J Epidemiol *108:161–175, 1978.)*

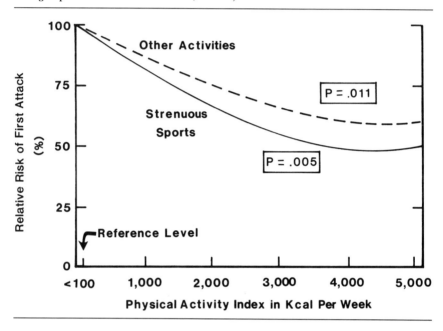

the physical activity epidemiologist should consider whether prescribed increases in physical activity for a population will be cost-effective in the reduction of that disease or health outcome. For example, the promotion of running may cost too much or may produce too many injuries bringing about the substantial cost savings associated with reduced rates of CHD. Although cost-effectiveness analyses are the domain of health economists, the physical activity epidemiologist will be responsible for providing the cost-effectiveness model with relevant information from population-based epidemiologic research. Such applications of epidemiologic data are useful to policymakers.

Using the results of epidemiologic research as a guide, Hatziandreu et al. [87] recently performed a cost-effectiveness analysis of physical activity and its effect on CHD. The analysis relied on the methodologic critique by Powell et al. [176] that established the consistency of the relative risk between physical activity and CHD at 1.9 (from a range of

1.5 to 2.4). However, the authors chose for their model the specific relationship of 2000 kcal/week that Paffenbarger et al. [161] found to result in a 50% reduction in CHD events. The authors developed a hypothetical cohort of 1000 35-year-old men, half of whom ran and the other half of whom performed no physical activity, and "followed" them for 30 years. In addition, data from the Framingham heart study set forth the most likely incidence data of fatal and nonfatal events of CHD [202]. Finally, the epidemiologic study by Koplan et al. [113] established the annual occurrence of a running injury that would result in a visit to a health care professional.

The authors allowed for direct costs (e.g., equipment, clothing, medical care of injuries) and benefits (savings from reduced CHD events and treatment costs) and indirect costs (time spent in running) and benefits (healthy time gained from running after CHD prevention). Their results revealed that subjects who were counseled by a physician to run would have fewer CHD events, and more quality-adjusted life years than those who performed no exercise. The cost of the quality-adjusted life years appeared similar to cost-effectiveness indices derived for other therapeutic or preventative maneuvers for CHD [87]. Further, the authors also indicated that if the effects of physical activity on other chronic diseases and conditions were included, the cost-effectiveness of physical activity, relative to public health in general, would have improved above the authors' estimates for CHD events alone.

The conclusion that running prescriptions made by physicians to middle-aged men are cost-effective could form the basis for guiding public health policy. Hence, Hatziandreu et al.'s analysis is a persuasive example of how epidemiologic data can guide the development of cost-effectiveness models. These models can help policymakers draft appropriate policy decisions for public health that are based on population-based research rather than on subjective opinion. Such data applications extend the utility of physical activity epidemiologic research beyond the identification of causal associations between physical activity and health outcomes.

SUMMARY AND CONCLUSION

This review was conducted to provide the reader with a brief overview of the science of epidemiology as applied specifically to physical activity as a behavior. Definitions were offered for epidemiology, for physical activity, and finally for physical activity epidemiology. In addition to considering epidemiologic concepts, this review stressed the importance of carefully measuring physical activity—perhaps the principal function of anyone who ultimately claims to be a physical activity epidemiologist. The breadth and scope of physical activity epidemiology are extensive, and there is fertile ground for continuing to apply physical activity epidemiology to exercise science well into the future. This chapter should provide the exercise scientist with a firm foundation to begin his or her trek into the realm of physical activity epidemiology.

REFERENCES

1. Albert M: Descriptive three year data study of outdoor and indoor professional soccer injuries. *Athletic Training* 18:218–220, 1983.
2. Albright JP, McAuley E, Martin RK, Crowley GT, Foster DT: Head and neck injuries in college football: an eight-year analysis. *Am J Sports Med* 13:147–152, 1985.
3. Aloia JF, Cohn FH, Tabu T, Abesanis C, Kalici N, Ellis I: Skeletal mass and body composition in marathon runners. *Metabolism* 12:1783–1796, 1978.
4. Aloia JF, Cohn SH, Ostuni JA, Cane R, Ellis K: Prevention of involutional bone loss by exercise. *Ann Intern Med* 89:356–358, 1978.
5. Aloia JF: Exercise and skeletal health. *J Am Geriatr Soc* 29:104–107, 1981.
6. Andersen KL, Masironi R, Rutenfranz J, Seliger V (eds): Habitual Physical Activity and Health (WHO Publication Series #6). Copenhagen, World Health Organization, 1978.
7. Aravanis C, Corcondilas A, Dontas AS, Lekos D, Keys A: The Greek islands of Crete and Confu. *Circulation* (suppl) 46:I88–I100, 1970.
8. Aravanis C, Dontas AS, Lekos D, Keys A: Rural populations in Crete and Confu, Greece. *Acta Med Scand Suppl* 460:209–230, 1966.
9. Baecke JAH, Burema J, Frijters JER: A short questionnaire for the measurement of habitual physical activity in epidemiological studies. *Am J Clin Nutr* 36:932–942, 1982.
10. Bailey DA, Shephard RJ, Mirwald RL: Validation of a self-administered home test of cardiopulmonary fitness. *Can J Appl Sport Sci* 1:67–78, 1976.
11. Baranowski T, Dworkin RJ, Cieslik CJ, Hooks P, Clearman DR, Ray L, Dunn JK, Nader PR: Reliability and validity of children's self-report of aerobic activity: Family Health Project. *Res Q Exerc Sport* 55:309–317, 1984.
12. Baranowski T: Methodologic issues in self-report of health behavior. *J School Health* 55:179–182, 1985.
13. Bell RQ: Adaptation of small wrist watches for mechanical recording of activities in infants and children. *J Exp Child Psychol* 6:302–305, 1968.
14. Birrer RB, Halbrook SP: Martial arts injuries. The results of a five year national survey. *Am J Sports Med* 16:408–410, 1988.
15. Blair SN, Cooper KH, Gibbons LW: Changes in coronary heart disease risk factors associated with increased treadmill time in 753 men. *Am J Epidemiol* 118:352–359, 1983.
16. Blair SN, Goodyear NN, Gibbons LW, Cooper KH: Physical fitness and incidence of hypertension in healthy normotensive men and women. *JAMA* 252:487–490, 1984.
17. Blair SN, Goodyear NN, Wynne KL, Saunders RP: Comparison of dietary and smoking habit changes in physical fitness improvers and nonimprovers. *Prev Med* 13:411–420, 1984.
18. Blair SN, Haskell WL, Ho P, Paffenbarger RJ Jr, Vranizan KM, Farquhar JW, Wood PD: Assessment of habitual physical activity by a seven-day recall in a community survey and in controlled experiments. *Am J Epidemiol* 122:794–804, 1985.
19. Blair SN, Jacobs DR, Powell KE: Relationships between exercise or physical activity and other health behaviors. *Public Health Rep* 100:172–180, 1985.

20. Blair SN, Kohl HW, Goodyear NN: Rates and risks for running and exercise injuries: studies in three populations. *Res Q Exerc Sport* 58:221–228, 1987.
21. Blair SN, Lavey RS, Goodyear N, Gibbons LW, Cooper KH: Physiological responses to maximal graded exercise testing in apparently healthy white women aged 18–75 years. *J Cardiac Rehabil* 4:459–468, 1984.
22. Blair SN: Risk factors and running injuries. *Med Sci Sports Exerc* 17:xii, 1985.
23. Blyth CS, Mueller FO: An epidemiologic study of high school football injuries in North Carolina, 1968–1972 (U. S. Consumer Product Safety Commission Publication 5203-0054). Washington, DC, U.S. Government Printing Office, 1974.
24. Blyth CS, Mueller FO: Football injury survey. Part III. Injury rates vary with coaching. *Physician Sportsmed* 2:45–50, 1974.
25. Bouchard C, Lesage R, Lortie G, Simoneau JA, Hamel P, Boulay MR, Perusse L, Theriault G, Leblanc C: Aerobic performance in brothers, dizygotic and monozygotic twins. *Med Sci Sports Exerc* 18:639–646, 1986.
26. Bouchard C, Tremblay A, Leblanc C, Lortie G, Savard R, Theriault G: A method to assess energy expenditure in children and adults. *Am J Clin Nutr* 37:461–467, 1983.
27. Bradfield RB: A technique for determination of usual daily expenditure in the field. *Am J Clin Nutr* 24:1148–1154, 1971.
28. Brand RJ, Paffenbarger RS Jr, Sholtz RI, Kampert JB: Work activity and fatal heart attack studied by multiple logistic risk analysis. *Am J Epidemiol* 110:52–62, 1979.
29. Breslow L, Buell P: Mortality from coronary heart disease and physical activity of work in California. *J Chronic Dis* 11:421–444, 1960.
30. Brooks C: Adult physical activity behavior: a trend analysis. *J Clin Epidemiol* 41:385–392, 1988.
31. Brooks CM: Adult participation in physical activities requiring moderate to high levels of energy expenditure. *Physician Sportsmed* 15:119–132, 1987.
32. Brunner D, Manelis G, Modan M, Levin S: Physical activity at work and the incidence of myocardial infarction, angina pectoris and death due to ischemic heart disease. An epidemiological study in Israeli collective settlements (kibbutzim). *J Chronic Dis* 27:217–233, 1974.
33. Bullen BA, Reed RB, Mayer J: Physical activity of obese and non-obese adolescent girls appraised by motion picture sampling. *Am J Clin Nutr* 14:211–223, 1964.
34. Buzina R, Keys A, Mohacek I, Hahn A, Brozek J, Blackburn H: Rural men in Dalmatia and Slavonia, Yugoslavia. *Acta Med Scand Suppl* 460:147–168, 1966.
35. Buzina R, Keys A, Mohacek I, Marinkovic M, Hahn A, Blackburn H: Five year follow-up in Dalmatia and Slavonia. *Circulation* (suppl) 46:I40–I51, 1970.
36. Caspersen CJ, Christenson GM, Pollard RA: Status of the 1990 physical fitness and exercise objectives—evidence from NHIS 1985. *Public Health Rep* 101:587–592, 1986.
37. Caspersen CJ, Pollard RA, Pratt SO: Scoring physical activity data with special consideration for elderly populations. In *Proceedings of the 21st National Meeting of the Public Health Conference on Records and Statistics: Data for an Aging Population, July 13–15, 1987.* (DHHS Pub. No. (PHS) 88-1214) Washington, DC, U.S. Department of Health and Human Services, 1987, pp 30–34.
38. Caspersen CJ, Pollard RA: Prevalence of physical activity in the United States and its relationship to disease risk factors. *Med Sci Sports Exerc* 19(suppl.):S7, 1987.
39. Caspersen CJ, Pollard RA: Validity of global self-reports of physical activity in epidemiology. *CVD Epidemiol Newsl* 43:15, 1988.
40. Caspersen CJ, Powell KE, Christenson GM: Physical activity, exercise, and physical fitness: definitions and distinctions for health-related research. *Public Health Rep* 100:126–131, 1985.

41. Caspersen CJ: Epidemiology of running injuries one year following a 10 km road race. *Med Sci Sports Exerc* 17:xii, 1985.
42. Caspersen CJ: Physical inactivity and coronary heart disease (guest editorial). *Physician Sportsmed* 15:43–44, 1987.
43. Cassel J, Heyden S, Bartel AG, Kaplan BH, Tyroler HA, Coroni JC, Hames CG: Occupation and physical activity and coronary heart disease. *Arch Intern Med* 128:920–928, 1971.
44. Cauley JA, LaPorte RE, Black-Sandler R: Measurement of physical activity in older populations. Paper presented at Society for Epidemiologic Research, Houston, TX, 1984.
45. Cauley JA, LaPorte RE, Sandler RB, Schramm MM, Kriska AM: Comparison of methods to measure physical activity in postmenopausal women. *Am J Clin Nutr* 45:12–22, 1987.
46. Cauley JA, LaPorte RE, Sandler RB: Measurement of physical activity in older populations. *Am J Epidemiol* 120:471–472, 1984.
47. Centers for Disease Control: Sex-, age-, and region-specific prevalence in selected states—the Behavioral Risk Factor Surveillance System. *MMWR* 36:195–204, 1987.
48. Centers for Disease Control: Protective effect of physical activity on coronary heart disease. *MMWR* 36:426–430, 1987.
49. Centers for Disease Control: Comprehensive plan for epidemiologic surveillance: Centers for Disease Control, August, 1986. Atlanta, GA, Centers for Disease Control, 1986.
50. Chapman JM, Goerke LS, Dixon W, Loveland DB, Phillips E: The clinical status of a population group in Los Angeles under observation for two to three years. *Am J Public Health* 47:33–42, 1957.
51. Chave SPW, Morris JN, Moss S: Vigorous exercise in leisure time and the death rate: a study of male civil servants. *J Epidemiol Community Health* 32:239–243, 1978.
52. Christensen CC, Frey HM, Foenstelie E, Aadland E, Refsum HE: A critical evaluation of energy expenditure estimates based on individual O_2 consumption/heart rate curves and average daily heart rate. *Am J Clin Nutr* 37:468–472, 1983.
53. Cumming GR, Glenn J: Evaluation of the Canadian Home Fitness Test in middle-aged men. *Can Med Assoc J* 117:346–349, 1977.
54. Dauncey MJ, James WPT: Assessment of the heart rate method for determining energy expenditures in man, using a whole-body calorimeter. *Br J Nutr* 42:1–13, 1979.
55. Dauncey MJ, Murgatroyd PR, Cole TJ: A human calorimeter for direct and indirect measurement of 24-h energy expenditure. *Br J Nutr* 39:557–566, 1978.
56. DeBacker G, Kornitzer M, Sobolski J, Dramaix M, Degré S, deMarneffe M, Denolin H: Physical activity and physical fitness levels of Belgian males aged 40–55 years. *Cardiology* 67:110–128, 1981.
57. Dishman RK, Sallis JF, Orenstein DR: The determinants of physical activity and exercise. *Public Health Rep* 100:158–171, 1985.
58. Donahue RP, Abbott RD, Reed DM, Yano K: Physical activity and coronary heart disease in middle-aged and elderly men: the Honolulu Heart Program. *Am J Public Health* 78:1–3, 1988.
59. Durnin JVGA, Ferro-Luzzi A: Conducting and reporting studies of human energy intake and output: suggested standards. *Hum Nutr Appl Nutr* 37:141–144, 1983.
60. Durnin JVGA, Namyslowski L: Individual variations in energy expenditure of standardized activities. *J Physiol* 143:573–578, 1958.
61. Durnin JVGA: Energy consumption and its measurement in physical activity. *Ann Clin Res* 14(suppl. 34):6–11, 1982.

62. Ekstrand J, Gillguist J, Moller M, Oberg B, Liljedahl SO: Incidence of soccer injuries and their relation to training and team success. *Am J Sports Med* 11:63–67, 1983.
63. Ekstrand J, Gillguist J: The frequency of muscle tightness and injuries in soccer players. *Am J Sports Med* 10:75–78, 1982.
64. Ekstrand J, Gillguist J: The avoidability of soccer injuries. *Int J Sports Med* 4:124–128, 1983.
65. Ekstrand J, Gillguist J: Soccer injuries and their mechanisms. A prospective study. *Med Sci Sports Exerc* 15:267–270, 1983.
66. Evang K, Andersen KL: Physical activity in health and disease. Oslo, Universitetsforlaget, 1966.
67. Farmer ME, Locke BZ, Mosciki EK, Dannenberg AL, Larson DB, Radloff LS: Physical activity and depressive symptoms: the NHANES I Epidemiologic Follow-up Study. *Am J Epidemiol* 128:1340–1351, 1988.
68. Fidanza F, Puddu V, Imbimbo B, Menotti A, Keys A: Five-year experience in rural Italy. *Circulation Suppl* 46:63–75, 1970.
69. Fidanza F, Puddu V, del Vecchio A, Keys A: Men in rural Italy. *Acta Med Scand (Suppl)* 460:116–146, 1966.
70. Foster FG, McPartland RJ, Kupfer DJ: Motion sensors in medicine: a report on reliability and validity. *J Inter-Am Med* 3:4–8, 1978.
71. Friedman M, Manwaring JH, Rosenman RH, Donlon G, Ortega P, Grube SM: Instantaneous and sudden death. Clinical and pathological differentiation in coronary artery disease. *JAMA* 225:1319–1328, 1973.
72. Frisch RE, Wyshak G, Albright NL, Albright TE, Schiff I, Jones KP, Witschi J, Shiang E, Koff E, Marguglio M: Lower prevalence of breast cancer and cancers of the reproductive system among former college athletes compared to non-athletes. *Br J Cancer* 52:885–891, 1985.
73. Garabrant DH, Peters JM, Mack TM, Bernstein L: Job activity and colon cancer risk. *Am J Epidemiol* 119:1005–1014, 1984.
74. Garcia-Palmieri MR, Costas R Jr, Cruz-Vidal M, Sorlie PD, Havlik RJ: Increased physical activity. A protective factor against heart attacks in Puerto Rico. *Am J Cardiol* 50:749–755, 1982.
75. Garrick JG, Gillien DM, Whiteside P: The epidemiology of aerobic dance injuries. *Am J Sports Med* 14:67–72, 1986.
76. Garrick JG, Requa RK: Epidemiology of women's gymnastics injuries. *Am J Sports Med* 8:261–264, 1980.
77. Garrick JG, Requa RK: Injuries in high school sports. *Pediatrics* 61:465–469, 1978.
78. Gayle RH, Montoye HJ, Philpot J: Accuracy of pedometers for measuring distance walked. *Res Q* 48:632–636, 1977.
79. Gerberich SG, Priest JD, Boen JR, Straub CP, Maxwell RE: Concussion incidence and severity in secondary school varsity football players. *Am J Public Health* 73:1370–1375, 1983.
80. Gerhardsson M, Norrell SE, Kirviranta H, Pedersen NL, Ahlbam A: Sedentary jobs and colon cancer. *Am J Epidemiol* 123:775–780, 1986.
81. Glagor S: Heart rate during 24 hours of usual activity for 100 normal men. *J Appl Physiol* 29:799–805, 1970.
82. Halpern B, Thompson N, Curl WW: High school football injuries: identifying the risk factors. *Am J Sports Med* 15:316–320, 1987.
83. Halverson CF, Waldrop MF: The relations of mechanically recorded activity level to varieties of preschool play behavior. *Child Dev* 44:678–681, 1973.
84. Hang Y-S, Peng S-M: An epidemiologic study of upper extremity injury in tennis players with a particular reference to tennis elbow. *J Formosan Med Assoc* 83:307–316, 1984.

85. Hartley HL, Herd A, Day W, Abusamia J, Howes B: An exercise testing program for large populations. *JAMA* 241:269–271, 1979.

86. Haskell WL, Taylor HL, Wood PD, Schrott H, Heiss G: Strenuous physical activity, treadmill exercise test performance and plasma high-density lipoprotein cholesterol. The lipid research clinics program prevalence study. *Circulation* 62(suppl IV):IV-53-IV-61, 1980.

87. Hatziandreu EI, Koplan JP, Weinstein MC, Caspersen CJ, Warner KE: A cost-effectiveness analysis of exercise as a health promotion activity. *Am J Public Health* 78:1417–1421, 1988.

88. Hayes D: Hockey injuries: how, why, where, and when? *Physician Sportsmed* 3:61–65, 1975.

89. Heady JA, Morris JN, Kagan A: Coronary heart disease in London busmen: a progress report with special reference to physique. *Br J Prev Soc Med* 15:143–153, 1961.

90. Hennekens CH, Rosner B, Jesse MJ, Drolette ME, Speizer FE: A retrospective study of physical activity and coronary deaths. *Int J Epidemiol* 6:243–246, 1977.

91. Herman B, Schmitz PI, Leyten AC, van Luijk JH, Frenken CWEM, deCoul AAWO, Schutte BPM: Multivariate logistic analysis of risk factors for stroke in Tilburg, The Netherlands. *Am J Epidemiol* 118:514–525, 1983.

92. Hoff GL, Martin TA: Outdoor and indoor soccer: injuries among youth players. *Am J Sports Med* 14:231–233, 1986.

93. Holme I, Helgland A, Hjermann I, Leren P, Lund-Larsen PG: Physical activity at work and at leisure in relation to coronary risk factors and social class: a 4-year mortality follow-up. The Oslo Study. *Acta Med Scand* 209:277–283, 1981.

94. Hornof Z, Napravnik C: Analysis of various accident rate factors in ice hockey. *Med Sci Sports* 5:283–286, 1973.

95. Horwitz RI, Feinstein AR: Methodologic standards and contradictory results in case-control research. *Am J Med* 66:556–562, 1979.

96. Husemann B, Neubauer MG, Duhme C: Sitzende tatigkeit und rektum-sigma-karzinom. *Onkologie* 4:1658–1671, 1980.

97. Iverson DC, Fielding JE, Crow RS, Christenson GM: The promotion of physical activity in the U.S. population: the status of programs in medical, worksite, community, and school settings. *Public Health Rep* 100:212–214, 1985.

98. Jacobs SJ, Berson BL: Injuries to runners: a study of entrants to a 10,000 meter race. *Am J Sports Med* 14:151–155, 1986.

99. Janda DH, Wojtys EM, Hankin FM: Softball sliding injuries. A prospective study comparing standard and modified bases. *JAMA* 259:1848–1850, 1988.

100. Jette M, Campbell J, Mongeon J, Routhier R: The Canadian Home Fitness Test as a predictor of aerobic capacity. *Can Med Assoc J* 114:180–182, 1976.

101. Jette M: The standardized test of fitness in occupational health: a pilot study. *Can J Public Health* 69:431–438, 1978.

102. Kahn HA: The relationship of reported coronary heart disease mortality to physical activity of work. *Am J Public Health* 53:1058–1067, 1963.

103. Kannel WB, Belanger A, D'Agostino R, Israel I: Physical activity and physical demand on the job and risk of cardiovascular disease and death: the Framingham Study. *Am Heart J* 112:820–825, 1986.

104. Kannel WB, Sorlie P: Some health benefits of physical activity: the Framingham Study. *Arch Intern Med* 139:857–861, 1979.

105. Kannel WB, Wilson PWF, Blair SN: Epidemiological assessment of the role of physical activity and fitness in development of cardiovascular disease. *Am Heart J* 109:876–885, 1985.

106. Kannel WB: Recent findings of the Framingham Study. *Resident Staff Physician* 24:56–71, 1978.

107. Kiburz D, Jacobs R, Reckling F, Mason J: Bicycle accidents and injuries among adult cyclists. *Am J Sports Med* 14:416–419, 1987.
108. Kiens B, Jorgensen I, Lewis S, Jensen G, Lithell H, Vessby B, Hoe S, Schnor P: Increased plasma HDL-cholesterol and apo A-1 in sedentary middle-aged men after physical conditioning. *Eur J Clin Invest* 10:203–209, 1980.
109. Klein PD, James WP, Wong WW, Irving CS, Murgatroyd PR, Cabrera M, Dallosso HM, Klein ER, Nichols BL: Calorimetric validation of the doubly-labeled water method for estimation of energy expenditure in man. *Hum Nutr Clin Nutr* 38C:95–106, 1984.
110. Klesges RC, Coates TJ, Molderhauer LM: The FATS: an observational system for assessing physical activity in children and associated parent behavior. *Behav Assess* 6:333–345, 1984.
111. Klesges RC, Klesges LM, Swenson A, Pheley M: A validation of two motion sensors in the prediction of child and adult physical activity levels. *Am J Epidemiol* 122:400–410, 1985.
112. Knuttgen HG: Force, work, power, and exercise. *Med Sci Sports* 10:227–228, 1978.
113. Koplan JP, Powell KE, Sikes RK, Shirley R, Campbell CC: An epidemiologic study of the benefits and risks of running. *JAMA* 248:3118–3121, 1982.
114. Koplan JP, Siscovick DS, Goldbaum G: The risk of exercise: a public health view of injuries and hazards. *Public Health Rep* 100:189–195, 1985.
115. Kramer MS, Boivin J-F: Toward an "unconfounded" classification of epidemiologic research design. *J Chronic Dis* 40:683–688, 1987.
116. Krauss J, Conroy C: Mortality and morbidity from injuries in sports and recreation. *Annu Rev Public Health* 5:163–192, 1984.
117. Kriska AM, Sandler RB, Cauley JA, LaPorte RE, Hom DL, Pambianco G: The assessment of historical physical activity and its relation to adult bone parameters. *Am J Epidemiol* 127:1053–1063, 1988.
118. LaPorte RE, Adams LL, Savage DD, Brenes E, Dearwater S, Cook T: The spectrum of physical activity, cardiovascular disease and health: an epidemiologic perspective. *Am J Epidemiol* 120:507–517, 1984.
119. LaPorte RE, Black-Sandler R, Cauley JA, Link M, Bayles C, Marks B: The assessment of physical activity in older women: analysis of the interrelationship and reliability of activity monitoring, activity surveys and caloric intake. *J Gerontol* 38:394–397, 1983.
120. LaPorte RE, Cauley JA, Kinsey CM, Corbett W, Robertson R, Black-Sandler R, Kuller LH, Falkel J: The epidemiology of physical activity in children, college students, middle aged men, menopausal females and monkeys. *J Chronic Dis* 35:787–795, 1982.
121. LaPorte RE, Kuller LH, Kupfer DJ, McPartland RJ, Matthews G, Caspersen C: An objective measure of physical activity for epidemiologic research. *Am J Epidemiol* 109:158–168, 1979.
122. LaPorte RE, Montoye HJ, Caspersen CJ: Assessment of physical activity in epidemiologic research: problems and prospects. *Public Health Rep* 100:131–146, 1985.
123. Langmuir AD: The surveillance of communicable diseases of national importance. *N Engl J Med* 268:182–192, 1963.
124. Lapidus L, Bengtssen C: Socioeconomic factors and physical activity in relation to cardiovascular disease and death. *Br Heart J* 55:295–301, 1986.
125. Last JM (ed): A Dictionary of Epidemiology. New York, Oxford University Press, 1983.
126. Leon AS, Blackburn H: The relationship of physical activity to coronary heart disease and life expectancy. *Ann NY Acad Sci* 301:561–578, 1977.

127. Leon AS, Connett J, Jacobs DR Jr, Rauramaa R: Leisure-time physical activity levels and risk of coronary heart disease and death: the Multiple Risk Factor Intervention Trial. *JAMA* 258:2388–2395, 1987.

128. Lie H, Mundal R, Erikssen J: Coronary risk factors and incidence of coronary death in relation to physical fitness. Seven-year follow-up study of middle-aged and elderly men. *Eur Heart J* 6:147–157, 1985.

129. Loosli AR, Requa RK, Ross W, Garrick JG: Injuries in slow-pitch softball. *Physician Sportsmed* 16:110–118, 1988.

130. Lorentzon R, Wedren H, Pietila T, Gustavsson B: Injuries in international ice hockey. A prospective, comparative study of injury incidence and injury types in international and Swedish elite ice hockey. *Am J Sports Med* 16:389–391, 1988.

131. Lorentzon R, Wedren H, Pietila T: Incidence, nature, and causes of ice hockey injuries. A three year prospective study of a Swedish elite ice hockey team. *Am J Sports Med* 16:392–396, 1988.

132. Lowry CB, Leveau BF: A retrospective study of gymnastics injuries to competitors and noncompetitors in private clubs. *Am J Sports Med* 10:237–239, 1982.

133. Magnus K, Matroos A, Strackee J: Walking, cycling, or gardening, with or without seasonal interruption, in relation to acute coronary events. *Am J Epidemiol* 110:724–733, 1979.

134. Marti B, Vader JP, Minder CE, Abelin T: On the epidemiology of runnning injuries: the Bern Grand-Prix Study. *Am J Sports Med* 16:285–294, 1988.

135. Maughan RJ, Miller JDB: Incidence of training-related injuries among marathon runners. *Br J Sports Med* 17:162–165, 1983.

136. McDonough JR, Hames CG, Stulb SC, Garrison GE: Coronary heart disease among negroes and whites in Evans county, Georgia. *J Chronic Dis* 18:443–448, 1965.

137. Menotti A, Puddu V: Ten-year mortality from coronary heart disease among 172,000, men classified by occupational physical activity. *Scand J Work Environ Health* 5:100–108, 1979.

138. Menotti A, Seccareccia F: Physical activity at work and job responsibility as risk factors for fatal coronary heart disease and other causes of death. *J Epidemiol Community Health* 39:325–329, 1985.

139. Michael M, Boyce WT, Wilcox AJ: Biomedical Bestiary: An Epidemiologic Guide to Flaws and Fallacies in the Medical Literature. Boston, Little, Brown, 1984.

140. Miller Brewing Company. *The Miller Lite Report on American Attitudes Towards Sports.* Miller Brewing Company, Milwaukee, 1983.

141. Montoye HJ, Taylor HL: Measurement of physical activity in population studies: a review. *Hum Biol* 56:195–216, 1984.

142. Montoye HJ, Washburn R, Servais S, Ertle LA, Webster JG, Nagle FJ: Estimation of energy expenditure by a portable accelerometer. *Med Sci Sports Exerc* 15:403–407, 1983.

143. Montoye HJ: Estimation of habitual physical activity by questionnaire and interview. *Am J Clin Nutr* 24:1113–1118, 1971.

144. Morgan K, Hughes AO, Philipp R: Reliability of a test of cardiovascular fitness. *Int J Epidemiol* 13:32–37, 1984.

145. Morris JN, Crawford MD: Coronary heart disease and physical activity of work: evidence of a national necropsy survey. *Br Med J* 2:1485–1496, 1958.

146. Morris JN, Everitt MG, Pollard R, Chave SPW: Vigorous exercise in leisure-time: protection against coronary heart disease. *Lancet* 2:1207–1210, 1980.

147. Morris JN, Hagan A, Pattison DC, Gardener MJ: Incidence and prediction of is-chemic heart disease in London busmen. *Lancet* 2:553–559, 1966.

148. Morris JN, Heady JA, Raffle PAB, Roberts CG, Parks JW: Coronary heart disease and physical activity of work. *Lancet* 265:1053–1057, 1111–1120, 1953.

149. Mortensen JM, Stevensen TT, Whitney LH: Mortality due to coronary disease analyzed by broad occupational groups. *Arch Ind Health* 19:1–4, 1959.
150. Mueller FO, Blyth CS: An update on football deaths and catastrophic injuries. *Physician Sportsmed* 14:139–142, 1986.
151. Mueller FO, Blyth CS: North Carolina high school injury study: equipment and prevention. *J Sports Med* 2:1–10, 1974.
152. Mueller JK, Gossard D, Adams F, Taylor CB, Haskell WL: Assessment of prescribed increases in physical activity: application of a new method for microprocessor analysis of heart rate. *Am J Cardiol* 57:441–445, 1986.
153. Nagle FS, Balke B, Naughton JP: Gradational step tests for assessing work capacity. *J Appl Physiol* 20:745–748, 1965.
154. Nathan M, Goedeke R, Noakes TD: The incidence and nature of rugby injuries experienced at one school during the 1982 rugby season. *S Afr Med J* 64:132–137, 1983.
155. Nilsson S, Roaas A: Soccer injuries in adolescents. *Am J Sports Med* 6:358–361, 1978.
156. Olson OC: The Spokane study: high school football injuries. *Physician Sportsmed* 7:75–82, 1979.
157. Paffenbarger RS Jr, Hale WE: Work activity and coronary heart disease mortality. *N Engl J Med* 292:545–550, 1975.
158. Paffenbarger RS Jr, Hale WE, Brand RJ, Hyde RT: Work-energy level, personal characteristics, and fatal heart attack: a birth-cohort effect. *Am J Epidemiol* 5:200–213, 1977.
159. Paffenbarger RS Jr, Hyde RT, Wing AL: Physical activity and incidence of cancer in diverse populations: a preliminary report. *Am J Clin Nutr* 45:312–317, 1987.
160. Paffenbarger RS Jr, Hyde RT, Wing AL, Hsieh C-C: Physical activity, all-cause mortality, and longevity of college alumni. *N Engl J Med* 314:605–614, 1986.
161. Paffenbarger RS Jr, Hyde RT, Wing AL, Steinmetz CH: A natural history of athleticism and cardiovascular health. *JAMA* 252:491–495, 1984.
162. Paffenbarger RS Jr, Wing AL, Hyde RT, Jung DL: Physical activity and incidence of hypertension in college alumni. *Am J Epidemiol* 117:245–256, 1983.
163. Paffenbarger RS Jr, Wing AL, Hyde RT: Physical activity as an index of heart attack risk in college alumni. *Am J Epidemiol* 108:161–175, 1978.
164. Pashby TJ: Eye injuries in Canadian hockey. Phase III. Older players now at most risk. *Can Med Assoc J* 121:643–644, 1979.
165. Passmore R, Durnin JVGA: Human energy expenditure. *Physiol Rev* 35:801–840, 1955.
166. Patrick JM, Bassey ES, Irving JM, Blecher A, Fentem PH: Objective measurements of customary physical activity in elderly men and women before and after retirement. *Q J Exp Physiol* 71:47–58, 1986.
167. Paul O, Lepper MH, Phelan WH, Dupertuis GW, MacMillan A, McKean H, Park H: A longitudinal study of coronary heart disease. *Circulation* 28:20–31, 1963.
168. Persky V, Dyer AR, Leonas J, Stamler J, Berkson DM, Lindberg HA, Paul O, Shekelle RB, Lepper MH, Schoenberger JA: Heart rate: a risk factor for cancer? *Am J Epidemiol* 114:477–487, 1981.
169. Peters RK, Cady LD Jr, Bischoff DP, Bernstein L, Pike MC: Physical fitness and subsequent myocardial infarction in healthy workers. *JAMA* 249:3052–3056, 1983.
170. Pettrone FA, Ricciardelli E: Gymnastic injuries: the Virginia experience 1982–1983. *Am J Sports Med* 15:59–62, 1987.
171. Pollock ML, Gettman LR, Milesis CA, Bah MD, Durstine L, Johnson RB: Effects of frequency and duration of training on attrition and incidence of injury. *Med Sci Sports* 9:31–36, 1977.

172. Pomrehn PR, Wallace RB, Burmeister LF: Ischemic heart disease mortality in Iowa farmers: the influence of life-style. *JAMA* 248:1073–1076, 1982.
173. Pooling Project Research Group: Relationship of blood pressure, serum cholesterol, smoking habit, relative weight and ECG abnormalities to incidence of major coronary events: final report of the pooling project. *J Chronic Dis* 31:202–306, 1978.
174. Powell KE, Kohl HW, Caspersen CJ, Blair SN: An epidemiologic perspective of running injuries. *Physician Sportsmed* 14:100–114, 1986.
175. Powell KE, Paffenbarger RS Jr: Workshop on epidemiologic and public health aspects of physical activity and exercise. *Public Health Rep* 100:118–126, 1985.
176. Powell KE, Thompson PD, Caspersen CJ, Kendrick JS: Physical activity and the incidence of coronary heart disease. *Annu Rev Public Health* 8:253–287, 1987.
177. Punsar S, Karvonen MJ: Physical activity and coronary heart disease in populations from east and west Finland. *Adv Cardiol* 18:196–207, 1976.
178. Raven PB: ACSM and its science. *Sports Med Bull* 23:3, 1988.
179. Reiff GG, Montoye HJ, Remington RD, Napier JA, Metzner HL, Epstein FH: Assessment of physical activity by questionnaire and interview. In Karvonen MJ, Barry AJ, (eds): Physical Activity and the Heart. Springfield, IL, Charles C Thomas, 1967, pp 336–372.
180. Robey JM, Blyth CS, Mueller FO: Athletic injuries: application of epidemiologic methods. *JAMA* 217:184–189, 1971.
181. Rosenman RH, Bawol RD, Oscherwitz M: A 4-year prospective study of the relationship of difficult habitual vocational physical activity to risk and incidence of coronary heart disease in volunteer federal employees. *Ann NY Acad Sci* 301:627–641, 1977.
182. Rosenman RH, Brand RJ, Jenkins CD, Friedman M, Straus R, Wurm M: Coronary heart disease in the Western Collaborative Group Study: final follow-up experience of a 8½ years. *JAMA* 233:872–877, 1975.
183. Ross CE, Hayes D: Exercise and psychologic well-being in the community. *Am J Epidemiol* 127:762–771, 1988.
184. Rothenberger LA, Chang JI, Cable TA: Prevalence and types of injuries in aerobic dancers. *Am J Sports Med* 16:403–407, 1988.
185. Roux CE, Goedeke R, Visser GR, van Zyl WA, Noakes TD: The epidemiology of schoolboy rugby injuries. *S Afr Med J* 71:307–313, 1987.
186. Sackett DL: Bias in analytic research. *J Chronic Dis* 32:51–63, 1979.
187. Sallis JF, Haskell WL, Wood PC, Fortmann SP, Rogers T, Blair SN, Paffenbarger RS, Jr.: Physical activity assessment methodology in the Five-City Project. *Am J Epidemiol* 121:91–106, 1985.
188. Sallis JF, Nader PR, Rupp JW, Atkins CJ, Wilson WC: San Diego surveyed for heart-healthy foods and exercise facilities. *Public Health Rep* 101:216–219, 1986.
189. Salonen JT, Lakka T: Assessment of physical activity in population studies—validity and consistency of the methods in the Kupoio ischemic heart disease risk factor study. *Scand J Sports Sci* 3:89–95, 1987.
190. Salonen JT, Puska P, Tuomilehto J: Physical activity and risk of myocardial infarction, cerebral stroke and death: a longitudinal study in Eastern Finland. *Am J Epidemiol* 115:526–537, 1982.
191. Salonen JT, Slater JS, Tuomilehto J: Leisure time and occupational physical activity: risk of death from ischemic heart disease. *Am J Epidemiol* 127:87–94, 1988.
192. Sandelin J, Santavirta S, Lattila R, Vuolle P, Sarna S: Sports injuries in a large urban population: occurrence and epidemiological aspects. *Int J Sports Med* 9:61–66,1988.
193. Saris W: The assessment and evaluation of daily physical activity in children: a review. *Acta Paediatr Scand Suppl* 318:37–48, 1985.

194. Saris WHM, Snel P, Backe J, van Waesberghe F, Binkhorst RA: A portable miniature solid-state heart rate recorder for monitoring daily physical activity. *Biotelemetry* 4:131–140, 1977.

195. Schlesselman JJ: "Proof" of cause and effect in epidemiological studies: criteria for judgement. *Prev Med* 16:195–210, 1987.

196. Schoeller DA, Webb P: Five day comparison of the doubly labeled water method with respiratory gas exchange. *Am J Clin Nutr* 40:153–158, 1984.

197. Schoeller DA, van Santen E: Measurement of energy expenditure in humans by doubly labeled water method. *J Appl Physiol* 53:955–959, 1982.

198. Schoeller DA: Energy expenditure from doubly labeled water: some fundamental considerations in humans. *Am J Clin Nutr* 38:999–1005, 1983.

199. Schoenborn CA: Health habits of U.S. adults, 1985: the 'Alameda 7' revisited. *Public Health Rep* 101:571–580, 1986.

200. Scragg R, Stewart A, Jackson R, Beaglehole R: Alcohol and exercise in myocardial infraction and sudden coronary death in men and women. *Am J Epidemiol* 126:77–85, 1987.

201. Shapiro S, Weinblatt E, Frank CW, Sager RV: The HIP study of incidence and prognosis of coronary heart disease: preliminary findings on incidence of myocardial infarction and angina. *J Chronic Dis* 18:527–558, 1965.

202. Shurtleff D: Section 30. Some characteristics related to the incidence of cardiovascular disease and death. Framingham study, an 18-year follow-up. In Kannel WB, Gordon T (eds): *The Framingham Study: An Epidemiologic Investigation of Cardiovascular Disease* (DHEW Pub No. (NIH) 74-599). Bethesda, MD, Public Health Service, 1976.

203. Siconolfi SF, Cullinane EM, Carleton RA, Thompson PD: Assessing $\dot{V}O_2max$ in epidemiologic studies: modification of the Astrand-Rhyming test. *Med Sci Sports Exerc* 14:335–338, 1982.

204. Siconolfi SF, Garger CE, Lasater TM, Carleton RA: A simple valid step test for estimating maximal oxygen uptake in epidemiologic studies. *Am J Epidemiol* 121:382–390, 1985.

205. Siconolfi SF, Lasater TM, Snow RC, Carleton RA: Self-reported physical activity compared with maximal oxygen uptake. *Am J Epidemiol* 122:101–105, 1985.

206. Siscovick DS, Weiss NS, Fletcher RH, Schoenbach BJ, Wagner EH: Habitual vigorous exercise and primary cardiac arrest: effect of other risk factors on the relationship. *J Chronic Dis* 37:625–631, 1984.

207. Siscovick DS, Weiss NS, Hallstrom AP, Inui TS, Peterson DR: Physical activity and primary cardiac-arrest. *JAMA* 248:3113–3117, 1982.

208. Slater CH, Green LW, Vernon SW, Keither VM: Problems in estimating the prevalence of physical activity from national surveys. *Prev Med* 16:107–118, 1987.

209. Sobolski J, Kornitzer M, DeBacker G, Dramaix M, Abramowicz M, Degre S, Denolin H: Protection against ischemic heart disease in the Belgian Physical Fitness Study: physical fitness rather than physical activity? *Am J Epidemiol* 125:601–610, 1987.

210. Sobolski JC, DeBacker G, Degre S, Kornitzer M, Denolin H: Physical activity, physical fitness and cardiovascular disease: design of a prospective epidemiologic study. *Cardiology* 67:35–51, 1981.

211. Sopko G, Jacobs DR, Taylor H: Dietary measures of physical activity. *Am J Epidemiol* 120:900–911, 1984.

212. Spain DM, Bradess VA: Occupational physical activity and the degree of coronary atherosclerosis in "normal" men. A postmortem study. *Circulation* 22:239–242, 1960.

213. Stamler J, Lindberg HA, Berkson DM, Shaffer A, Miller W, Poindexter A, Colwell M, Hall Y: Prevalence and incidence of coronary heart disease in strata of the labor force of a Chicago industrial corporation. *J Chronic Dis* 11:405–420, 1960.
214. Stephens T, Jacobs DR, White CC: The descriptive epidemiology of leisure-time physical activity. *Public Health Rep* 100: 147–158, 1985.
215. Stephens T: Exercise and mental health in the United States and Canada: evidence from four population surveys. *Prev Med* 17:35–47, 1988.
216. Stephens T: Secular trends in adult physical activity: exercise boom or bust? *Res Q Exercise Sport* 58:94–105, 1987.
217. Sullivan JA, Gross RH, Grana WA, Garcia-Moral CA: Evaluation of injuries in youth soccer. *Am J Sports Med* 8:325–327, 1980.
218. Sutherland GW: Fire on ice. *Am J Sports Med* 4:264–268, 1976.
219. Szklo M: Design and conduct of epidemiologic studies. *Prev Med* 16:142–149, 1987.
220. Tator CH, Edmonds VE: National survey of spinal injuries in hockey players. *Can Med Assoc J* 130:875–880, 1984.
221. Taylor CB, Coffey T, Berra K, Jaffaldano R, Casey K, Haskell WL: Seven-day activity and self-report compared to a direct measure of physical activity. *Am J Epidemiol* 120:818–824, 1984.
222. Taylor CB, Kraemer HC, Bragg DA, Miles LE, Rule B, Savin WM, De Busk RF: A new system for long-term recording and processing of heart rate and physical activity in outpatients. *Comput Biomed Res* 15:7, 1982.
223. Taylor HL, Blackburn H, Keys A, Parlin RW, Vasquez C, Punchner T: Five-year follow-up of employees of selected U.S. railroad companies. *Circulation* 41(Suppl I):I20–I39, 1970.
224. Taylor HL, Buskirk ER, Remington RD: Exercise in controlled trials of the prevention of coronary heart disease. *Fed Proc* 32:1623–1627, 1973.
225. Taylor HL, Jacobs DR, Schucker B, Knudsen J, Leon AS, DeBacker G: A questionnaire for the assessment of leisure time physical activities. *J Chronic Dis* 31:741–755, 1978.
226. Taylor HL, Klepetar E, Keys A, Parlin W, Blackburn H, Puchner T: Death rates among physically active and sedentary employees of the railroad industry. *Am J Public Health* 52:1697–1707, 1962.
227. Taylor HL, Parlin RW, Blackburn H, Keys A: Problems in the analysis of the relationship of coronary heart disease to physical activity or its lack, with special reference to sample size and occupational withdrawal. In Evang K, Andersen KL (eds): *Physical Activity in Health and Disease.* Oslo, Universitetsforlaget, 1966, pp 242–261.
228. Thacker SB, Berkelman RL: Public health surveillance in the United States. *Epidemiol Rev* 10:164–190, 1988.
229. Thompson N, Halpern B, Curl WW, Andrews JR, Hunter SC, McLeod WD: High school football injuries: evaluation. *Am J Sports Med* 15:117–124, 1987.
230. Thompson PD, Funk EJ, Carleton RA, Sturner WQ: Incidence of death during jogging in Rhode Island from 1975 through 1980. *JAMA* 247:2535–2538, 1982.
231. Tryon W: *Behavioral Assessment in Behavioral Medicine.* New York, Springer, 1985.
232. Vena JE, Graham S, Zielezny M, Swanson MK, Barnes RE, Nolan J: Lifetime occupational exercise and colon cancer. *Am J Epidemiol* 122:357–365, 1985.
233. Vena JE, Graham S, Zielezny M, Brosure J, Swanson MK: Occupational exercise and risk of cancer. *Am J Clin Nutr* 45:318–327, 1987.
234. Walter SD, Hart LE, Sutton JR, McIntosh JM, Gauld M: Training habits and injury experience in distance runners: age- and sex-related factors. *Physician Sportsmed* 16:101–113, 1988.
235. Walter SD, Sutton JR, McIntosh JM, Connolly C: The aetiology of sports injuries, a review of methodologies. *Sports Med* 2:47–58, 1985.

236. Warnold T, Lenner RA: Evaluation of the heart rate method to determine the daily energy expenditure in disease. A study of juvenile diabetics. *Am J Clin Nutr* 30:304–315, 1977.
237. Washburn RA, Adams L, Haile G: Physical activity assessment for epidemiologic research: the utility of two simplified approaches. *Prev Med* 16:636–646, 1987.
238. Washburn RA, Chin MK, Montoye HJ: Accuracy of pedometer in walking and running. *Res Q Exercise Sport* 51:695–702, 1980.
239. Washburn RA, Montoye HJ: The assessment of physical activity by questionnaire. *Am J Epidemiol* 123:563–576, 1986.
240. Washburn RA, Montoye HJ: Validity of heart rate as a measure of mean daily energy expenditure (abstract). *Med Sci Sports Exerc* 16:196–197, 1984.
241. Wilhelmsen L, Bjure J, Ekstrom-Jodal B, Aurell M, Grimby G, Svardsudd K, Tibblin G, Wedel H: Nine years' follow-up of a maximal exercise test in a random population sample of middle-aged men. *Cardiology* 68(suppl 2):1–8, 1981.
242. Wilhelmsen L, Tibblin G, Aurell M, Bjure J, Ekstrom-Jodal B, Grimby G: Physical activity, physical fitness and risk of myocardial infarction. *Adv Cardiol* 18:217–230, 1976.
243. Wilson PWF, Paffenbarger RS, Morris JN, Havlik RJ: Assessment methods for physical activity and physical fitness in population studies: a report of a NHLBI Workshop. *Am Heart J* 111:1177–1192, 1986.
244. Wong TC, Webster JG, Montoye HJ, Washburn RA: Portable accelerometer device for measuring human energy expenditure. *IEEE Trans Biomed Eng* 28:467–471, 1981.
245. Wu A, Paganini-Hill AH, Ross RK, Henderson BE: Alcohol, physical activity and other risk factors for colorectal cancer: a prospective study. *Br J Cancer* 55:687–694, 1987.
246. Yach D, Botha JL: Epidemiological research methods: Part I. Why epidemiology? *S Afr Med J* 70:267–270, 1986.
247. Yach D, Botha JL: Epidemiological research methods: Part II. Descriptive studies. *S Afr Med J* 70:766–772, 1986.
248. Yach D, Botha JL: Epidemiological research methods: Part VII. Epidemiological research in health planning. *S Afr Med J* 72:633–636, 1987.
249. Yano K, Reed DM, McGee DL: Ten-year incidence of coronary heart disease in the Honolulu Heart Program. *Am J Epidemiol* 119:653–666, 1984.
250. Yasin NS, Alderson MR, Marr JW, Pattison DC, Morris JN: Assessment of habitual physical activity apart from occupation. *Br J Soc Prev Med* 21:163–169, 1967.
251. Yasin S: Measuring habitual leisure time physical activity by recall record questionnaire. In Karvonen MJ, Barry AJ (eds): *Physical Activity and the Heart*. Springfield, IL, Charles C Thomas, 1967, pp 372–373.
252. Zukel WJ, Lewis RH, Enterline PE, Painter RC, Ralston LS, Fawcett RM, Meredith AP, Peterson B: A short-term community study of the epidemiology of coronary heart disease. *Am J Public Health* 49:1630–1639, 1959.

13
Modeling Considerations in Motor Skill Acquisition and Performance: An Integrated Approach

PENNY McCULLAGH, Ph.D.
MAUREEN R. WEISS, Ph.D.
DIANE ROSS, Ph.D.

Visual demonstrations have been used extensively as an instructional technique for a variety of skills. In fact, social psychologists have long acknowledged modeling "to be one of the most powerful means of transmitting values, attitudes and patterns of thought and behaviors" [7]. Over the years a variety of terms including "imitation," "identification," "modeling," "vicarious learning," and "observational learning" have been employed to refer to the process of reproducing actions that have been executed by another individual. In general, the theoretical explanations for the modeling process have corresponded with the psychological orientations of the era and have moved from instinctual interpretations [133] through classical conditioning [63], reinforcement [95], and more recently cognitive interpretations [5–7, 129]. The primary theoretical basis for observational learning in the last two decades has been derived from Bandura's progressive reformulations of mediational–contiguity theory [5], social learning theory [6], and more recently the social cognitive analysis of observational learning [7].

Although Bandura's theory has generated a great deal of interest among social psychologists, surprisingly little theoretical research has been conducted examining the acquisition and retention of motor or sport skills [56]. This paucity of research is surprising considering the wide use of demonstrations as an instructional technique, and more recently the use of videotapes to enhance elite performance [132].

The integrated perspective proposed herein addresses pertinent issues from a multidisciplinary perspective within motor behavior. These include social psychological, developmental, and motor learning/control principles. We believe that the researchers in these motor behavior fields have not energetically pursued the study of modeling for a number of reasons.

First, Bandura's original theory was primarily designed for the acquisition and modification of social skills and behaviors. Motor learning researchers may not have pursued modeling since the process for acquiring motor skills may be markedly different from that of learning social skills [100] and the available theory was not viewed as viable. Also, motor learning researchers have demonstrated strong allegiance to tests of Adams' closed loop theory [1] and Schmidt's schema theory [119] to explain skill learning. Both theories rely heavily on the role of knowledge of results after movement as the primary source of information for improving performance. It is indeed interesting that just recently Adams [2], who sparked this long line of research, now claims that the skill acquisition literature "has featured instrumental learning operations at the expense of other learning paradigms" and has suggested that we focus attention on observational learning. Newell's [100] review on skill learning had previously recognized the role of demonstrations as a means of providing information prior to action but little scholarly interest was generated.

Second, observational learning did not receive much attention from motor development specialists because Bandura's original formulations did not include developmental considerations. Subsequent theoretical delineations [7, 154] speak to these issues and limited research in motor behavior [93, 147, 148] has recently emerged.

Finally, although Bandura's theory was employed by motor behavior researchers interested in social psychological variables that influence modeling, direct examination of the theory has been meager [103]. For example, Bandura hypothesized that model characteristics influence attention and therefore learning. Few studies have attempted to directly [156] or indirectly [89, 90] test this prediction although model characteristics have been manipulated and performance effects observed [57, 75].

It is our contention that modeling is an extremely viable topic for motor behavior researchers since it can potentially consolidate aspects of all three motor behavior subdisciplines. Modeling can be approached from a developmental perspective; it can incorporate principles of motor learning and movement control; and it can encompass social psychological variables that may influence the performer. However, few studies to date have incorporated aspects of the subdisciplines into modeling [e.g., 82].

The purposes of the present chapter are to propose a model of observational learning that consolidates aspects of the major motor behavior disciplines, review current research that examines issues related to the model, and finally propose hypotheses and directions for future research. The model presented in Figure 13.1 illustrates the multidimensionality of observational learning and will serve as the basis for discussion in this chapter.

A primary consideration in modeling is the impact of the observer on what is perceived in the demonstration and how this information is

FIGURE 13.1
Modeling considerations in skill acquisition and performance.

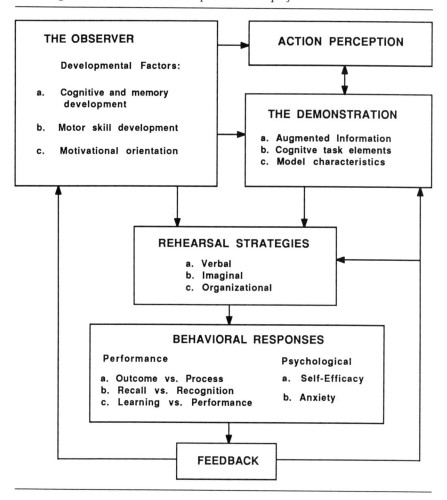

rehearsed. A second element that has received only limited attention in the motor behavior literature is action perception, which focuses on the perception of human motion. This is argued as an important aspect of modeling since observers must perceive the motions they are later required to reproduce. Within observational learning a number of factors may have a direct impact on the demonstration itself, and how well the movement is reproduced can be influenced by the rehearsal strategies employed by the learner. In addition, the level of analysis employed in determining the adequacy of the response on both reproduction and psychological factors is an important consideration when assessing the acquisition and subsequent performance of movement or sport skills. Finally, although full discussion is beyond the scope of the present chapter, brief mention will be made of feedback principles that may have impact on the modeling process.

THE OBSERVER

When addressing the role of the observer in the modeling of motor skills and behaviors, there are two questions of interest: (*a*) What characteristics of the observer influence the relationship between modeling and performance? And (*b*) what effects can observational learning have on the psychological (nonperformance) characteristics of the observer? The first question will be addressed with a focus on developmental factors as they influence the modeling process, with particular emphasis on cognitive differences, physical abilities, and motivational orientation. The second question is addressed in the Behavioral Response section.

Developmental Factors
When considering aspects of developmental modeling, knowledges from four perspectives must be integrated. These are *cognitive development*, or in general the way in which individuals process and assimilate information from the model; *memory development*, with a focus on rehearsal strategies; *motor skill development*, including the qualitative changes in motor skill acquisition and performance; and *social psychology*, with particular interest in the motives individuals have for attempting to reproduce modeled actions. There is very little research on modeling and motor skill acquisition from a developmental perspective, and one of the major reasons is a failure to integrate these areas of knowledge.

To better address the role of developmental factors in observational learning, Yando et al. [154] formulated a two-factor theory of imitation. Their consolidation of other modeling theories (e.g., Piaget, Bandura) was based on an extensive study of 4-, 7-, 10-, and 13-year-old children. They found that the age period from 4 to 7 years is a transitional stage in which a variety of related neurophysiological changes occur, resulting in increasingly more cognitive, perceptual, and motor organization. For example, evidence shows that the child's motor system comes under verbal system control during these years [41, 83] and that the predominance of visual systems in early years gradually gives way to symbolic and verbal representation at more advanced stages of development [18]. In a recent study [108], it was found that by age 3 years, children are influenced by both the motor and verbal aspects of modeling, suggesting that we must examine both the motor behaviors of models as well as how they verbally describe their behaviors when considering developmental issues.

In Yando et al.'s [154] two-factor theory of modeling, the cognitive–developmental factor addresses attention span and selective attention capabilities, memory capacity, coding capabilities and use of rehearsal strategies, and physical and motoric capabilities. Motivational orientation addresses the role of intrinsic incentives (e.g., model characteristics, competence-related motives) versus extrinsic incentives (e.g., avoidance of punishment, gain tangible reinforcement) in the modeling process. It is clear that their theory is markedly similar to Bandura's conceptualization. However, developmental factors are emphasized, particularly the qualitative differences on these factors with age. Little research has been conducted to test Yando et al.'s theory, but studies that have focused on cognitive–developmental factors in motor performance [45, 50, 147, 148] have lent credibility to Yando et al.'s theory.

COGNITIVE AND MEMORY DEVELOPMENT. A great deal of insight on cognitive and memory development has been provided by Thomas, Gallagher, and their associates [45–50, 134, 136, 152]. They have demonstrated age differences in information processing capabilities, particularly selective attention, visual processing speed, and control processes such as labeling, rehearsal, and organization. For example, attention to appropriate movement characteristics proceeds from overexclusiveness in which a limited number of cues are utilized (up to ages 5–6) to overinclusiveness in which both relevant and irrelevant task stimuli are assimilated (between about 6 and 11–12 years) and finally to selective attention (over 11–12 years) [47]. With speed of visual processing, older children process more information in the same time it takes younger children to process less information [134].

Control processes also differentiate the younger from the older child. Children less than 7 or 8 years of age do not tend to label or name modeled cues without prompting, or to engage in spontaneous rehearsal to help remember movements. Finally, younger children do not have the cognitive abilities to effectively and efficiently organize and chunk information as with grouping or recoding strategies. Labeling, rehearsal, and organization are strategies designed to facilitate moving information from short-term to long-term memory, thereby affecting the ability to retain and reproduce modeled skills [134]. Recent articles on the development of knowledge structures [43, 135] suggest that the ability to use memory strategies contributes to the development of a knowledge base which, in turn, can enhance decision making, motor control, and actual execution of motor skills and strategies.

In sum, this work by motor behavior researchers confirms earlier hypotheses about the use of verbal self-instructional skills in the execution of motor output [41, 83]. For example, Flavell's [41] production deficiency hypothesis underscored differences between younger and older children. Flavell stated that (a) an activity may be within a child's reach but spontaneous use of a verbal strategy to guide behavior is not used, (b) an increase in overt self-instruction occurs between the ages of 5 and 7 years, (c) spontaneous verbal strategies are seldom used under 6 years of age, and (d) tasks requiring sequential movements may be especially conducive to self-regulating speech. These points not only have salience for the modeling of motor skills but provide guidelines for practical applications as well. Fuson [44], in a review of the literature on verbal rehearsal strategies, summarized that the two major effects of rehearsal and self-instructional verbal strategies are attention focusing and retention facilitation.

Some studies have examined age differences in modeling [4, 30, 137], but few studies to date have examined cognitive–developmental factors in modeling from an information processing perspective [93, 147, 148]. Findings from these various studies, however, provide a great deal of insight and a starting place for further developmental inquiry.

Feltz [30] was interested in differences between children and adults as well as number of demonstrations on a balance task and found that both form and outcome scores differentiated the age groups. In addition, when subjects were asked to describe the demonstration which they saw, children were able to describe only one component of form correctly, as compared to the three components identified by the adults. Feltz concluded that children's performance was probably lower because of attentional and/or retentional deficits, and that a model who verbalized skill components may have facilitated both cognitive and execution capabilities.

Weiss [147] has investigated the interaction between age level and instructional type on modeling of a motor skill sequence. Ages of children were chosen on the basis of cognitive–developmental criteria as suggested by Yando et al.'s theory and the verbal rehearsal literature. Thus, 4- to 5- and 7- to 8-year-old children were randomly assigned to instructional type conditions (verbal model, silent model, or no model) and verbal self-instruction condition (presence or absence of instructions to use this strategy). Results revealed an interaction between age and model type, with older children benefiting equally from either model condition, but younger children performing best under a verbal model only. The findings offered support for Yando et al.'s theory that cognitive–developmental differences such as attention, retention, and verbal–cognitive abilities play a critical role in the modeling process. Specifically, the verbal or "show and tell" model appeared to enhance selective attention and retention of the modeled skills by younger children.

In a subsequent study, Weiss and Klint [148] assigned younger (5-0 to 6-11 years) and older (8-0 to 9-11 years) children to one of four instructional groups. Again, a motor skill sequence served as the task. Quantitative results indicated that the verbal rehearsal only and model plus rehearsal groups performed significantly better than the verbal model and control groups, regardless of age. However, qualitative analyses indicated that although the verbal model plus rehearsal and verbal rehearsal only groups were best for either age group, the two groups of children went about remembering the motor sequence in markedly different ways. When asked "How did you try to remember the order of the skills?", younger children responded, "I thought in my head," "I thought hard," "I don't know," and "Used my brain." Older children most frequently referred to strategies such as: "I thought about what I had done and what was left to do," "Saying it over in my mind," and "I pictured in my mind the order of the skills."

These and other verbal descriptions and behavioral indicants suggested that older children were more planful in devising memory strategies to help subsequent performance. The frequency with which remembering strategies were used and the quality of the strategies themselves signified cognitive–developmental differences between younger and older children. In sum, however, verbal rehearsal appeared to be the critical component of demonstrations for children. The use of a retention design, however, may have uncovered whether the model plus rehearsal condition may have emerged as a superior instructional method to verbal rehearsal only.

Finally, McCullagh et al. [93] designed a dance sequence in which children ages 5-0 to 6-6 and 7-6 to 9-0 years of age either saw a visual demonstration with verbal cues or received a verbal explanation. Following these manipulations, subjects either verbally or did not verbally rehearse the sequence before execution. Both quantitative (sequencing) and qualitative (form) performance were measured. Results revealed that for both age groups, the visual model resulted in better qualitative performance than verbal instructions, but verbal instructions were conducive to better sequencing scores than a visual model. The lack of an age by model type or rehearsal interaction might be attributed to the nature of the modeling conditions in that both entailed verbal cues which perhaps facilitated attention and/or retention for both age groups, but were of particular help for the younger children. In sum, these few studies demonstrate that an understanding of cognitive and memory development differences in children provides a great deal of insight into the ability of children to reproduce modeled actions.

MOTOR SKILL DEVELOPMENT. Inherent in all modeling theories is the ability of the observer to physically reproduce the modeled action. Even if the learner possesses the cognitive capabilities for symbolically organizing the visual demonstration, unless these thoughts can be translated to action, modeling will have no visible effects. Burwitz and Borrie [19] contend that many of the equivocal findings with regard to the effect of modeling on motor performance may be attributed to naive subjects not possessing the requisite skills for replicating the model's actions. In fact, little to date is known about the role of skill or experience on observational learning.

The notion of physical abilities in the modeling process necessarily contends that such factors as strength, endurance, coordination, timing, and balance must be required to reproduce movements demonstrated by a model. A good example is the Feltz [30] study described earlier. Children performed more poorly than adults on a balance task, and were also unable to remember as many of the model's actions. Although many (91%) were able to recall the important quickness component of the model, only 49% actually reproduced it. Thus, the age differences in modeling in this study could have been due, at least in part, to the larger repertoire of physical skills and abilities on the part of the adults. Thus, in order to maximize modeling effects, children may require more practice time than adults.

Insight regarding children's capabilities for physically reproducing motor skills can be obtained from a recent review of the motor development literature [144]. Fundamental motor skill development can be viewed from two perspectives. Using the total body approach (associated with researchers at Michigan State University), research has shown that at age 6, only 60% of boys and 60% of girls were able to perform two out of eight fundamental motor skills at a mature level (boys: running, throwing; girls: running, skipping). Using a component approach (associated with the researchers at the University of Wisconsin) to ask the same question revealed that by age 13, only 29% of girls but 82% of boys had reached the advanced level of humerus action in the overarm throw. The common findings from both approaches seem to suggest that while children can at least minimally reproduce fundamental motor skills to some degree, there is a tremendous amount of variability in the quality of movements among age groups as well as between and within genders.

However, few modeling studies have assessed modeling effects on qualitative changes in motor skills such as form or technique [30, 90, 93, 113], but have instead focused on performance outcome such as distance, height, and time. What researchers and practitioners are really interested in, however, is the quality of movement such as the technique of a movement, maturity of a fundamental motor skill, or the overall coordination of body parts in relation to a skill sequence. If we really want to assess the child's ability to reproduce modeled actions, then we must measure the extent to which they qualitatively produce, rather than quantitatively perform modeled skills. These issues of outcome versus process are considered further in a discussion of response considerations later in this chapter.

Finally, other factors to consider with regard to the role of physical abilities in modeling include physical maturity, body size and composition, and experience participating in organized sport. For example, since early-maturing children tend to perform motor skills better than do late maturers, it is perhaps logical to suggest that early maturers may benefit more from modeling strategies due to their richer cognitive and physical repertoire. Children of various body sizes or compositions may be more inclined to reproduce certain modeled tasks better than others (e.g., a small, thin child versus a large child executing a cartwheel). Finally, recent evidence seems to suggest that years of experience participating in organized sport contributes to an overall knowledge base and a repertoire of movements needed for more advanced skills and strategies [43, 135, 143]. Thus, children who have had youth sport opportunities may be at an advantage in modeling new motor skills based on these characteristics. However, physical maturity, body type, and sport experience factors remain to be tested with regard to their influence on the relationship between modeling and motor performance.

MOTIVATIONAL ORIENTATION. The second factor of Yando et al.'s [154] developmental theory of modeling dealt with the intrinsic/extrinsic motives observers hold for modeling behavior. That is, even if a child selectively attends to task relevant cues, verbally rehearses required skill components, and possesses the requisite physical abilities to reproduce modeled actions, matching behaviors may not occur because of a lack of desire or motivation. Thus, incentives need to be considered in the observational learning of motor skills.

Yando et al. [154] address the possible intrinsic and extrinsic motives that may guide an observer's behavior. Extrinsic motives refer to the rewards or punishments that may occur as a result of modeling or not modeling behavior. The focus here, however, is on intrinsic motives in the observational learning process, which have been primarily couched in competence-related motives [60, 61, 149] and affective or attachment-related motives (primarily characteristics of the model in relation to the observer).

Competence motives refer to the individual's desire to have an effect on the environment, be good at something, or simply do something well. When individuals engage in mastery attempts which are perceived as "successful," positive affect, enhanced self-esteem, and perceptions of internal control result [60, 61]. These characteristics are then predictive of future motivated behavior. From the perspective of modeling, the central notion would be to meet competence or intrinsic motives by demonstrating optimal challenges for the observer to emulate. Yando et al. [154] refer to this as the "cutting edge hypothesis": Skills or tasks which are just beyond the reach of the observer's current level are ideal for modeling to affect skill acquisition and performance. To date, however, no studies have examined the challenge of the demonstrated task in relation to physical capabilities for reproducing the skills. Such potential "optimal challenge modeling" studies could include (a) varying the task difficulty variable (e.g., easy, optimal, difficult) in relation to observer's capabilities, (b) varying the type of instructional strategy (e.g., autocratic vs. problem-solving style), (c) varying the spacing of demonstrations and physical practice, and (d) varying the emphasis on learning versus performance goals.

Most studies addressing the issue of modeling and motivation, whether developmental or nondevelopmental in nature, have focused on attachment motives or, rather, the model/observer relationship. Thus, the characteristics of the model can have a motivational effect on the observer by the perceived bond that exists. One of the key model characteristics, especially in research with children, is the similarity of the model to the observer, which could include such factors as age, gender, status, and competence.

The use of peer models, in particular, has been a popular area of study with regard to motivational effects. The underlying tenet of a peer model is that individuals will be motivated to emulate modeled actions because of the vicarious involvement of a similar other. Specifically, a peer model may not be constraining with regard to ability as an adult might be. For example, Feltz [31] used a peer model along with an adult model to teach a 12-year-old mentally retarded child to execute a modified forward dive. The peer model was a friend of the subject, held in high esteem and similar in age and IQ. Although it was not possible from the design of this study to tease out the effects of the adult and peer model, the student was able to master the skill in four sessions and was able to sustain performance at a 3-week follow-up test.

Brody and Stoneman [16, 17] conducted two studies to examine how age-similar and -dissimilar (younger or older) peers influenced acquisition and performance of nonmotor behaviors via modeling. In the first study [16], results revealed that children selectively imitated same age and older models (> 2 years) when they were juxtaposed with a younger peer. In a subsequent study [17] children were exposed to models that varied in age (same or younger) and competence (same, lower, or no information provided). Results revealed that in the absence of competence information, observers modeled actions of same-age peers more frequently than younger models, and in the presence of competence and age information, modeling was primarily influenced by information regarding the model's competence (i.e., younger model with same-age competence over a same-age model with younger competence).

Finally, in a recent study by Schunk et al. [122], peer models who varied in either mastery or coping behavior were examined in relation to children's performance on mathematical skills. A mastery model was one who demonstrated faultless performance on the math skills, while the coping model initially demonstrated (verbalized) the typical fears and deficiencies of observers but gradually improved his or her performance. Results indicated that the observers rated themselves as more similar to the coping model and demonstrated higher self-efficacy, skill, and training performance than observers of a mastery model. Since self-efficacy is predictive of motivated behavior in the form of choice, effort, and persistence, the use of similar, and in this case coping, models has the effect of maximizing the modeling–performance relationship.

ACTION PERCEPTION

Traditional View

From the perspective of Bandura's social learning theory [5–7], the model is considered to contain information which can be acquired through visual observation. This information is then transformed into symbolic codes which can be cognitively rehearsed and which function to mediate the desired response. That is, the cognitive representation guides response execution and functions as the standard against which performance feedback is compared so that response adjustments are possible. Bandura postulates the requirement of four subprocesses which govern the acquisition of cognitive representations: attention, retention, motoric reproduction, and motivation/reinforcement.

One of the major distinctions between social learning theory and action systems views [72, 73, 104, 112] is the requirement of translation and mediation. Once observed behaviors are cognitively represented, they can be translated into action. During actual motoric reproduction, visual monitoring of the response provides the information for comparison with the cognitive representation so that, through mediation, mismatches are corrected and retention improved. It has been demonstrated that concurrent visual monitoring of a series of movements performed outside the visual field facilitates future reproductions of that action if an adequate cognitive representation had been previously developed [21, 22]. At the same time, the more accurate the cognitive representation, the more skilled are reproductions of the modeled actions [23].

Bandura's theory rests on a mediation function between the content of the cognitive information and the motor output. Action theorists have no need to postulate such a mediation function since it is the perception of the content of the environment as viewed by the mover which determines the motor response directly. Social learning theory is mechanistic and follows the traditional information processing perspective [5, 7].

There are specific and clearly defined predictions which are testable. For example, the type of information processed is dependent on the observer's attention to relevant cues in the modeled behavior and thus determines the accuracy of the cognitive representation [20, 89, 90]. The quality and clarity of the input will influence the translation of conception into action and rehearsal strategies will affect the retention process differentially as well as other predictions discussed in this chapter. To date, social learning theory is certainly the most popular theoretical explanation for observational learning effects.

Action Perception Theory
The application of action perception theory to motor skills and observational learning is relatively recent and has been rather limited, probably due to the strength of mechanistic approaches to learning movement skills such as Thorndike's [138] behavioristic views and information processing concepts [1, 119]. The study of perception in psychology paralleled the theoretical work in motor skills. Gibson [52] was the spokesperson for the position of direct visual perception as opposed to the classical indirect perspective of perception which, while no longer popular, still has its strong supporters [e.g., 58]. However, it is the notion of direct perception which has theoretical implications for developing explanations for observational learning. Since vision is the most heavily relied on sensory modality for environmental information and appears to be intimately related to the motor system, examination of how vision relates to action perception may aid in understanding observational learning.

DIRECT PERCEPTION. The position of Gibson [52] and those who followed his view of visual perception [e.g., 26, 70, 71], is that the stimulus itself contains all the information necessary for three-dimensional perception, and therefore it is not necessary to determine how retinal images are translated by the observer into percepts and then into action/movements. In contrast, the classical perspective has been termed indirect. Indirect perception requires additional levels of information transformation to explain the relationship between external events and perception. For example, in Whiting's [150] information processing model, which posits perceptual mechanisms, translatory mechanisms, and movement mechanisms, the basic notion of indirect perception and movement is articulated in a motor skills context. Gibson [52], on the other hand, stated that the essence of the study of perception should focus on *what* is perceived rather than *how* it is perceived.

From the direct perception view it follows that the perceiving beings' navigation through the environment is based on changes in the optic array [53, 54]. That is, movement relative to the environment results in an optic flow pattern at the eye. The structure of the flow pattern is dependent on the form of the movement and the structure or organization of the environment. It is the spatial and temporal components of the optic flow pattern which give valuable information to the perceiver [see 39]. For example, as the head moves forward in a stable environment, the visual field tends to expand or the eye perceives an outward-flow pattern, but movement backward away from the stationary environment results in a contraction of the visual array [140]. However, if the environment is moving toward a stationary head and eye position, the visual array will expand but there will be a deletion of clarity of those items behind the approaching object. Thus, there is an invariant pattern of change for every type of movement (e.g., linear, circular). It is the invariant characteristics in the optical flow pattern that are of interest to action perception theorists [125].

PERCEPTION AND MOVEMENT. A theory of action perception articulated by Turvey [140] and Kugler et al. [73] emphasizes an ecological viewpoint whereby action is examined in its natural context. "Adaptation to an environment is synonymous with the evolution of special biological and behavioral features that are compatible with special features of the environment" [42]. Thus, an organism exhibits skilled motor behavior as it adapts to the environment in which the movement occurs and which determines its behavior. The movement becomes the property of a physically constrained system [125]. However, for the movement to be coordinated in the environment there must be reciprocity between the action and perception.

From this point of view, action is thought to be executed through the control of groups of muscles referred to as "coordinative structures" [12, 141]. These muscle groups function together as a unit and are sensitive to constraints in the environment, and individual commands to specific muscles (as proposed by Pew [109] and Schmidt [119]) are not a conceivable mode of functioning. Given the number of possible combinations of specific muscles and possible tension values and contraction speeds, it would be impossible for the system to respond as efficiently and effectively as it would if all parameters had to be specified by the biological system. The solution to this "degrees of freedom" problem is to conceptualize the system as functioning through coordinative structures [see reference 142 for a clear discussion of this solution]. Thus, the concept of action perception posits that visual perception of environmental constraints during biological motion results in alterations (tuning) of the coordinative structures [39, 139, 142]. This alteration is thought to be produced by "varying a minimal number of parameters to produce a maximal amount of behavioral change" [39].

One of the lines of evidence to demonstrate the power of the visual system is in the "moving room" experiments [79, 80]. In these situations, Lee uses a large bottomless box suspended just above the floor. Subjects, both adults and infants, standing in the center of the box unconsciously and unavoidably produce postural adjustments when the room sways. Subjects either sway excessively or lose their balance. The only source of information to elicit these changes is visual since neither the floor nor the individual moves prior to the movement correction. Lee has further explained the role of vision in orienting, body-centered activities, and locomoting: the basic components of motor skills, particularly sport skills [77, 78]. For example, one need only think of how it feels to step off a curb that is unexpected. The motor system is not prepared for the slight change in elevation and responds rather drastically. However, if visual perception of the environment is available prior to stepping off the curb, alteration or tuning of the movement pattern occurs automatically.

Research Implications
The view that perception is action and action is perception suggests alternate ways of studying the field of observational learning. Newell, Morris, and Scully [103] in a strongly critical perspective of the observational learning research state that the important question of *what* information should be conveyed through modeling has not been studied. Rather the question of *how* to display the desired behavior has been the thrust of previous work. Newell [101] has also suggested that the action systems perspective lends itself to the study of coordination, control, and skill in the learning of motor tasks. He states that coordination can be considered as the topological quality (kinematics) of the action while control can be thought of as the scalar value (speed) of the movement. Thus, skill requires that an optimal value be assigned to the controlled variables. If in the initial stages of learning it is the coordination function which is to be learned, then perhaps the appropriate relative motion patterns should be provided in any demonstration [101]. Under these conditions data from Newell and Walter [105] suggest it may also be important that the response contingent feedback be in the same format.

In an attempt to identify what is critical in the demonstration for the observer, Johansson [71] has shown (using the point-light technique which provides relative motion information in the absence of structural cues) that observers can differentiate a human walk from a wooden puppet walk. But how are observers able to do this? According to Cutting [25] events such as walking have an underlying structure regardless of the surface contours. It is the perception of invariance in the underlying structure of the event which gives rise to the ability to distinguish accurately the two forms of walking. Both topographic invariants and dynamic invariants provide the essential characteristics of structural relations in space and structural relations in time. Cutting [25] defines topographic invariants as "structural properties in space that hold over the course of the event," and dynamic invariants as "rules that govern the nature of change over the course of the event".

Some very interesting work has recently been done by Scully [124–126]. Using the point-light technique Scully [124] has shown that observers can perceive and thus judge both technical execution and aesthetic qualities in balance beam routines almost as well as they do from the natural performance. Evidently the kinematics of transformational information provided in the point-light display were sufficient to evaluate performance of a known skill. This phenomenon was evidenced in all three groups of judges who had varying experience levels.

In a well-designed series of experiments, Scully [125] attempted to determine in a sport skill context if the topological properties of the relative motion patterns are invariant and if the scaling of these relative motion patterns can be noted. Relative motion in this context was considered to be the displacement pattern of the limbs, while absolute motion was defined as the speed of the total movement (e.g., fast, medium, or slow). To test these concepts Scully used the overarm throw and the overarm bowl because the two patterns of movement are similar and yet distinct. Observers were asked to classify seven relative motion patterns comprised of one real action pattern of each skill, two abstraction patterns of each skill (e.g., an overarm throw with less whiplike action of the elbow), and one ambiguous pattern. These seven relative patterns were presented at five speeds ranging from very slow to very fast. Observers viewing the point-light displays were able to classify correctly the real movement patterns 100% of the time and the abstractions of the bowl or throw 92–97% of the time. They were able to do this regardless of the speed of the movement presentation. Thus, the topological characteristics were perceived as invariant even though the absolute motion varied.

In Experiment 2 the speed of point-light displays were varied. Three point-light speeds were used. For the real action patterns, there was no perception problem at all three speeds. However, observers perceived the abstraction patterns differently. Hence, the relative motion of the movement pattern is invariant across abstractions of the movement pattern, but the scaling factor or perception of absolute motion appears to have boundary limits for categorization. These studies seem to link together the notion of the relationship between direct action and perception and lead to a greater understanding of what in the demonstration may be essential in observational learning. Since in the Scully experiments it was the relative motion pattern which was critical, one is led to the conclusion that static demonstrations (still pictures) provide little information regarding coordination of the pattern [126].

Future research from this perspective should be directed toward determining how the learner reproduces the observed action pattern. Since changes in relative motion provide the critical features for individuals to distinguish movement patterns, the dependent variables should be the topographical characteristics (kinematics) rather than the goal outcome. If, as suggested [101], the control factor is the scaling function, then future studies should determine if demonstrations containing scaling information do assist in the reproduction of movement control. Lastly, if being skilled means optimizing the control variables, then it needs to be shown that this too can be learned through observational learning as, perhaps, the results of both Hatze [62] and Howell [68] suggest.

THE DEMONSTRATION

When teaching someone a novel skill or when attempting to modify one's existing skill level through demonstrations, elements contained within the demonstration may have an influence on a performer's subsequent responses. We have identified three elements of the demonstration that have been shown to influence performance levels: (a) Augmented information may be provided in addition to the visual information inherent in the demonstration, (b) the cognitive elements of the task may influence the extent of modeling effects, and (c) the characteristics of the demonstrator or model may influence performance.

Augmented Information

Typically, augmented information is used to refer to information that is provided to subjects after movement. As noted by Newell et al. [103], however, augmented information need not be restricted to the feedback situation and they use the term in its broadest sense to refer to any information not inherent in the task that conveys information to a learner. The issue to be addressed here is what information, in addition to a demonstration, may be useful for skill acquisition and performance. For example, what modalities are important for skill learning, and are verbal cues in addition to visual information important? If we presume that a demonstration provides useful information to a learner then can the limits of the demonstration be enhanced by additional information?

When providing learners with a demonstration we typically think of using visual demonstrations; however, for some motor skills an auditory demonstration may be effective. Newell [99, Experiment 1], designed an experiment to determine if subjects could develop recognition memory for a timing movement from auditory demonstrations in the absence of physical practice with knowledge of results. Increasing the number of sound demonstrations led to better recognition memory. Other researchers have similarly supported the efficacy of auditory demonstrations [157].

More recently, Doody et al. [27] investigated the potency of various modalities for enhancing the cognitive representation induced by a model in a timing skill and compared demonstrations to knowledge of results.

Knowledge of results has long been held as the most important variable for motor learning, and these authors questioned whether demonstrations were as potent a source of information for enhancing the cognitive representation. Control subjects physically practiced the timing skill and received knowledge of results (KR) after each attempt while subjects in the demonstration groups received 10 physical practice trials interspersed with 50 auditory, visual, or auditory plus visual demonstrations. All modeling groups performed better than the physical practice with KR group during an immediate retention test, leading these authors to claim support for the effectiveness of modeling over KR. In addition to these findings there were also differences between the modalities. The visual model was the least effective for reproducing the timing task. A subsequent experiment by McCullagh and Little [92] further examined the role of modalities in demonstrations and found a similar ordering of demonstration groups. A visual model was not very useful for the reproduction of a timing skill. Contrary to Doody et al. [27], however, these authors found that KR resulted in less error than the demonstration groups. The findings from all of these experiments suggest that at least for the timing tasks employed, visual demonstrations, although intuitively appealing as an information source, may not be the optimum mode for all presentations. Perhaps the modality of presentation interacts with the type of task employed. Auditory demonstrations may be best for tasks that involve timing or sequencing whereas visual demonstrations may be best for learning the spatial or qualitative aspects of the task. Limited support for this notion has been derived from recent experiments [64, 93, 148] although further experimentation is needed before conclusions can be reached.

A second way to enhance the information provided in a demonstration is by providing verbal cues in addition to the demonstration. Recent experiments have addressed this issue [2, 113]. Roach and Burwitz [113] tested Bandura's notion that verbal cues when used in conjunction with demonstrations may act as mediator for enhancing the cognitive representation and may also aid retention. Although these authors did not assess retention they did find enhanced performance in the condition that received verbal cues in addition to modeling, concluding that verbal directing cues may enhance the observer's attention and subsequent performance.

Adams [2] also examined the role of verbal cues in addition to demonstrations. Adams' [1] closed loop theory relied heavily on the role of KR after movement for learning. It was his contention that by providing subjects with error information they become actively engaged in the learning process, develop a hypothesis for future movements, and determine the satisfactoriness of their learning after receiving KR on their next trial. Adams [2] reasoned, therefore, that a learner who views demonstrations of someone learning forms a cognitive representation but the viewer who also receives the model's KR will become actively involved in the learning process and be better equipped to match the cognitive representation against the error information (this argument holds, of course, only for tasks in which the outcome is not self-evident). Results produced a slight advantage for subjects who viewed a learning model and also received their KR over a group who viewed the learning model but did not receive their KR and a physical practice control group.

McCullagh and Caird took this notion one step further [91] to alleviate the problems of previous experiments [2, 27] which had confounded modeling and KR. Both prior experiments had provided subjects with demonstrations and then with KR about their own movements. Thus the potency of demonstrations as a learning tool could not be assessed. In addition, the viability of an exemplary or correct model with a learning sequence or variable model was compared. The findings suggested that KR and demonstrations by a learning sequence model produced superior performance during both acquisition and retention tests. All of the above findings suggest that augmented information, whether it be information from specific modalities or the addition of verbal information with demonstrations can enhance performance.

Cognitive Elements

What exactly is learned by viewing a demonstration? An experiment by Martens et al. [85] suggests we learn the cognitive components or strategies of the task. To test this notion their subjects viewed either a correct, incorrect, or learning sequence model, and in addition to assessing performance scores, ratings of strategies employed by subjects were obtained. The results clearly demonstrated that modeling affected the strategies adopted by subjects, which in turn affected the level of their performance. Other experiments have produced findings in support of this notion [19, 90].

Although to date, researchers have not experimentally tested a direct link between mental imagery and modeling, innuendos have been made that the processes governing these factors may be similar [29, 35, 64, 117]. In modeling, you observe someone perform, encode and rehearse this information, and then reproduce a response. In imagery, you typically think about what you are to perform, encode and rehearse this information, and then reproduce a response. Studies have shown that mental imagery is more effective in improving cognitive as opposed to motor task components [46, 98, 116, 117, 130, 153] and a meta-analysis of the research [35] has supported this general notion. If modeling can be viewed as a form of covert rehearsal that primarily influences performance because task components are symbolically coded and if these representations provide the internal standard upon which reproduction is based, then the parallels between modeling a mental imagery may not be that distant.

Housner [64, 65] has provided some data that speak to the role of imagery in conjunction with modeling. It was his contention that imaginal coding strategies are similar to imagery and therefore people identified as having high ability to image should benefit more from modeling than people who have low imaging ability. Free recall as well as serial recall of performance was assessed, and imagery ability was found to affect only free recall [65]. The author discussed these findings by relying on the work of Paivio [106] and suggested that visual imagery may be important for recognition or free-recall situations whereas verbal processes may be more important for tasks that require temporal ordering of items. Preliminary evidence from a developmental study on modeling supports this contention [93].

Although the cognitive–motor hypothesis has received direct experimental testing [116, 117] for mental practice, to date it has received only indirect support in the modeling literature. Similar to an early study by McGuire [94], both Feltz [30] and McCullagh [90] found that modeling assisted subjects in attaining the correct task strategies. Unfortunately, few studies have attempted to assess this component of performance. More discussion on this issue will occur when rehearsal and response considerations are discussed.

Model Characteristics
The final aspect of the demonstration which is important to modeling concerns who demonstrates and what they say and do when they demonstrate. Within Bandura's theory [5] model characteristics were originally hypothesized to influence the attentional phase of observational learning. It was presumed that observers would differentially focus their attention to relevant cues dependent on model attributes. Although there have been few direct tests of this hypothesis, numerous studies found performance differences dependent on model characteristics such as competence [11], prestige [87], status level [75, 89], age [10], social power [97], and similarity [57, 90]. Yussen and Levy [155] directly measured children's visual attention after observing either a warm or neutral model and found that children paid more attention to a warm model. McCullagh [89, 90] conducted two experiments to examine the attention–model characteristic relationship and found that model characteristics influenced performance but did not appear to be a result of attentional factors. The effect of model characteristics in observational learning settings seems clear. Model characteristics do affect performance. However, whether these differences are due to attentional or motivational differences is unclear and whether learning is affected as suggested by Bandura has not been clearly demonstrated [89, 90].

The role the model plays in providing a demonstration has recently been combined with self-efficacy theory [6]. According to self-efficacy theory, individual performance levels are determined by an individual's cognitive beliefs in their own personal competence levels. Feltz [32, 33] has previously provided reviews on this topic, and the role of modeling in modifying efficacy and anxiety will be further elaborated upon in the discussion of psychological responses to modeling.

REHEARSAL STRATEGIES

During the discussion of the observational learning process it has been shown that there are benefits from variables which appear to assist the memory coding process. As stated previously, Bandura's theory posits that modeling experiences are maintained in memory through the mediation of symbols [5, 6]. The evidence suggests that the beneficial effect of rehearsal strategies depends on (*a*) meaningfulness of the stimulus in the case of verbal and numeric associations [8, 9, 69], (*b*) extent of experience with the stimulus in imaginal rehearsal [35, 59, 117], and (*c*) organizational structure in combination with physical practice [13, 74, 137].

Verbal Rehearsal

To determine the role of symbolic coding and rehearsal processes, Bandura and Jeffery [8] tested the effects of both numeric codes and letter codes associated with unidirectional movements. Directional movements to the left were associated with odd numbers and those to the right with even numbers, while progressively longer length movements were associated with increasingly larger numeric values. In using letter code symbols, vowels were associated with movements to the right and consonants with movements to the left. The ability to rehearse the symbolic code [e.g., BAD or 134] enhanced the retention of the desired movement sequence. When elementary school aged children were required to retain a specific sequence of gross motor activities they had observed, those who had attached verbal labels to the movements displayed superior retention [147, 148]. When verbal labels were attached to demonstrated motoric responses from the manual language of the deaf, retention was better [51]. This response suggests that symbolic coding mediated a task defined primarily as a spatial task.

It has also been shown that not only attachment of a verbal code to movement is important, but also the content of the rehearsal code is an important aspect of retention. In tasks which required either the construction of three-dimensional forms using wooden rods and joints [69] or reproduction of a particular modeled pattern of downward and lateral action combinations [9], retention was better when there was an organizational structure to the verbal codes. For example, the letters TBSNSB, corresponding to directional movements, were better retained when the coding structure was a sentence coding condition, e.g., "Tall boys stand near small boys" (9). It appears that under some conditions, attaching meaningful verbal labels to modeled movements provides rehearsal strategies for the reproduction of the movements. It is not known to what extent direct application to sport skills is possible. Likewise, the relationship of verbal label rehearsal to imaginal rehearsal has not been investigated.

Imaginal Rehearsal
If observing motor skills results in some cognitive representation of the skill then it should be possible to rehearse that skill through a mental process without motorically performing the skill. It may be that at highly skilled performance levels, the observation process itself is a mental rehearsal of the action. However, most often imaginal rehearsal is thought to occur without the presence of the stimulus event. The individual is thought to reinstate the entire movement by "thinking" of it or "mentally practicing." Various theories have been proposed to explain how this process is possible by defining the way that information is stored in memory [14].

One such view states that the mental representation is in the form of propositions or a propositional network [76, 110]. That is, memory codes are in an abstract form that contains relationships among concepts [14]. Lang suggests that the content of propositions includes the logical relationship among concepts. When an image is formed the visual information, motor activity, and emotions associated with the image are reinstated [76]. Thus, imaginal rehearsal of a motor skill would include the entire elaboration of the associated propositional network.

On the other hand, the dual code theory posits that information is represented in memory in the form of verbal codes or visual codes. The verbal codes are thought to store information which is auditory in nature while the visual codes are considered to represent spatial relationships. Basic to this notion is the assumption that memory systems are connected directly to the auditory and sensory modalities. Both Paivio [106, 107] and Finke [37, 38], among others, are proponents of this view. In a recent article, Finke has written that there appear to be some common neural mechanisms between imagery and visual perception. In one study, subjects were asked to view a transparent cylinder in which four identifiable animals were hanging at different heights. After the animals had been removed from the cylinder subjects were asked to form mental images of what they had seen. The clear cylinder was then physically rotated and subjects were asked to rotate their images in the same rotational direction and then to draw what they imaged. There was a clear correspondence reported between the rotated image drawings and the actual rotated three-dimensional spatial relationship of the hanging objects within the cylinder. As a result of these findings and a number of other similar results, Finke [38] concluded,

> When a person decides to create a mental image of a particular object, the kind of image that can be fashioned depends on the knowledge the person has about the object, such as its size, color and shape. Then once the image is formed it can begin to function in some respects like the object itself, bringing about the activation of certain types of neural mechanisms at lower levels in the visual system.

Finke's statements, when placed in a motor skills context, suggest that the more elaborate the cognitive representation (through experience and observational learning) the more effective the imaginal rehearsal should be. On the basis of a meta-analysis of the imaginal or mental practice literature, Feltz and Landers [35] concluded that the effects of imaginal rehearsal depend on the type of task. It might be that the content of highly cognitive tasks is more visually oriented and therefore results in greater mental elaboration than tasks primarily motor in nature. Thus cognitive imaginal rehearsal requires fewer practice trials to be beneficial.

However, the potency of imaginal rehearsal may depend on certain individual difference characteristics [59]. Statistical differences have been shown to exist between subjects classified as high or low imagers [66, 67], or as either predominantly visual or kinesthetic imagers [84]. Performance differences as a function of image vividness have also been reported by other researchers [111, 117, 127, 128]. Since it has not been shown that there are individual differences in observational learning ability, perhaps those persons who are high vivid visual imagers might benefit to a greater extent from observing a visual model than would those individuals who are classified as predominantly kinesthetic imagers. This line of inquiry could possibly link the attributes of imagery to the study of individual differences in observational learning and provide greater theoretical understanding of the associations among visual perception, action perception, and observational learning.

Organizational Considerations

SPACING OF DEMONSTRATIONS. The question of when and how often the learner should observe the model to maximize the learning effect has not had theoretical importance. In practice one or two demonstrations are usually given so that the learner has an idea of the movement and the expected outcome with additional demonstrations given as warranted. However, in experimental studies it has been shown that observation of the model before and during practice is beneficial, depending on the task and the age of the performer [3, 4, 74, 137]. The optimal number of spaced demonstrations is not known but the number is perhaps affected by the nature of the skill and the frequency or length of practice sessions [30].

In an attempt to determine the relative importance of observational learning and physical practice, Bird et al. [13] interspersed modeling throughout the entire acquisition phase while systematically manipulating the ratio of modeling to physical practice. They found that skill retention accuracy was superior for those subjects who spent a greater proportion of time in observation of a correct model than in physical practice with knowledge of results. Those subjects who had no physical practice displayed very little learning while those subjects who had no observational learning displayed significant forgetting after a 24-hour retention interval. The authors concluded that to maximize retention, a combination of modeling and physical practice was necessary. Further research examining the relative versus absolute frequency of demonstrations in the absence of KR and in combination with KR will reveal the contribution of each information source to skill learning.

VARIABILITY OF OBSERVATION PRACTICE. The notion that the content of the modeled demonstration contains task-relevant information which facilitates cognitive representational development is central to Bandura's theory. One means of manipulating task relevant information is to vary the content of the demonstration. In the first of four experiments, Martens et al. [85] found that those subjects who observed either a correct model or a learning sequence model prior to and during practice were significantly better than a no model control group but not different from each other. Other investigations [15, 91] that have varied the demonstrations have found that exposing subjects to a number of different responses during the demonstration period enhances performance.

Observational learning researchers may glean important insight from [119] schema theory. Although this theory did not speak to modeling effects, Schmidt postulated that a variety of movement responses will assist learners in developing a schema or rule that allows them to generalize their learning to novel responses. Limited evidence [15, 91] suggests that the same type of concept may be viable for modeling.

THE RESPONSE

Within Bandura's original formulation of modeling, very little consideration was given to motor reproduction or actual assessment of the skill. Since the theory was primarily designed for the acquisition of social behavior, many of the response categories that were being assessed were dichotomous (i.e., either the behavior was exhibited or it was not). However, when assessing motor performance or sport skills, we are interested not only in whether an act is executed, but in the quality and accuracy of the executed movements. There are two major categories of response considerations. The first category addresses performance responses and addresses three issues: (*a*) Does modeling differentially affect movement outcome versus movement execution or form? (*b*) Does modeling differentially affect recall and recognition processes? And (*c*) Does modeling affect learning or performance? The second category examines the effects of modeling on psychological (nonperformance) responses and addresses how modeling (*a*) influences self-efficacy and (*b*) may modify anxiety.

Performance Responses

OUTCOME VERSUS PROCESS. When providing learners with a demonstration two important aspects of the skill to be learned can be conveyed: the goal or outcome of the task and the movement pattern required to execute the skill efficiently. Most investigators have assessed the potency of modeling effects by assessing movement outcome as opposed to measuring whether the learner exhibits the same movement patterns as the model. Recently, however, a few studies have attempted to assess components of movement form as well [21–23, 30, 82, 90]. What we expect learners to reproduce may be related to the cognitive components of the task discussed earlier in the chapter.

Feltz [30] assessed both movement outcome and form as rated by judges for subjects learning a balance task. Her findings indicated that form was a better determinant of modeling effects than performance outcome. McCullagh [90] also assessed both outcome and form scores on the same task and found that control group subjects who received no demonstrations were able to reach the same level of performance as demonstration subjects when outcome was assessed. When form was measured, however, the control group was not executing the correct form. This study once again elucidates the importance of measuring more than outcome when assessing modeling effects.

Another way to assess movement execution or form besides using judges' ratings is through the use of two- or three-dimensional kinematic analysis (i.e., displacement, velocity, and acceleration profiles) of the movement pattern. By employing such techniques, a precise comparison can be made between the model's execution and the learner's execution of the skill. Relatively few studies have used these techniques, but those that have have produced some interesting findings [131, 151].

Southard and Higgins [131] investigated the role of practice and demonstrations in the striking pattern used for a racquetball serve. Subjects were assigned to one of four experimental groups and practiced under their designated conditions for 5 days. The findings indicated that both the practice and combination groups (demonstration plus practice) changed their limb configurations from pre- to posttest, whereas the demonstration group was no better than the control group in successfully changing these form components. The authors concluded that providing a demonstration was not sufficient for changing constrained movement patterns whereas practice allows subjects to adopt the appropriate kinematic characteristics of the movement.

A study by Whiting et al. [151], however, showed enhanced performance for demonstration subjects over control subjects. Experimental group subjects viewed a model during acquisition of a slalom-type ski movement, whereas control group subjects practiced without the benefit of demonstrations for a 5-day acquisition period. The model's performance was videotaped and the frequency, amplitude, and fluency of the movements were recorded with a Selspot motion analysis system so that an adequate comparison could be made between the model and the subjects. The results indicated that the subjects did not reach the performance level of the model but demonstration subjects were significantly more fluent and produced more consistent movements than control subjects.

The limited findings generated thus far clearly indicate the need to assess both response execution and response outcome when determining modeling effects. For example, in the Southard study, it would have been theoretically important if outcome or accuracy had been assessed in addition to execution. Also, it would have been informative if the movement components of the model had been clearly measured and described to determine how closely the subjects approximated the model's movements. Combining these variables with stage of practice may provide insight on how subjects use and perceive demonstration information early and late in practice.

RECALL VERSUS RECOGNITION. A primary difference between motor learning theories of skill acquisition and Bandura's view of observational learning lies in the distinction between recall and recognition. Adams' [1] closed loop theory of motor learning and Schmidt's [119] schema theory both posit two separate memory states: one that produces the movement (recall) and one that evaluates the outcome (recognition). Bandura, on the other hand, suggests that the cognitive representation that is generated by observing a model "provides the internal model for response production and the standard for response correction" [7]. Thus, according to Bandura, both recall and recognition are governed by the same mechanism. While motor learning researchers have for years attempted to experimentally demonstrate the independence of recall and recognition [e.g., 145], observational learning researchers have not attempted to make this distinction although a review of the literature suggests that modeling may differentially affect these processes. In fact, research by Carroll and Bandura [21–23] has consistently attempted to assess the effects of modeling on recall and recognition but have not proclaimed a need to separate these processes theoretically.

In their most recent study Carroll and Bandura [23] examined the role of visual guidance in observational learning. They assessed recall through reproduction accuracy of a nine-component wrist–arm paddle motion. Recognition was assessed by two different measures. Subjects were shown photographs of the nine correct movement components individually and were also shown an incorrect component. The strength of the cognitive representation produced from modeling was assessed by the number of correctly chosen components. In addition, subjects were asked to arrange photographs of the nine movement components into the correct order. The manipulation of whether subjects concurrently or separately matched their movements with the model and also whether they could visually monitor their own performances did have an affect on reproduction accuracy but did not affect the recognition measures. The correlations between the recognition measures and reproduction performance although significant ($r = .34–.64$) were not extremely high, suggesting that perhaps recall and recognition did not develop at the same rate.

In the study previously discussed by Newell [99], subjects were provided with auditory demonstrations and recall and recognition were assessed for a ballistic timing skill. It was Newell's contention that if the two memory states were independent, then it should be possible to develop one memory mechanism independently of the other. The findings indicated that increasing the number of auditory demonstrations increased recognition memory but since demonstration subjects were more accurate in their movement productions even on their first active attempt, it was concluded that the demonstrations also influenced recall.

While the task employed by Newell was extremely simple, it could be argued that demonstrations may serve a useful function in learning to recognize complex skills as well. In other words, it may take extended practice to achieve an increasingly perfected movement but with the aid of demonstrations, subjects may be able to recognize their own errors earlier in the learning process. Recognition of one's own errors could perhaps be further enhanced by providing subjects with videotaped feedback of their own movement coupled with demonstrations of the correct movement so they can match discrepancies. Within the observational learning paradigm, subjects are typically required to perform this conception matching process based on their memory of the demonstration as well as memory of their own movements.

LEARNING VERSUS PERFORMANCE. According to Schmidt [120], learning is "a set of processes associated with practice or experience leading to relatively permanent changes in the capability for responding." Although Bandura made a distinction between learning and performance in his original theoretical formulation, few motor behavior studies, especially those dealing with social psychological variables, have attempted to make this distinction. Schmidt has clearly outlined the procedures for using transfer designs to assess whether the effects of particular variables are relatively transient (called performance variables) or relatively permanent (called learning variables).

The procedure for transfer designs requires the manipulation of independent variables during an initial acquisition phase followed by performance under a common level of the independent variable during the transfer phase. The transfer phase should occur after the independent variable manipulations have had time to dissipate. Transfer designs in motor behavior research vary in the length of this rest period from minutes to days.

Although Bandura had originally postulated that attention and retention processes affected learning whereas motor reproduction and motivation affected performance, few motor behavior studies test these predictions or differentiate between learning and performance. In fact, many studies use the terms interchangeably and therefore incorrectly. Recently, however, investigators have attempted to separate learning and performance effects.

McCullagh [89, 90] examined the influence of model status and model similarity and in both experiments employed a transfer design. In support of previous investigations [57, 75] that had manipulated model characteristics, performance differences were found for the status and similarity manipulations. However, both experiments found the effects of modeling to be rather short lived since no group differences were evident during the transfer phases.

In assessing the potency of modeling with videotape feedback and physical practice, Ross et al. [114] assessed both immediate and delayed retention using a transfer design. In this experiment all experimental groups performed similarly during acquisition but differential group effects were found during the transfer phases, suggesting that learning had been effected. In a subsequent experiment using the same timing task [27] it was similarly found that the modality of model presentations (visual/auditory) affected performance during transfer, suggesting learning differences.

It can be concluded that model characteristics affect performance but not learning and that augmented information such as modality of presentations affects learning. However, since only limited research has been conducted in these areas, these conclusions are offered cautiously. Additional research is definitely warranted to determine which variables produce only transient performance effects and which affect long-term learning.

Psychological Responses

Although modeling has been primarily viewed as an instructional strategy for teaching motor skills, it has also been shown to have a powerful effect on social and psychological behaviors of the observer. Such behaviors include self-efficacy, anxiety, motivation, attributions, and aggression. The major issue addressed here revolves around what the model does and says that influences subsequent observer behavior. The characteristics of self-efficacy and anxiety will be discussed.

SELF-EFFICACY. By far, the majority of studies on the social psychological effects of modeling have examined self-efficacy changes. Self-efficacy is defined as the strength of a person's conviction that he or she can execute the behavior needed for successful performance [7]. The studies examining self-efficacy changes have employed participant modeling, similar models, and model talk to modify efficacy.

Participant modeling uses a three-step approach: (*a*) demonstration by a model, (*b*) guided physical practice, and (*c*) gradual removal of the guidance. A number of studies have strongly supported the use of participant models in augmenting self-efficacy of observers and subsequently performance of motor skills [31, 36, 88, 146]. This modeling technique appears to function as a means of providing social support and allaying performance fears. For example, Feltz et al. [36] compared participant, live, and videotaped modeling on performance of a high-avoidance skill. Subjects received one of the modeling instructions for four acquisition trials, after which performance was measured on a second set of four trials without guidance. Results revealed that subjects in the participant modeling group reported significantly higher self-efficacy and performance scores than the two other modeling conditions.

Studies using models perceived as similar to the observer have also shown a relationship between modeling and self-efficacy [24, 55, 57, 122]. For example, in the Gould and Weiss study [57], female subjects viewed a similar model (nonathletic female), a dissimilar model (athletic male), or no model performing on a leg extension task. Results supported a model similarity hypothesis in that subjects who viewed the female model reported higher self-efficacy levels and performed better than did subjects in the other two groups. Corbin et al. [24] conducted an experiment in an aerobic exercise environment in which subjects either viewed and listened to three vicarious success presentations from similar models or viewed and listened to rules and strategies for exercising. After the month-long program, results showed that adherence to activity and changes in pre- to post-experimental self-efficacy were significantly greater in the treatment as compared to the control group.

Verbalizations made by a model have been examined with regard to self-efficacy in observers [57, 121, 123, 159]. One underlying hypothesis is that the model verbally persuades the observer into thinking that he or she can do it. For example, Zimmerman and Ringle [159] found that children exposed to a confident (high self-efficacy statements) as compared to a pessimistic (low self-efficacy statements) model resulted in higher self-efficacy estimates and persistence on a puzzle task. Schunk and Rice [123] found that models who verbalized strategies for better reading skills affected both reading comprehension and self-efficacy in comparison to mere visual models.

In sum, a variety of modeling strategies including participant modeling, similar models, and verbalizing models have had simultaneous effects on both performance and self-efficacy. Of course, the effect of enhancing self-efficacy is to positively influence motivated behavior in the form of choosing to participate, exerting effort and persistence in attempts at mastering skills.

ANXIETY. Modeling has also been found to be an effective strategy for reducing anxiety in a variety of social evaluative or fearful situations [81, 88, 118, 146]. Lewis [81] examined the effectiveness of modeling and physical practice in reducing anxiety and fear, and enhancing children's approach behavior toward water activities. She found that a combination of a coping model (who gradually demonstrated improvement) plus actual physical practice was better than a model only or practice only for improving self-report and instructor ratings of fear. Weinberg et al. [146] compared participant and live model groups on anxiety, self-efficacy, and performance on a horizontal bar gymnastics task. Subjects in the participant modeling group performed significantly better and reported less performance anxiety and higher self-efficacy than did subjects in the model only condition.

These studies demonstrate that modeling can be used as a strategy to concurrently reduce anxiety and enhance performance in physical activities. Although this aspect of modeling has not been a steady research topic, the nature of sport may be especially conducive to examination of modeling effects on anxiety reduction. Many sport skills may pose an element of fear or danger (e.g., gymnastics, swimming). It may be that observers possess the physical skills to reproduce what has been demonstrated, but their fears, anxieties, or confidence about negative performance consequences may create avoidance behaviors. The use of participant, positive self-talk, similar, and coping models may benefit the observer by appealing to his or her perceptions of competence and thus approach, effort, and persistence in the activity.

FEEDBACK

Although discussion of feedback considerations is outside the realm of this chapter, the potency of providing feedback within motor skill acquisition is well recognized and a brief discussion of how feedback can serve as a modeling stimulus is warranted. For example, when learners are provided with a videotape of their previous movement before their next movement, this information serves not only as feedback from the last movement, but also as a demonstration (although perhaps not a correct one) for their next movement. Thus the distinction between information prior to movement and information subsequent to movement becomes somewhat blurred. In addition, some studies [21–23] have provided subjects with concurrent videotape information, thus providing learners with information during movement. Surprisingly little research has been conducted on the role of videotape feedback in motor skill acquisition. A meta-analysis [115] suggested that verbal directing cues in conjunction with videotape feedback was important for enhancing performance and that experienced subjects benefited more than beginners from this sort of information.

Another paradigm that has examined the use of videos for skill enhancement is the self-modeling literature. Dowrick [28] defines self-modeling as "observation of oneself on videotapes that show only desired target behaviors," and readers are referred to this book for a discussion of this literature. Besides providing subjects with videotape feedback, subjects can be provided with kinematic information about their movements such as force/time curves [68], position/time graphs [62], or kinematic feedback [102, 104]. The effects of task-specific feedback in combination with modeling is an area of investigation which needs further research and has both theoretical and sport skill application potential.

CONCLUDING REMARKS

Modeling or observational learning has not received prolonged and systematic study in motor behavior or sport. Bandura's theoretical formulations have generated extensive research in other disciplines; however, the proposal that four subprocesses (attention, retention, motor reproduction, and motivation) govern movement behaviors has not been enthusiastically tested in motor performance. The present chapter proposes an organizational scheme that incorporates aspects of the major motor behavior disciplines and presents concepts that will, it is hoped, lead to empirical testing and new theoretical developments.

One final consideration is a discussion of *relationships* among the variables specified in the model. Probably the most obvious relationship exists between the observer and the other categories specified. For example, the cognitive and motor skill capabilities of the observer can affect how the demonstration will be perceived, rehearsed, and subsequently executed. It is likely that the ability to select relevant cues from the demonstration display is a function of both the experience and developmental level of the observer. In addition, the demonstration could be modified to enhance the modeling process dependent on developmental level. Augmented verbal cues or verbal rehearsal strategies may be more important for children or for learners who are inexperienced with the task. Thus, the developmental level of the observer will influence what is perceived, what aspects of the demonstrations are important, and how the information is rehearsed.

Aspects of the demonstration are likely to interact with rehearsal strategies. For example, cognitive task elements may be better retained in memory by inducing learners to use imaginal strategies. Providing augmented information such as verbal directing cues in a demonstration may induce learners to verbally rehearse the movements. However, the type of rehearsal strategy employed may also influence the execution. As previously discussed, visual demonstrations may be best for qualitative performance whereas verbal descriptions or auditory demonstrations may be best for the correct ordering of movement sequences.

All factors, including that which is perceived, the motivational and developmental level of the observer, and the demonstration and its subsequent rehearsal, will impact performance execution. In many modeling studies subjects are asked to recall and reproduce the task outcome while the actual execution (movement process) or the subjects' ability to recognize error (either their own or someone else's) is ignored. Both of these latter responses should be more carefully assessed in future research. In addition, the long-term impact of modeling variables is often overlooked at the expense of assessing only performance and not learning. It should also be recognized that modeling can influence psychological responses that may in turn influence the performance response. Increases in self-efficacy and reduction of anxiety have both been shown to be mediators of performance. To effectively determine the impact of modeling, a multilevel analysis of response execution is needed.

A final consideration is the role of feedback in the modeling process. With the increasing availability of videotapes and computer movement analysis systems, it is possible to provide performers with either ongoing or instantaneous response feedback. Such information serves not only as feedback about the last movement but also as a demonstration before the next movement. The ability of subjects to meaningfully use this information may be influenced by all the previous components discussed. Furthermore, the aspects of performance and psychological responses emphasized in the feedback could influence elements perceived in the demonstration and how this information is rehearsed.

We have neglected the role of extrinsic feedback and a discussion of how it may affect components of the model presented in Figure 13.1. For example, an instructor could provide verbal cues directing attention to relevant task components, thus modifying how the observer perceives the action. Or extrinsic feedback could focus on movement execution as opposed to outcome, thus producing differential motivational and performance levels. While we recognize the importance of providing subjects with error information after movements, motor skill researchers have for years examined this question. The present chapter has been limited to the importance of modeling as a variable in skill learning, and we urge researchers to determine the importance of demonstrations independent of other potent modifiers of behavior.

The status of the research at the present time precludes making many practical applications. One obvious extension would be using videotapes of skilled performers or videotape feedback to modify sport skills. Such techniques are increasingly evident [132] in practice; while it is intuitively appealing to presume that watching videotapes of skilled movement executions could assist individuals to improve their own performance, scientific evidence to support this notion is severely lacking [29]. Additional theoretical development and applied field research are needed before the parameters of modeling can be well documented for practical application.

ACKNOWLEDGMENTS

This chapter is based on a symposium by Penny McCullagh, Maureen Weiss, and Diane Ross at the North American Society for the Psychology of Sport and Physical Activity, Vancouver, in 1987.

We would like to thank Stephen A. Wallace for comments on an early draft of this chapter. In addition we would like to recognize the technical assistance of Elizabeth Bitzer, Jeffrey Caird, and Amy Meriweather and the word-processing assistance of Barbara Miller.

REFERENCES

1. Adams JA: A closed-loop theory of motor learning. *J Mot Behav* 3:111–150, 1971.
2. Adams JA: Use of the model's knowledge of results to increase the observer's performance. *J Hum Mov Stud* 12:89–98, 1986.
3. Anderson DF, Gebhart JA, Pease DG, Ludwig DA: Effects of age temporal placement of a modeled skill on children's performance on a balance task. *Percept Mot Skills* 55:1263–1266, 1982.
4. Anderson DF, Gebhart JA, Pease DG, Rupnow AA: Effects of age, sex, and placement of a model on children's performance on a ball-striking task. *Percept Mot Skills* 57:1187–1190, 1983.
5. Bandura A: *Principles of Behavior Modification*. New York, Holt, Rinehart and Winston, 1969.
6. Bandura A: *Social Learning Theory*. Englewood Cliffs, NJ, Prentice Hall, 1977.
7. Bandura A: *Social Foundations of Thought and Action: A Social Cognitive Theory*. Englewood Cliffs, NJ, Prentice-Hall, 1986.
8. Bandura A, Jeffery RW: Role of symbolic coding and rehearsal processes in observational learning. *J Pers Soc Psychol* 26:122–130, 1973.
9. Bandura A, Jeffery RW, Bachicha DL: Analysis of memory codes and cumulative rehearsal in observational learning. *J Res Pers* 7:295–305, 1974.

10. Bandura A, Kapers CJ: Transmission of patterns of self-reinforcement through modeling. *J Abnorm Soc Psychol* 69:1–9, 1964.
11. Baron RA: Attraction toward the model and model's competence as determinants of adult initiative behavior. *J Pers Soc Psychol* 14:345–351, 1970.
12. Bernstein N: *The Coordination and Regulation of Movements.* Oxford, Pergamon Press, 1967.
13. Bird AM, Ross D, Laguna P: *The Observational Learning of a Timing Task.* Arlington, VA, ERIC Documentation Reproduction Service, 1983, pp 269–370.
14. Bird AM, Cripe BK: *Psychology and Sport Behavior.* St. Louis, MO, Times Mirror/Mosby, 1986.
15. Bird AM, Rikli R: Observational learning and practice variability. *Res Q Exercise Sport* 54:1–4, 1983.
16. Brody GH, Stoneman Z: Selective imitation of same-age, older, and younger peer models. *Child Dev* 52:717–720, 1981.
17. Brody GH, Stoneman A: Peer imitation: an examination of status and competence hypotheses. *J Genet Psychol* 146:161–170, 1986.
18. Bruner JS: The course of cognitive growth. *Am Psychol* 19:1–15, 1964.
19. Burwitz L, Borrie A: Observational learning of a complex motor skill under extended practice. Unpublished paper, 1987.
20. Bush RL: The effects of observational learning on selected volleyball skills. Master's thesis, California State University, Fullerton, CA, 1987.
21. Carroll WR, Bandura A: The role of visual monitoring in observational learning of action patterns: making the unobservable observable. *J Mot Behav* 14:153–167, 1982.
22. Carroll WR, Bandura A: The role of visual monitoring and motor rehearsal in observational learning of action patterns. *J Mot Behav* 17:269–281, 1985.
23. Carroll WR, Bandura A: Translating cognition into action: the role of visual guidance in observational learning. *J Mot Behav* 19:385–398, 1987.
24. Corbin CB, Laurie DR, Gruger C, Smiley B: Vicarious success experience as factor influencing self-confidence, attitudes, and physical activity of adult women. *J Teach Phys Educ* 4:17–23, 1984.
25. Cutting JE: Six tenets of event perception. *Cognition* 10:71–78, 1981.
26. Cutting JE, Proffitt DR: Gait perception as an example of how we may perceive events. In Walk R, Pick HL Jr (eds): *Intersensory Perception and Sensory Integration.* New York, Plenum, 1981, pp 32–47.
27. Doody SG, Bird AM, Ross D: The effect of auditory and visual models on acquisition of a timing task. *Hum Movement Sci* 4:271–281, 1985.
28. Dowrick PW: Self-modeling. In Dowrick JPW, Biggs SJ (eds): *Using Video: Psychological and Social Applications.* New York, Wiley & Sons, 1983, pp 105–124.
29. Druckman D, Swets JA: *Enhancing Human Performance: Issues, Theories and Techniques.* Washington, DC, National Academy Press, 1983.
30. Feltz DL: The effect of age and number of demonstrations on modeling form and performance. *Res Q Exercise Sport* 53:291–296, 1982.
31. Feltz DL: Teaching a high-avoidance motor task to a retarded child through participant modeling. *Educ Training Mentally Retarded* 15:152–155, 1982.
32. Feltz DL: Self-efficacy as a cognitive mediator of athletic performance. In Straub WF, Williams JM (eds): *Cognitive Sport Psychology.* New York, Sport Science Association, 1984, pp 191–198.
33. Feltz DL: Self-confidence and sport performance. In Pandolf KB (ed): *Exercise and Sport Sciences Reviews.* New York, McMillan, 1988, vol 16, pp 423–457.
34. Feltz DL, Landers DM: Informational and motivational components of a model's demonstration. *Res Q* 48:525–533, 1977.

35. Feltz DL, Landers DM: The effects of mental practice on motor skill learning and performance: a meta-analysis. *J Sport Psychol* 5:25–57, 1983.
36. Feltz DL, Landers DM, Raeder U: Enhancing self-efficacy in high avoidance motor tasks: a comparison of modeling techniques. *J Sport Psychol* 1:112–122, 1979.
37. Finke RA: Levels of equivalence in imagery and perception. *Psychol Rev* 87:113–132, 1980.
38. Finke RA: Mental imagery and the visual system. *Sci Am* 254:88–95, 1986.
39. Fitch HL, Tuller B, Turvey MT: The Bernstein perspective: III. Tuning of coordinative structures with special reference to perception. In Kelso JAS (ed): *Human Motor Behavior: An Introduction*. Hillsdale, NJ, Erlbaum, 1982, pp 271–181.
40. Flavell JH: Spontaneous verbal rehearsal in a memory task as a function of age. *Child Dev* 37:283–299, 1966.
41. Flavell JH: Developmental studies of mediated memory. In Reese HW, Lipsilt LP (eds): *Advances in Child Development and Behavior* (Vol. 5). New York, Academic Press, 1970.
42. Fowler CA, Turvey MT: Skill acquisition: an event approach with special reference to searching for the optimum of a function of several variables. In Stelmach GE (ed): *Information Processing in Motor Control and Learning*. New York, Academic Press, 1978, pp 1–40.
43. French KE, Thomas JR: The relation of knowledge development to children's basketball performance. *J Sport Psychol* 9:15–32, 1987.
44. Fuson KC: The development of self-regulating aspects of speech [a review]. In Zivin G (ed): *The Development of Self-Regulation Through Private Speech*. New York, Wiley, 1979.
45. Gallagher JD: Adult–child motor performance differences: a developmental perspective control processing deficits. Unpublished doctoral dissertation, Louisiana State University, Baton Rouge, LA, 1980.
46. Gallagher JD: The effects of developmental memory differences on learning motor skills. *J Phy Ed Rec Dance* 53:36–37, 1982.
47. Gallagher JD: Influence of developmental information processing abilities on children's motor performance. In Straub W, Williams J (eds): *Cognitive Sport Psychology*. Lansing, NY, Sport Science Association, 1984, pp 153–157.
48. Gallagher JD, Hoffman S: Memory development and children's sport skill acquisition. In Gould D, Weiss MR (eds): *Advances in Pediatric Sport Sciences*: Vol. 2, *Behavioral Issues*. Champaign, IL, Human Kinetics, 1987, pp 187–210.
49. Gallagher JD, Thomas JR: Rehearsal strategy effects on developmental differences for recall of a movement series. *Res Q Exercise Sport* 55:123–128, 1984.
50. Gallagher JD, Thomas JR: Developmental effects of grouping and recoding on learning a movement series. *Res Q Exercise Sport* 57:117–127, 1986.
51. Gerst MS: Symbolic coding processes in observational learning. *J Pers Soc Psychol* 19:9–17, 1971.
52. Gibson JJ: *The Perception of the Visual World*. Boston, Houghton Mifflin, 1950.
53. Gibson JJ: *The Senses Considered as Perceptual Systems*. Boston, Houghton Mifflin, 1966.
54. Gibson JJ: *The Ecological Approach to Visual Perception*. Boston, Houghton Mifflin, 1979.
55. Gould D: The influence of motor task types on model effectiveness. Unpublished doctoral dissertation, University of Illinois, Champaign, Urbana, IL, 1978.
56. Gould D, Roberts GC: Modeling and motor skill acquisition. *Quest* 33:214–230, 1982.
57. Gould D, Weiss M: The effects of model similarity and model talk on self-efficacy and muscular endurance. *J Sport Psychol* 3:17–29, 1981.
58. Gregory RL: *Eye and Brain*, ed 2. London, World University Library, 1972.

59. Hall C, Goss S: Imagery research in motor learning. In Goodman D, Wilberg RB, Franks IM (eds): *Differing Perspectives in Motor Learning, Memory, and Control*. Amsterdam, North-Holland, 1985, pp 139–154.
60. Harter S: Effectance motivation reconsidered. *Hum Dev* 21:34–64, 1978.
61. Harter S: A model of intrinsic mastery motivation in children: individual differences and developmental change. In Collins WA (ed): *Minnesota Symposium on Child Psychology*. Hillsdale, NJ, Erlbaum, 1981, vol 14, pp 215–255.
62. Hatze H: Biomechanical aspects of a successful motion optimization. In Komi PV (ed): *Biomechanics V-B*. Baltimore, MD, University Park Press, 1976, pp 5–12.
63. Holt EB: *Animal Drive and the Learning Process*. New York, Holt, 1931.
64. Housner LD: The role of visual imagery in recall of modeled motoric stimuli. *J Sport Psychol* 6:148–158, 1984.
65. Housner LD: The role of imaginal processing in the retention of visually presented sequential motoric stimuli. *Res Q Exercise Sport* 55:24–31, 1984.
66. Housner L, Hoffman SJ: Imagery and short-term motor memory. In Roberts GC, Newell KM (eds): *Psychology of Motor Behavior and Sport*. Champaign, IL, Human Kinetics, 1978, pp 182–191.
67. Housner L, Hoffman SJ: Imagery ability in recall of distance and location information. *J Mot Behav* 13:207–223, 1981.
68. Howell ML: Use of force–time graphs for performance analysis in facilitating motor learning. *Res Q* 27:12–22, 1956.
69. Jeffery RW: The influence of symbolic and motor rehearsal in observational learning. *J Res Pers* 10:116–127, 1976.
70. Johansson G: *Configurations in Event Perception*. Uppsala: Almquist & Wiksell, 1950.
71. Johansson G: Spatio-temporal differentiation and integration in visual motion perception. *Psychol Res* 38:379–393, 1976.
72. Kugler PN, Kelso JAS, Turvey MT: On the concept of coordinative structures as dissipative structures: I. Theoretical lines of convergence. In Stelmach GE, Requin J (eds): *Tutorials in Motor Behavior*. Amsterdam, North Holland, 1980, pp 3–47.
73. Kugler PNN, Kelso JAS, Turvey MT: On the control and coordination of naturally developing systems. In Kelso JAS, Clark JE (eds): *The Development of Movement Control and Coordination*. New York, Wiley, 1982, pp 5–78.
74. Landers DM: Observational learning of a motor skill: temporal spacing of demonstrations and audience presence. *J Mot Behav* 7:281–287, 1975.
75. Landers DM, Landers DM: Teacher versus peer models: effects of model's presence and performance level on motor behavior. *J Mot Behav* 5:129–139, 1973.
76. Lang PJ: A bio-informational theory of emotion imagery. *Psychophysiology* 16:495–512, 1979.
77. Lee DN: The functions of vision. In Pick HL Jr, Saltzman E (eds): *Modes of Perceiving and Processing Information*. Hillsdale, NJ, Erlbaum, 1978, pp 159–170.
78. Lee DN: Visuo-motor coordination in space–time. In Stelmach GE, Requin J (eds): *Tutorials in Motor Behavior*. Amsterdam, North-Holland, 1980, pp 281–295.
79. Lee DN, Aronson E: Visual proprioceptive control of standing in human infants. *Percept Psychophys* 15:529–532, 1974.
80. Lee DN, Lishman JR: Visual proprioceptive control of stance. *J Hum Mov Stud* 1:87–95, 1975.
81. Lewis S: A comparison of behavior therapy techniques in the reduction of fearful avoidance behavior. *Behav Ther* 5:648–655, 1974.
82. Little WS, McCullagh P: A comparison of motivational orientation and modeled instructional strategies: the effects of knowledge of performance and knowledge of results on form and accuracy. *J Sport Exerc Psychol*, in press.

83. Luria A: *Speech and the Development of Mental Processes in the Child*. London, Stapes Press, 1959.
84. Mahoney MJ, Avener M: Psychology of the elite athlete: an exploratory study. *Cognit Ther Res* 1:135–141, 1977.
85. Martens R, Burwitz L, Zuckerman J: Modeling effects on motor performance. *Res Q* 47:277–291, 1976.
86. Matteson R, Ross D: Knowledge of results and goal modeling effects on a linear position task. *Perspectives* 6:42–50, 1984.
87. Mausner B: Studies in social interaction III. Effect of variation in one partner's prestige on the interaction of observer pairs. *J Appl Psychol* 37:391–393, 1953.
88. McAuley E: Modeling and self-efficacy: a test of Bandura's model. *J Sport Psychol* 7:283–295, 1985.
89. McCullagh P: A model status as a determinant of attention in observational learning and performance. *J Sport Psychol* 8:319–331, 1986.
90. McCullagh P: Model similarity effects on motor performance. *J Sport Psychol* 9:249–260, 1987.
91. McCullagh P, Caird J: A comparison of exemplary and learning sequence models and the use of model knowledge of results to increase learning and performance. *Psychol Mot Behav Sport* 116, 1988.
92. McCullagh P, Little WS: The potency of information provided by various modalities in modeling in comparison with knowledge of results. *Psychol Mot Behav Sport* 42, 1987.
93. McCullagh P, Stiehl J, Weiss MR: Developmental considerations in modeling: the role of visual and verbal models and verbal rehearsal in skill acquisition. *Psychol Mot Behav Sport* 115, 1988.
94. McGuire WJ: Some factors influencing the effectiveness of demonstration films: repetition of instructions, slow motion, distribution of showings, and explanatory narrations. In Lumsdaine AA (eds): *Student Responses in Programmed Instructions*. Washington, DC, National Academy of Sciences, National Research Council, 1961, pp 187–207.
95. Miller NE, Dollard J: Social learning and imitation. New Haven, CT, Yale University Press, 1941.
96. Minas SC: Mental practice of a complex perceptual–motor skill. *J Hum Mov Stud* 4:102–107, 1978.
97. Mischel W, Grusec J: Determinant of the rehearsal and transmission of neutral and aversive behaviors. *J Pers Soc Psychol* 3:197–205, 1966.
98. Morrisett LN: The role of implicit practice on learning. Unpublished doctoral dissertation, New Haven, CT, Yale University, 1956.
99. Newell KM: Motor learning without knowledge of results through the development of a response recognition mechanism. *J Mot Behav* 8:209–217, 1976.
100. Newell KM: Skill learning. In Holding D (ed): *Human Skills*. New York, Wiley & Sons, 1981, pp 203–226.
101. Newell KM: Coordination, control and skill. In Goodman D, Wilberg RB, Franks IM (eds): *Differing Perspectives in Motor Learning, Memory, and Control*. Amsterdam, North-Holland, 1985, pp 295–317.
102. Newell KM, Quinn JT Jr, Sparrow WA, Walter CB: Kinematic information feedback for learning a rapid arm movement. *Hum Mov Sci* 2:255–269, 1983.
103. Newell KM, Morris LR, Scully DM: Augmented information and the acquisition of skills in physical activity. In Terjung RL (ed): *Exercise and Sport Sciences Reviews*. New York, MacMillan, 1985, pp 235–261.
104. Newell KM, Sparrow WA, Quinn JT Jr: Kinetic information feedback for learning isometric tasks. *J Hum Mov Stud* 11:113–123, 1985.

105. Newell KM, Walter CB: Kinematic and kinetic parameters as information feedback in motor skill acquisition. *J Hum Mov Stud* 7:235–254, 1981.
106. Paivio A: *Imagery and Verbal Processes.* New York, Holt, Rinehart & Winston, 1971.
107. Paivio A: Psychophysiological correlates of imagery. In McGuigan FJ, Schoonover RA (eds): *The Psychophysiology of Thinking: Studies of Covert Processes.* New York, Academic Press, 1973, pp 263–295.
108. Patrick K, Richman CL: Imitation in toddlers as a function of motor and verbal aspects of modeling. *J Genet Psychol* 146:507–518, 1986.
109. Pew RW: Human perceptual–motor performance. In Kantowitz BH (ed): *Human Information Processing: Tutorials in Performance and Cognition.* Hillsdale, NJ, Erlbaum, 1974, pp 1–40.
110. Pylyshyn ZW: What the mind's eye tells the mind's brain: a critique of mental imagery. *Psychol Bull* 80:1–22, 1973.
111. Rawlings EI, Rawlings IL: Rotary pursuit tracking following mental rehearsal as a function of voluntary control of visual imagery. *Percept Mot Skills* 38:302, 1974.
112. Reed ES: An outline of a theory of action systems. *J Mot Behav* 14:98–134, 1981.
113. Roach NK, Burwitz L: Observational learning in motor skill acquisition: the effect of verbal directing cues. In Watkins J, Burwitz L (eds): *Sports Science: Proceedings of the VIII Commonwealth and International Conference on Sport, Physical Education, Dance, Recreation and Health.* London, E & FN Spon, 1986, pp 349–354.
114. Ross D, Bird AM, Doody SG, Zoeller M: Effect of modeling and videotape feedback with knowledge of results on motor performance. *Hum Mov Sci* 4:149–157, 1985.
115. Rothstein AL, Arnold RK: Bridging the gap: application of research on videotape feedback and bowling. *Mot Skills Theory Prac* 1:35–62, 1976.
116. Ryan ED, Simons J: Cognitive demand, imagery, and frequency of mental rehearsal as factors influencing acquisition of motor skills. *J Sport Psychol* 3:35–45, 1981.
117. Ryan ED, Simons J: What is learned in mental practice of motor skills: a test of the cognitive–motor hypothesis. *J Sport Psychol* 5:419–426, 1983.
118. Sarason IG: Test anxiety and the self-disclosing coping model. *J Consult Clin Psychol* 43:148–153, 1975.
119. Schmidt RA: A schema theory of discrete motor skill learning. *Psychol Rev* 82:225–260, 1975.
120. Schmidt RA: *Motor Control and Learning: A Behavioral Emphasis.* Champaign, IL, Human Kinetics, 1988.
121. Schunk DH: Modeling and attributional effects on children's achievement: a self-efficacy analysis. *J Educ Psychol* 73:93–105, 1981.
122. Schunk DH, Hanson AR, Cox CD: Peer-model attributes and children's achievement behaviors. *J Educ Psychol* 79:54–61, 1987.
123. Schunk DH, Rice JM: Strategy self-verbalization: effects on remedial readers' comprehension and self-efficacy. Paper presented at the annual meeting of the American Psychological Association, Toronto, August 1984.
124. Scully DM: Visual perception of technical execution and aesthetic quality in biological motion. *Hum Mov Sci* 5:185–206, 1986.
125. Scully DM: Visual perception of biological motion. Unpublished doctoral dissertation, Urbana-Champaign, IL, University of Illinois, 1987.
126. Scully DM, Newell KM: Observational learning and the acquisition of motor skills: toward a visual perception perspective. *J Hum Mov Stud* 12:169–187, 1985.
127. Sheehan PW: Functional similarity of imaging to perceiving: individual differences in vividness of imagery. *Percept Mot Skills* 23:1011–1033, 1966.
128. Sheehan PW: Visual imagery and the organizational properties of perceived stimuli. *Br J Psychol* 58:247–252, 1967.

129. Sheffield FN: Theoretical considerations in the learning of complex sequential tasks from demonstrations and practice. In Lumsdaine AA (ed): *Student Response in Programmed Instruction.* Washington, DC, National Academy of Sciences–National Research Council, 1961, pp 13–32.

130. Smyth MM: The role of mental practice in skill acquisition. *J Mot Behav* 7:199–206, 1975.

131. Southard D, Higgins T: Changing movement patterns: effects of demonstration and practice. *Res Q Exercise Sport* 58:77–80, 1987.

132. Sportsmediscope. *U.S.O.C. Sports Medicine and Science Division Newsletter* 7(3):1, 1988.

133. Tarde G: *The Laws of Imitation.* New York, Holt, 1903.

134. Thomas JR: Acquisition of motor skills: information processing differences between children and adults. *Res Q* 51:158–173, 1980.

135. Thomas JR, French KE, Humphries CA: Knowledge development and sport skill performance: directions for motor behavior research. *J Sport Psychol* 8:259–272, 1986.

136. Thomas JR, Gallagher JD: Memory development and motor skill acquisition. In Seefeldt V (ed): Contributions of physical activity to human well-being. Reston, VA, AAHPERD Publications, 1986, pp 125–139.

137. Thomas JR, Pierce C, Ridsdale S: Age differences in children's ability to model motor behavior. *Res Q* 48:592–597, 1977.

138. Thorndike EL: *Educational Psychology.* New York, Columbia University, 1914.

139. Tuller B, Fitch HL, Turvey MT: The Bernstein perspective: II. The concept of muscle linkage or coordinative structure. In Kelso JAS (ed): *Human Motor Behavior: An Introduction.* Hillsdale, NJ, Erlbaum, 1982, pp 253–270.

140. Turvey MT: Preliminaries to a theory of action with reference to vision. In Shaw RE, Bransford J (eds): *Perceiving, Acting, and Knowing.* Hillsdale, NJ, Erlbaum, 1977, pp 211–265.

141. Turvey MT: Contrasting orientations to the theory of visual information processing. *Psychol Rev* 84:67–88, 1977.

142. Turvey MT, Fitch HL, Tuller B: The Bernstein perspective: I. The problems of degrees of freedom and context-conditioned variability. In Kelso JAS (ed): *Human Motor Behavior: An Introduction.* Hillsdale, NJ, Erlbaum, 1982, pp 239–252.

143. Ulrich BD: Perceptions of physical competence, motor competence, and participation in organized sport: their interrelationships in young children. *Res Q Exercise Sport* 58:54–67, 1986.

144. Ulrich BD: Developmental perspectives of motor skill performance in children. In Gould D, Weiss M (eds): *Advances in Pediatric Sport Sciences: Vol 2. Behavioral Issues.* Champaign, IL, Human Kinetics, 1987, pp 167–186.

145. Wallace SA, McGhee RC: The independence of recall and recognition in motor learning. *J Mot Behav* 11:141–151, 1979.

146. Weinberg RS, Sinardi M, Jackson A: Effect of modeling and bar height on anxiety, self-confidence and gymnastic performance. *Int Gymnast Tech Suppl* 8:11–13, 1982.

147. Weiss MR: Modeling and motor performance: a developmental perspective. *Res Q Exercise Sport* 54:190–197, 1983.

148. Weiss MR, Klint KA: "Show and tell" in the gymnasium: an investigation of developmental differences in modeling and verbal rehearsal of motor skills. *Res Q Exercise Sport* 58:234–241, 1987.

149. White R: Motivation reconsidered: the concept of competence. *Psychol Rev* 66:297–333, 1959.

150. Whiting HTA: *Acquiring Ball Skills.* Philadelphia, Lea & Febiger, 1969.

151. Whiting HTA, Bijlard MJ, den Brinker BPLM: The effect of the availability of a dynamic model on the acquisition of a complex cyclical action. *Q J Exp Psychol* 39A:43–59, 1987.
152. Winther KT, Thomas JR: Developmental differences in children's labeling of movement. *J Mot Behav* 13:77–90, 1981.
153. Wrisberg CA, Ragsdale MR: Cognitive demand and practice level: factors in the mental rehearsal of motor skills. *J Hum Mov Stud* 5:201–208, 1979.
154. Yando R, Seitz U, Zigler E: *Imitation: A Developmental Perspective.* New York, Wiley, 1978.
155. Yussen SR, Levy NM: Effects of warm and neutral models on the attention of observational learners. *J Exp Child Psychol* 20:66–72, 1975.
156. Yussen SR: Determinants of visual attention and recall in observational learning by preschoolers and second graders. *Dev Psychol* 10:93–100, 1974.
157. Zelaznik HN, Spring J: Feedback in response recognition and production. *J Mot Behav* 8:309–312, 1976.
158. Zelaznik HN, Shapiro DC, Newell KM: On the structure of motor recognition memory. *J Mot Behav* 10:313–323, 1978.
159. Zimmerman BJ, Ringle J: Effects of model persistence and statements of confidence on children's self-efficacy and problem solving. *J Educ Psychol* 73:485–493, 1981.

14
The Tradition of the "Six Things Non-Natural": Exercise and Medicine from Hippocrates through Ante-Bellum America

JACK W. BERRYMAN, Ph.D.

INTRODUCTION

Cary Kimble has shown that since the 1960s we have seen a revival of "interest among many Americans in 'lifestyle' health care: jogging and bicycling, health foods, special diets, sports and exercise, yoga and meditation, health spas, reformed smoking and drinking habits" [59, pp 72–73]. Kimble noted that Robert Rodale's *Prevention* magazine, with a circulation of 2,225,000 in 1980, was the fastest growing U.S. magazine except for *People*. In addition, books such as the *Better Homes and Gardens Family Medical Guide*, Fixx's *The Complete Running Book*, Eshelman and Winston's *The American Heart Association Cookbook*, and Morehouse and Gross's *Total Fitness in 30 Minutes a Week*, dominated the *New York Times* best-seller list during the 1970s. These have been replaced by *Jane Fonda's Workout* and Pearson and Shaw's *Life Extension: A Practical Scientific Approach*, among numerous others, and a multitude of diet books in the 1980s. John Naisbitt in his own best-seller *Megatrends*, published in 1982, believed that the recent trend of individuals promoting and improving their own health was the "triumph of the new paradigm of wellness, preventive medicine and wholistic care over the old model of illness, drugs, and surgery, and treating systems rather than the whole person" [74, p 147]. He substantiated his point with statistics of millions of exercising Americans, changing diets, health foods, and fitness equipment sales.

More recently, in 1988, at a regional hearing to provide input for improving public health by the year 2000 organized by the U.S. Public Health Service and the National Academy of Sciences's Institute of Medicine, Dr. Mark Oberle from the Centers for Disease Control in Atlanta testified that "we could be pushing ahead with high-tech medicine when the dollars would be better put to use in a preventive strategy that reduces the burden of illness on society." Additional testimony by Dr. Peter Pulrang, medical consultant for Washington State's Department of Social and Health Services' Bureau of Parent and Child Health, suggested that "the idea is to figure out how to prevent things from happening rather than just treating them after the fact" [*Seattle Post-Intelligencer*, December 4, 1988, p B-3].

These few examples of America's changing health care system as well as the thoughts of health care professionals, are only the tip of the iceberg when it comes to providing examples of the "new era" in medicine. No one living in American society during the 1980s can avoid noticing the increased interest in popularizing a preventive form of health behavior. Much like the lessons taught during the ancient period, we are told to breathe fresh air, eat proper foods, drink the right beverages, exercise, get adequate sleep, have a bowel movement a day, and take into account the emotions when analyzing our overall well-being. These "laws of health," which are presently so effectively disseminated throughout the population via a system of public and private schools as well as an elaborate media network of published materials, tapes, films, videos, television, and radio, were usually referred to as the "six things non-natural" before the mid-19th century. While we have benefited immensely from technological advances in the communications process during the 20th century, the primary method of health popularization from the ancient period through the 1850s was the published book. Accordingly, the primary objective of this chapter is to review the book literature pertaining to the "six things non-natural" and to explain their critical role in hygiene education before 1860.

This chapter is developed chronologically with an emphasis on the key authors and their books representing the non-natural theme. These primary sources are supplemented by appropriate secondary literature. The book coverage begins with the origins of the non-naturals in the ancient period, resumes in the 16th and 17th centuries in western Europe with the revival of the theme during the Renaissance, and continues through the 18th century Enlightenment period when the non-natural tradition is expanded. Beginning with the 19th century, books by American physicians and American editions of European publications are surveyed. These publications, all dealing with preventive medicine and hygiene, are divided into two groups representing 30-year time periods. The first group of books were published between 1800 and 1830 and the second group between 1831 and 1860. This section is followed by a final cluster of books, also published between 1830 and 1860. They represent a literature which began using the term "physical education," which at the time embodied the non-natural tradition.

In each of these books from the ancient period through ante-bellum America, it is shown that much of the content, structure, and message was attributable to the non-natural tradition. Consequently, numerous medical books had entire sections or chapters devoted to exercise. In addition, just as physicians decided to write individual works on air, diet, sleep, evacuations, or passions of the mind, several physicians published treatises on exercise.

The final portion of the chapter is devoted to a survey of the literature that attempted to explain the use and history of the "six things non-natural" term. This is followed by a review of some recent historical studies utilizing the non-natural concept. Finally, since our major focus within the non-naturals is exercise, a brief analysis of the historical literature pertaining to exercise is included.

Today, research has shown quite convincingly that exercise, one of the original six non-naturals, is good for one's health and that insufficient exercise can be detrimental to overall bodily functioning. Although adequate data to support these conclusions are fairly recent in historical terms, the recognition of the necessity for sufficient exercise for healthy living dates back to at least Hippocrates (460–370 B.C.) and Galen (129–210 A.D.). The concept of medicine articulated by these two ancient physicians became known as the "humoral theory."

Galen, who borrowed much from Hippocrates, structured his "theory" around the naturals (of, or with nature—physiology), the non-naturals (things not innate—hygiene), and the contra-naturals (against nature—pathology). Crucial to this theory were the six non-naturals: (*a*) air, (*b*) food and drink, (*c*) motion and rest, (*d*) sleep and wake, (*e*) excretions and retentions, and (*f*) passions of the mind [123]. The non-naturals needed to be utilized in moderation as to quantity, quality, time, and order; for if taken in excess or put into an imbalance, disease would result. Regulation of the six non-naturals could also influence the naturals, especially the qualities (hot, cold, moist, and dry) and the humors (blood—hot and moist, phlegm—cold and moist, yellow bile—hot and dry, and black bile—cold and dry). Therefore, along with drugs and surgery, the non-naturals were critical therapy for a variety of disease states. Exercise then, as part of motion and rest in the "non-natural" tradition, was incorporated in much of the early regimen, hygiene, and preventive medicine literature and, to a lesser extent, the literature of therapeutic medicine. While exercise was also recommended as therapy for a variety of ailments and as a cure for gout, dyspepsia, and consumption among others, the focus of this chapter is on exercise as prophylaxis rather than exercise as treatment.

Classical Greek preventive hygiene was part of formal medical training through the 18th century and continued on in the American health reform literature of the first half of the 19th century. During the latter period, an effort was made to popularize the "laws of health" as the non-naturals came to be known. Their maintenance and balance were something that each individual was responsible for. Accordingly, "self-help," "self-regulation," "self-management," "health behavior," and "personal health" were highly popular terms used in the preventive medicine literature of the 19th century [92]. Today, we use the terms "wellness" and "lifestyle alteration" in much the same way.

ORIGINS OF THE "NON-NATURAL" TRADITION WITH THE ANCIENT PHYSICIANS

Historians are in agreement that the close connection between exercise and medicine dates back to three ancient physicians: Herodicus (ca. 480–?), Hippocrates (460–370 B.C.), and Galen (129–210 A.D.). The first to study "therapeutic gymnastics," or "gymnastic medicine" as it was often called, was the Greek physician and former *paidotribes*, Herodicus. As a wrestling and boxing instructor, he realized that his weakest students could be made strong through exercise [78, 65]. Blundell [9] noted that Herodicus believed that it was "just as important to provide against diseases in the healthy man as to cure him who was already attacked." In the mind of Herodicus, physicians "recognized bodily exercise as part of their duties under the designation of 'Conservative Medicine' or 'Hygiene'" [9, p 32]. The anonymous author of a biographical sketch of Herodicus in *Rees' Encyclopaedia* [91] in 1819 reported that he was "a master of a school of exercise, or *gymnasium*" and that he devoted his career to "gymnastic medicine" whereby he set out to "ascertain the regulations of it most conducive to its proper end, according to the difference of age, constitution, and disorder of the patient, and to the climate, season, & c." [91, Vol. 17]. Cyriax [30] blamed Herodicus for causing a feud between physicians and gymnasts because "the physicians accused the gymnasts of usurping the functions of medical men" [30, p 181].

Most historians credit the interest of Hippocrates in exercise and diet to the influence of Herodicus. Hippocrates has been universally honored as "the father of scientific medicine" and physicians still take the "Hippocratic oath." He is given credit as the chief compiler of some 87 treatises on Greek medicine known as the "Corpus Hippocraticum" [86, 30, 65, 78]. In addition, the humoral theory of medicine mentioned earlier in the chapter is attributable to Hippocrates [2].

Although somewhat confusing, it appears that Hippocrates authored two separate works on regimen—*Regimen in Health*, with nine very short chapters, and *Regimen*, composed of four long sections or books [49]. The first seven chapters of *Regimen in Health* offer advice on the preservation of health and are directed to "the layman." Advice is given on what to drink and eat at certain times of the year. Hippocrates also suggested rapid walking in winter and slow in summer, recommended emetics and clysters for the bowels, and devoted a chapter to "athletes in training" [49, pp 45–59].

Regimen, the longer of his two works, was probably written sometime around 400 B.C. and once it is read, it becomes clear why Hippocrates has been called "the father of preventive medicine" [49, p 1]. In Book 1, we are told,

> Eating alone will not keep a man well; he must also take exercise. For food and exercise, while possessing opposite qualities, yet work together to produce health. For it is the nature of exercise to use up material, but of food and drink to made good deficiencies. And it is necessary, as it appears, to discern the power of various exercises, both natural exercises and artificial, to know which of them tends to increase flesh and which to lessen it; and not only this, but also to proportion exercise to bulk of food, to the constitution of the patient, to the age of the individual, to the season of the year, to the changes in the winds, to the situation of the region in which the patient resides, and to the constitution of the year. [49, p 229]

Still in Book 1, instructions are given to "take sharp runs so that the body may be emptied of moisture" [49, p 283] and to take walks after dinner. Much of Book 2 is devoted to exercise and training. Hippocrates classified exercises as natural (sight, hearing, voice, thought, and walking) and violent (running, wrestling, sparring, and ball games among others.) He also discussed the value of "running in a cloak" to increase body heat, swinging the arms while running, and how to avoid "fatigue pains" for "men out of training" [49, pp 353–359]. In Book 3, Hippocrates explained his invention of the prevention of disease:

> The discovery that I have made is how to diagnose what is the overpowering element in the body, whether exercises overpower food or food over-powers exercises; how to cure each excess, and to insure good health so as to prevent the approach of disease, unless very serious and many blunders be made. [49, p 367]

Later in the same book, he elaborated on his discovery:

> This discovery reflects glory on myself its discoverer, and is useful to those who have learnt it. . . . It comprises prognosis before illness and diagnosis of what is the matter with the body, whether food over-powers exercise, whether exercise overpowers food, or whether the two are duly proportioned. For it is from the overpowering of one or the other that diseases arise, while from their being evenly balanced comes good health. [49, p 383]

Much of the remainder of Book 3 is devoted to the proper food and exercises for each of the four seasons.

Just as Herodicus influenced Hippocrates, Hippocrates was a major influence on the career of Claudius Galenus or Galen, a physician in Rome during the 2nd century A.D. Galen authored numerous works of great importance to medical history, but for our purposes, his book *On Hygiene*, is of most interest. Galen was the dominating authority in the field of medicine at least through the Renaissance, and his works were widely read among physicians and educated laymen alike [1]. As a physician, Galen followed Hippocrates and borrowed from him the concepts of the four cardinal humors and the elementary qualities. And, as we have seen, when their balance was upset, disease resulted. As a hygienist, Galen the physician would try to maintain normal equilibrium by prescribing various orderings of the non-naturals, among other preventives and therapies. Galen himself admitted that until the age of 28 he suffered from a variety of illnesses. But after that, he discovered that there was "an art of health" [11, p 230]. Overall, Galen regarded exercise as one branch of hygiene and hygiene as part of the science of medicine.

On Hygiene provides the best collection of Galen's views on exercise and health. The book, called *Hygieina* in Greek and *De sanitate tuenda* in Latin, was translated by Thomas Linacre into French in 1517 [102]. It was not translated into English until Robert M. Green did so in 1951 [43]. Probably written around 180 A.D., *On Hygiene* was not directed to physicians but toward the educated layman. As Sigerist said, "It was a scientific work intended for educated people who were studying medicine as amateurs, to be sure, without the intention of ever practising the art" [102, p 6]. The book was divided into six books. Galen does not include the non-naturals as a term in *On Hygiene* but does subject the inevitable causal factors of disease to a fourfold classification: (*a*) things taken (food, drink, drugs), (*b*) things eliminated (bodily secretions and excretions), (*c*) things done (massage, walking, riding, exercise, sleep, watch, and coitus), and (*d*) things happening from without [89, p 341].

Most of the material on exercise was in the first three books. Book 1, "The Art of Preserving Health," was composed of 15 chapters. Chapter 8 was entitled "The Use and Value of Exercise" and dealt mainly with the need for motion in all ages. Whether by sailing, riding on horseback, driving, or via cradles, swings, and arms, everyone, even infants, Galen said, needed exercise [43, p 25]. Other chapters pertained to bathing and massage, fresh air, beverages, and evacuations. "Exercise and Massage" was the title of Book 2 and it comprised 12 chapters. Chapter 2, "Purposes, Time, and Methods of Exercise and Massage," included some very important material on the role exercise played in Galen's conception of hygiene. For example, in reference to the type and definition of exercise, Galen said,

> To me it does not seem that all movement is exercise, but only when
> it is vigorous. But since vigor is relative, the same movement might

be exercise for one and not for another. The criterion of vigorousness is change of respiration; those movements which do not alter the respiration are not called exercise. But if anyone is compelled by any movement to breathe more or less or faster, that movement becomes exercise for him. This therefore is what is commonly called exercise or gymnastics. [43, pp 53–54]

He saw the uses and values of exercise as follows:

The uses of exercise, I think, are twofold, one for the evacuation of the excrements, the other for the production of good condition of the firm parts of the body. For since vigorous motion is exercise, it must needs be that only these three things result from it in the exercising body—hardness of the organs from mutual attrition, increase of the intrinsic warmth, and accelerated movement of respiration. These are followed by all the other individual benefits which accrue to the body from exercise; from hardness of the organs, both insensitivity and strength for function; from warmth, both strong attraction for things to be eliminated, readier metabolism, and better nutrition and diffusion of all substances, whereby it results that solids are softened, liquids diluted, and ducts dilated. And from the vigorous movement of respiration the ducts must be purged and the excrements evacuated. [43, p 54]

Space does not permit elaboration in this review essay, but Galen's ideas about the proper time for exercise, factors to consider before exercise, the varieties of exercise, the different qualities of exercises, and the places for exercise, are truly amazing and quite perceptive. Book 3 entitled "Apotherapy, Bathing, and Fatigue," has a chapter on "Bathing After Exercise" and one on "Exercise After Sex Relations." In all, Galen's *On Hygiene* was a masterful document with far-reaching ramifications.

RENAISSANCE MEDICINE AND A REVIVAL OF THE "NON-NATURALS" IN 16TH AND 17TH CENTURY EUROPE

"Orthodox Greek hygiene," as Smith [104] called it, or the "regimen of the non-naturals," flourished as part of the revival of Galenic medicine as early as the 13th century. The leading medical schools of the world, Italy's Salerno, Padua, and Bologna, taught hygiene to their students as part of general instruction in the theory and practice of medicine. The works of Hippocrates and Galen dominated a system whereby "the ultimate goal was to be able to practise medicine in the manner of the ancient physicians" [18, p 341]. In fact, Galen's influence had become so strong that Bylebyl referred to the 16th century as "the golden age of Galenism." He noted that thanks to the work of the scholars, translators and book publishers Galen's works were more widely available, and in more complete and accurate form, than previously, and thanks to the dedication of his followers they were also more highly admired, more thoroughly studied, and probably better understood, than at anytime before or since. [18, p 340]

Padua, Bylebyl [18] claimed, was so dedicated to the classical tradition that they continued to teach medical theory from the works of Hippocrates and Galen through the mid-1700s.

At the same time physicians were learning about the non-naturals in their medical education, the early vestiges of the "self-help" movement were beginning in western Europe. Classical medicine also informed physicians and the lay public alike that responsibility for disease and health was not the province of the gods. Each individual either independently or in counsel with his or her physician had a moral responsibility for the preservation and attainment of health. As the 16th century progressed, "laws of bodily health were expressed as value prescriptions" [15, p 208]. Accordingly, as Paul Slack concluded in his study of medical literature in Tudor England, "regimens, textbooks and collections of remedies dominated the list of medical best-sellers between 1485 and 1604" [103, p 247]. In reference to the same literature, which Smith aptly called "medical advice books," she noted,

for individuals who sought some means of rational and prudential control for reasons of simple survival or personal enlightenment, there were the medical advice books. These vernacular works were written ostensibly for the lay individual. . . . For a large number of people they could well have been a far more familiar source of information than the personal advice of the trained physician. . . . One of the most obvious facts relating to the medical advice books is that they are published in English, and were on the face of it accessible to all those who could actually read—not just those who could read Latin. [104, pp 250–251]

In a very real sense then, non-natural regimen, the major component of the "advice book", became more and more important in one's management of the body and in the ideas of proper health behavior. In addition, all aspects of the non-natural tradition began to enter into the common language of life itself.

Regimen also became important during the Renaissance in a literature which Gruman [44] identified as "prolongevity hygiene." Gruman defined it as "the attempt to attain a markedly increased longevity by means of reforms in one's way of life" [44, p 221]. Central to the writings on longevity was the belief that any individuals who decided to live a temperate life, especially with reforms in their habits of diet and exercise, could extend their longevity in a significant manner. Beginning with the writing of Cornaro in 1558, the non-natural tradition achieved increasing attention from those wishing to live longer and more healthy lives.

Thomas Elyot's (1490–1546) *Castel of Helthe,* published in the 1530s and most likely in 1539, was the "originator and chief representative" of the genre of publications dealing with regimen as part of the new 16th century medical advice literature [103, p 250]. Its contents and style, built on the Galenic traditional regimen and the *Regimen sanitatis Salerni* (to be discussed later), served as a model for additional advice books for at least another century. Elyot's work was the first manual of popular or "domestic" medicine in the vernacular designed to provide the poor with simple instructions on how to keep well.

Although not a physician, Elyot had studied medicine with Thomas Linacre, England's most eminent physician at that time, who himself had trained at Padua and, as noted earlier, translated Galen's *On Hygiene* in 1517. In his preface, Elyot explained he "was not all ignorante in phisycke" since the physician to Henry VIII (Linacre) had read "unto me the workes of Galene" [33, p 4]. Elyot, like Galen before him, and like others writing about the non-naturals after him, improved his own poor health with proper attention to regimen. Toward the end of his book when discussing certain "grievous diseases," Elyot said, "I my selfe was by the space of foure years continually in this discrasy, . . . at the last felynge my selfe very feeble, and lacking appetite and slepe, as I happned to reade the bokes of Galene. . . . I perceyved that I had ben long in an errour" [33, p 79].

Elyot intended his book to be a fortress against disease, thus the title of *Castel of Helthe.* The content was devoted almost entirely to the "thynges naturall, thynges not naturall, and thynges against nature" [33, p 1]. The "thynges not Naturall be soo called, by cause they be no portion of a naturall body, as they be which be called Naturall things: but yet by the temperance of them, the body beinge in healthe, is therin preservyd" [33, p 13]. After sections on "Of meate and drinke" and "Of sleape and watche," Elyot included a part on "The commoditie of exercise, and the tyme when it should be used." Galen's influence is obvious when Elyot states,

> Every meuving is not an exercise, but only that whiche is vehement, thence wherof is alteration of the breath or mynde of a man. Of exercise do procede two commodities, evacuation of excrements, and also good habite of the body, for Exercise beinge a vehement motion, therof nedes must ensue hardness of the members. [33, pp 43–44]

He also included material on friction and rubbing before exercise, the diversities of exercises, and the use of the voice as a form of exercise.

The *Castel of Helthe* went through at least 15 editions by 1610 and far surpassed Elyot's earlier work, *The Boke Named The Governour*, in popularity. This latter work, written in 1531, also included a substantial amount of information and advice on exercise [10, pp 17–22].

Christobal Mendez (1500–1561), who received his medical training at the University of Salamanca, was the first physician to write a printed book devoted to exercise. A resident of the city of Jaen in Spain and later Seville, Mendez published his *Libro del Exercicio Corporal* or *Book of Bodily Exercise* [72] in 1553. Much of the contents seem to be based on his own experience and those of his acquaintances; however Mendez does refer to Aristotle, Celsus, Galen, and Pliny, among a few other ancient authors. But his debt to Galen is obvious since he made reference to him twice in the first three pages and identified Galen's three parts of medicine as "prevention, restoration and preservation." In regard to the latter, Mendez said, "The last group we may say is healthy, and to preserve health must do our exercises" [72, p 3]. Although *Book of Bodily Exercise* [72] does not appear to have had a very wide readership, Mendez's ideas on the subject of exercise were novel and preceded developments in exercise physiology and sports medicine thought to be unique to the early 20th century.

The book was divided into four treatises, each with several chapters. The first treatise dealt with exercise and its benefits; the second showed the divisions of exercise, including which is best; the third explained the common exercises and the advantages of each; and the fourth pertained to the best time for exercise. In chapter 3 of the first treatise, dealing with "Exercise Is the Easiest Way to Preserve Health," Mendez, in keeping with the non-natural tradition, said, "The physician must organize his patient's life and the things called un-natural such as eating and drinking, evacuation and retention, sleep and vigil, movement and rest, and the passions of the soul and the alteration of the air" [72, pp 6–7]. Also in the first treatise in Chapter 10, believing as the humoral theorists did that the physician had to clear away excess moisture in the body, Mendez wrote of the popularity of vomiting, bloodletting, purging, sweating, and urination. Then, after explaining the ill effects of each method, he noted,

> Having considered this, we realize that exercise was invented and used to clean the body when it was too full of harmful things. It cleans without any of the above-mentioned inconvenience and is accompanied by pleasure and joy (as we will say). If we use exercise under the conditions which we will describe, it deserves lofty praise as a blessed medicine that must be kept in high esteem. [72, p 22]

In the remaining three treatises, some of the subjects Mendez addressed were exercises for women, walking as the most beneficial exercise, exercises for youth, injuries from exercise, and exercise for the handicapped.

As noted earlier, Luigi Cornaro (1467–1565), a nonphysician resident of Padua, was the most influential proponent of prolongevity hygiene [44]. Cornaro discovered that he was in very poor health when he was in his late 30s and, through his knowledge of Galenic medical theory, blamed his condition on eating and drinking to excess as he lived in the fashion of the nobility during the early years of the 16th century in Italy. He reformed his life-style and adopted the regimen of a "sober life" whereby he avoided intemperance, preserved health and happiness, and attained a ripe and enjoyable old age [114]. Putting his habits into words at the age of 83, Cornaro published *Trattato della Vita Sobria (Treatise on a Sober Life)* in 1558, which was followed 3 years later by *Compendio della Vita Sobria (Compendium of a Sober Life)* [102].

In *Treatise on a Sober Life* [28], Cornaro recommended moderation in everything with more emphasis on diet than the other non-naturals. Since the book was written by a layman, who "practiced what he preached," for laymen, it had a certain appeal and persuasive power lacking in other books of the period. It was translated and published in French, Dutch, and German, although the English editions were the most popular. The first English edition was published in 1634 and the first American edition was published in Philadelphia in 1793. The 1826 London edition was listed as the 36th [102].

Another Italian physician and graduate of Padua, Girolamo Cardano (1501–1576), published *De sanitate tuenda (Care of Health)* in Rome in 1560 [34]. Possessing the same title as Galen's earlier work, which was translated as *On Hygiene*, others have referred to Cardano's book as *On Safeguarding the Health*. And while he admitted that Galen, "whose very high position and virtue have been conspicuous, has necessarily had great influence with me," Cardano said Galen's treatise was "too pedantic" and "wanders from the point, goes far afield and lingers on irrelevancies" when it came to his discussion of massage and exercise [20, pp 234–235]. The book was written in Latin with two editions appearing in 1580 and 1582 [34, p 282].

Care of Health was composed of six volumes with the material on exercise in Volume 4 on "Old Age." In this section Cardano discussed exercise as a factor in "quickening the spirits," the value of exercise for increasing the appetite, aiding digestion, and resisting illness and disease, and different physical activities for various age groups [34, pp 285–286]. We also learn from his autobiography *De Vita Propria Liber (The Book of My Life)* published in 1575, that he had been ill for much of his early life and exercised himself with swords and shields, running, jumping, and walking while fully armed [20, pp 26–27]. Exercise, combined with the other parts of the non-natural tradition, assisted in his recovery.

In "Manner of Life," Chapter 8 of his autobiography, Cardano reported, "There are seven principal genera of things: air, sleep, exercise, food, drink, medication, and preservative" [20, p 31]. Although not identical to our original list of the "six things non-natural," it is clear Cardano's philosophy of regimen and hygiene was based on them.

The third Italian physician in our review to write about exercise was Hieronymus Mercurialis (1530–1606) or Girolamo Mercuriale, as his name is sometimes written. Mercuriale's book, *De arte gymnastica aput ancientes (The Art of Gymnastics Among the Ancients)*, was published in Venice in 1569 and went through several editions. Although the book never moved beyond its original Latin language, it was still an effective transmitter of Galenic doctrine. Mercuriale quoted Galen relentlessly throughout the book and really provided more of a descriptive compilation of ancient material than an original work. Most of Book 1 is devoted to the gymnasia and thermae in Greece and Rome; Book 2 included dancing, Roman ball games and Olympic events; Book 3 dealt with more recreative activities like fishing, swimming, and hunting; in Book 4 Mercuriale examined the pros and cons of exercise while surveying the opinions of past notables; and Books 5 and 6 provided information on the effects of different exercises, when they ought to be done, and who should do them. Again, much of this was taken directly from Galen [71, 35].

Mercuriale was educated at Padua and taught medicine at Padua, Bologna, and Pisa while writing extensively in the field of medicine on subjects ranging from dermatology and pediatrics to gynecology. He had acquired such a reputation that he was called to Vienna to attend Emperor Maximilian II in 1573. In all, Mercuriale used nearly 200 works from Greek and Roman authors in his *Art of Gymnastics* and in so doing, helped further the non-natural tradition. That a physician of his stature wrote what appears to be the first illustrated book on exercise and medicine has had extensive ramifications [9]. Joseph, in his article on medical gymnastics, wrote, "In reality, all the books on gymnastics of the next centuries are based on this standard work" [57, p 1045].

English physician Thomas Cogan authored *The Haven of Health* [23], which was first published in London in 1584. Cogan directed his espistle to students whom, because of their sedentary ways, he believed were susceptible to sickness. He based his work on that of Elyot and the School of Salerno but it was the non-natural tradition of Hippocrates and Galen that formed the real basis of his work. In his opening message, "To the Reader," Cogan wrote,

> But wise Englishmen I trust will use the old English fashion still: and follow the rule of Hip. approved by Galen, and by common experience in mens bodies found most wholesome: Such as have

written of the preservation of health before me, for the most part have followed the divisio of Galen of things not natural, which be six in number. [23, p iii]

He then divided his chapters into (*a*) "Labour or Exercise," (*b*) "Meate," (*c*) "Drinke," (*d*) "Sleep" and (*e*) "Venus."

Cogan particularly liked "Tenise" as an exercise for students because it exercised "all parts of the body alike, as the legges, armes, neck, head, eyes, backe and loynes, and delighteth greatly the minde, making it lusty and cheerful." He went on to praise colleges for erecting "Tenis-courts for the exercise of their Schollers" [23, p 4]. He also emphasized that "exercise must be used in a good and wholesome aire . . . faire and cleare . . . lightsome and open . . . not stinking or corrupted" [23, p 7]. Almost at the end of the book, Cogan left a message to the student to "practice in your life, this short lesson":

Ayre, labour, food, repletion,
Sleepe, and Passions of the minde,
Both much and little, hurt a like,
Best is the meane to finde. [23, p 265]

Cogan's book, like that of Elyot, was not directed toward physicians. It was a major representative of the medical advice literature of 16th century England.

Although probably written in the late 13th or early 14th century, the Latin *Regimen Sanitatis Salernitanum* is included in the 17th century literature since it was not popularized until John Harington (1561–1612) translated it into English in 1607. Under the title *The Englishmans Doctor. Or the Schoole of Salerne. Or Physicall Observations for the Perfect Preserving of the Body of Man in Continuall Health* [48], the book is thought to be an accumulation of all the hygienic wisdom from Salerno's medical school. Clearly based on Galen's physiology, it was widely read. It was printed and reprinted repeatedly and Sigerist claimed that "never has there been a more successful medical book" [102, p 22].

Besides the fact that the contents were addressed to the physician and layman alike, the book was also very popular because it was written in verse. Early editions have over 360 verses, while more recent editions have included additional ones accumulated over the years. It included simple and common-sense rules applying to sleep, rest and exercise, effects of foods and drinks, as well as the "foure humors" and "foure Elements" [102, pp 30–31]. For several centuries, the *Regimen Sanitatis Salernitanum* provided rules on personal hygiene in a very attractive and readable form modeled after the old non-natural tradition.

In his chapter, "Pathology at Mid-Century," in Debus's *Medicine in 17th Century England,* L. J. Rather [90] called Robert Burton's (1577–1640) "entertaining discussion of the six non-naturals in the *Anatomy of Melancholy* . . . the best treatment of the subject in English" [90, p 102]. Burton, without formal medical credentials, wrote this very popular treatise in 1621. For Burton, melancholy was used to signify the disease known by many as "melancholia," but also made use of the term to refer to the melancholy humor (black bile). Throughout the book, he emphasized the importance of rectifying any disturbances or imbalances in the "six non-natural things" [52, pp 95–97]. Accordingly, sections of the book were devoted to the topics of "passions," "sleeping and waking," and "exercise." A large section was called "Exercise rectified of Body and Mind" as Part 2, Sec. 2, Memb. 4. Here, Burton referred to numerous authorities in the field but used Galen's writings most heavily [16, pp 336–356].

Although it was first published in 1564, Ambroise Pare's (1510–1590) classic work *Surgery* [79] did not appear in English translation until 1634. Pare (sometimes written as Parey) was a famous surgeon and served as the court physician for two different kings in his native France. His book does not include as much on exercise as the others reviewed, but it is included as an example of how powerful and popular the non-natural tradition was in the medical community. Part 1, "An Introduction or Compendious Way to Chirurgery" was divided into several chapters pertaining to the medical theory of the period. Beginning with Chapter 12, which was devoted to "Of Things Not Naturale" and continuing through several more chapters, Pare elaborated on each of the non-naturals and how it contributed to good health. Chapter 15 was entitled "Of Motion and Rest" and included information on the uses of exercise, the best time for exercise, the qualities of exercise, and "what discommodities proceed from idleness" [79, pp 34–35]. Pare also used the common form for listing the non-naturals whereby each was preceded by "of," as popularized by Elyot in his *Castel of Helthe.*

The final book to be covered in this section is Friedrich Hoffmann's (1660–1742) *Fundamenta Medicinae* which he published in 1695 [51]. A distinguished German physician, Hoffmann was appointed the first professor of medicine at Halle University around 1694. Although Hoffmann wrote on such diverse medical topics as personal hygiene, physiology, pathology, pediatrics, and medical ethics, *Fundamenta Medicinae* was his most distinguished work. It combined "the old and the new, Galenic teachings and new mechanical philosphy," directed toward students. Hoffmann organized the small book along the lines of the tradition of "Institutes" which involved relatively succinct instruction in a compendium form. The "Institutes" normally covered physiology, pathology, semeiology, hygiene, and therapeutics [51, pp ix–xi]. The fourth section,

"Medical Hygiene," included chapters devoted to (a) "Of the general rules for maintaining health," (b) "Of the various uses and abuses of the six non-naturals," and (c) "Of special rules to be observed in diets" [51, pp 103–113]. Later in his career, Hoffmann wrote several essays on bodily exercise and the preservation of health. Johann C. F. Guts Muths (1759–1839) referred to the work of Hoffmann several times in his classic work on *Gymnastics for the Young*, published in 1793, in Germany [63, 62].

ENLIGHTENMENT MEDICINE AND THE EXPANSION OF THE "NON-NATURAL" THEME IN 18TH CENTURY EUROPE

Although Galenism and the humoral theory of medicine were affected by new ideas from the fields of anatomy and physiology in particular, the non-natural tradition in the form of hygiene and regimen continued to flourish in 18th century Europe. Individual treatises continued to be written focusing on health preservation via "self-help," living long, and in some instances, specific books focusing on exercise as a therapy for certain diseases. Generally using the term "medical gymnastics," the authors looked to exercise as a cure as well as for the rehabilitation of body parts, particularly the limbs. This literature is outside the realm of this chapter, but a few of the dominant works are mentioned. Finally, some physicians during the 18th century began to look at exercise and the other non-naturals as viable alternatives to the heroic therapeutic practices of bleeding, purging, and drugging. Realizing that the "cure" could be worse than the disease, some physicians advocated nonintervention tactics which revolved around guiding and monitoring health behavior.

Books on health for the layman generally fell into two broad categories through the end of the 18th century. The first group comprised regimen and long life and were written for the educated and leisured classes. The non-natural message was directed to wealthy and sedentary city dwellers, generally aristocratic and professional men who tended to overeat and overdrink. Regimen was presented as a way to counteract the "diseases of civilization" where excess, intemperance, and inactivity abounded. In most instances, this literature was sort of a "religio-medical" prescription for regularity and sober living. And since those individuals to whom the literature was directed could afford physicians and regular medical attention, very little in the way of therapy or the description of specific diseases was included. These were books to read and contemplate.

The second group of books were health manuals generally consisting of material on health preservation as well as information on diseases and their cure. They included the typical non-natural guidance but also included "recipes" or lists of medicines and their applications for home or self-treatment. This literature was more directed to the middle classes rather than the idle rich or working poor, and the physicians that authored these handbooks often spoke out against drugging and the use of medical men. Instead, they recommended using one's own intuition, relying more on nature, and a proper ordering and balancing of the six non-naturals. Scepticism of the heroic healers combined with a commitment to self-sufficiency and a concern for the family group led the authors of this literature to value prevention in the form of hygiene and regimen over treatments by physicians. Because of this basic philosophy and their prospective audience, terms like "easy and natural," "prevention," and "domestic" were incorporated in their titles.

While the literature on the uses of exercise or "medical gymnastics" as a cure are outside the purview of this chapter, three important works were written during this time period and represented a new form of therapy which would continue on into the 19th century and, in some instances, beyond. Francis Fuller's (1670–1706) *Medicina Gymnastica: or, A Treatise Concerning the Power of Exercise* [40] was published in London in 1704 and had gone into nine editions by 1777. Not a physician himself, Fuller based many of his ideas on his own experiences as well as the influence of Thomas Sydenham, one of Britain's most famous physicians. Joseph-Clement Tissot's (1747–1826) *Medicinal and Surgical Gymnastics* [64] was first published in Paris in 1780 and was translated into several other languages by the 1790s. The third book was written by John Pugh (dates unknown) in London in 1794 and was titled *A Physiological, Theoretic and Practical Treatise on the Utility of the Science of Muscular Action for Restoring the Power of the Limbs* [87]. Pugh was an anatomist and included a chapter "On the necessity and importance of exercise" in which he quoted several individuals, including Hippocrates, Galen, and Cornaro.

The first division of health literature for the layman devoted to regimen and long life is represented by five publications: *The Ladies Library* [69], George Cheyne's *An Essay of Health and Long Life* [22], John Armstrong's *The Art of Preserving Health* [4], the *Encyclopedie* [24], and James Mackenzie's *The History of Health, and the Art of Preserving It* [67]. The *Ladies Library*, "written by a Lady," published in three volumes in London in 1714, was a compilation of material written both earlier and contemporary on all aspects of the proper life of the 18th century woman. Major chapters were entitled "Employment," "Recreation," "The Wife," "The Mother," and "The Mistress." It went through eight editions in English and two in French, and was translated into Dutch before 1772. The influence of the non-natural tradition was clearly evident when the author summarized the hygienic recommendations of the work as a "few and easie observable Rules; Plenty of *open* Air, *Exercise* and *Sleep*, plain *Diet*, no *Wine* or *strong Drink*, and very little or no *Physick*" [69, p 372].

George Cheyne's (1671–1743) *An Essay of Health and Long Life* was published in London in 1724 and by 1745 had gone through 10 editions and translations in French, Dutch, Latin, and German. Cheyne himself turned to regimen after he had grown to 445 pounds. The author of numerous medical works, Cheyne was a respected physician, a member of the Royal Society, and included John Wesley among his elite patients [113, 70, 108, 109]. His message was directed to the London affluent and the health problems of intellectuals, professional men, and the aristocracy. *An Essay of Health and Long Life* followed the Galenic doctrine very closely and in his introduction Cheyne said, "And that I might write with some Order and Connexion, I have chosen to make some Observations and Reflections on the Non-Naturals . . . they seem to me, the best general Heads for bringing in those Observations and Reflections I am to make in the following Pages" [22, p 3]. Not surprising then, Chapter 1 is entitled "Of Air," Chapter 2 "Of Meat and Drink," Chapter 3 "Of Sleeping and Watching," and Chapter 4 "Of Exercise and Quiet." In the latter chapter, Cheyne recommended walking as the "most natural" and "most useful" exercise while riding was the "most manly" and "most healthy" [22, p 94]. He also advocated exercises in the open air like tennis and dancing and recommened cold baths and the use of the "flesh brush" to promote perspiration and improve circulation.

The *Art of Preserving Health* [4] by John Armstrong (1709–1779), was first published in London in 1744 and by 1757 had been reprinted five times, including a United States edition in Philadelphia in 1745. By 1830, it had been reprinted 13 times. The book was divided into four books, one devoted to air, one to diet, one to exercise, and one on passions. Like the *Regimen Sanitatis Salernitanum*, Armstrong presented his rules for health in verse form. Book 3 on "Exercise" offered,

Toil, and be strong. By toil the flaccid nerves
Grow firm, and gain a more compacted tone;
The greener juices are by toil subdu'd,
Mellow'd, and subtiliz'd; the vapid old
Expell'd, and all the rancour of the blood. [4, p 89]

Armstrong also wrote about the joys of nature and the healthfulness of hunting and fishing. As the chapters indicated, Armstrong was continuing the non-natural tradition in his guide to the preservation of health.

The *Encyclopedie*, a dictionary of the sciences and arts, was directed by the philosopher Diderot and the mathematician D'Alembert in collaboration with the most prominent scientists of the mid-18th century. Coleman [24, 25] called the entries on "health," "hygiene," and the "non-naturals" "a medical doctrine for the bourgeoisie" and viewed the *En-*

cyclopedie as a true representative of Enlightenment thought. Originally published in 1751 in Paris, it went through several editions. Arnulfe D'Aumont, a graduate of Montpellier and a professor at the medical school in Valence, authored the articles as noted above. Jean Noel Halle, a member of the medical faculty at Paris, authored the entry on "hygiene" in editions after 1780. In this section, Halle identified the substance of hygiene as "the things which mankind uses or handles, improperly called non-natural, and their influence on our constitution and organs" [54, p 124]. Halle also identified "public hygiene" as compared to "private hygiene," and said hygiene can vary "depending on whether one attends to man collectively or in a society or whether he is viewed as an individual" [24, p 414]. The *Encyclopedie*, like the other literature in this classification, went primarily into the hands of the educated members of the bourgeoisie and nobility. Yet as Coleman so aptly explained in reference to Enlightenment thought, "the doctrine of the non-naturals as a guide to correct hygienic practice was wholly consonant with this striking reorientation of Western thought" [24, p 419].

James Mackenzie's (1680–1761) book *The History of Health, and the Art of Preserving It* [67] was published in Edinburgh in 1758. Mackenzie was a Fellow of the Royal College of Physicians in Edinburgh and wrote a book that was designed to be casual and relaxed reading for an educated elite. His book was a history and review of the rules related to the preservation of health and thus devoted a considerable amount of space to the non-naturals. In Chapter 6 on Hippocrates, Mackenzie noted, "I shall endeavor, *first*, to range in order all his precepts and remarks on the *six articles necessary to life*, vulgarly called the Non-Naturals" [67, p 81]. Other major portions of the book were devoted to "Motion and Rest" and "Of Exercise." In his introduction, Mackenzie credited Galen with originating the term "non-naturals" and explained that in their "proper use and regulation of which the art of preserving health principally consists" [67, pp 4–5].

The second division of health literature for the layman usually consisted of information on the preservation of health but also included lists of diseases and medicines for them. More directed to the middle classes and designed to be used rather than studied and contemplated, this literature is also represented in this chapter by five publications: John Wesley's *Primitive Physic* [118], William Buchan's *Domestic Medicine* [12], Bryan Cornwell's *The Domestic Physician, or Guardian of Health* [29], Bernard Faust's *Catechism of Health* [37], and *The Art of Preventing Diseases, and Restoring Health* by George Wallis [115].

John Wesley's (1703–1791) *Primitive Physic* [118], first published in 1747, was influenced to a large degree by George Cheyne, and as Turner suggested, "There was an obvious attraction between Wesley's religious asceticism and Cheyne's view of the Christian importance of maintaining the body in good health through sober living, regular hours, exercise and temperance" [109, p 265]. However, through Wesley's book, Cheyne's ideas probably reached a much wider audience. In his preface Wesley noted, "The power of exercise, both to preserve and restore health, is greater than can well be conceived; especially in those who add temperance thereto" [118, p iv]. Later in the preface, Wesley reported, "For the sake of those who desire, through the blessing of God, to retain the health which they have recovered, I have added a few plain, easy rules, chiefly transcribed from Dr. Cheyne." [118, p vii] Wesley then proceeded to discuss each of the six non-naturals, including two pages devoted to exercise. The second part of *Primitive Physic* was devoted to "A Collection of Recipes" for a multitude of ailments since Wesley believed "simple remedies are in general the most safe for simple disorders, and sometimes do wonders under the blessing of God" [118, p xi]. Through an American edition published as early as 1793 and through numerous English editions, Wesley's faith in the non-natural tradition was spread from chapel to chapel and throughout the congregations of Methodism in Western Europe and the United States.

Domestic Medicine [12] by William Buchan (1729–1805) was the classic of classics. Aimed at individual and family improvement via proper regimen, Buchan's book contained rules for the healthy as well as the sick. It was written for the layman as a substitute for the deficiencies of medical care and was so popular that it achieved a lifespan of 144 years. First published in 1769 in Edinburgh where Buchan was educated, *Domestic Medicine* appeared in new editions and reprints every few years in Britain through 1846. The first American edition appeared in Philadelphia in 1771. The book was translated into French, Spanish, Italian, German, Russian, and Swedish. The last edition appeared in Boston in 1913 [61, 8].

While Buchan did not use the term non-naturals, he acknowledged his debt to Cheyne and divided his book into the six classical headings. For example, Chapter 4 was "Of Air," Chapter 5 "Of Exercise," Chapter 6 "Of Sleep," and Chapter 10 "Of the Passions." Chapter 1, "Of Children," included a portion devoted to "Of the Exercise of Children" in which Buchan said,

Of all the causes which conspire to render the life of man short and miserable, none have greater influence than the want of proper Exercise. . . . Sufficient exercise will make up for several defects in nursing; but nothing can supply the want of it. It is absolutely necessary to the health, the growth, and the strength of children. [12, p 43]

In Chapter 5 Buchan exclaimed,

Inactivity never fails to induce a universal relaxation of the solids, which disposes the body to innumerable diseases. When the solids are relaxed neither the digestion nor any of the secretions can be duly performed. . . . Weak nerves are the constant companions of inactivity. Nothing but exercise and open air can brace and strengthen the nerves, or prevent the endless train of diseases which proceed from a relaxed state of these organs. [12, pp 85–86]

Other portions of *Domestic Medicine*, like *Primitive Physick*, dealt with numerous remedies for ills ranging from "dropsy" to rheumatism. In the realm of therapy, Buchan was particularly against the use of drugs and where possible, advocated herbal medicines. Before the term was popular, Buchan seemed to be practicing "holistic medicine" [99].

Bryan M. L. Cornwell (dates unknown) followed the Wesley and Buchan models in his book *The Domestic Physician, or Guardian of Health* [29], published in London in 1788. In his preface, Cornwell quoted Galen's definition of medicine as "the art of preserving present health, and of retrieving it when lost" [29, p v]. Also in the preface, Cornwell explained that medicine was "divided into five principal branches" and said that "the fourth branch considers the remedies, and their use, whereby life may be preserved; whence it is called hygiene: its objects are what we strictly call non-natural" [29, pp viii–ix]. Part 1 of the book, "On the Causes of Diseases," had chapters entitled "Of Air," "Of Exercise," "Of Sleep," and "Of the Passions." Part 2 was devoted to "Of the Knowledge and Cure of Diseases."

German physician Bernard Christoph Faust (1755–1842) wrote *Catechism of Health for the Use of Schools, and for Domestic Instruction* [37] in 1794. It was a small booklet of 92 pages designed to teach the elements of hygiene to children. More than 150,000 copies were sold in a few years and it was translated into several different languages. An edition "Published for the use of the Citizens of the United States" was printed in New York in 1798 [101]. *Catechism of Health* was divided into two major parts, "Of Health" and "Of Disease." The first incorporated the usual non-natural divisions, with chapters on "Of Air," "Of Food," "Of Exercise and Rest," and "Of Sleep." Each of the chapters was arranged with a question-and-answer format.

The first popular text devoted solely to preventive medicine to be published in the United States was written by London physician George Wallis (1740–1802). *The Art of Preventing Diseases, and Restoring Health* [115] was published in New York in 1793 with a second edition in 1794. In the style of Buchan, the book was directed to a wider audience than those manuals presented in our first division. Wallis quoted Hippocrates, Galen, Hoffmann, and Cornaro, among others, and wrote of the "non-naturals" in his "Explanatory Preface." Section 3 was devoted to "Of the

Non-Naturals" and spanned some 24 pages with two on "Exercise and Rest." Wallis concluded his "Non-Naturals" section almost apologetically by saying,

> What we have here delivered, perhaps may be by some thought of too trivial consequence; and is by many too much, even in the practice of medicine, neglected—still will be found, on experience, worthy of very close atttention: for the knowledge from thence to be collected, and properly, as we shall soon have occasion to shew, forms one part of medicine, comprehending that which is stiled—prophylactic or preventive. [115, pp 88–89]

Regarding exercise in particular, Wallis emphasized the importance of activities that incorporated the mind because when "the mind is exhilirated" it "will communicate agreeable sensations, and give firmness to the moving powers" [157, p 76].

AMERICAN EDITIONS AND UNITED STATES PHYSICIANS: THE "NON-NATURALS" IN ANTE-BELLUM AMERICA

Nineteenth century America was fertile ground for both the non-natural tradition and the general hygiene movement, which were finding their way into the United States via American editions of western European medical treatises or through books on hygiene written by American physicians. The United States between 1800 and 1860 was a rapidly changing land with a large percentage of its inhabitants residing in the northeastern cities. While Americans still looked to Europe for guidance in several realms, including medical practice, the young country was also trying to stand on its own merits and demonstrate "independence" in all walks of life.

Part of this latter trend was the concern for the physical degeneracy of the American people, particularly city dwellers. Comparisons with their European counterparts, especially England, generally showed that urbanites were in poor health and lacked the basic rudiments of proper hygiene. Health of the new nation became part of a general reform movement with nationalism as the primary motivator.

The "self-help" era was also in full bloom during ante-bellum America. Individual reform writers wrote about "self-improvement," "self-regulation," the "responsibility for personal health," and "self-management." It was suggested that the responsibility for disease resided with each individual and that if one got sick, it was his or her own fault. Personal health, the reformers claimed, could be improved and disease prevented by obeying the "natural laws." If individuals ate too much, slept too long, or did not get enough exercise, then they could only blame themselves for illness. By the same token, they could also dictate their own good health [112, 73, 21, 77].

Others took the doctrine of "natural laws" further when they suggested that morality resulted from individual hygienic improvements. These Christian reformers saw "natural law" as the dictate of God and believed that healthfulness and Godliness went hand-in-hand. If one chose to violate the "laws," then illness or death would follow. For those who obeyed and followed the principles of health, they would be rewarded by God with a long and wholesome life under his watchful eye [119].

Prevention literature and hygiene instruction were also popular in American medical practice before 1860 because there still were not many known cures. It was an era when many laymen and physicians alike still had much faith in nature. In fact, the term "natural" was used in the medical literature to signify a state of well-being. As such, improvements in public health measures, a reliance on and trusting of nature, and plans for educating the public on living habits, each received attention in the medical literature [116].

The medical literature also contained hygienic instructions and recommendations for individual aspects of the non-natural tradition as part of the opposition to "heroic" healing practices. Drugging, bleeding, and purging were often viewed as being more dangerous than the disease they were enlisted to cure. Sleep, diet, exercise, herbs, and water, among others, were recommended either individually or wholly as alternative medicines [121, 98].

Although numerous health care books were written for the layman during the ante-bellum period, only a few are reviewed in this chapter. Because of their numbers and for organizational purposes, the first group of books have publication dates between 1800 and 1830. Six representative books are covered in this section. They include A. F. M. Willich's *Lectures on Diet and Regimen* [122], Shadrach Ricketson's *Means of Preserving Health, and Preventing Diseases* [93], James Thacher's *American Modern Practice; Or, A Simple Method of Prevention and Cure of Diseases* [107], James Ewell's *The Medical Companion, or Family Physician* [36], John Gunn's *Domestic Medicine* [45], and Edward Hitchcock's *Dyspepsy Forestalled and Resisted* [50].

Willich's (dates unknown) book, directed to "the most rational means of preserving health and prolonging life," was designed "for the use of families" and was first published in London in 1799. Two editions were sold out that first year and in 1800 it went into its third edition. The first New York edition appeared the next year in 1801. It was simple enough for families to use yet formal enough for physicians. As the title suggests, Willich's lectures in England during the winter of 1798 made up the bulk of the contents. He indicated his intent in the "Postscript":

My design, in these Lectures, has not been to lay down particular rules for the distinction and treatment of diseases, but rather for their prevention, and, conse-quently, for the preservation of health. [122, p 454]

Also in his "Postscript," Willich indicated his reliance on the non-naturals when he said that "we cannot effect a favorable change in the nature and progress of a disease, whether chronic or acute, without due attention to food, drink, air, sleep, exercise, or rest & c." [122, p 455].

The chapter arrangement included the typical non-natural topics. Chapter 1 dealt with "On the Means of Preserving Health and Prolonging Life" and some of the other chapters were as follows: "Of Air and Weather," "Of Food," "Of Exercise and Rest," "Of Evacuations," and "Of the Passions and Affections of the Mind." Willich's chapter on exercise began with the idea of the necessity of motion:

Motion, or bodily exercise, is necessary to the preservation of health, which is promoted, while the bounds of moderation are not exceeded. Too violent exercise, or a total want of it, are attended with equal disadvantages. [122, p 303]

He included information on specific kinds of exercises (active and passive), the time for exercise, and the duration of exercise. The essential advantages of exercises included increased bodily strength, improved circulation of the blood and all other fluids, aid in necessary secretions and excretions, help in clearing and refining the blood, and removal of obstructions. In all, the chapter spanned 20 pages.

Shadrach Ricketson (1768–1839), a New York physician, is credited with writing "the first American text on hygiene and preventive medicine" [97, p 140]. Published in 1806, Ricketson's book was titled *Means of Preserving Health, and Preventing Diseases: Founded Principally on an Attention to Air and Climate, Drink, Food, Sleep, Exercise, Clothing, Passions of the Mind, and Retentions and Excretions* [93]. His dependence on the non-natural tradition is obvious from the title. The book was well-received by other physicians and contained material from his own experiences as well as quotations from other medical writers.

Like most of the other books examined, Ricketson's chapter structure followed each of the non-naturals. Chapter 5 was devoted to "Exercise" and, like Willich's, covered about 20 pages. Ricketson quoted from Cheyne's *Essay on Health* as well as various encyclopedias. In his opening statement, he explained,

A certain proportion of exercise is not much less essential to a healthy or vigorous constitution, than drink, food, and sleep; for we see, that people, whose inclination, situation, or employment does not admit of exercise, soon become pale, feeble, and disordered. [93, p 152]

Ricketson went on to say that "exercise promotes the circulation of the blood, assists digestion, and encourages perspiration" [93, p 152]. He also warned of the destructiveness of "high living and strong drink" and noted that "idleness and luxury create more diseases than labour and industry" [93, p 153].

James Thacher (1754–1844), a Boston physician and author of *The American New Dispensatory* and *Observations on Hydrophobia*, published *American Modern Practice* [107] in Boston in 1817. Thacher's ability and knowledge of American medicine was illustrated in his introduction, titled "Historical Sketch of Medical Science, and the Sources and Means of Medical Instruction in the United States." This 65-page survey was then followed by four books. The first book dealt with the means of preserving health and obtaining longevity, with chapters including "Of the Nonnaturals," "Of Air or Atmosphere," "Exercise," "Of the Passions," and "Of Sleep" among others. The other three books pertained to diseases, with Book 2 focusing on children. A small portion of it dealt with "Of the Exercise of Children."

Thacher credited Willich's book for information on the "nonnaturals." In Chapter 2 on "Exercise," he made reference to Galen and Sydenham and said that "the position is universally established, that exercise should be ranked as among the most important agents which we can employ, for the preservation of life and health" [107, p 77]. He recommended walking, running, leaping, riding, swimming, and fencing as active exercises and referred to "friction" as "a kind of exercise that remarkably contributes to the health of sedentary persons" [107, p 80]. In his concluding statement, Thacher warned of the old non-natural theme of balance and moderation for all aspects of regimen, including exercise:

Although bodily exercise is an essential requisite for the preservation of health, this should not exceed the bounds of moderation; as too violent exercise, and to a total want of it, are attended with equal disadvantages.[107, p 80]

The Medical Companion, or Family Physician [36], by James Ewell (1773–1832), was written in the best tradition of Buchan, Wesley, Cornwell and others where part of the book dealt with the preservation of health and the remainder addressed specific ailments and offered advice for treatment. Ewell practiced medicine in Savannah, Georgia and then moved to Washington, D.C., when he wrote the book. Originally published in 1882, *The Medical Companion* had reached its eighth edition by 1834.

The first major section, "On Hygiene; Or the Art of Preserving Health," was divided into parts devoted to each of the non-naturals. In a brief introduction Ewell said,

I shall now show, that by due attention to the 'Non-naturals,' *air, food, exercise, sleep, evacuations,* and *passions,* we may go far to preserve this fabric in good health from the cradle to the grave. Nay, so wonderful is the body and its resources, its powers of renovation; and so sovereign are the virtues of the Non-naturals, that thousands are the instances of persons who, after having their health apparently ruined by an *abuse* of them, have on returning to a wise and temperate use, recovered their health, and attained to a most active and happy old age.[36, p 65]

The section "Of Exercise" included warnings about inactivity and the power of "daily exercise in the open air." Also included was material on the value of exercise in cold climates and the ability of the body's physiological system to resist cold.

Like Buchan's *Domestic Medicine,* John C. Gunn's (1800–1863) *Gunn's Domestic Medicine, Or Poor Man's Friend* [45] was a classic. Written and originally published in Knoxville in 1830, the book went through many editions until it was revised and enlarged in 1857. By 1876, the book had reached 160 editions, and by the time the last recorded edition was issued in 1920, it had achieved 234 printings. Gunn dedicated the book to President Andrew Jackson and directed much of the book to a southwestern population, mainly residents of Tennessee. Part of the text dealt with prevention and part dwelled on diseases and a "Dispensatory, or Classification of Medicines" for the "home doctors" he was writing for. Evidently, the book was also used quite frequently as a basic reference for physicians on the frontier which increased Gunn's popularity throughout much of the West [68].

It was clear that Gunn adhered to the non-natural tradition when he noted in his introduction that "The greatest number of diseases and infirmities are of our own begetting; because we have infringed the healthy laws of nature" [45, p 13]. This was followed by a lengthy section called "Of the Passions." Gunn's part on "Exercise" recommended temperance, exercise, and rest and valued nature's way over traditional medical treatment.

Exercise, for the purpose of producing perspiration, and throwing off the excrementitious or bad matter from the system, is much better than any merely medical means; not only because it is the means which nature herself prescribes, but because, unlike medical drugs generally, it strengthens instead of weakening the system. [45, p 108]

He also recommended exercise for women and claimed that all of the "diseases of delicate women" like "hysterics and hypochondria, arise from want of due exercise in the open, mild, and pure air" [45, p 109]. Finally, in an interesting statement for the 1830s if not the 1980s, Gunn recommended a training system for all:

> The advantages of the *training system*, are not confined to pedestrians or walkers—or to pugilists or boxers alone; or to horses which are trained for the chase and the race track; they extend to man in all conditions; and were training introduced into the United States, and made use of by physicians in many cases instead of medical drugs, the beneficial consequences in the cure of many diseases would be very great indeed. [45, p 113]

The final book to be reviewed as one of the six representational health care books published between 1800 and 1830 is Edward Hitchcock's (1793–1864) *Dyspepsy Forestalled and Resisted: Or Lectures on Diet, Regimen, and Employment; Delivered to the Students of Amherst College, Spring Term, 1830* [50]. Much like Willich's *Lectures on Diet and Regimen* [122], Hitchcock divided his book into nine different "lectures." A second edition was published in nearby Northampton in 1831 by the Amherst College professor of chemistry and natural history. Hitchcock later became president of the college.

Whereas books by Gunn amd others were directed to the general population, Hitchcock directed his "lectures" to college students who did not understand good health practices. As Allmendinger has noted, "The student lived without family restraints or collegiate custom, a potential victim of his own ignorance or intemperance" [3, p 105]. Accordingly, Hitchcock provided guidance in "self-regulation" with information on alcohol, narcotic substances, study time, recreation, rules for diet, and the physical and mental effects of dyspepsy. He quoted Galen, Cheyne, Cornaro, and Wallis and devoted two lectures in Part 2 on "Regimen" to the various non-naturals. Lecture 6 was totally given to exercise and spanned some 30 pages. Lecture 7 included advice on air, clothing, cleanliness, evacuations, sleep, manners, and the imagination and passions. Hitchcock was particularly fond of "physical education" and included the transcript of an "Address on the Physical Culture Adapted to the Times Delivered Before the Mechanical Association in Andover Theological Seminary, September 21, 1830" as the final portion of the book.

Four books are representative of the health care literature published in the United States between 1831 and 1860. Although many more existed, the four chosen are some of the more important ones and appeared at different times throughout the period. These are Andrew Combe's *The Principles of Physiology Applied to the Preservation of Health* [26], Robley Dunglison's *On the Influence of Atmosphere and Locality; . . . Exercise, Sleep . . . On Human Health* [32], Sylvester Graham's *Lectures on the Science of Human Life* [41], and John King's *The American Family Physician: or Domestic Guide to Health* [60].

Andrew Combe's (1797–1847) *The Principles of Physiology Applied to the Preservation of Health, and to the Improvement of Physical and Mental Education* [26] was another classic work with far-reaching ramifications. One scholar, in commenting on Combe's book, said American health reformers cited it "as theologians cited the Bible." It was originally published in Edinburgh in 1834 where Combe served as personal physician to the Queen of Scotland. There was a New York edition that same year and by the 1843 New York edition, it was in its seventh Edinburgh edition. It was included in the Harper Brothers Home Library series selling for 50 cents, which increased its availability considerably. Like other health manuals reviewed, Combe's book was designed to help people help themselves live a comfortable and healthy life. As Cooter said, "Combe's works were eminently sensible and readable, offering cogent discussion on the structures and functions of the body and the rational regimen necessary for maintaining health" [27, p 75].

There was much on the value of exercise spread through several of Combe's 11 chapters, but Chapter 4 on the "Nature of the Muscular System" and Chapter 5 on the "Effects of, And Rules For, Muscular Exercise" contained the most important information on the topic. After discussing the physiological effects of muscular exercise on the human body, Combe elaborated on the best time for exercise and the different kinds of exercise. He recommended walking, riding, dancing, gymnastics and "callisthenic exercises," fencing, shuttlecock, and reading aloud. Combe particularly disapproved of the different exercises often prescribed for the two sexes and suggested that the exercises for women should not differ that radically from men. In this regard he suggested "club exercise" for women [26, pp 131–154].

Robley Dunglison (1798–1869) was a professor of hygiene and medical jurisprudence at the University of Maryland and is credited with writing "the first American textbook on preventive medicine prepared for use by medical students" [97, p 147]. His book *On the Influence of Atmosphere and Locality; Change of Air and Climate; Seasons; Food; Clothing; Bathing; Exercise; Sleep; Corporeal and Intellectual Pursuits, & c. & c. on Human Health; Constituting Elements of Hygiene* [32] was a testimony to Dunglison's strong belief in the importance of the non-naturals. He paid tribute to Combe and his book and noted in the preface that: "Hygiene is, therefore, a part of *practical* medicine. It teaches the course to be adopted in the way of prophylaxis or preservation" [32, p iii]. Chapter

5 was called "Exercise" and Dunglison's opening statement was, "There is no hygienic agency of more importance than the due exercise of the body" [32, p 425]. He discussed the topic for the next 18 pages in considerable detail.

The life and contributions of Sylvester Graham (1794–1851) are widely known as a result of the fine work of Shryock [100], Nissenbaum [76], and Whorton [120]. Graham argued for self-improvement and asked each individual to become "a healthy animal." His message of a "physiology of subsistence" was directed primarily to the middle classes [112]. Graham published several books, including his lengthy *Lectures on the Science of Human Life* [41] in 1839. As a Presbyterian minister rather than a physician, Graham's impact on American health reform was impressive.

Volume 2 of Graham's *Lectures* [41] included a major portion devoted to diet in which he compared vegetables and flesh, gave the proper times for eating and the frequency, and discussed quantities of food along with what to drink. This material encompassed more than 600 pages. The remaining 50 pages dealt with the other non-naturals of sleep, air, exercise, and evacuations. For exercise, Graham said, "Indeed, exercise may truly be considered the most important natural *tonic* of the body" [41, p 652]. Later, Graham noted that "exercise in order to be most beneficial, must be enjoyed" [41, p 655]. He also discussed the benefits of walking, running, leaping, dancing, swimming, and riding on horseback.

The last book discussed in this section is included because of its lateness chronologically and the fact that it maintained a style of health care first popularized by Buchan. John King (1813–1893), a professor at the Eclectic College of Medicine in Cincinnati, published *The American Family Physician; Or Domestic Guide to Health* [60] in 1860. Like other books of this type, King structured the contents around chapters devoted to each of the non-naturals. Intended for "the most uneducated," King presented "the greatest amount of useful information, in *plain* and *familiar* language, free from the mysterious and incomprehensible *medical terms*, in which physicians endeavor to hide their art" [88, p iii]. Chapter 9 was devoted to exercise and included information on the rules for exercise, sailing, walking, running, dancing, swimming, friction, and gymnastics. Like so many before him, King divided exercises into passive and active.

LEARNING THE "LAWS OF HEALTH": THE "NON-NATURALS" EMBODIED IN THE TERM "PHYSICAL EDUCATION"

The basic rudiments of the hygiene movement, or the non-natural tradition itself, found further expression in ante-bellum America through a new literature devoted to "physical education." In the early 19th century, a number of physicians began to use the term "physical education" in journal articles, speeches, and book titles to represent the task of teaching children the "laws of health." As Willich [122] explained in 1801, "by *physical education* is meant the bodily treatment of children; the term *physical* being applied in opposition to *moral*" [122, p 60]. He continued in his section "On the Physical Education of Children" to discuss stomach ailments, bathing, fresh air, exercise, dress, and diseases of the skin among various other topics [122, pp 60–73]. Similarly, Dr. John G. Coffin's editorship of the *Boston Medical Intelligencer, Devoted to the Cause of Physical Education and to the Means of Preventing and of Curing Diseases* from 1826 to 1828 represented a definition of "physical education" much broader than exercise or gymnastics. "Physical education," then, implied educating about one's *physical* body rather than exercising the body in a gymnasium or elsewhere. Knowledge about one's body was deemed crucial to a well-educated and healthy individual by several physicians whom, as Whorton has suggested, "dedicated their careers to birthing the modern physical education movement" [120, p 282].

The writings on "physical education" by four of these physicians are reviewed as representative of this ante-bellum American trend. These include Charles Caldwell's *Thoughts on Physical Education* [19], John C. Warren's *Physical Education and the Preservation of Health* [117], Miles M. Rodgers' *Physical Education and Medical Management of Children* [96], and Elizabeth Blackwell's *The Laws of Life, with Special Reference to the Physical Education of Girls* [7].

A former student of the well-known physician Benjamin Rush, Charles Caldwell (1772–1853) held a prominent position in Lexington's Transylvania University Medical Department. Although he wrote on a variety of medical topics, his *Thoughts on Physical Education* [19] gained him national recognition. Originally a speech delivered to a teacher's convention in his hometown in 1833, *Thoughts on Physical Education* was published as a book the following year by Marsh, Capen and Lyon of Boston. It was later published in Edinburgh in 1836 and again in 1844.

Caldwell explained the relationship of physical education to moral and intellectual education and reminded his audience that "physical education is far more important than is commonly imagined. Without a due regard to it . . . man cannot attain the perfection of his nature" [19, p 26]. Later in the book, Caldwell defined "physical education" as

> that scheme of training, which contributes most effectually to the development, health, and perfection of living matter.—As applied to man, it is that scheme which raises his whole system to its summit of perfection. . . . Physical education, then, in its philosophy and practice, is of great compass. If complete, it would be tantamount to an entire system of Hygeiene. It would embrace every thing, that,

by bearing in any way on the human body, might injure or benefit in its health, vigor, and fitness of action. [19, pp 28–29]

As an example of this "scheme of training" for maximum health, Caldwell said a sound nursery education for children should consist of "the judicious management of diet, cleanliness, clothing, atmospherical temperature, respiration, muscular exercise, sleep, and the animal passions" [19, p 34].

John C. Warren (1778–1856) was a professor of anatomy and surgery at Harvard University and was quite interested in exercise and health from the 1820s on. He gave several addresses on the topic of "physical education," one of which was published in 1845 as *Physical Education and the Preservation of Health* [117]. A second edition appeared in 1846. The book was divided into several sections focusing on such topics as digestion, exercise, sleep, ventilation, and the external use of water. Warren's adherence to the non-natural tradition and its philosophy of the individual's duty to obey the "laws of nature" is exhibited by his concluding advice:

When, by the combined influence of nature and education, the constitution has become developed in its full power and strength, it depends on the individual to retain health and avoid disease. In other words, it may be considered as a general law, that health may be preserved to a late period of life by the use of those things, which are friendly, and the avoidance of those which are noxious. Most diseases are the consequences of violations of the laws of nature, sometimes the result of ignorance, more frequently of inattention. [117, p 90]

That Warren's definition of "physical education" included more than just physical development became clear when he noted, "Exercise is so material to physical education, that it has sometimes been used synonymously, though it really constitutes only a part of it" [117, p 33].

Physical Education and Medical Management of Children. For the Use of Families and Teachers [96], published in 1848 by upstate New York physician Miles M. Rodgers (dates unknown), exhibited through its title that "physical education" was part of the overall "medical management of children." In his introduction, Rodgers lamented the fact that "a general knowledge of the laws of life and health form[ed] no part of a popular system of education" [96, p 10]. He went on to say, "The study of our own natures is perhaps the most elevating and ennobling subject which can engage the mind" [96, p 10]. The non-natural tradition was also evident in Rodgers's book, since he devoted sections of Chapter 2 to "Air," "Sleep," "Exercise," "Diet," and "Drinks."

Elizabeth Blackwell's (1821–1910) treatise *The Laws of Life, With Special Reference to the Physical Education of Girls* [7] was published in 1852 and serves as a final example of the idea that "physical education" as a term embodied the basic components of the non-natural tradition. While Blackwell was the first woman in the United States to graduate from medical school, she also had an impact on history through a variety of publications and lectures devoted to hygiene. As was common for the 1850s, physicians that wrote about "physical education" based much of their analysis on anatomy and physiology. Blackwell was no exception and discused the "law of exercise" and how movement was important for blood flow, organ health, and muscle tone. She blamed a lack of understanding of the laws of health for the impaired health of American girls and actively campaigned for physical education instruction in schools and colleges.

THE "SIX THINGS NON-NATURAL" AND THE HISTORY OF THE TERM

As explained in the introduction, the non-natural tradition was inherent to humoral theory and Galenic medicine. Withington [123] provided a detailed analysis of the naturals, non-naturals, and contra-naturals and presented the complicated material in a clear manner. The role of exercise and rest in the theory related to its effects on the qualities and humors in particular. It was believed that excessive rest would increase cold and moisture, whereas excessive exercise would at first heat the body and then be followed by cold and dryness. Moderate exercise would maintain warmth. Various baths were also part of this division. Baths of different temperatures and contents (sweet, salt, bitter, etc.) were recommended for their coolness, dryness, or heating capabilities. Since causes for disease were seen to be due to heat, cold, dryness, or moisture, exercise and the other non-naturals played important roles in therapy. Regulating the six non-naturals along with drug prescription and surgery were all within the physicians' realm. However, the non-naturals also played a significant role in hygiene. Those liable to illness or those wishing to maintain their healthfulness were provided a regimen whereby the six non-naturals were regulated to ensure a constant proper balance.

It was medical historian L. J. Rather, in his book on Jerome Gaub (1705–1780) [88] in 1965, who first began exploring the origins, meaning, and use of the term "non-naturals." In his discussion of two of Gaub's essays published in 1747 and 1763, Rather noted that "physicians of Gaub's day still held to some aspects of the Galenical tradition of medical treatment with great persistence. Down to the end of the 18th century they continued to write books, monographs, and dissertations on the six non-naturals" [88, pp 16–17]. Later in the book, Rather explained that "the conception of the non-naturals is especially set forth by Galen, although he does not use the term" [88, p 82]. Curious about the term, Rather then provided some additional information in his footnotes. Gaub himself believed that "the term indicates their position midway between things in accord with nature (*secundum naturam*) and against nature (*contra naturam*)" [88, p 82]. Galen's *Ars medica* also contained some relevant passages. Rather explained that the

> conserving causes (*phylaktika aitia*) of health and disease include both necessary and non-necessary factors, the former being those which cannot be avoided and therefore the more important. They are numbered by Galen as follows: (1) air, (2) motion and rest, (3) sleeping and waking, (4) that which is taken in, (5) that which is excreted or retained, (6) the emotions or passions. Whether they are good or bad for the health depends on their various relations with other things. [88, p 212]

Finally, Rather suggested that Levinus Lemnius (1505–1568), in reference to a passage in Galen's *Ars medica*, provided another explanation of the term. Lemnius noted, "Galen's conserving causes are termed non-naturals by later physicians not because they are praeternatural but because they are things external rather than within us" [88, p 213].

His interest piqued by the non-natural dilemma that surfaced in his book on Gaub, Rather published an article on the subject in which he investigated "the origins and fate of a doctrine and a phrase" [89]. He explained that the concept or doctrine referred to the "six categories of factors that operatively determine health or disease, depending on the circumstances of their use or abuse, to which human beings are unavoidably exposed in the course of daily life. Management of the regimen of the patient, that is, of his involvement with these six sets of factors, was for centuries the physician's most important task" [89, p 337]. Rather also noted that the "*phrase* 'six things non-natural' makes its debut early in the history of Western European medicine. It plays an important role for six centuries or more. Then, early in the 19th century, it bows out, departs from the scene, and is forgotten" [89, p 337]. Although the term itself was not used, Rather was clear to point out that "medical involvement with the factors designated by the phrase remains as active as ever, but they are now subsumed under the rubric of physical and moral (or mental) hygiene" [89, p 337]. He concluded that "the term and phrase were introduced into the Western European medical vocabulary in Latin translations of Arabic works largely based on Galen" [89, p 341].

After Rather's initial article in *Clio Medica* in 1968, several other historians of medicine began researching and writing about the term in the medical history literature of the early 1970s. Jarcho's essay appeared in the *Bulletin of the History of Medicine* in 1970 [53]. Here, like Rather, he traced the concept to Galen's *Ars medica*. The following year, the same issue of the *Bulletin* included articles on the non-naturals by Niebyl [75] and Bylebyl [17]. Both authors attributed their interest in the topic to Rather and Jarcho. Niebyl suggested that Joannitius, a translator of Galen's works into Arabic, obtained the non-naturals term from Galen's pulse books "rather than from an imperfect recollection of the list of necessary causes in the *Ars medica*, as suggested by Rather" [75, p 488]. And, important for the purposes of this chapter, Niebyl asserted that "although the humoral aspect of ancient doctrine gradually disappeared, the regimen of the non-naturals continued to play a dominant role in medicine, especially in the more popular hygiene literature" [75, p 491]. Bylebyl, through further reading of Galen's writings on the pulse, discovered that Galen had in fact written, "First is change of [the pulse] according to nature. Second is [change] which is neither according to nature, nor entirely against nature. Third is [change] which is against nature." In a later discussion, Bylebyl said, "Galen referred to the second category several times as non-natural causes" [17, p 483]. Bylebyl also noted that "from the kinds of things he placed in these three categories it also appears that the non-naturals are activities which are more or less optional and not harmful in themselves, as distinct from unavoidable circumstances and activities which are either essential for life (the naturals) or intrinsically pathological (the praeternaturals)" [17, p 484]. Temkin's book on Galenisim as a medical philosophy [106] also devoted some attention to the non-natural tradition and its origins.

The final article published in the 1970s was by Burns [15]. He referred to the earlier work of Rather, Jarcho, Niebyl, and Temkin and called the non-naturals "a paradox in the western concept of health" [15, p 202]. Burns noted that in the Galenic tradition, "physicians were needed by those suffering from praeternatural conditions. As prognosticators and therapists, they were expected to discern the nature of the imbalance among the naturals or were between the naturals and non-naturals" [15, p 203]. Also, as hygienists, "physicians were expected to protect their patients from harm by attending especially to the non-naturals. Prescribing a proper regimen of non-naturals would secure a group of healthy clients attuned to the beneficient purposes of nature" [15, p 204]. The paradox, as Burns saw it, resided in the fact that since the latter decades of the 19th century when physicians devoted themselves to disease rather than to health, "the traditional obligation of physicians to act as hygienists" disappeared along with the idea of the non-naturals [15, p 210].

RECENT HISTORICAL STUDIES USING THE "NON-NATURAL" CONCEPT

On the basis of the previous section, it is not surprising to learn that medical historians did not begin to include the non-naturals in their research plans until the early 1970s. Once the term, its origins, and its significance were better understood, however, it did not take long for historians to begin to produce some important publications. Burnham [14], in his recent book, explained why historians were attracted to the topic:

> Implicit in the historians' interest in the non-naturals was the striking and amusing fact that the specific content in the modern obsession with the health of body and mind closely resembled those ancient teachings about the non-natural elements essential to life. In the late 20th century and in Roman times both, health writers believed that health was profoundly determined by those elements: air, food, and drink, movement and rest, evacuation and retention, and harmonious 'passions of the soul.' The continuities were perfectly explicit. . . . By the 1980s only the term had disappeared from much of the health advice popularizers were still passing on. [14, p 46]

While some historians like Rather [90], Riley [94, 95], and Jackson [52] acknowledged the existence of the non-naturals, or the "laws of health" like Verbrugge [111], others have done significant research on the non-natural tradition or its individual components.

Coleman's work on the *Encyclopedie* [24] explained the origins of the modern hygiene movement in 18th century France and the non-naturals were central to this research. At the outset, he explained that "during the 18th century both conception and action with regard to the health of the individual were identified with the use of the Galenic-Arabic 'six things non-natural.' The use of the non-naturals was essential to the definition of health advocated by Enlightenment authors, notably Arnulfe d'Aumont writing in the *Encyclopedie*" [24, p 399]. In fact, in his essay on "Hygiene," d'Aumont stated,

> These conditions are essentially defined by the proper use of *six things* which we call, following the ancients, *non-natural*. They become natural when our use of them benefits health and contra-natural when their use is harmful to the animal economy. . . . The rules which must be stated regarding their good and bad effects constitute practical medicine, that is, hygiene. [24, p 405]

Lawrence's [61] article included a discussion of the non-naturals as used in Buchan's *Domestic Medicine* and Burnham [13] devoted considerable attention to the role of the non-naturals in the popular health literature in the United States. Smith [104] explained how the non-naturals were incorporated into the self-help literature of late 18th century England; Dannenfeldt [31] just published an article on the theory and practice of sleep as one of the non-naturals during the late Renaissance, and Lomax [66] discussed the non-naturals as the basis for instruction in health and human physiology in the American school system during the 19th century.

EXERCISE AND THE "NON-NATURALS" IN THE HISTORICAL LITERATURE

Although numerous books and articles have been written about the history of exercise, medical gymnastics, and physical education, one is struck by the paucity of information concerning the relationship between exercise, medicine, and good health. Not until Haley's book [47] in 1978 did any historian studying exercise even mention the non-naturals. He referred to "natural law" and the "laws of nature" and then noted that "physicians increasingly turned to hygiene and to the *res non-naturals*— air, water, food, sleep— as the basis of their therapeutics" [47, pp 15–17]. Finney [38], writing in 1966 about medical theories of vocal exercise, referred to Galen's "six eminently sensible rules" and listed the traditional six. While she did not use the non-naturals as a term, it is clear she was aware of the concept. Whorton's *Crusaders for Fitness* [120], published in 1982, included the best description and analysis of the non-naturals and their role in American health reform during the first half of the 19th century. While not yet published, Virginia Smith's essay on "regimenical literature in Britain from 1700–1850, with special reference to exercise" [105] examined the household book literature on regimen and exercise within the context of the non-naturals.

At least two authors writing about the history of exercise included the term "non-naturals" in their articles, but it was because it was mentioned in a book they were quoting. Fletcher [39] quoted Giorgio Baglivi (1669–1707) who referred to the "six non-natural things." Then in a note, Fletcher said that "in medieval medicine, the six 'non-natural' things (things which caused health or disease and were not actual parts of the human parts) were meat and drink, retention and evacuation, air, exercise, sleep and waking, and passions of the mind" [39, p 38]. Licht [65] noted that "Rhazes was the first Arab physician to write a book on hygiene" and it stated "health is preserved by a just measure of exercise and the other non-naturals" [65, p 9].

Most of the remaining literature reviewed in this final section is devoted to the history of physical education and the key individuals and important developments which assisted in that profession's growth. Exercise in one form or another is their major focus, but invariably most of the authors looked toward educational literature rather than medical history for information. There has been commendable work done listing what exercises people performed, explaining systems of exercise, and identifying major proponents of exercise, but very little research into the origins of the medical rationale for exercise. Most historians have looked to the "humanistic educators" of the Renaissance as a source of interest in the body rather than to the role exercise played in the non-natural medical tradition. Even those who have looked at the influence of medicine seem surprised that the topic of exercise would be discussed by a physician or appear in a medical publication. In reality, much of the interest in exercise came from the non-natural tradition and those educators espousing exercise were doing so as a result of medicine's influence.

Leonard and Affleck [63] do not mention Hippocrates or Galen but refer to Cardano (1501–1576) and Mecurialis (1530–1606). They wrote about "physical training advocated by writers on education" [63, p 64] and devoted an entire chapter to Locke and Rousseau. In the same chapter, they also noted that "a number of medical writers had been directing attention to the importance of bodily exercise in the restoration and preservation of health" [63, p 64] and devoted some space to Friedrich Hoffmann (1660–1742) and Clement Joseph Tissot (1750–1826). Joseph's four articles published in 1949 [55–58] are filled with valuable information on exercise in both education and medicine. He used many original works and dealt with most of the leading individuals from the 16th to the 18th century. The four-article series is one of the most important cursory views of the topic. Hackensmith [46] briefly referred to Galen and Mecurialis but included very little on medical writers and their influence on physical education. Brailsford [10] had a chapter entitled "Exercise, Education and Social Attitudes, 1600–1650" and one entitled "The Motion of Limbs." A major section of the latter chapter was devoted to "Medicine and Exercise." Here, he devoted considerable attention to Robert Burton, Francis Fuller, and John Locke. Brailsford's analysis is excellent and he does a good job with the medicine and exercise relationship. Finally, Van Dalen and Bennett [110] noted that Galen "devoted considerable attention to the influence of exercise and diet upon health" [110, p 77]. Later, in their discussion of the Enlightenment, they stated, "Medical men began to study anatomy and physiology, and a number of treatises appeared concerning exercises and their influence on health" [110, p 187].

Some of the best work to be done on exercise, health, and medicine was authored by John Betts and Roberta Park. While neither dealt directly with the role of exercise in the non-natural tradition, both were keenly aware of the significant role played by medicine in the popularization of exercise. Bett's 1968 article on "Mind and Body in Early American Thought" [5] was quite inclusive and mentioned most of the major medical works and their authors during the first 50 years of the 19th century. While we now know that a medical rationale for exercise was developed before the 19th century, or the Enlightenment for that matter, Betts was still not incorrect when he said,

In the quarter century between 1820 and 1845 educators, physicians, and reformers had begun to develop a philosophical rationale concerning the relationship of physical to mental and spiritual benefits derived from exercise, games, and sports. From the diffusion of ideas developed by the medical profession under the influence of the Enlightenment and by educators and reformers affected by the romantic spirit, Americans were alerted to the threat against their physical and mental powers that came from the confinements of the home and school and the more sedentary habits of the city. [5, p 805]

Betts's article "American Medical Thought on Exercise as the Road to Health, 1820–1860" [6] also quite inclusive and informative, concluded in much the same way as his earlier article:

A scientific and medical rationale for the movement toward health reform, physical education, field sports, athletics, and exercise for the masses had nonetheless been laid by scores of conscientious, observant, and informed physicians in the decades prior to the Civil War. [6, p 152]

Again, while Betts was not really wrong, the rationale being promulgated was nothing more than a continuation of the value of exercise for good hygiene as stipulated by the non-natural tradition.

Roberta Park has written more authoritatively about the history of health and exercise than any other individual. Although she has published extensively, only six of her articles are dealt with here. The first reviewed is the most important one for our purposes since in it she dealt with the writings of 18th century physicians and informed laymen on health and exercise [80]. Here, although she does not refer to the term or concept of the non-naturals, Park summarized her research in a sound and accurate manner:

During the 1700s a substantial number of works were written by physicians and informed laymen who expressed concern for the maintenance and restoration of health and/or for hygiene and the role of exercise and active recreations in the growth and development of children. The publication of popular medical texts in the vernacular, rather than the traditional Latin, and the translation of several of these works into other languages enabled an increasingly literate citizenry to become acquainted with the ideas presented. Those who read such works could hardly escape their message— active physical exercise, along with proper diet, rest, and similar care, could be a powerful means for achieving, preserving, and even restoring, health. [80, p 763]

Park also wrote about New England Transcendentalists and their attitudes toward health and exercise [81], concerns for health and exercise in the English educational reform movement of 1640–1660 [82], and the concern for the physical education of American women during the ante-bellum period [83]. A major part of the latter research dealt with "various medical and quasi-medical contributions" and in that section Park made reference to "the laws of health" [83, p 23]. While not dealing with the reasons why, Park said that "both doctors and laymen authored books and pamphlets on the general subject of health, many of which devoted considerable attention to matters of hygiene and physical education" [83, p 24]. Additional articles by Park dealt with the "healthful regimens" of the 16th and 17th century Utopian authors [84] and the American hygienic and educative interests in athletics and physical education between 1856 and 1906 [85].

Eleanor English [34, 35] has also written about exercise, health, and the influence of a few key Renaissance physicians. She discussed the writings of Girolamo Cardano (1501–1576) and Thomas Elyot (1490–1546) in her 1982 article and added Christobal Mendez (1500–1561) and Hieronymus Mecurialis (1530–1606) to her 1984 essay. In analyzing the writing of the four physicians, it is clear that English was not aware of the non-natural tradition or the role exercise played in it. She credited "the Italian humanists who advocated an educational curriculum (*studia humanitatis*) which brought forth the harmonious development of the whole man (*l'uomo universale*)— intellectually, morally, and physically" for introducing "the concept of exercise as being necessary for physical and mental development" [34, p 283]. Later, in the same article referring to Cardano's *Care of Health* (1560) and the appearance of materials on exercise, she suggested that "by this inclusion of a treatise on exercise in a medical work, an unusual occurrence, exercise was given status among medical concerns" [34, p 288].

Two recent books provide an informed treatment of exercise, health, and the American medical community. Whorton [120], already mentioned, wrote eruditely and convincingly about the ante-bellum health reform movement and was fully aware of the role and importance of the non-natural tradition. Early in his book, in reference to Jacksonian "hygienic optimism," Whorton explained that "as modern as that optimism was, it borrowed heavily from ancient ideas about health." He went on to say that the "rules of healthful living" were

> formally codified as part of medical thought by Galen. . . . Galenic answers to virtually all medical questions dominated theory and practice into the 1600s, but while most features of Galenism were cast aside during that century, the code of hygiene retained its hold. It was, after all, solidly founded on experience, ordered around the individual's careful regulation of those factors of existence over which he had control: air, food and drink, sleep and watch, motion and rest, evacuation and repletion, and passions of the mind. Attention to these 'six non-naturals,' as they had come to be confusingly called, had been urged by medical writers throughout the late Middle Ages and Renaissance, but the matter seemed to assume new importance during the mid-1700s. [120, pp 14–15]

Lastly, Harvey Green's *Fit for America: Health, Fitness, Sport, and American Society* [42] covered the century between the 1830s and the 1930s and offered insights into a variety of topics like diet, dress, sanitation, nervousness, ventilation, exercise, sport, and therapies utilizing water and electricity.

POSTSCRIPT

After this review of the literature of the non-naturals, their place in the history of medicine, and the dominant position exercise had in that structure, it should be evident that the contemporary discussions of wellness, preventive medicine, and exercise prescription are simply the latest flowering of a tradition dating to antiquity. This cordial and growing relationship between exercise and medicine in the 1980s is neither new nor unique. We are simply rekindling a practice once popular but abandoned.

REFERENCES

1. Ackerknecht EH: Aspects of the history of therapeutics. *Bull Hist Med* 36:389–419, 1962.
2. Ackerman L: *Health and Hygiene: A Comprehensive Study of Disease Prevention and Health Promotion.* New York, Ronald Press, 1943.
3. Allmendinger DF Jr: *Paupers and Scholars: The Transformation of Student Life in Nineteenth-Century New England.* New York, St. Martin's Press, 1975.

4. Armstrong J: *The Art of Preserving Health*. London, T. Cadell and W. Davies, 1795.
5. Betts JR: Mind and body in early American thought. *J Am Hist* 54:787–805, 1968.
6. Betts JR: American medical thought on exercise as the road to health, 1820–1860. *Bull Hist Med* 45:138–152, 1971.
7. Blackwell E: *The Laws of Life, with Special Reference to the Physical Education of Girls*. New York, George P. Putnam, 1852.
8. Blake JB: From Buchan to Fishbein: the literature of domestic medicine. In Risse GB, Numbers RT, Leavitt JW (eds): *Medicine Without Doctors: Home Health Care in American History*. New York, Science History Publications, 1977, pp 11–30.
9. Blundell JWF: *The Muscles and Their Story, From the Earliest Times; Including the Whole Text of Mercurialis, and the Opinions of Other Writers Ancient and Modern, on Mental and Bodily Development*. London, Chapman & Hall, 1864.
10. Brailsford D: *Sport and Society: Elizabeth to Anne*. London, Routledge & Kegan Paul, 1969.
11. Brock AJ: (trans. and annot.) *Greek Medicine: Being Extracts Illustrative of Medical Writers From Hippocrates to Galen*. London, J. M. Dent & Sons, 1929.
12. Buchan W: *Domestic Medicine: Or, a Treatise on the Prevention and Cure of Diseases, by Regimen and Simple Medicines*. Boston, Joseph Bumstead, 1813.
13. Burnham JC: Change in the popularization of health in the United States. *Bull Hist Med* 58:183–197, 1984.
14. Burnham JC: *How Superstition Won and Science Lost: Popularizing Science and Health in the United States*. New Brunswick, NJ, Rutgers University Press, 1987.
15. Burns CR: The nonnaturals: a paradox in the western concept of health. *J Med Philos* 1:202–211, 1976.
16. Burton R: *The Anatomy of Melancholy*. New York, AC Armstrong and Son, 1885.
17. Bylebyl JJ: Galen on the non-natural causes of variation in the pulse. *Bull Hist Med* 45:482–485, 1971.
18. Bylebyl JJ: The school of Padua: humanistic medicine in the sixteenth century. In Webster C (ed): *Health, Medicine and Mortality in the Sixteenth Century*. Cambridge, Cambridge University Press, 1979, pp 335–370.
19. Caldwell C: *Thoughts on Physical Education: Being a Discourse Delivered to a Convention of Teachers in Lexington KY, on the 6th and 7th of November, 1833*. Boston, Marsh, Capen & Lyon, 1834.
20. Cardan [Cardano] J: *The Book of My Life* (trans. from the Latin by Jean Stoner). New York, EP Dutton, 1930.
21. Cassedy JH: Why self-help? Americans alone with their diseases, 1800–1850. In Risse GB, Numbers RL, Leavitt JW (eds): *Medicine without Doctors: Home Health Care in American History*. New York, Science History Publications, 1977, pp 31–48.
22. Cheyne G: *An Essay of Health and Long Life*. New York, Edward Gillespy, 1813.
23. Cogan T: *The Haven of Health, Chiefly Made for the Comfort of Students, and Consequently for All Those That Have a Care for Their Health, Amplified Upon Fine Wordes of Hippocrates, Written Epid. 6. Labour, Meate, Drinke, Sleepe, Venus*. London, Bonham Norton, 1596.
24. Coleman W: Health and hygiene in the *Encyclopedie*: a medical doctrine for the bourgeosie. *J Hist Med* 29:399–421, 1974.
25. Coleman W: The people's health; medical themes in eighteenth-century French popular literature. *Bull Hist Med* 51:55–74, 1977.
26. Combe A: *The Principles of Physiology Applied to the Preservation of Health, and to the Improvement of Physical and Mental Education*. New York, Harper & Brothers, 1843.
27. Cooter R: The power of the body: the early nineteenth century. In Barnes B, Shapin S (eds): *Natural Order: Historical Studies of Scientific Culture*. London, Sage Publications, 1979, pp 73–92.

28. Cornaro L: *The Art of Living Long. A New and Improved English Version of the Treatise by the Celebrated Venetian Centenarian Louis Cornaro with Essays by Joseph Addison, Lord Bacon, and Sir William Temple*. Milwaukee, William F. Butler, 1905.

29. Cornwell B: *The Domestic Physician, or Guardian of Health*. London, Printed for the Author, 1788.

30. Cyriax RJ: A short history of mechano-therapeutics in Europe until the time of Ling. *Janus* 19:178–240, 1914.

31. Dannenfeldt KH: Sleep: theory and practice in the late Renaissance. *J Hist Med* 41:415–441, 1986.

32. Dunglison R: *On the Influence of Atmosphere and Locality; Change of Air and Climate; Seasons; Food; Clothing; Bathing; Exercise; Sleep; Corporeal and Intellectual Pursuits, & c. on Human Health; Constituting Elements of Hygiene*. Philadephia, Carey, Lea & Blanchard, 1835.

33. Elyot T: *The Castel of Helthe. Together with the Title Page and Preface of the Edition of 1539. With an introduction by Samuel A Tannenbaum*. New York, Scholar's Facsimiles & Reprints, 1937.

34. English EB: Girolamo Cardano and *de sanitate tuenda*: a Renaissance physician's perspective on exercise. *Res Q* 53:282–290, 1982.

35. English EB: Sport, the blessed medicine of the Renaissance. Paper presented at the North American Society for Sport History, Louisville, KY, 1984.

36. Ewell J: *The Medical Companion, or Family Physician: An Essay on Hygiene, or the Art of Preserving Health, Without the Aid of Medicine*. Philadelphia, Carey, Lea & Blanchard, 1834.

37. Faust BC: *Catechism of Health for the Use of Schools, and for Domestic Instruction* (Trans. by JH Basse). Dublin, C. Dilly, 1794.

38. Finney G: Medical theories of vocal exercise and health. *Bull Hist Med* 50:395–406, 1966.

39. Fletcher GF: The history of exercise in the practice of medicine. *J Med Assoc GA* 72:35–40, 1983.

40. Fuller F: *Medicina Gymnastica: or, a Treatise Concerning the Power of Exercise, with Respect to the Animal Oeconomy; and the Great Necessity of it, in the Cure of Several Distempers*. London, John Matthews, 1705.

41. Graham S: *Lectures on the Science of Human Life* (2 vols). Boston, March, Capen, Lyon and Webb, 1839.

42. Green H: *Fit for America: Health, Fitness, Sport, and American Society*. New York, Pantheon Books, 1986.

43. Green RM: *A Translation of Galen's Hygiene* (De sanitate tuenda). Springfield, IL, Charles C Thomas, 1951.

44. Gruman GJ: The rise and fall of prolongevity hygiene: 1558–1873. *Bull Hist Med* 35:221–229, 1961.

45. Gunn JC: *Gunn's Domestic Medicine: A Facsimile of the First Edition with an Introduction by Charles E Rosenberg*. Knoxville, University of Tennessee Press, 1986.

46. Hackensmith CW: *History of Physical Education*. New York, Harper & Row, 1966.

47. Haley B: *The Healthy Body and Victorian Culture*. Cambridge, MA, Harvard University Press, 1978.

48. Harington J (Trans.): *The School of Salernum*. New York, Paul B. Hoeber, 1920.

49. Hippocrates: *Regimen* (trans. by WHS Jones). Cambridge, MA, Harvard University Press, 1967.

50. Hitchcock E: *Dyspepsy Forestalled and Resisted: Or Lectures on Diet, Regimen and Employment; Delivered to the Students of Amherst College, Spring Term, 1830*. Amherst, MA, JS & C Adams, 1831.

51. Hoffmann FH: *Fundamenta Medicinae. Translated, and with an Introductionn by LS King*. New York, American Elsevier, 1971.

52. Jackson SW: *Melancholia and Depression: From Hippocratic Times to Modern Times*. New Haven, CT, Yale University Press, 1986.

53. Jarcho S: Galen's six non-naturals: a bibliographic note and translation. *Bull Hist Med* 44:372–377, 1970.

54. Jordanova LJ: Earth science and environmental medicine: the synthesis of the late Enlightenment. In Jordanova LJ, Porter RS (eds): *Images of the Earth: Essays in the History of the Environmental Sciences*. Bucks, England, British Society for the History of Science, 1979, pp 119–146.

55. Joseph LH: Physical education in the early Middle Ages. *Ciba Symp* 10:1030–1033, 1949.

56. Joseph LH: Gymnastics during the Renaissance as a part of the humanistic educational program. *Ciba Symp* 10:1034–1040, 1949.

57. Joseph LH: Medical gymnastics in the sixteenth and seventeenth centuries. *Ciba Symp* 10:1041–1053, 1949.

58. Joseph LH: Gymnastics in the pre-revolutionary eighteenth century. *Ciba Symp* 10:1054–1060, 1949.

59. Kimble C: In pursuit of well-being. *Wilson Q* 4:60–74, 1980.

60. King J: *The American Family Physician: Or Domestic Guide to Health. Prepared Expressly for the Use of Families, in Language Adapted to the Understanding of the People*. Indianapolis, IN, Streight & Adams, 1860.

61. Lawrence CJ: William Buchan: medicine laid open. *Med Hist* 19:20–35, 1975.

62. Leonard FE: The beginnings of modern physical training in Europe. *Am Phys Educ Rev* 9:89–110, 1904.

63. Leonard FE, Affleck GB: *A Guide to the History of Physical Education*, ed 3. Philadelphia, Lea & Febiger, 1947.

64. Licht E, Licht S: *A Translation of Joseph-Clement Tissot's Gymnastique Medicinale et Chirurgicale with a Facsimile of the Original French and Facsimiles of Eighteenth-Century Translations into German, Italian, and Swedish*. New Haven, CT, Elizabeth Licht, 1964.

65. Licht S: History [of therapeutic exercise]. In Basmajian JV (ed): *Therapeutic Exercise*, ed 4. Baltimore, Williams & Wilkins, 1984, pp 1–44.

66. Lomax ER: The introduction into the school curriculum of instruction in health and human physiology. Unpublished paper, 1987.

67. Mackenzie J: *The History of Health, and the Art of Preserving It: Or, An Account of All That Has Been Recommended by Physicians and Philosophers, Towards the Preservation of Health, from the Most Remote Antiquity to This Time*. Edinburgh, William Gordon, 1759.

68. McClary BH: Introducing a classic: Gunn's *Domestic Medicine*. *Tenn Hist Q* 45:210–216, 1986.

69. McCoy RF: Hygienic recommendations of the *Ladies Library*. *Bull Hist Med* 4:367–372, 1936.

70. McCrae T; George Cheyne, an old London and Bath physician (1671–1743). *Johns Hopkins Hosp Bull* 15:84–94, 1904.

71. McIntosh PC: Hieronymus Mercurialis *De Arte Gymnastica*: classification and dogma in physical education in the sixteenth century. Unpublished paper, 1980.

72. Mendez C: *Book of Bodily Exercise* (Trans. by Guerra F; ed. by Kilgour FG). New Haven, CT, Elizabeth Licht, 1960.

73. Morantz RM: Making women modern: middle-class women and health reform in 19th-century America. In Leavitt JW (ed): *Women and Health in America: Historical Readings*. Madison, WI, Univeristy of Wisconsin Press, 1984, pp 346–358.

74. Naisbitt J: *Megatrends: Ten New Directions Transforming Our Lives*. New York, Warner Books, 1984.

75. Niebyl PH: The non-naturals. *Bull Hist Med* 45:486–492, 1971.
76. Nissenbaum S: *Sex, Diet, and Debility in Jacksonian America: Sylvester Graham and Health Reform.* Westport, CT. Greenwood Press, 1980.
77. Numbers RL: Do-it-yourself the sectarian way. In Risse GB, Numbers RL, Leavitt JW (eds): *Medicine Without Doctors: Home Health Care in American History.* New York, Science History Publications, 1977, pp 49–72.
78. Olivova V: Scientific and professional gymnastics. In Olivova V (ed): *Sports and Games in the Ancient World.* New York, St. Martin's Press, 1984, pp 135–144.
79. Pare A: *The Collected Works of Ambroise Pare* (Trans. by Johnson T). Pound Ridge, NY, Milford House, 1968.
80. Park RJ: Concern for health and exercise as expressed in the writings of 18th century physicians and informed laymen (England, France, Switzerland). *Res Q* 47:756–767, 1976.
81. Park RJ: The attitudes of leading New England transcendentalists toward healthful exercise, active recreations and proper care of the body: 1830–1860. *J Sport Hist* 4:34–50, 1977.
82. Park RJ: The advancement of learning: expressions of concern for health and exercise in English proposals for educational reform—1640–1660. *Can J Hist Sport P E* 8:51–61, 1977.
83. Park RJ: Embodied selves: the rise and development of concern for physical education, active games and recreation for American women, 1776–1865. *J Sport Hist* 5:5–41, 1978.
84. Park RJ: Strong bodies, healthful regimens, and playful recreations as viewed by utopian authors of the 16th and 17th centuries. *Res Q* 49:498–511, 1978.
85. Park RJ: Physiologists, physicians, and physical educators: nineteenth century biology and exercise, *hygienic* and *educative. J Sport Hist* 14:28–60, 1987.
86. Precope J: *Hippocrates on Diet and Hygiene.* London, Williams, Lea & Co., 1952.
87. Pugh J: *A Physiological, Theoretic and Practical Treatise on the Utility of the Science of Muscular Action for Restoring the Power of the Limbs.* London, C. Dilly, 1794.
88. Rather LJ: *Mind and Body in Eighteenth Century Medicine: A Study Based on Jerome Gaub's De regimine mentis.* Berkeley, University of California Press, 1965.
89. Rather LJ: The 'six things non-natural': a note on the origins and fate of a doctrine and a phrase. *Clio Med* 3:337–347, 1968.
90. Rather LJ: Pathology at mid-century: a reassessment of Thomas Willis and Thomas Sydenham. In Debus AG (ed.): *Medicine in Seventeenth Century England.* Berkeley, University of California Press, 1974, pp 71–112.
91. Rees A. et al: *The Encyclopaedia: Or, Universal Dictionary of Arts, Sciences, and Literature.* London: Longman, Hurst, Rees, Orme & Brown, 1819.
92. Reiser SJ: Responsibility for personal health: a historical perspective. *J Med Philos* 10:7–17, 1985.
93. Ricketson S: *Means of Preserving Health, and Preventing Diseases: Founded Principally on an Attention to Air and Climate, Drink, Food, Sleep, Exercise.* New York, Collins, Perkins, 1806.
94. Riley JC: The medicine of the environment in eighteenth-century Germany. *Clio Med* 18:167–178, 1983.
95. Riley JC: *The Eighteenth-Century Campaign to Avoid Disease.* New York, St. Martin's Press, 1987.
96. Rodgers MM: *Physical Education and Medical Management of Children. For the Use of Families and Teachers.* Rochester, NY, Erastus Darrow, 1848.
97. Rogers FB: Shadrach Ricketson (1768–1839): Quaker hygienist. *J Hist Med* 20:140–150, 1965.

98. Rosenberg CE: The therapeutic revolution: medicine, meaning, and social change in nineteenth-century America. In Vogel MJ, Rosenberg CE (eds): *The Therapeutic Revolution: Essays in the Social History of American Medicine.* Philadelphia, University of Pennsylvania Press, 1979, pp 3–25.

99. Rosenberg CE: Medical text and social context: explaining William Buchan's *Domestic Medicine. Bull Hist Med* 57:22–42, 1983.

100. Shryock RH: Sylvester Graham and the popular health movement, 1830–1870. *Miss Vall Hist R* 18:172–183, 1931.

101. Sigerist HE: Faust in America. *Med Life* 41:192–207, 1934.

102. Sigerist HE: *Landmarks in the History of Hygiene.* London, Oxford University Press, 1956.

103. Slack P: Mirrors of health and treasures of poor men: the uses of the vernacular medical literature of Tudor England. In Webster C (ed): *Health, Medicine and Mortality in the Sixteenth Century.* Cambridge, Cambridge University Press, 1979, pp 237–271.

104. Smith G: Prescribing the rules of health: self-help and advice in the late eighteenth century. In Porter R (ed): *Patients and Practitioners: Lay Perceptions of Medicine in Pre-Industrial Society.* Cambridge, Cambridge University Press, 1985, pp 249–282.

105. Smith V: Household books: regimenical literature in Britain 1700–1850, with special reference to exercise (unpublished paper). Cambridge, Wellcome Unit for the History of Medicine, 1987.

106. Temkin O: *Galenism: Rise and Decline of a Medical Philosophy.* Ithaca, Cornell University Press, 1973.

107. Thacher J: *American Modern Practice; or, a Simple Method of Prevention and Cure of Diseases, According to the Latest Improvements and Discoveries, Comprising a Practical System Adapted to the Use of Medical Practitioners of the United States.* Boston, Ezra Read, 1817.

108. Turner BS: The discourse of diet. *Theory, Cult Soc* 1:23–32, 1982.

109. Turner BS: The government of the body: medical regimens and the rationalization of diet. *Br J Soc* 33:254–269, 1982.

110. Van Dalen DB, Bennett BL: *A World History of Physical Education: Cultural, Philosophical, Comparative.* Englewood Cliffs, NJ, Prentice Hall, 1971.

111. Verbrugge MH: The social meaning of personal health: the Ladies' Physiological Institute of Boston and vicinity in the 1850s. In Reverby S, Rosner D (eds): *Health Care in America: Essays in Social History.* Philadelphia, Temple University Press, 1979.

112. Verbrugge MH: Healthy animals and civic life: Sylvester Graham's physiology of subsistence. *Rev Am Hist* 9:359–364, 1981.

113. Viets HR: George Cheyne, 1673–1743. *Bull Hist Med* 23:435–452, 1949.

114. Walker WB: Luigi Cornaro, a renaissance writer on personal hygiene. *Bull Hist Med* 28:525–534, 1954.

115. Wallis G: *The Art of Preventing Diseases, and Restoring Health, Founded on Rational Principles, and Adapted to Persons of Every Capacity.* New York, Samuel Campbell, 1794.

116. Warner JH: *The Therapeutic Perspective: Medical Practice, Knowledge, and Identity in America, 1820–1885.* Cambridge, Harvard University Press, 1986.

117. Warren JC: *Physical Education and the Preservation of Health.* Boston, William D. Ticknor, 1846.

118. Wesley J: *Primitive Physic: Or, An Easy and Natural Method of Curing Most Diseases.* Philadelphia, Parry Hall, 1793.

119. Whorton JC: Christian physiology: William Alcott's prescription for the millenium. *Bull Hist Med* 49:466–481, 1975.

120. Whorton JC: *Crusaders for Fitness: The History of American Health Reformers.* Princeton, NJ, Princeton University Press, 1982.

121. Whorton JC: The first holistic revolution: alternative medicine in the nineteenth century. In Stalker D, Glymour C (eds): *Examining Holistic Medicine.* New York, Prometheus Books, 1985.
122. Willich AFM: *Lectures on Diet and Regimen: Being a Systematic Inquiry into the Most Rational Means of Preserving Health and Prolonging Life: Together with Physiological and Chemical Explanations, Calculated Chiefly for the Use of Families, in Order to Banish the Prevailing Abuses and Prejudices in Medicine.* New York, T and J Swords, 1801.
123. Withington ET: *Medical History from the Earliest Times, A Popular History of the Healing Art.* London, Scientific Press, 1894.

Index

Page numbers in *italics* denote figures; those followed by "t" denote tables

561